Neuroimaging of Human Memory

Linking cognitive processes to neural systems

Neuroimaging of Human Memory

Linking cognitive processes to neural systems

Edited by

Frank Rösler

Charan Ranganath

Brigitte Röder

Rainer H. Kluwe

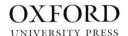
OXFORD
UNIVERSITY PRESS

OXFORD

UNIVERSITY PRESS

Great Clarendon Street, Oxford ox2 6DP

Oxford University Press is a department of the University of Oxford.
It furthers the University's objective of excellence in research, scholarship,
and education by publishing worldwide in

Oxford New York

Auckland Cape Town Dar es Salaam Hong Kong Karachi
Kuala Lumpur Madrid Melbourne Mexico City Nairobi
New Delhi Shanghai Taipei Toronto

With offices in

Argentina Austria Brazil Chile Czech Republic France Greece
Guatemala Hungary Italy Japan Poland Portugal Singapore
South Korea Switzerland Thailand Turkey Ukraine Vietnam

Oxford is a registered trade mark of Oxford University Press
in the UK and in certain other countries

Published in the United States
by Oxford University Press Inc., New York

© Oxford University Press, 2009

A catalogue record for this title is available from the British Library
Data available

Library of Congress Cataloging in Publication Data
Data available

Typeset in Minion by Cepha Imaging Private Ltd., Bangalore, India
Printed in Italy
on acid-free paper by

L.E.G.O. S.p.A.

ISBN 978–0–19–921–7298

10 9 8 7 6 5 4 3 2 1

Contents

Contributors

Zara M. Bergström
Memory and Consciousness Research
Group, Department of Neurology,
Faculty of Medicine,
Otto von Guericke University,
Magdeburg, Germany.

Christian Büchel
NeuroImage Nord, Department of
Systems Neuroscience,
University Medical Center
Hamburg-Eppendorf,
Germany.

Bradley R. Buchsbaum
Helen Wills Neuroscience Institute and
Department of Psychology, University of
California, Berkeley, CA, USA.

Mark D'Esposito
Helen Wills Neuroscience Institute and
Department of Psychology, University of
California, Berkeley, CA, USA.

Emrah Düzel
Institute of Cognitive Neuroscience,
University College London,
London, UK.

Guillén Fernández
Donders Institute for Brain, Cognition
and Behaviour, Dept. of Neurology,
Radboud University Nijmegen,
Nijmegen, The Netherlands.

Dara G. Ghahremani
Department of Psychiatry & Biobehavioral
Sciences, University of California,
Los Angeles, Los Angeles, CA, USA.

Sebastian Guderian
Laboratory of Neuropsychology, National
Institute of Mental Health, National
Institutes of Health, Bethesda, MD, USA.

Adam Hampshire
Medical Research Council Cognition
and Brain Sciences Unit, 15,
Cambridge, U.K.

Alumit Ishai
Institute of Neuroradiology,
University of Zurich,
Zurich, Switzerland.

Theodor Jäger
Experimental Neuropsychology Unit,
Department of Psychology,
Saarland University,
Saarbrücken, Germany.

Matthew R. Johnson
Interdepartmental Neuroscience Program,
Yale University, New Haven, CT, USA.

Marcia K. Johnson
Interdepartmental Neuroscience Program,
and Department of Psychology,
Yale University, New Haven, CT, USA.

Patrick Khader
Experimental and Biological Psychology,
Philipps-University Marburg,
Marburg, Germany.

Rainer H. Kluwe
Helmut-Schmidt-University Hamburg,
Hamburg, Germany.

Kevin S. LaBar   Center for Cognitive
Neuroscience,
Duke University, Durham, NC, USA.

Elena Magno
Memory and Consciousness Research
Group, Department of Neurology,
Faculty of Medicine,
Otto von Guericke University,
Magdeburg, Germany.

Gerasimos Markopoulos
Memory and Consciousness Research
Group, Department of Neurology,
Faculty of Medicine,
Otto von Guericke University,
Magdeburg, Germany.

Axel Mecklinger
Experimental Neuropsychology Unit,
Department of Psychology, Saarland
University, Saarbrücken, Germany.

Ehren L. Newman
Department of Psychology, Princeton
University, Princeton, NJ, USA.

Kenneth A. Norman
Department of Psychology, Princeton
University, Princeton, NJ, USA.

John P O'Doherty
Division of Humanities and Social
Sciences and Computation and Neural
Systems Program,
California Institute of Technology,
Pasadena, CA, USA.

Adrian M. Owen
Medical Research Council Cognition
and Brain Sciences Unit,
Cambridge, U.K.

Ken A. Paller
Interdepartmental Neuroscience Program
and Department of Psychology,
Northwestern University,
Evanston, IL, USA.

Russell A. Poldrack
Department of Psychology,
University of California, Los Angeles,
Los Angeles, CA, USA.

Bradley R. Postle
Department of Psychology, University of
Wisconsin-Madison,
Maidson, WI, USA.

Joel R. Quamme
Department of Psychology, Princeton
University, Princeton, NJ, USA.

Charan Ranganath
Center for Neuroscience,
University of California at Davis,
Davis, CA, USA.

Paul J. Reber
Department of Psychology,
Northwestern University, Evanston,
IL, USA.

Alan Richardson-Klavehn
Memory and Consciousness Research
Group, Department of Neurology,
Faculty of Medicine,
Otto von Guericke University,
Magdeburg, Germany.

Brigitte Röder
Biological Psychology and
Neuropsychology,
University of Hamburg,
Hamburg, Germany.

Frank Rösler
Experimental and Biological Psychology,
Philipps-University Marburg,
Marburg, Germany.

Michael D. Rugg
Center for the Neurobiology of Learning
and Memory and Department of
Neurobiology and Behavior,
University of California Irvine,
Irvine, CA, USA.

Jon S. Simons
Department of Experimental Psychology,
University of Cambridge,
Cambridge, UK.

Catherine M. Sweeney-Reed
Memory and Consciousness Research
Group, Department of Neurology,
Faculty of Medicine,
Otto von Guericke University,
Magdeburg, Germany.

Indira Tendolkar
Donders Institute for Brain, Cognition
and Behaviour, Dept. of Psychiatry,
Radboud University Nijmegen,
Nijmegen, The Netherlands.

Rolf Ulrich
Cognitive and Biological Psychology,
University of Tübingen,
Tübingen, Germany.

Joel L. Voss
Interdepartmental Neuroscience Program
and Department of Psychology,
Northwestern University,
Evanston, IL, USA.

Carmen E. Westerberg
Interdepartmental Neuroscience Program
and Department of Psychology,
Northwestern University,
Evanston, IL, USA.

Maria Wimber
Memory and Consciousness Research
Group, Department of Neurology,
Faculty of Medicine, Otto von Guericke
University, Magdeburg, Germany.

Andrew P. Yonelinas
Department of Psychology, University of
California Davis, Davis, CA, USA.

Abbreviations and acronyms

a.k.a.	as known as		
ACC	Anterior Cingulate Cortex		
BA	Brodmann Area	mPFC	medial Prefrontal Cortex
BOLD	Blood Oxygenation Level Dependent (Signal)	MTL	Medial Temporal Lobe
		MTLC	Medial Temporal Lobe Cortex
CA1, 2, 3	Cornu Ammonis fields 1, 2, 3 (cell structures of the hippocampus proper)	MVPA	Multi-Voxel Pattern Analysis
		NIRS	Near-Infrared Spectroscopy
		OFC	Orbito-Frontal Cortex
CFE	Categorical Fluency Effect	PCT	Probabilistic Classification Task
CLS	Complementary Learning Systems	PCu	Precuneus
COVIS	Competition between Verbal and Implicit Systems (model)	PD	Parkinson's Disease
		PET	Positron Emission Tomography
CS	Conditioned Stimulus	PFC	Prefrontal Cortex
DCM	Dynamic Causal Modeling	PMC	Premotor Cortex
DLPFC	Dorsolateral Prefrontal Cortex	PPA	Parahippocampal Place Area
Dm	Difference based on subsequent memory	PPC	Posterior Parietal Cortex
		PTSD	Posttraumatic Stress Disorder
EEG	Electroencephalogram	RB	Rule Based (learning)
ERP	Event-related Potential	RL	Reversal Learning
FA	False Alarm	ROI	Region of Interest
FDR	False Discovery Rate	RSC	Retrosplenial Cortex
FFA	Fusiform Face Area	RT	Response time
fMRI	functional Magnetic Resonance Imaging	SAC	Source of Activation Confusion
		SARSA	State-Action-Reward-State-Action
HCS	Healthy Control Subjects	SCR	Skin Conductance Response
HMM	Hidden Markov Model	SEM	Structural Equation Modeling
IFG	Inferior Frontal Gyrus	SFG	Superior Frontal Gyrus
II	Information Integration (learning)	SN	Substatia nigra
IOG	Inferior Occipital Gyrus	SPL	Superior Parietal Lobule
IPS	Intra-Parietal Sulcus	SPM	Statistical Parametric Mapping
ISI	Inter-Stimulus Interval	STG	Superior Temporal Gyrus
LFP	Local Field Potential	STR	Short Term Retention
LOP	Levels of Processing	UCS	Unconditioned Stimulus
LOFC	Lateral Orbito-Frontal Cortex	VLPFC	Ventrolateral Prefrontal Cortex
LTD	Long-Term Depression	V4	Visual (cortex area) 4
LTM	Long-Term Memory	VT	Ventral Temporal
LTP	Long-Term Potentiation	VTA	Ventral Tegmental Area
MEM	Multiple-Entry, Modular model of memory and cognition	WM	Working Memory
MEG	Magnetoencephalography		
MFG	Middle Frontal Gyrus		
MOG	Middle Occipital Gyrus		

Chapter 1

Introduction: Neuroimaging of human memory

Frank Rösler, Charan Ranganath, Brigitte Röder, and Rainer H. Kluwe

The goals of this book

The advent of functional neuroimaging has brought about dramatic changes in the field of cognitive psychology. However, despite considerable technical, methodological, and theoretical advances in neuroimaging research, the potential value of imaging data for cognitive theories is not undisputed. Some have criticized the lack of *a priori* hypotheses and the atheoretical approach guiding some imaging studies (e.g. Grafman, Partiot, & Hollnagel, 1995, p. 349). More generally, several researchers have asked: *Why is it useful for understanding the cognitive system to know which brain regions are active in association with a particular task? What additional information can neuroimaging studies provide to extend cognitive theories about the principles how the 'mind' works?* (see Uttal, 2001; Coltheart, 2006). These questions formed the initial impetus for what eventually developed into this book.

The purpose of this book is not to provide a forum for theoretical or philosophical debates between psychologists and neuroimaging researchers on the validity and usefulness of imaging data. Although such dialogues can be useful and informative, these topics have been covered in detail elsewhere (e.g. special issues of Cortex 2006, 42 (3) or PNAS 1998, 95 (3); Uttal, 2001; Henson, 2005). Instead, our goal is to provide a cogent and accessible introduction to the rapidly expanding body of imaging research on human memory, along with thoughtful appraisals of the significance of these findings with regard to fundamental psychological questions. Apart from summarizing findings and methodological approaches, we hope to increase the sensitivity of active researchers and interested consumers of brain-imaging results to the challenges inherent in attempting to relate psychological and biological concepts. We hope that, as a consequence, this book can make a step towards the formidable task of developing comprehensive theories of memory that bridge brain and behaviour.

The whole enterprise was started when Frank Rösler (FR) and Rainer H. Kluwe (RHK) had a dispute with colleagues of the Wilhelm-Wundt-Society[1] about the merits of

---

[1] The Wilhelm-Wundt-Society (Wilhelm-Wundt-Gesellschaft, WWG) is a professional organization of psychologists in Germany dedicated to advance basic research in experimental psychology.

brain-imaging tools for cognitive psychology. This debate motivated FR and RHK to promote a broader discourse by providing better information to critics of cognitive neuroimaging, and by prompting imaging researchers to critically evaluate the status of their own field. Shortly after that, Charan Ranganath and FR had an informal talk at a conference of the Memory Disorders Research Society (MDRS),[2] where they agreed that discussions about brain-imaging methods in cognitive psychology often seem to be based on incomplete information. They agreed that it would be helpful to present material about brain-imaging results in a more concise manner so that researchers and students who want to be better informed do not have to go to the many journals where original papers are scattered around. Rather, they thought, the best of this research should be assembled in a volume that provides a concise and up-to date overview.

The editors then set forth to the task of assembling a group of contributors to discuss the potential value of neuroimaging research for theories of memory and also to consider to what extent brain-imaging research on memory has profited from progress in cognitive psychology. To this end, the editors and contributors, along with another 80 attendees (graduate students, post-docs, and scientists) met for a conference in 2006 at the Philipps-University in Marburg, Germany. With the invitation, the contributors were asked to present a first draft of a chapter for the planned book which outlined the potential value of their research for psychological theories of memory. More specifically, each contributor was asked to provide answers to the following questions: *Can results from neuroimaging constrain, support, or falsify psychological theories of memory?* and *How is research on the biological bases of memory guided by psychological theory?* The quality of these presentations was outstanding, and the ideas presented in these talks stimulated a great deal of discussion amongst the contributors and attendees of the conference. Following the meeting, all but three of the invited speakers finalized their contributions, which were then sent out for peer review to provide additional feedback. In addition to these chapters, the book contains four integrative commentary chapters. Four leading scientists in the field – Mark D'Esposito, Andy Yonelinas, Mick Rugg, and Alan Richardson-Klavehn – were asked and thankfully agreed to provide these discussion chapters on the basis of the contributions of the four sections of the book.

The organization of the volume

Section A of the book summarizes some general epistemological problems relevant for imaging research. These issues are discussed by two of the editors, Frank Rösler & Charan Ranganath, and by Rolf Ulrich. Both chapters address, from a more general

---

The society's membership is limited by 30 active members and by invitation only. (http://hermes.psych.uni-halle.de/wwg)

[2] The Memory Disorders Research Society (MDRS) is a professional society dedicated to the study of memory and memory disorders. Membership in the society is by invitation only, and is open only to individuals with a faculty appointment. The society meets once every year. (http://www.memory-disorders.org)

perspective, the question of how to uncover unobservable cognitive mechanisms, and they discuss epistemological problems connected with this enterprise. While Rösler and Ranganath tackle this problem in close relation to the prevailing discussion and the available evidence on brain-imaging research on cognitive functions, Ulrich introduces an additional perspective. He outlines how mathematical formalization of psychological theories helps to delineate hypothetical constructs and intervening variables that mediate between input and output. This approach can, as it is hoped, improve mappings between the unobservable entities and the observable biosignals in more precise statements, as is usually the case with heuristic psychological theories.

The remaining four sections of the book cover specific areas of human memory research that have been extensively studied with modern brain-imaging techniques: *Part 2: Learning and consolidation*, *Part 3: Working memory control processes and storage*, *Part 4: Long-term memory representations*, and *Part 5: Retrieval control processes*. These groupings of topics are somewhat arbitrary and should not be taken as a theoretical statement regarding the nature of memory processes, but rather as a means of organizing the chapters in a manner that could allow some broader connections to be made. Each section comprises four to five original papers in which leading scientists summarize their own and the work of others on a particular subject area, and an integrative commentary in which a leading scientist evaluates these contributions with respect to the overall scope of the book.

Learning and consolidation

This section concerns changes in functional brain activity, which can either be expected from theories of learning, or which are empirically observed and, therefore, can inform theories of learning. Christian Büchel and John O'Doherty both review recent work on classical conditioning, reinforcement learning, and reward processing in uncertain situations. These studies help to delineate areas in the brain whose activity can be mapped onto hypothetical constructs suggested by psychological theories of learning, e.g. the Rescorla–Wagner model, or the actor–critic model. Core concepts are prediction error, probability estimates, and action-related reward expectations. The results show that expected value seems not to be coded on a single continuum – as suggested by some utility theories – but rather that gains and losses are handled by the system as qualitatively distinct states, or that, on the other hand, avoidance of punishment (experience of safety signals) has the same biological effects as actual positive reward (experience of appetitive signals). This latter prediction was made a long time ago in order to explain the extinction resistance of avoidance learning, but it could never be proved convincingly on the basis of behavioural data alone (Gray, 1975). Moreover, O'Doherty presents data which substantiate strategy shifts in reward-learning situations showing that participants switch between exploitation and exploration and that these two states, predicted by a mathematical model of behaviour, are functionally related to the activity dominance of distinct brain areas – the striatum and the prefrontal cortex.

The next two chapters by Dara G. Ghahremani & Russell A. Poldrack and by Paul Reber focus on the question of whether brain-imaging data can decide between unitary vs. multiple memory systems, i.e. whether information is stored, consolidated, and retrieved always within one and the same biological substrate or whether distinct systems are involved depending on the type of material or task. Three issues intensely debated in experimental psychology and neuropsychology are addressed in these chapters and in each case data from brain-imaging studies strongly support the notion of multiple rather than unitary memory systems. The issues are (explicit) declarative memory vs. (implicit) skill memory, learning of prototypes vs. exemplars in categorization tasks, and (explicit) rule based vs. (implicit) information integration learning. Ghahremani and Poldrack provide evidence for the inverse relationship between medial temporal lobe structures and basal ganglia during different stages of learning, but also in distinct tasks which allow an explicit or a more implicit learning strategy. Paul Reber extends this scenario by reviewing data showing that category learning not only recruits regions that have been previously implicated in learning and memory processes (e.g. medial temporal lobes and basal ganglia), but also regions implicated in perceptual processing (e.g. occipital cortex). These findings clearly support psychological theories claiming distinct mechanisms for different types of learning (e.g. explicit/declarative vs. implicit/nondeclarative learning) and they provide a basis for understanding how these systems are modified due to experience. In addition, these findings challenge traditional views that fragment the mind into stages that are dedicated either to perception or to memory.

Finally, Guillén Fernández & Indira Tendolkar summarize evidence on *Declarative memory consolidation* that has been accumulated since the seminal paper of Müller and Pilzecker (1900). Much that has been learned and hypothesized on memory consolidation in the meantime comes from neuropsychology and animal work. However, recent neuroimaging tools made it possible to test specific predictions that follow from consolidation theory – that hippocampal activity during retrieval is reduced with increasing remoteness of the learning situation, and that replay takes place during sleep such that short-script engrams held in MTL are used to reactivate the full engram in cortical areas in order to modify synaptic connectivity.

The section is concluded by the integrative commentary of Alan Richardson-Klavehn and colleagues. In addition to specific comments on the preceding five chapters, the authors pick up the more general theme of how interlacing experimental psychology with neuroimaging tools can facilitate scientific progress. In so doing, they put special emphasis on the problem of distinguishing between theories of unitary or multiple memory systems and on how the research standard of functional dissociations between memory measures and memory systems may depend on specific contextual constraints. They also support their arguments in favour of the neuroimaging approach with data from their own research, specifically, on the dissociation between priming and conscious recollection (see also Part 5 of this volume) and on retrieval inhibition.

Working memory: Control processes and storage

Contributions to this section focus on mechanisms that control information flow during encoding and retrieval, processes which maintain items in an active state, and processes that enable flexible tuning or binding of task-relevant information.

Mark Johnson and Marcia Johnson review the MEM (multiple entry, modular framework, see Johnson, 1983) model of cognition which comprises a set of hierarchically ordered levels of perceptual and reflective sub-systems of information processing. The hierarchy reflects the distinction between bottom-up (perceptual) and top-down (reflective) processes which, in part, correlates with automatic vs. controlled (attention consuming) functions (Schneider & Shiffrin, 1977). The framework has been used to guide brain-imaging studies in identifying biological bases of hypothesized processes as refreshing, noting, or rehearsing of information, or of initiating actions. The results show that these functions, sometimes subsumed under the umbrella term 'executive functions' may be implemented in part by different regions of the prefrontal cortex (PFC). The research program shows that different component processes are associated with different patterns of activity in the PFC. The chapter illustrates how imaging research can help constrain models that aim to explain cognitive control processes not only with respect to memory, but also in a variety of other cognitive domains. As eloquently stated by the authors, 'We do not need neuroimaging to ask what we mean by terms such as executive function, working memory, cognitive control, or reflection, and many elegant cognitive-behavioural experiments have helped clarify such concepts. However, the further agenda of linking cognitive processes to brain function provides one way of deconstructing those concepts for a more specific level of analysis, and may therefore result in a more complete science of cognition.'

This idea is also emphasized in the chapter of Adrian Owen and Adam Hampshire who focus on working-memory functions represented within the mid-ventrolateral frontal cortex (VLPFC). In their chapter, they first summarize a series of studies providing strong evidence that the VLPFC is closely related to intentional encoding and retrieval of information in working memory. However, additional brain-imaging findings with different tasks (e.g. reversal learning or intrinsically guided attentional shifts in recognition memory tasks) modified and enlarged this perspective by suggesting that VLPFC functions are not only relevant for working memory encoding and retrieval per se but that they serve a more general goal, i.e. a flexible allocation of attentional resources. Thus, control of attentional resources seems to be one of the core functions of PFC structures that finds its expression in regulating input and output information flow but also in fore- and backgrounding of information in working memory (see also Oberauer & Kliegl, 2006).

A similar view is put forward in Brad Postle's chapter, which argues that brain-imaging studies may suggest a new theory of working memory (see also Postle, 2006). Rather than assuming that working memory comprises a set of highly specific and narrowly defined modules (e.g. buffer structures, as phonological loop, visuo-spatial scratch pad, etc.), it is suggested that working memory is an emergent property of a hierarchically interacting set of neural networks whose main function is the allocation of attentional resources among sensory-, representation-, and action-related brain areas. Postle backs this claim by experiments that were guided by the 'what and where' distinction of the visual system and that revealed distinct interactions between visual and non-visual areas of the brain, i.e. they revealed that working memory tasks involved not only highly specialized networks located within the visual system but also networks within the action system (e.g. the frontal and supplementary eye fields or the basal ganglia). Thus, in keeping with findings suggesting links between perception and action (Keysers & Gazzola, 2007; Schütz-Bosbach & Prinz, 2007), Postle's data show that spatial working memory may be an emergent property of interactions between visual-perception and action.

All three chapters directly address the questions of how brain-imaging data can inform psychological theories and vice versa. First, they illustrate how clever experimentation guided by psychological theories can lead to results that feed back to the theory (e.g. the finding that visual working memory tasks involve an activation of motor areas suggests the need to modify the definition of how visuo-spatial information is encoded in working memory). Second, they show that a strict distinction between purely psychological and neural theories becomes somewhat obsolete in this field of research, and that imaging findings can substantially modify our ideas about psychological processes.

Charan Ranganath brings into focus another aspect of brain-imaging research on working memory. Traditionally, working memory (WM) has been seen as distinct from long-term memory (LTM) and the two topics have generally been studied in isolation. However, results from a series of experiments by Ranganath and his coworkers have shown that WM and LTM may be closely interrelated, both functionally and neuroanatomically. For example, the data has led many to question neuropsychological dissociations between WM and LTM, by revealing that the hippocampus contributes to WM maintenance as well as to LTM formation. Moreover, activity during WM maintenance is predictive of subsequent LTM performance. These imaging results support an alternative view, namely that WM and LTM differ less with respect to the involved neuroanatomical structures but more with respect to activation states and the specific interactive pattern of involved brain areas. Another line of research described in the chapter focuses on using concepts from psychological studies of memory encoding to understand the roles of different regions of the prefrontal cortex in WM and LTM. Drawing from psychological theories that posit distinctions between item-specific and relational encoding processes, Ranganath suggests that the ventrolateral prefrontal cortex may implement control processes that support item-specific encoding, whereas the dorsolateral and ventrolateral prefrontal cortices may support relational encoding. This work is an excellent example of the synergistic effects of using psychological theories to guide imaging studies.

In their integrative commentary chapter, Bradley Buchsbaum and Mark D'Esposito tie the threads of the four chapters together to one rope and put the findings into the broader perspective of how brain-imaging tools have provided new insights and modified theories on memory. In particular, they stress the point that psychological distinctions between functionally encapsulated modules handling either WM or LTM encoding and retrieval or being specialized on specific sub-processes have to be questioned on the basis of brain-imaging data. They cite Joaquin Fuster, who picked up and elaborated on Karl Lashley's claim (Lashley, 1950) by saying that 'Memory is a functional property, among others, of each and all of the areas of the cerebral cortex, and thus all cortical systems' (Fuster, 1995). And, one might continue the theme by saying that, therefore, it is essential to study the brain in close relationship to psychological ideas about functions, because, otherwise, an incomplete or even an incorrect picture of memory might result.

Long-term memory representations

The key question in this section is what brain-imaging data can tell about how information is represented in long-term memory and how it is reactivated in distinct tasks. Psychological research supports the idea that there exist content-specific memories (e.g. dual code theory of semantic and pictorial information, Paivio, 1986), however, behavioural data did not provide a clear cut answer to whether there are distinct types of representations or not (Kosslyn, 1994). Moreover, as already outlined above, traditional psychological research made a strict distinction between short-living working memory and permanent long-term memory contents (Baddeley, 1990), while more recently, a functional overlap of the two storage forms has been proposed (Cowan, 1995). Brain-imaging research provides many pieces of evidence that address the question of code-specific long-term memory representations and that also show a close overlap between neural networks activated during both WM and LTM tasks. These findings have an immediate influence on how models about LTM codes and about storage and retrieval are formulated.

Alumit Ishai's chapter provides a concise overview of studies that use fMRI to delineate category-specific memory representations. Earlier studies (e.g. Ishai, Ungerleider, Martin, & Haxby, 2000) made a strong claim that distinct anatomical areas in the occipital and the inferior temporal lobe are specifically activated when exemplars of distinct categories are processed in recognition memory tasks. More recent work, however, that is summarized in this chapter shows that these activation patterns are only in part due to memory-specific processes. Another strong influence seems to be the particular task performed by the participants. By contrasting tasks that have a high perceptual vs. a high imagery component, it was shown by the author and by others that these activation patterns in the inferior temporal lobe are primarily evoked when perceptual processing dominates, whereas activation in these areas is much weaker during imagery tasks in which information has to be retrieved from long-term memory. The chapter also discusses how face-specific activation patterns in the FFA and other brain areas are modulated by the emotional expression of a perceived face, again highlighting the task dependence of such category-related activation patterns. In sum, A.I. concludes from these results that recognition memory may be mediated by activation in a distributed neural system that includes regions in visual cortex, where stimulus-specific representations are stored; areas in parietal cortex, where visual similarity to familiar prototypes is processed; memory-related areas in parietal and prefrontal cortices, where novel items are classified as a match or a mismatch based on their similarity to familiar prototypes; and the hippocampus, where veridical memory traces are recovered.

Patrick Khader and Frank Rösler review behavioural, neurophysiological, and neuroimaging studies that reveal dissociations between storage or retrieval of clearly distinct, global stimulus categories (e.g. verbal vs. spatial, or motor vs. visual representations), of less distinct stimulus categories (spatial vs. object information), and of fine-grained distinctions within object categories (e.g. faces vs. buildings vs. tools vs. chairs vs. houses, etc.). These results clearly show that material-specific cortical networks exist which are systematically activated during LTM retrieval. However, these networks overlap substantially with areas that are also activated during perceptual and working memory tasks. Therefore, the findings are compatible with information processing models of memory storage and retrieval assuming that memory traces are encoded as connectivity changes within modality-specific projection areas, and that recognition and recall are to be seen as re-instantiations of activity patterns within these very areas. Studying the question of 'where' long-term memories are represented does also contribute to the question of 'how' this is accomplished. In particular, the findings are at variance with the traditional psychological distinction between perceptual and motor processing of information on the one side and memory on the other. Rather, the very same areas which are relevant for online information processing seem also to be the storage sites where long-term engrams are formed and reactivated.

The next chapter of Kenneth Norman and colleagues serves two purposes. On the one hand, it expands on the question of how and where in the brain memory representations are stored and reactivated in that the authors not only look for macro patterns of activation that extend over brain areas of the size of Brodmann areas but rather they analyse the whole pattern of voxels and relate the complete pattern to specific contents or states of memory retrieval. On the other hand, the chapter has a strong methodological focus because it presents a relatively novel and innovative method for the analysis of fMRI results. The authors review their work on multi-voxel pattern analysis (MVPA) or, more generally, on multivariate biosignal pattern analysis. After a short introduction to the method, three examples are presented to show how it can be used to delineate and distinguish between memory-related brain states. The first two examples exploit multivariate information from fMRI data, the third from EEG data. The results prove that multivariate brain activation pattern analysis can be used to successfully distinguish between (i) states in which distinct categories are reactivated during recall, (ii) between states in which recognition decisions are either based on familiarity or recollection judgments, and finally, (iii) between states in which prime-target relations are either positively or negatively primed. The chapter covers the question of how brain-imaging data can inform psychological theories and it also demonstrates that psychology provides a theoretical basis for studying highly specific hypotheses about brain activation patterns. The problems associated with this approach of reverse inference are explicitly addressed, and the possible advantages and future perspectives are outlined too.

From the very beginning, research on memory has been guided by the information-processing paradigm (Lachman, Lachman, & Butterfield, 1979). For example, issues of representations, storage, and retrieval have been studied independently from emotional and motivational influences. It is only recently that these modulating influences, whose strong impact on memory has been long known by clinical psychologists, has been integrated into psychological and neuroscience research programs. Kevin LaBar summarizes how advances in functional neuroimaging have opened a new window into understanding how the human brain encodes and retrieves memories of emotionally salient events. Initial neuroimaging studies in humans have provided support for the hypothesis that arousal benefits memory through the modulating effect of the amygdala on consolidation processes mediated by the hippocampus. Moreover, neuroimaging studies have revealed characteristics of emotional memory that were not predicted by animal models, including sex differences in brain lateralization, valence-specific memory modulation effects, and contributions of medial temporal lobe regions to emotional memory retrieval. Recent developments in event-related designs and functional connectivity analysis have helped to specify the neural correlates of emotion–memory interactions in greater detail. Applications to the domain of autobiographical memory have elucidated how emotion affects neural activity during recall of events from the remote personal past. Ultimately, these lines of research promise to provide novel insights into the dysregulation of emotional memories in affective disorders that lead to intrusive traumatic recollection and mood-congruent biases (e.g. Elbert, Rockstroh, Kolassa, Schauer, & Neuner, 2006).

Andrew Yonelinas integrates the issues touched in these chapters in his commentary, and broadens the perspective again towards epistemological issues discussed in Part 1. He points out that the approaches pursued in imaging research can be allocated to one of three categories – exploratory studies, validation studies, and hypothetico-deductive studies. The first two types of studies belong to the 'forward inference' domain, the third to the 'reverse inference' domain (see Part 1, Chapter 2). A.Y. stresses how each of these approaches can and does advance the field. In addition, he gives a convincing example from his own research of how brain-imaging results that relate source recollection and familiarity to distinct parts of the temporal lobe can motivate new behavioural experiments and consequently have an impact on theories of recognition memory.

Control processes during encoding and retrieval

This part covers processes relevant for information retrieval from memory, as source monitoring, familiarity, recollection, and processes relevant for encoding of information into memory.

The two chapters of Axel Mecklinger and Theodor Jäger and Ken Paller together with his colleagues Joel Voss and Carmen Westerberg, respectively, summarize research on the familiarity/recollection distinction relevant for recognition memory. The main focus is on ERP effects that support a functional distinction between recognition decision states. In this respect the chapters are special, because their main focus is not on anatomical differences as disclosed by fMRI, but on temporal differences as disclosed by the time-sensitive measures of event-related brain potentials.

Mecklinger and Jäger provide a comprehensive and well-balanced account of the topic of recollection by reviewing work from other labs as well as their own. They report novel studies of recognition of morphed faces that nicely illustrate how states of familiarity and recollection can be experimentally manipulated, and how these two distinct states are reliably associated with distinct signatures in the ERP. By so doing, they explicitly address the question on how brain-imaging data, or more generally phrased, biological data can help to inform psychological theories of memory.

Ken Paller and colleagues also focus on how distinct states of recognition memory can be functionally characterized in recordings of event-related brain potentials. In contrast to much of the work published in this field, Paller *et al.* not only consider recollection and familiarity as two distinct states but they also include priming effects in their discussion. Behaviourally, all three outcomes of a memory test situation indicate that something has been stored by the system but the three states differ with respect to their degree of consciousness. Recollection reveals that a participant is fully conscious of the fact that she remembers an item and also that she remembers specific details of the storage situation. Familiarity indicates only consciousness about having encountered an item before, without remembering any details. Finally, priming is a behavioural improvement in processing of an item on repeated exposure that can be observed even when participants are unaware of having previously processed the item. From a psychological perspective, these three states might be seen as lying on a continuum of recognition memory activity. The interesting point, however, is that ERPs show clear latency and topographic differences between the three states. This is another convincing example of how neuroimaging data can help to sharpen psychological concepts/constructs by suggesting that there is not a one-dimensional continuum of recognition memory processes but, most likely, that there exist qualitatively distinct processes. Moreover, seen from a wider perspective, the work in this field supports the idea that brain-imaging methods can help to objectify the somewhat vague distinction between conscious and non-conscious processing.

In the next chapter, Jon Simons also addresses the question *to what extent humans do have access to the context in which a memory was formed?* The chapter presents a comprehensive summary of research done by the author and his co-workers on prefrontal cortex function in relation to source monitoring during memory retrieval. In the past, this process has been specifically related to memory retrieval but here it is discussed in a broader context and related to other functions/constructs that are not so closely tied to the domain of memory, but more to the domain of executive and other 'higher' control functions. Among others, these are reality monitoring, control of internally and externally generated context, prospective memory, mentalizing, and attention regulation between input (cues) and central representations. With regard to the main objective of the book, the argument rests primarily on the logic of reverse inference, and by using this strategy, the author integrates various results by referring to the 'gateway' hypothesis. In short, this hypothesis says that the medial anterior PFC enables attention regulation between stimulus-dependent and stimulus-independent 'thought'. Such an attentional bias seems to lie at the heart of source monitoring during memory retrieval.

The last chapter by Emrah Düzel and Sebastian Guderian elaborates on the question of how pre-stimulus brain states during encoding have an effect on later memory performance. They comprehensively summarize recent findings on that topic and they also provide explanations of how these influences might be understood on the basis of neuroanatomical connections and functional mechanisms, such as the calculation of prediction errors or the evaluation of novelty. In this respect, they address how imaging tools can advance our understanding of learning and memory by not only looking at 'hot spots' in the brain, but also by relating these spots to *dynamic* changes observable in the MEG or EEG as transient oscillations.

Based on the material presented in this section Michael Rugg picks up again in his integrative commentary some of the broader epistemological issues touched on in Part 1 and in other sections of the book. But rather than just reiterating some of the points mentioned before, he brings into focus some additional problems that are still unsettled when it comes to mapping psychological and biological measures and constructs onto each other. For example, when the mapping problem is addressed (Henson, 2005; Rösler and Ranganath, Chapter 2), it is usually not clearly distinguished on the psychological side between process and content, or, in words more specifically applicable to the domain of memory, between representation and operation. Tacitly, it is assumed that an activation dissociation observed within the same task for different materials is due to different representations that are stored or reactivated within different networks. On the other hand, if a dissociation is observed within the same task at different stages, e.g. during initial and late phases of learning, it is assumed that distinct processes or operations are involved. Rugg is completely right in pointing out that such implicit conclusions have to be spelled out more explicitly in future research.

A word of thanks

The whole enterprise could not have been completed without the help and support of many individuals and institutions. First of all, we thank the German Research Foundation (Deutsche Forschungsgemeinschaft, DFG, http://www.dfg.de/en/) and the Alexander von Humboldt Foundation (http://www.humboldt-foundation.de/) for generous financial support. The DFG had supported a research group on 'dynamics of cognitive processes' at the Philipps-University of Marburg and in the course of this had provided money for scientific meetings. The Alexander von Humboldt Foundation had provided the money for the Max-Planck-Prize for international cooperation awarded to FR in 2002. By means of these two grants most of the costs of the conference held in Marburg in preparation of the book could be covered. This conference was also supported by the Wilhelm-Wundt society. All this financial support is greatly acknowledged.

We thank all the contributors and discussants for providing and reshaping their highly readable chapters. We very much appreciate their extra efforts, in addition to the routine scientific work, and we thank them, in particular, for their discipline in keeping to deadlines. Without these efforts nothing could have been accomplished. Many thanks to our outside peer reviewers Jan Born, Leun Otten, Tobias Sommer, and Hubert Zimmer, who, in addition to the 'inside' peer reviewers, helped with thoughtful comments to sharpen the focus of the chapters. Finally, we thank Carol Maxwell at Oxford University Press who accompanied the project with enthusiasm and support and, last but not least, Aline Jakobi who invested many hours of secretarial effort to check references and other formal issues, and who helped to standardize the layout of the manuscripts.

References

Baddeley, A. D. (1990). *Human Memory – Theory and Practice*. Erlbaum: Hove and London.

Coltheart, M. (2006). What has functional neuroimaging told us about the mind (so far)? *Cortex, 42*(3), 323–331.

Cowan, N. (1995). *Attention and Memory – An Integrated Framework*. New York: Oxford University Press.

Elbert, T., Rockstroh, B., Kolassa, I.-T., Schauer, M., & Neuner, F. (2006). The influence of organized violence and terror on brain and mind: a co-constructive perspective. In: P. B. Baltes, P. Reuter-Lorenz, & F. Rösler, (Eds), *Lifespan Development and the Brain* (pp. 326–349). Cambridge: Cambridge University Press.

Fuster, J. M. (1995). *Memory in the Cerebral Cortex*. Cambridge, MA: MIT Press.

Grafman, J., Partiot, A. & Hollnagel, C. (1995). Fables of the prefrontal cortex. *Behavioral and Brain Sciences, 18*, 349–358.

Gray, J. A. (1975). *Elements of a Two-Process Theory of Learning*. London: Academic Press.

Henson, R. N. A. (2005). What can functional neuroimaging tell the experimental psychologist? *Quarterly Journal of Experimental Psychology. A, Human Experimental Psychology, 58*(2), 193–233.

Ishai, A., Ungerleider, L. G., Martin, A., & Haxby, J. V. (2000). The representation of objects in the human occipital and temporal cortex. *Journal of Cognitive Neuroscience, 12*(Suppl. 2), 35–51.

Johnson, M. K. (1983). A multiple-entry, modular memory system. *The Psychology of Learning and Motivation: Advances in Research and Theory, 17*, 81–123.

Keysers, C., & Gazzola, V. (2007). Integrating simulation and theory of mind: from self to social cognition. *Trends in Cognitive Sciences, 11*(5), 194–196.

Kosslyn, S. M. (1994). *Image and the Brain: The Resolution of the Imagery Debate*. Cambridge, MA: MIT Press.

Lachman, R., Lachman, J. L., & Butterfield, E. C. (1979). *Cognitive Psychology and Information Processing*. Hillsdale, NJ: Erlbaum.

Lashley, K. D. (1950). In search of the engram. *Symposia of the Society for Experimental Biology, 4*, 454–482.

Müller, G. E. & Pilzecker, A. (1900). Experimentelle Beiträge zur Lehre vom Gedächtnis, *Zeitschrift für Psychologie, 1*, 1–300.

Oberauer, K., & Kliegl, R. (2006). A formal model of capacity limits in working memory. *Journal of Memory and Language, 55*, 601–626.

Paivio, A. (1986). *Mental Representations*. New York: Oxford University Press.

Postle, B. R. (2006). Working memory as an emergent property of the mind and brain. *Neuroscience, 139*(1), 23–38.

Schneider, W., & Shiffrin, R. M. (1977). Controlled and Automatic Human Information Processing: I. Detection, Search, and Attention. *Psychological Review, 84*, 1–66.

Schütz-Bosbach, S., & Prinz, W. (2007). Perceptual resonance: action-induced modulation of perception. *Trends in Cognitive Sciences, 11*(8), 349–355.

Uttal, W. R. (2001). *The New Phrenology: The Limits of Localizing Cognitive Processes*. London, Cambridge, MA: The MIT Press.

Part 1

Setting the stage

Chapter 2

On how to reconcile mind and brain

Frank Rösler and Charan Ranganath

Introduction

Neurophysiological methods have been used to study cognition for over a century, but until recently, these methods have had a limited impact on the field of psychology. However, beginning with the pioneering positron emission tomography (PET) studies of Posner, Petersen, Fox, and Raichle (1988) and continuing through the subsequent explosion of research using event-related functional magnetic resonance imaging (FMRI), there has been a growing dialogue between neuroimaging researchers and cognitive psychologists. Initially, many psychologists expressed skepticism about the utility of these methods, and even now, there are many who remain unconvinced that functional neuroimaging can provide information that would be useful to constrain or develop psychological theories. A growing number of psychologists, however, are not only interested in learning about functional imaging results, but actively using imaging techniques to test their theories. In this chapter, we will first critically evaluate the validity of arguments used to discount the utility of functional imaging. Next, we will present some epistemological arguments to highlight the mutual interdependence of cognitive neuroscience and cognitive psychology. Consideration of these points suggests that although there are conceptual and methodological challenges that psychologists must address before the potential benefits of neuroimaging can be realized, imaging data is nonetheless a powerful tool to reconcile concepts of mind and brain, so that we may move beyond the so-called 'black box' models of cognition.

Uncovering the unobservable

Ultimately, cognitive psychologists and neuroimaging researchers want to understand how the mind works, but they sometimes do not agree on the methods that are feasible to make progress in this enterprise. To illustrate such disagreements, consider a statement by Randy Buckner, a pioneer in the field of cognitive neuroimaging (Buckner, 2000, p. 817): 'A primary challenge for the cognitive neuroscience of human memory is the development and application of methods that link mnemonic processes with their underlying neural bases. Providing one kind of link, functional neuroimaging methods offer a means to visualize brain areas active during cognitive operations in awake, healthy human.' This is in stark contrast, to more skeptical points of view as, e.g. expressed by Van Orden & Paap (1997): 'What has functional neuroimaging told us about the mind so far?', 'Nothing, and it never will: the nature cognition is such that this technique in principle cannot provide evidence about the nature of cognition'; (see Coltheart, 2006 for more arguments of this kind).

As a matter of fact, disagreement between biologically minded and behaviourally minded scientists is not a new development. More than 30 years ago, when experimental psychologists had just started to use event-related brain potentials to study the mind (McCallum & Knott, 1976), these researchers faced many of the same criticisms that brain imagers currently face. Looking somewhat deeper into this issue reveals a fundamental philosophical question of how to reconcile mind and body. In general, pure cognitive psychology involves manipulation of 'input' variables and the measurement of observable 'output' variables, as response times or error rates of overt behaviour (finger movements, eye movements, spoken utterances). These two observables (input and output) are then related by making more or less sophisticated assumptions about unobservable intervening variables, their number, their quality and their dynamics (see Figure 2.1). In the weakest formulation, the intervening variables have the status of heuristic assumptions, and in the strongest formulation, they are pinned down to mathematical statements that make very precise predictions about unobserved hypothetical processes (see Ulrich this volume). This is a valuable

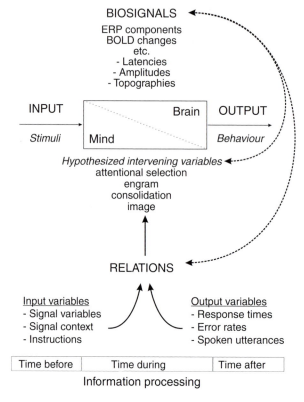

Figure 2.1 Research approach of cognitive psychology (lower part without the dashed lines) and cognitive neuroscience (see text for explanation).

and challenging intellectual enterprise that can provide deep insights into the mechanics of the mind (Scarborough & Sternberg, 1998; see Miyake & Shah, 1999 for memory-specific examples). The fact remains, however, that all these intervening processes and variables are purely hypothetical (MacCorquodale & Meehl, 1948) and they may not describe how the human brain actually works. For instance, it is possible to explain psychological phenomena by assuming that there are stages through which information is passed on sequentially (Sternberg, 1969), but evidence from neuroscience suggests that this may not be a biologically plausible assumption (Van Essen & Drury, 1997; Lamme, Super, Landman, Roelfsema, & Spekreijse, 2000).

Physiological measures (PET, fMRI), on the other hand, provide statements about blood flow changes and their relation to neural and/or energy consumption processes within cortical areas (Moonen & Bandettini, 2000). As such, they do not bear any direct relationship to psychological constructs or intervening variables. For example, the dependent measure in FMRI studies, blood oxygenation level dependent (BOLD) signal, is psychologically empty as long as one does not know the particular task in which it was recorded. In other words, simply knowing that a particular brain area is more active now than a few seconds earlier, or that it is more active in situation A but not in situation B, does not necessarily reveal about which function might have caused this activation change. However, to put this argument into perspective, response times (which essentially reflect downstream measures that emerge from activity in the primary motor cortex) are equally empty if one does not know the experimental context. Thus, whether one is considering behavioural or imaging data, insight into the functional significance of an effect is only achieved by considering the experimental context and by considering the findings relative to what would be predicted on the basis of competing theories that relate input, intervening, and output variables.

Of course, biological measures, unlike response time measures, more directly index the brain processes that mediate between input and output. Thus, in the context of well-planned experiments, biological data can be reliably and systematically related to the very processes that cognitive psychologists want to get a hand on but which are unobservable to them in principle. Nonetheless, a common argument presented by skeptics is that the study of cognitive processes and the study of brain function represent two levels of description that are incommensurable. For example, one common claim is that the software (cognition) cannot be understood by studying the hardware (neurobiology). This position rests on two presuppositions: (1) the computer software/hardware distinction is a valid analogy for the human mind, and (2), that a one-to-one mapping of psychological (hypothetical constructs, intervening variables) and biological terms (activation states of neural networks) is impossible.

Hardware, software, or wetware?

Ulrich's chapter in this volume presents an elaborate illustration of the software-hardware analogy. The general argument is that one will not understand a complex computer program by measuring electrical currents or energy consumptions of certain hardware modules of a notebook (the CPU, the cache, the graphic chip, or the disc controller).

If one accepts the validity of this analogy, however, this conclusion is not so clear cut. A computer programmer might use a high-level scripting language to perform some computations, but ultimately, the execution of these computations requires the instantiation of a particular pattern of 'activity' in the hardware. Furthermore, a program that is written to work with some kinds of hardware may not be able to run on a computer with a different hardware configuration. In some sense, the most appropriate aspect of the software–hardware analogy is that computer hardware performs computations in a manner that is hidden from the user, much as the interface between cognition and behaviour is not directly observable by cognitive psychologists.

A more critical concern with the software–hardware analogy is, however, that it presents an inaccurate portrayal of the human brain. Typical multiple purpose computers have a fixed hardware configuration consisting of a limited number of integrated circuits (processing modules). The brain is built from 100 billion neurons that are highly interconnected (Nauta & Feirtag, 1986) and *whose number and connectivity changes* due to environmental influences (Shaw & McEachern, 2001; Baltes, Reuter-Lorenz, & Rösler, 2006). It is a gigantic associative network (Aertsen & Braitenberg, 1992), and unlike a computer, it is not brought to 'life' by uploading software programs. The functional principles of the brain and its distinguishable modules (e.g. sensory or motor cortices) do not result from a software running on the neuronal hardware but rather these functions emerge from the connectivity pattern of the neurons. 'Wetware' would be a more appropriate term to adequately describe the situation. For instance, in the visual cortex, the functional features of neurons (receptive fields) are not realized as software nor are they established as genetically-predetermined hardware. The functional features of simple, complex and hyper-complex cells develop due to a very close interaction between genetic predispositions and environmental influences (Black, Jones, Nelson, & Greenough, 1998; Rosenzweig, Krech, Bennett, & Diamond, 1962; Hubel, Wiesel, & LeVay, 1977). During a critical window of development, the connectivity pattern of the neurons changes due to the encountered input and at the end of this plastic period the functional features emerge from the specific connectivities of the neurons. In other words, the interconnected set of neurons acquires by its connectivities features of a filter that selectively responds to certain properties of the (visual) environment. Such filter features can be described abstractly as kind of a software routine (e.g. a Fourier-transformation), but this does not take place in the strict sense (Westheimer, 1986). In biological reality, it is a wetware filter (Sejnowski, 1981), and the function cannot be seen as separate from the neural network and its specific connectivities.

This does not only hold for neural networks close to the input or output side of the system but applies as well to higher cognitive functions as a decision between two input signals that gives rise to one or another response (e.g. up- or downward movement of the eyes). Such a decision can be described abstractly on a functional level as applying Bayes formula and by assuming that somewhere between input and output a module must exist that evaluates the evidence, calculates priors and conditional probabilities, and based on these calculations sends a signal to the output module that triggers the response. In biological reality, however, the computations appear to be implemented by neural networks that – by subtracting firing rates of antagonistically interconnected neurons – can compute the relative likelihood of the evidence for the one or the other option (Gold & Shadlen, 2001). Although the output of the system may give the impression that there is a software Bayes calculator implemented somewhere, measurements of neural firing patterns reveal that the brain only needs to compare the relative signal strength between two sets of neurons to provide the correct output. Thus, a cognitive theory about decision-making of a monkey or a human may make the correct predictions about behaviour in given conditions, but the assumed mediating processes that are derived from input–output relationships may not exist in biological reality at all. Rather, wiring principles can exist that produce the correct behaviour according to Bayes rule but in a much simpler manner. With such more complex functions it is most likely that the system acts as a cascaded wetware filter that samples evidence and combines this evidence in order to maximize the likelihood of specific input–output relationships.

However, if the system is functioning more like a hierarchically organized bank of filters with feedforward and feedback connections rather than like a software program running on a multiple purpose computer, the features of the system, its 'mechanics', and dynamics, cannot be understood realistically without considering the wetware and the built-in principles that transform input into output.

Mapping psychology onto biology and vice versa

Even if one dismisses the software–hardware metaphor as inadequate and accepts instead that cognitive functions result from specific wetware configurations, one can still argue that biological variables are useless for understanding how the mind works, because the concepts and tools used in the study of the mind and those used in the study of the brain cannot be mapped onto each other. This argument, however, can only be defended in final consequence, if one holds a dualistic position about mind and brain, or soul and body, in the tradition of Descartes. It seems there are only few scientists left in the 21st century who would subscribe to such a strong dualistic position. Rather, the majority adhere to a monistic position in that they assume only one ontological entity which can be described and studied from different perspectives – introspectively and with subjective and objective *psychological* terms and methods and also from the outside with physiological, more generally, *physical* terms and methods. We presume that even very dogmatic cognitive psychologists are most likely not ontological dualists but, if cornered on this issue, would describe themselves as ontological monists and, possibly, as methodological dualists. However, accepting ontological monism and conceding methodological dualism, one is forced to assume that there exists, at least in principle, a one-to-one mapping of psychological and physiological states (terms). A thought, a memory content, a perceptual entity, more generally, each cognitive state must have a unique physiological equivalent that becomes manifest in an activation pattern within the neural wetware. Of course, accepting this equivalence as a matter of principle, it is not automatically implied that such mappings are possible given the terms, variables, and measurement procedures available today within the two domains.

We think that such a mapping is possible, but one has to be aware of two empirical problems that might obscure the exact nature of psychophysiological relationships. First, the descriptive terms and categories on both sides of the equation may apply to distinct levels of observation. Second, the measurement tools might not allow identifying phenomena with sufficient resolution.

Distinct hierarchical levels

On the biological side, the hierarchy of anatomic observables starts with the organism as the most comprehensive level, covers subcategories as the brain, the hemispheres, Brodmann areas, Nuclei, subcortical entities, cell assemblies, neural networks, neurons, synapses, and ends at the most fine-grained level with subsynaptic entities as ion channels, etc. With respect to functional variables that can be measured by means of the available physiological tools, the categories follow by and large the same hierarchy. And the measures at issue in the present context – event-related brain potentials and BOLD responses – belong most likely to the level as described by Brodmann areas or subcortical nuclei, sometimes to levels of finer grain as narrowly circumscribed cell assemblies (e.g. stripes in the visual cortex, e.g. Pfeuffer *et al.,* 2002). On the psychological side, hierarchies of cognitive processes/representations are less obvious, although there is some agreement. For example, in language, graphemes, morphemes, words, sentences, texts form a hierarchy, and in vision, elementary features (edges, colour, movement, etc.), combinations of these features (objects), and combinations of objects (scenes) also form a hierarchy. However, it has to be admitted that the hierarchies and the categories are not as straightforwardly defined as on the biological, especially the anatomical side. So the logical question is whether a psychologically defined intervening entity – e.g. an engram of a spatial location or an object – can be mapped onto a biological activation state such that both biological and psychological descriptions do correspond. To date, nobody will claim that one-to-one mappings between corresponding hierarchical levels are already given on the basis of our current psychobiological knowledge. Currently, this is still an empirical question, but the available tools as brain electrical potentials (EEG, ERP) and blood flow changes (BOLD) can provide answers to this question. The criterion is the amount of explained overlapping variance of the two sets of data and the precision of predictions for both sets of variables. These predictions have to be based on a theory that integrates biological *and* psychological terms and their relationships to input and output (see Ulrich this volume). Such a theory must, of course, explicitly relate hypothesized intervening variables to input manipulations, as well as to both measured variables – behavioural and biological. If properly handled on the theoretical level, such a psychobiological theory will have fewer degrees of freedom for formulating arbitrary intervening variables than a pure psychological theory that is not bounded by biological constraints.

Henson (2005) discussed in detail the subtleties of the mapping problem and stressed the kind of chicken–egg situation that exists here. On one hand, one needs the correct categories for the terms to be mapped onto each other, but on the other hand, in many areas, the critical goal is to use psycho-physiological data to help determine the psychological categories (function to structure deduction, forward inference, see Henson, 2005).

For example, if we want to relate memory representations to physiological activation states, we may start with the presupposition that each and every representation must have a physiological counterpart expressed by a pattern of neural activations (the two sides of the coin). However, what is the basic entity of a memory representation on the psychological side and its physiological counterpart? To address this question we have to start somewhere and by continuous experimentation we will have to refine our definition on both sides. Take faces as an example: We may assume for a start that faces are stored as wholistic entities, as exemplars and, possibly also as prototypes, we may also assume that on a subordinate level elementary features of faces and their relations are represented in memory, and on a superordinate level that faces are part of an integrated, more comprehensive representation of a person that includes voice, body appearance, personality traits, gait, etc. We can design experiments to find evidence for all of these representational levels, and we can then try to relate the findings for each level to biological activation patterns in narrowly circumscribed brain areas (e.g. FFA), in broadly defined areas as the inferior temporal lobe and lateral occipital cortex, or in an interconnected network of areas that is scattered over several macro-anatomical regions (Gauthier *et al.*, 2000; Khader, Burke, Bien, Ranganath, & Rösler, 2005; Yago & Ishai, 2006; Dricot, Sorger, Schiltz, Goebel, & Rossion, 2008; Miki, Watanabe, Honda, Nakamura, & Kakigi, 2007). Empirical work has shown that there are regions in the brain that can be mapped onto the conceptual level of objects, others that can be mapped onto the conceptual level of features, but that within these regions most likely more fine grained features are represented and reflected in the brain activation patterns (see Norman this volume). The correct mappings are for sure not disclosed by one single experiment but, as it is usually the case in all empirical sciences, by a sequence of experiments that will continuously sharpen the categories on both sides and their reciprocal mapping. At the beginning, there will be most often *many-to-one* mappings from psychology to biology, i.e. many distinct psychological functions will be related to one physiological-anatomical entity. But with increasing knowledge, the picture will become much sharper on both sides.

Measurement resolution

Another issue that can restrict mapping of neural and psychological concepts is the reliability and validity of the behavioural and neural data used to make these links. If one is using a behavioural measure that is influenced by more than one cognitive process, this can result in inconsistencies in mapping between processes and brain systems. For instance, initial PET and FMRI studies of recognition memory used simple yes/no recognition tests, but a great deal of research suggests that recognition judgments can be supported by recollection, familiarity, or both processes. More recent studies have therefore used behavioural methods to tease apart recollection and familiarity, and these studies have shown reliable neural dissociations between the two (Diana, Yonelinas, & Ranganath, 2007).

Conceding that there are phenomena and descriptive terms involved on each side of the psychophysiological equation that belong to distinct hierarchical levels, the mutual mapping of these terms can be further restricted by the limited resolution of available measurement tools and the limited specificity of concepts.

It is conceivable that psychological phenomena that are seen as equivalent on the behavioural or subjective level nevertheless do have distinct biological bases. This would result in a one-to-many mapping from psychology to biology. For example, a behavioural deficit as loss of access to specific memory contents can have different biological causes. It can be due either to the fact that areas containing the memory representations or that structures enabling access to these representations are lost after a stroke. Behaviourally, the two causes might be indistinguishable. In this case, the psychological phenomenon would not be defined and measured specific enough to allow a one-to-one mapping.

Of course, methodological limitations in the measurement of neural activity also can make it difficult to associate psychological processes with neural activity patterns. For instance, an imaging study might find that two subjectively distinct events may be indistinguishable on the biological level, but this result could occur if the resolution of our biological measurements is not fine enough to reveal the biological differences between these two distinct psychological states. A similar situation would result, if measurement resolution is sufficient but if the measures are not appropriate for detecting the critical differences. For instance, the two states do not differ in terms of overall BOLD signal, but instead in terms of synchronization in activity across different regions, or in terms of the relative timing of activity within a region.

The limitations described above are related to technical-methodological limitations of currently available behavioural and biological measurement tools. Believing in scientific progress, one is on safe ground to expect that substantial refinements on both sides will be available in the near future. Who had expected 40 years ago that it would someday be possible to dissociate activation patterns in the human brain with a precision of a few millimeters and to relate these activations to distinct functions? Moreover, current developments in improving our understanding of network and pattern analysis in an active brain (e.g. Norman *et al.* this volume, Friston, Ashburner, Kiebel, Nichols, & Penny, 2007, Part 7), will help to differentiate better between distinct neural phenomena. These methods capitalize on the fact that cognitive processes are most likely not realized exclusively within narrowly circumscribed brain regions, but instead result from the interaction of large sets of interconnected neural ensembles. In these networks, the same ensemble may be involved in several processes because the connectivity directions and the weighting of the element can vary too. Thus, identifying interconnected patterns of activity may reveal one-to-one mappings between processes and neural networks that could not be revealed by analyses of overall brain activation magnitudes.

Conclusion

In this chapter, we have briefly touched some of the epistemological problems that have to be kept in mind if brain-imaging methods are to be used to advance our understanding of cognitive processes. This analysis makes it clear that neither a purely functional approach ignoring biological concepts nor a purely biological approach ignoring psychological concepts will advance the field. As outlined above, the software–hardware metaphor is probably inadequate in describing the relationship between cognition and brain function. The concept of wetware (i.e. the idea that functions and their biological bases are inseparably interconnected) seems to be more appropriate. Highly complex information processing routines as described in psychology emerge as new properties from the interconnectivity of billions of neurons, and not as software routines running on a fixed hardware. Therefore, the functions will be better understood if they are studied in close relation to their biological bases.

Having said this, it is also clear that to make progress in this respect, all available methodological tools should be used and their mutual interdependence and individual advantages should be exploited. That is, behavioural, brain-imaging, lesion, electrophysiological, and neurochemical approaches should all be used with the goal of converging on models that can explain behavioural phenomena both at the functional and neural levels. And with respect to the topic of this book, good brain-imaging studies must inevitably rest on behavioural experiments that are derived from convincing cognitive theories, however, on the other hand, convincing theories about the mind must consider both biological and behavioural facts.

Acknowledgements

A first draft of this chapter was written while FR spent a sabbatical at the Institute of advanced study Berlin (Wissenschaftskolleg zu Berlin). The fruitful discussions with Béatrice Longuenesse from NYU during that time had substantial impact on framing some of the ideas summarized in this chapter and her input is greatly acknowledged.

References

Aertsen, A. & Braitenberg, V. (1992). *Information Processing in the Cortex*. Berlin-Heidelberg-New York: Springer.

Baltes, P. B., Reuter-Lorenz, P., & Rösler, F. (2006). *Lifespan Development and the Brain*. Cambridge: Cambridge University Press.

Black, J. E., Jones, T. A., Nelson, C. A., & Greenough, W. T. (1998). Neuroplasticity and the developing brain. In: N. Alessi, J. T. Coyle, S. I. Harrison, & S. Eth (Eds), *The Handbook of Child and Adolescent Psychiatry* (Vol. 6, pp. 31–53). New York: John Wiley & Sons.

Buckner, R. (2000). Neuroimaging of memory. (Gazzaniga, M. S.), *The new cognitive neurosciences* (2nd edn). Cambridge, MA: MIT Press.

Coltheart, M. (2006). What has functional neuroimaging told us about the mind (so far)? *Cortex, 42*(3), 323–331.

Diana, R. A., Yonelinas, A. P., & Ranganath, C. (2007). Imaging recollection and familiarity in the medial temporal lobe: a three-component model. *Trends in Cognitive Sciences, 11*(9), 379–386.

Dricot, L., Sorger, B., Schiltz, C., Goebel, R., & Rossion, B. (2008). The roles of "face" and "non-face" areas during individual face perception: Evidence by fMRI adaptation in a brain-damaged prosopagnosic patient. *Neuroimage, 40*(1), 318–332.

Friston, K., Ashburner, J., Kiebel, S., Nichols, T., & Penny, W. (2007). *Statistical Parametric Mapping – The Analysis of Functional Brain Images*. Amsterdam: Elsevier.

Gauthier, I., Tarr, M. J., Moylan, J., Skudlarski, P., Gore, J. C., & Anderson, A. W. (2000). The fusiform "face area" is part of a network that processes faces at the individual level. *Journal of Cognitive Neuroscience, 12*, 495–504.

Gold, J. I. & Shadlen, M. N. (2001). Neural computations that underlie decisions about sensory stimuli. *Trends in Cognitive Sciences, 5*(1), 10–16.

Henson, R. N. A. (2005). What can functional neuroimaging tell the experimental psychologist? *Quarterly Journal of Experimental Psychology. A, Human Experimental Psychology, 58*(2), 193–233.

Hubel, D. H., Wiesel, T. N., & LeVay, S. (1977). Plasticity of ocular dominance columns in monkey striate cortex. *Philosophical Transactions of the Royal Society of London. Series B: Biological Sciences, 278*(961), 377–409.

Khader, P., Burke, M., Bien, S., Ranganath, C., & Rösler, F. (2005). Content-specific activation during associative long-term memory retrieval. *Neuroimage, 27*, 805–816.

Lamme, V. A., Super, H., Landman, R., Roelfsema, P. R., & Spekreijse, H. (2000). The role of primary visual cortex (V1) in visual awareness. *Vision Research, 40*(10–12), 1507–1521.

MacCorquodale, K. & Meehl, P. E. (1948). On a distinction between hypothetical constructs and intervening variables. *Psychological Review, 55*, 95–107.

McCallum, W. C. & Knott, J. R. (Eds) (1976). *The Responsive Brain*. Bristol: John Wrigth and Sons, Ltd.

Miki, K., Watanabe, S., Honda, Y., Nakamura, M., & Kakigi, R. (2007). Effects of face contour and features on early occipitotemporal activity when viewing eye movement. *Neuroimage, 35*(4), 1624-1635.

Miyake, A. & Shah, P. (Eds) (1999). *Models of Working Memory*. Cambridge,UK: Cambridge University Press.

Moonen, C. T. W. & Bandettini, P. A. (Eds) (2000). *Functional MRI*. Berlin: Springer.

Nauta, W. J. H. & Feirtag, M. (1986). *Fundamental Neuroanatomy*. New York: Freeman.

Pfeuffer, J., van de Moortele, P. F., Yacoub, E., Shmuel, A., Adriany, G., Andersen, P., Merkle, H., Garwood, M., Ugurbil, K., & Hu, X. (2002). Zoomed functional imaging in the human brain at 7 Tesla with simultaneous high spatial and high temporal resolution. *Neuroimage, 17*(1), 272–286.

Posner, M. I., Petersen, S. E., Fox, P. T., & Raichle, M. E. (1988). Localization of cognitive operations in the human brain. *Science, 240*(4859), 1627–1631.

Rosenzweig, M. R., Krech, D., Bennett, E. L., & Diamond, M. C. (1962). Effects of environmental complexity and training on brain chemistry and anatomy: A replication and extension. *Journal of Comparative and Physiological Psychology, 55*, 429–437.

Scarborough, D. & Sternberg, S. (Eds) (1998). *Methods, Modes, and Conceptual Issues*. (Vol. 4). Cambridge, MA: MIT-Press (Bradford book).

Sejnowski, T. J. (1981). Skeleton filters in the brain. In: G. E. Hinton, & J. A. Anderson (Eds), *Parallel Models of Associative Memory* (pp. 189–212). Hillsdale, NJ: Erlbaum.

Shaw, C. A. & McEachern, J. C. (Eds) (2001). *Toward a Theory of Neuroplasticity*. Philadelphia: Taylor & Francis.

Sternberg, S. (1969). The discovery of processing stages: extensions of Donders' method. *Acta Psychologica, 30*, 276–315.

van Essen, D. C. & Drury, H. A. (1997). Structural and functional analyses of human cerebral cortex using a surface-based atlas . *Journal of Neuroscience, 17*(18), 7079–7102.

van Orden, G. C. & Paap, K. R. (1997). Functional neuroimages fail to discover pieces of mind in the parts of the brain. *Philosophy of Science, 64*, S85–S94.

Westheimer, G. (1986). The eye as an optical instrument. In: K. H. Boff, L. Kaufman, & J. P. Thomas (Eds), *Sensory Processes and Perception* (pp. 4.1–4.20). New York: Wiley.

Yago, E. & Ishai, A. (2006). Recognition memory is modulated by visual similarity. *Neuroimage, 31*(2), 807–817.

Chapter 3

Uncovering unobservable cognitive mechanisms: The contribution of mathematical models

Rolf Ulrich

Introduction

Perhaps only a few cognitive psychologists like mathematical models and the reasons for the general dislike are manifold. In fact, I have heard several colleagues claiming that one does not need mathematical models to advance cognitive psychology. Other colleagues, who appear open-minded towards mathematical models, often pose the following question: Why do we actually need these models? The answer to this question is perhaps less obvious to the readership of this book than the answer to the question 'why do we need brain-imaging techniques?' I think, however, the question 'why do we need mathematical models?' addresses some fundamental issues and this article tries to analyze this meta-theoretical question.

The main thesis put forward in this article is that mathematical models are indispensable if we want to understand cognition, because these models benefit from the deductive power of mathematics. This power allows one to chain several logical steps, which enables complex inferences. In contrast, verbal theories usually do not permit such complex inferences. Even more crucial, inferences in verbal theories usually rely on intuition. From research on intuitive reasoning, however, it is known that this intuitive reasoning can lead to false conclusions.

Of course, I do not want to create the impression that mathematical models are the silver bullet to knowledge. We cannot do without verbal theories, because they have several advantages. First, the content of verbal theories is usually relatively easy to communicate. Second, and perhaps more important, we often have only a vague idea about certain psychological phenomena. It is impossible to express such vague ideas in the language of mathematics. In particular, we usually need verbal theories when a new research field is emerging. At an early stage of such an enterprise, only a few results are available which are often not well understood. Only rough theoretical ideas are likely to advance such an initial stage. By contrast, successful mathematical models require a rather robust data basis. Finally, there is no doubt that great verbal theories exist not only in psychology but also in other fields of science (e.g. the theory of biological evolution by Charles Darwin).

Despite these advantages of verbal theories, I am strongly convinced that verbal theories are often insufficient to explain cognitive phenomena in a satisfactory way. In order to support this statement, it is useful to explain briefly the goal of cognitive psychology, before the merits of mathematical models can be outlined. Because this issue is so fundamental and thus not restricted to memory models (i.e. the main topic of this book), I approach this meta-theoretical issue from a rather general perspective without referring to specific memory models. Actually, I will also use an example from our current research on temporal cognition to support and illustrate some general claims.

The goal of cognitive psychology

What is the major goal of cognitive psychology? The answer to this question is rooted in the history of cognitive psychology itself. Cognitive psychology emerged in the sixties as a counter-movement to behaviourism. To put it simply, psychologists were no longer pleased with the way in which behaviourists had tried to explain psychological phenomena. Behaviourists kept away from *mentalistic concepts* in explaining such phenomena. For example, a concept like 'semantic memory' would have struck a behaviourist as a mentalistic concept since it is not an observable entity. Thus, any concept that was unobservable and thus not available to experience was considered metaphysical and thus unscientific. In short, behaviourists focused on observable behaviour and not on the cognitive mechanisms that underlie such behaviour – the real was restricted to the observable (e.g. Skinner, 1950).[1]

In philosophy, theories that ignore such unobservable mechanisms are called *black-box theories* (e.g. Bunge, 1967a, 1967b). These theories focus on the functional relationship between certain input and output variables of a system (Figure 3.1). Although these theories try to describe this relationship in a systematic way, they do not suggest a mechanism from which this relationship emerges. In psychology, the independent variables define the input, and the dependent variables define the output. For example, in a memory study, one might manipulate the length of a retention interval. The interval duration would define the input variable. Then, the percentage of recognized items would be the dependent variable and thus define the output. Note that the input is not necessarily equated with stimulus input and the output not with a response, although psychologists often define a black box in this way (e.g. Luce, 1993).

Black-box theories can be regarded as empirical generalizations about some stable experimental effects. In former times, these generalizations were termed 'laws' and named according to the person who discovered the empirical generalization: For example, Weber's law or the law of forgetting by Ebbinghaus. These laws may be qualitative or

---

[1] The classical view of behaviourism is that theories about behaviour should be entirely stated in terms of observables. By contrast, in neobehaviourism it was appropriate to postulate internal structures (e.g., memory, drive) of an organism. Thus neobehaviourism permitted the limited use of theoretical concepts that went beyond the observable. For example, neobehaviourists such as Hull passed the observable by introducing *hypothetical constructs* to enhance their theories with 'surplus meaning' (see MacCordquodale & Meehl, 1948).

Black-Box Theory

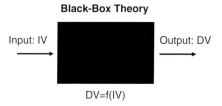

Input: IV   Output: DV

DV=f(IV)

Figure 3.1 The logical structure of black-box theories. These theories describe the functional relationship between independent variables (IV) and dependent variables (DV), i.e. these theories are low-level laws. They do not propose a mechanism from which this relationship emerges.

quantitative, that is, expressed as a formula. This difference, however, is not important here. Both are low-level laws.

Empirical generalizations by themselves do not provide any insight into the mechanisms within the black box. Therefore, these low-level laws have no explanatory power, although they may be very useful for prediction and thus are indispensable for applied research. In short, these laws are themselves in need of explanation. They have a low level of abstraction, because they often summarize single facts, which can be observed. These laws contain terms that are used to describe the data. When laws are formulated quantitatively, they usually also include one or more empirical constants.

For example, consider Weber's law. It claims that the just noticeable difference JND increases linearly with stimulus magnitude S, that is, $JND = k \cdot S$. The empirical constant $k > 0$ is called the Weber fraction, which usually is less than 1 and depends on the stimulus type. Note that this law by itself does not suggest an explanation why JND is linearly related to S. An example of a low-level law from memory research was provided by Bousfield and Sedgwick (1944). These authors asked their subjects to recall, for instance, as many birds they can remember. They noted that the mean number of words $N(t)$ recalled by time t could be described by an exponential growth function, i.e. $N(t) = c \cdot [1 - \exp(-a \cdot t)]$, with empirical constants $c > 0$ and $a > 0$. Although, this function describes the temporal course of free recall, it does not provide by itself an explanation of this observed relationship between $N(t)$ and t (see Albert, 1968; McGill, 1963; Ulrich & Dietz 1985; Vorberg & Ulrich, 1987 for models that can account for this relationship).

In summary, then, black-box theories do not reveal cognitive mechanisms, because they only focus on the relationship between input and output variables of a system. Cognitive psychology, however, wants to uncover these hidden mechanisms. Thus, cognitive psychology should strive to open the black box and search for the mechanisms from which these low-level laws emerge. More specifically, cognitive psychologists must map the observables onto deeper structures. These structures, however, cannot be directly observed, because these mechanisms are beyond our direct experience.

Other sciences, like physics, make similar efforts in order to develop better explanations about physical phenomena. For example, the concept of an electron is beyond our experience, though it is a very important concept for explaining an immense number of physical phenomena. Hence, the aim *to explain the observable with the unobservable* is not only the driving force of research in cognitive psychology and not only restricted to the explanation of psychological phenomena.

Theories that provide some insight into the black box are called *glass-box theories*. Such theories provide an internal mechanism that accounts for the observed input–output relationship between dependent and independent variables. These theories aim at a deeper explanation by exposing the modus operandi behind this relationship. So how can one open the black box in order to make the unobservable observable?

A thought experiment

At this point, some cognitive neuroscientists may want to turn to imaging techniques. In fact, a well-known neuroscientist – whose name will not be of interest here – has claimed that these techniques enable us to read the mind like a book. Sure, these techniques are enormously useful to investigate the neural correlates of cognitive processes, and the data from this research can be useful to inform theories of cognition. However, these techniques by themselves cannot replace theories about cognitive processes. I shall demonstrate this point with the following thought experiment.

Several software packages are installed in my laptop computer. One that fascinates me most is a package that carries out symbolic calculations. This program masters tough mathematical problems. For example, it rearranges equations, solves for an unknown, integrates, and so on. For me this program is magic. Although I can interact with this program at the level of the user interface, I have not the slightest idea how this software produces these fascinating results in almost an eye blink. How can I disclose the magic behind this fancy program?

First, as a fan of cognitive neuroscience, I could put my laptop into a special scanner that registers its heat radiation while it performs these mathematical operations. The result would be a heat radiation scan (Figure 3.2, upper left panel). On the basis of this scan, I might figure out all the active components of my laptop while it processes my request. Of course, I would subtract from this scan the heat radiation in a resting condition in order to get rid of task-unspecific radiation, such as the heat radiation of the power supply.

Second, as a fan of single-cell recording, I could implant dozens of electrodes in the electrical components of my laptop and record the electrical activity (Figure 3.2, lower left panel). I even could store this information and perform an offline data analysis on these recordings, such as coherence or cross-correlation analysis. I could use all of the fancy software packages for this measure and try to gain insights into my laptop.

Third, as a fan of event-related brain potentials, I could put several surface electrodes on my laptop (Figure 3.2, upper right panel). I could ask my laptop to do the same operation repeatedly. Then I would time-lock these waveforms to the input signal or to the response of my laptop in order to compute event-related potentials. Perhaps a dipole analysis might point to a specific component that is significantly involved in these computations.

Finally, as a fan of animal models, I might use a hammer and introduce an experimental lesion on my laptop (Figure 3.2, lower right panel). If I am lucky, I will succeed in

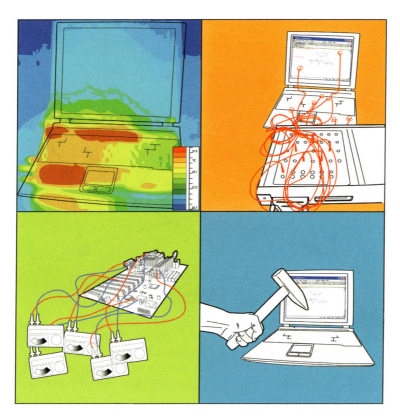

Figure 3.2 Illustrations of the thought experiment. Upper left panel: Heat radiation scan. Upper right panel: Event-related potentials. Lower left panel: Single-unit recording. Lower right panel: Experimental lesion.

inducing a specific lesion. Perhaps it would no longer allow me to do these symbolic calculations but I might still use my word processor.

It does not require a lot of imagination to see that none of these fancy neuroscience techniques can directly unravel the hidden mechanisms of this symbolic math program. Although we tried very hard to measure as near as possible to the place where these mechanisms are localized, these measurements are by themselves useless to gain insights in the mechanisms that underlie the performance of this fancy program. These techniques by themselves do not open a 'window' to cognitive events. Another problem is that measures in the brain sciences are usually noisy, which complicates matters even more. In short, then, these methods by themselves cannot turn on the light within the black box and so unravel the cognitive mechanisms behind human performance.

Glass-box theories

In order to advance the understanding about the inner workings of the black box, one needs some plausible basic assumptions, that is, *axioms* about the mechanisms in this box (Figure 3.3). Such axioms are the key feature of any glass-box theory. Most importantly,

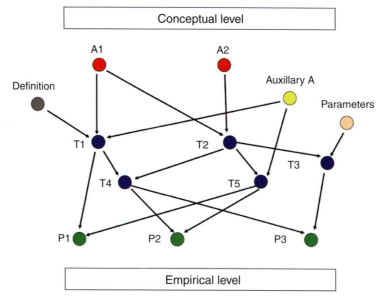

Figure 3.3 The logical structure of a glass-box theory. This structure denotes a network of inferences from the top to the bottom of the figure. It starts with initial assumptions about a mechanism (red nodes). This defines the conceptual level of the glass-box theory. These assumptions together with auxiliary assumptions (Aux) and definitions (D1 and D2) are combined to derive theorems (blue nodes: T1, T2, and T3). These theorems constitute the middle level of this network. Further combinations of these theorems lead to theorems at the lower level of this structure (green nodes). These are low-level theorems or predictions about certain input–output relations of a system. These theorems at this level may also account for already existing low-level laws.

these axioms usually include *theoretical terms*. These terms denote things that we can imagine and which, we assume, represent true aspects of reality (for example, terms like electron, black holes, mental lexicon, and semantic memory). In contrast to empirical concepts, like 'dog', 'green', or 'hot', theoretical terms are *transempirical*, because they are not grounded in our perceptions. These concepts are stimulus-free creations of our minds because they go beyond our experience.

Usually, the referents of theoretical terms cannot be perceived like a chestnut tree or a certain colour. Although, things like bacteria or certain stellar objects (e.g. Mars' Moons) cannot be perceived directly, instruments such as a microscope or a telescope enable a visual experience of these things. One can therefore name a chestnut tree, the colour red, bacteria, or Mars' Moons as observable objects because they induce perceptual experience. According to this definition, electrons would be unobservable. Nevertheless, one may consider all things as observable that can be detected with instruments even though these things do not result in a direct perceptual experience. With this very broad definition, electrons and even neutrinos are often loosely said to be 'observable', even though, these objects do not produce direct perceptual experience

(Shapere, 1982). Such entities may be observed indirectly by a hypothetical inference employing data, hypotheses, and background information, and hence this inference can be called an indirect observation at best (Bunge, 1967b; Shapere, 1982). So, it is difficult to draw an exact line between things that are observable and those that are unobservable. Nevertheless, it usually happens that theoretical terms describe things (e.g. objects, causal relationships, states) that are unobservable, at least for the time being (Adam, 2002). For example, think of the concept 'interference' or 'depth of processing' in memory research. It is difficult to imagine that the referents of these terms produce a perceptible experience and so can be looked at directly like at a chestnut tree. Thus, the theoretical terms that are included by the basic assumptions of a glass-box theory are not directly observable and hence these assumptions cannot be tested without the inferential structure of a glass-box theory.

These assumptions that include theoretical terms are the starting point of any glass-box theory. The next step can be very tough, because one needs to combine these basic assumptions in a logical manner to derive testable predictions, that is, theorems from these basic assumptions. The result of this activity yields a network of logically connected theorems. The basic assumptions form the highest level of this network; this is the conceptual level. The theorems at the middle level of this network are usually not directly testable and can be conceived as an intermediate deductive result. Further logical combinations of these intermediate theorems and auxiliary assumptions will finally lead to testable predictions. These theorems at the lowest level of the network can be linked to experience, and they constitute the empirical level of the glass-box theory. If the theory is true, these low-level theorems must be in agreement with the observed input-output relationships, that is, with the low-level laws in a certain domain of research.

Such a glass-box theory not only provides a relatively deep level of explanation of psychological phenomena, it also has the potential to link phenomena that have previously been viewed in isolation. Therefore, a glass-box theory also has the power to integrate a number of seemingly unconnected facts. For example, Newton's theory of mechanics highlights this point. This theory is based on only a few axioms and it connects a set of originally disconnected low-level laws on motion, such as Galilei's law of falling bodies, Kepler's law of planetary motion, Huygen's law of oscillation, and tidal phenomena. Cognitive psychologists have also successfully developed glass-box theories in order to account for a set of originally unconnected psychological phenomena and low-level laws. Raaijmakers and Shiffrin's (1981) memory model, for instance, successfully related several low-level laws from the extensive literature on free recall. This model provides a set of some axioms, which describe a memory mechanism that might underlie free recall performance (see also Raaijmakers & Shiffrin, 2002). In short, then, glass-box theories aim at a deeper understanding of certain phenomena by specifying the underlying mechanisms. In addition, such theories' networks of theorems also generate conceptual coherence among a set of seemingly unconnected phenomena, and therefore such theories systematize knowledge within a certain domain of research, such as free recall performance.

The role of mathematics

The inferential process of building a network of theorems from some basic assumptions is a crucial aspect of every glass-box theory. This process of combining one or more assumptions in order to derive a 'new' conclusion from these assumptions is called *deduction*. Without deduction, we cannot open the black box. Therefore, the construction of glass-box theories requires deductive reasoning. This, however, can be a painful business.[2] As we know from research on thinking, humans easily fail on even simple deductive reasoning problems (Hogarth, 2001; Kahneman, Slovic, & Tversky, 2005). For example, take the following syllogism:

Assumption 1:	All artists are psychologists.
Assumption 2:	Some psychologists are neuroscientists.
Conclusion:	Therefore, some neuroscientists are artists.

One might be inclined to suppose that this conclusion follows logically from the two assumptions. This, however, is not true. Such reasoning would be incorrect and not lead to a correctly deduced theorem. In this case it is likely that we would distrust our reasoning, because our intuition might warn us that this conclusion could be wrong.

In verbal theories, one often needs to rely on one's intuitions when deriving predictions from a set of assumptions. Almost all textbooks in cognitive psychology, however, suggest that we should not rely too much on our intuitive reasoning, because intuitions may be illusory and wrong, even when our intuitions are very strong. A nice illustration for this point is provided by the Monty Hall problem.

Assume that you stand in front of three closed doors in a TV show. The doors are labeled one, two, and three, respectively. Behind one of the doors is an attractive prize, for example, a Porsche. Behind the two other doors are gag prizes, for example, goats. Suppose you pick Door 1. It remains closed and the show master knows what is behind Door 1. Now the show master opens one of the other two doors, say Door 3, to reveal a goat. He then gives you the opportunity to switch to Door 2. Should you stick with Door 1 or switch to Door 2?

Many people insist that the remaining two Doors 1 and 2 are equally likely to hide the Porsche. They do not even question this belief. However, the probability is 2/3 that the Porsche is behind Door 2 and only 1/3 that it is behind Door 1. So, one would be better in the long run to switch to Door 2. This is one of several examples from probability theory, which shows that our intuitive reasoning is sometimes quite wrong and that we should not rely on our intuitions to validate the outcome of our reasoning process.

---

[2] To come up with a set of basic assumptions in glass-box theories is certainly the most creative part in building such theories. We do not know much about this creative process. Some might argue that this part is even more demanding than the subsequent deduction process. I think this is a matter of taste; perhaps both parts are usually difficult.

This is the stage where mathematics comes in. In order to derive valid conclusions (i.e. theorems) from a set of initial assumptions, one is often required to rely on mathematics or computer simulations[3] to generate valid conclusions in order to maintain logical coherence. In fact, and perhaps not surprisingly, validly derived conclusions can often be quite counterintuitive. This will be demonstrated in the following section.

In short, we unquestionably need intuitions to arrive at some plausible initial assumptions in our glass-box theory. Hence, we should take care and not employ intuition to derive invalid conclusions from a set of valid assumptions. Thus if one wants to derive predictions from a set of assumptions, one should certainly not appeal to intuition in order to avoid the costs of analytical thinking. Even strong intuitions can be misleading as the above textbook examples may already demonstrate.

An example of a mathematical model

In this section, I shall demonstrate the power of mathematical models with a simple example from our own research on crossmodal timing (Ulrich, Nitschke, & Rammsayer, 2006). This example also demonstrates that even conceptually simple assumptions may entail counterintuitive predictions, which one would not arrive at without the deductive power of mathematics.

The prediction of this mathematical model concerns the performance of an observer in a temporal discrimination task. In each trial of this task, two stimuli are delivered to an observer one after the other. The first stimulus is called the standard and it has a fixed duration, say 100 ms. The second stimulus is called the comparison and it can be shorter or longer than the standard. The observer is asked at the end of each trial to judge whether the comparison was shorter or longer than the standard.

In these experiments, the so-called difference limen (DL) is the dependent variable. This DL indicates how much the experimenter needs to prolong the comparison duration in order to yield 75% correct judgments. For a 100-ms standard, the magnitude of DL could be 10 ms or about 10% of the standard duration. When discrimination performance is high, DL is relatively small.

Now consider the discrimination performance in a crossmodal discrimination task. In congruent trials of this task, both the standard and the comparison are auditory ($A - A$) or both are visual ($V - V$). By contrast, in incongruent trials, one stimulus is auditory and the other stimulus is visual. In half of all incongruent trials, the visual stimulus precedes the auditory one and in the other half, this order is reversed ($V - A$ and $A - V$, respectively). Therefore, there are four trial types ($V - V$, $A - A$, $V - A$, and $A - V$) and for each type, one can determine a subject's DL.

---

[3] One may also use a numerical computer simulation to assess the predictions of set of axioms. Not all assumptions of a glass-box theory will lead to mathematically tractable theorems. In this case, numerical simulations are required to assess the behaviour (i.e., the predicted low-level laws at the empirical level) of the assumed mechanism. Thus a broader definition of mathematical models may include computer simulations as well.

Let us first focus on congruent trials and anticipate the discrimination performance for these trials. Since it is well-known that the temporal resolution of the auditory system is better than the one of the visual system, one would expect a smaller DL for $A - A$ trials than for $V - V$ trials, that is, $DL(V - V) > DL(A - A)$. Next, consider the discrimination performance on incongruent trials. Here two alternative predictions come to one's mind and each of the two appears plausible. First, one might reason that crossmodal discrimination should always be worse than intramodal discrimination, i.e. $DL(A - V) = DL(V - A) > DL(V - V) > DL(A - A)$ (Figure 3.4, top left panel). For example, one might assume that modality specific timing mechanisms enhance intramodal comparisons. Therefore, it should be harder to discriminate temporal information between two different modalities rather than within a single modality. Second, one might disagree with this prediction and instead insist that the discrimination performance on incongruent trials should be equal to the average of the two DLs in the congruent trials, i.e. $DL(A - V) = DL(V - A) = [DL(V - V) + DL(A - A)] / 2$ (Figure 3.4, top right panel). Note that both predictions assume that $DL(A - V) = DL(V - A)$, that is, that the presentation order of the two sensory modalities does not influence the discrimination performance. Interestingly, however, these predictions do not agree with the observed data. Although the data agree with the prediction $DL(V - V) > DL(A - A)$, they clearly show that the presentation order of the two sensory modalities matters, because an order effect was obtained, i.e. $DL(A - V) > DL(V - A)$ (Figure 3.4, lower panel).

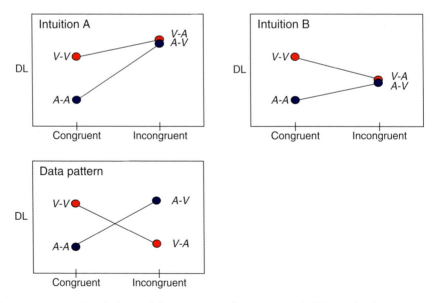

Figure 3.4 Expected and observed data pattern. Difference limen (DL) for each of the congruent trials (V–V and A–A) and incongruent trials (V–A and A–V). Top left panel: The expected data pattern for Intuition A. Top right panel: The expected data according to Intuition B. Bottom panel: A sketch of the observed data pattern.

We did not understand this data pattern well before we developed a simple model to account for another aspect of crossmodal discrimination performance unrelated to this issue. By accident, however, we also checked that model with regard to this unexpected order effect, and to our surprise, it made the correct prediction, although we did not invoke any post-hoc assumption to 'account for' this effect.

In order to appreciate the deductive power of this model, I need to explain the main steps of deriving its prediction. First, one needs a basic idea of how subjects may accomplish this discrimination task. According to pacemaker-counter models (see Creelman, 1962; Ulrich et al., 2006), a pacemaker generates pulses during each of the two stimulus intervals and a counter registers the pulses generated in each of the two intervals. Specifically, let the number of pulses counted during the first time interval t_1 be denoted by $N(t_1)$. Likewise, let $N(t_2)$ be the number of pulses counted during the second time interval, t_2. Now, according to this model, a subject will perceive the second interval to be longer than the first one if $N(t_2) > N(t_1)$ holds. In this case, we assume, the subject will respond that the second interval appears longer than the first interval. Due to random noise, the number of pulses in each interval varies from trial to trial and this already accounts for the finding that these duration judgements are sometimes inconsistent. Specifically, we assume that the interval between two successive pulses represents a random variable with a certain mean μ and a certain standard deviation σ (see Rammsayer & Ulrich, 2001).

Second, we also need some background knowledge for the model. For example, we already know that auditory stimuli are perceived as longer than visual ones of the same duration (Goldstone & Goldfarb, 1964). This is usually explained by assuming that auditory stimuli are arousing and that this arousal increases the pulse generation rate of the pacemaker (Penney, Gibbon, & Meck, 2000; Wearden, Edwards, Fakhri, & Percival, 1998). Clearly, this accounts for the finding that auditory stimuli are perceived as longer than visual stimuli. In addition, this also explains why temporal discrimination is better for auditory than for visual stimuli, because a higher pace rate results in a finer temporal resolution of the internal clock.

Further background information comes from probability theory. Specifically, it is known from probability theory how the number of pulses $N(t)$ in a certain time interval t varies across trials. We need not to go into this technical yet important aspect. It suffices to know that the number of pulses is distributed approximately normally with a mean of $E[N(t)] = t/\mu$ and a variance of $Var[N(t)] = t \cdot \sigma^2/\mu^3$ that depend on the duration t of the stimulus and on the mean μ and the standard deviation σ of the interpulse time. In deriving the predictions of our pacemaker-counter model, we incorporated these results from probability theory.

The third step is crucial. After one has specified the initial assumptions, it is necessary to combine these in order to realize the predictions that are implied by this set of initial assumptions. Mathematics is required at this step for at least two reasons. First, it provides a tool to combine two or more complex assumptions. Second, it ensures logical coherence and thus avoids false conclusions. For the above pacemaker-counter model, the details of this deductive process are presented somewhere else (Ulrich et al., 2006;

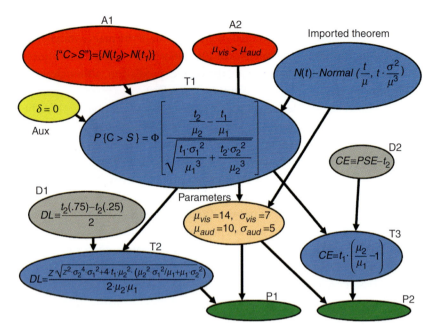

Figure 3.5 The logical structure of the pacemaker accumulator model. It shows the initial assumptions of the mechanism assumed in this model (A1 and A2), auxiliary assumptions (Aux), and definitions (D1 and D2) that are combined to derive theorems (T1, T2, and T3). Further combinations of these theorems lead to theorems at the lower level of this structure (P1 and P2), which are separately depicted in Figure 3.6.

Rammsayer & Ulrich, 2001). Figure 3.5 summarizes the outcome of this process by depicting the logical structure of this model. The basic assumptions of the model are shown in red. The intermediate theorems are coloured with blue and the derived low-level theorems are green. Yellow denotes auxiliary assumptions such as assumptions about parameter values. The green circles at the bottom represent the predictions (shown in Figure 3.6, upper panel), and these can be compared with the data (Figure 3.6, lower panel), that is, with the psychophysical results of our crossmodal discrimination experiment.

By comparing both panels in Figure 3.6, it can be seen that this simple model can account for the observed data pattern. As one expects, it correctly predicts that temporal performance is better in $A - A$ than in $V - V$ trials. Surprisingly and most crucially, however, the model correctly predicts the observed order effect $DL(A - V) > DL(V - A)$, that is, it fully accounts for the observed crossover interaction. It is intuitively difficult to grasp why this prediction follows from the model's basic assumptions, although no specific ad-hoc assumptions were included to 'predict' this order effect.[4] In addition, the model also correctly predicts that when the standard is increased from 100 to 1,000 ms, DL should become larger. More important, however, the prediction is qualitatively the same

---

[4] Readers interested in a possible intuitive explanation for this prediction should consult Ulrich *et al.* (2006).

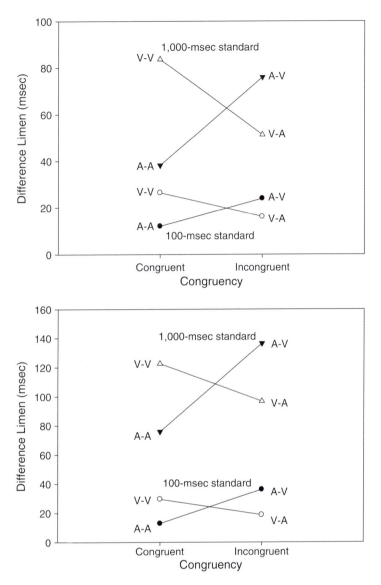

Figure 3.6 Upper panel: Predicted DL as a function of congruency (congruent vs. incongruent trials), of sensory modality of standard stimulus, and of standard duration. (Adapted from Figure 2 in Ulrich *et al.*, 2006). Lower panel: Observed DL as a function of congruency (congruent vs. incongruent trials), of sensory modality of standard stimulus, and of standard duration. (Adapted from Figure 3 in Ulrich *et al.*, 2006).

as for the 100-ms standard. This demonstration shows that even simple models can produce striking counterintuitive predictions. That is, we often do not (immediately) understand the implications of even very simple assumptions. In this case, we used a simple counting mechanism to address an intriguing order effect in a crossmodal temporal discrimination task.

A small side trip is in order. Recent research in cognitive neuroscience has proposed a two-system theory for duration perception (Lewis & Miall, 2003). It has been suggested that the system mediating the perception of very brief durations – in the milliseconds range – is different from the system mediating the perception of longer durations. A review of several brain-imaging studies by Lewis and Miall (2003) led these authors to conclude that frontal brain regions are involved in the perception of long intervals whereas motor regions are involved in the perception of short intervals. They have thus argued that the system mediating short intervals relies on automatic mechanisms without cognitive control, while the other system that processes longer intervals requires active processing and is under direct cognitive control. The present analysis, however, does not support the hypothesis that two different mechanisms operate on short and long temporal intervals. In light of the above analysis and other psychophysical research (Rammsayer & Ulrich, 2005), it seems plausible to conclude instead that the same timing mechanism operates at both time ranges. Nevertheless it is possible that different copies of the same timing mechanism are hosted by different brain regions. Each copy could mediate the processing of durations in a specific time range. Hence, this short side issue may illustrate that mathematical models of cognitive mechanisms can enhance the interpretation of brain imaging results.

Concluding remarks

Cognitive psychology strives for a better understanding of the mechanisms that underlie human performance. Unfortunately, however, these mechanisms are not directly observable. Therefore these mechanisms need to be described by glass-box theories employing transempirical terms, such as mental lexicon or central bottleneck process. In contrast to behaviourists, cognitive psychologists are realists because they assume that the entities, states, and processes described by correct theories about such hidden mechanisms do really exist. This view is called *scientific realism* in the philosophy of science (e.g. Hacking, 1983; Van Fraassen, 1980), and it is not only restricted to cognitive psychology but applies to other natural sciences as well. By contrast, behaviourists are anti-realists because they deny the existence of things that cannot be observed. This anti-realist tradition has been around for a long time and is usually called positivism, a name that was coined by the French philosopher Auguste Comte (see Hacking, 1983). In short, positivism claims that nothing can be known to be real except what might be observed. Thus a cognitive psychologist can not be a positivist; otherwise he missed his calling.[5]

Cognitive psychologists need certain research tools to uncover these hidden cognitive mechanisms. For example, brain-imaging techniques have become a major tool of cognitive

---

[5] Scientific realism assumes that transempirical concepts that are postulated by glass-box theories may really exist and thus are true given that data support the predictions of these theories. The view of instrumentalism, however, holds that such concepts and theories are merely useful instruments in explaining and predicting phenomena. Thus, instrumentalists deny the existence of transempirical concepts and that the truth of glass-box theories is evaluable (e.g., Gadenne, 2004). This position of instrumentalism is not popular in the cognitive sciences, since most scientists in this field do not deny the reality of transempirical concepts.

psychologists in the last 15 years or so for unraveling these mechanisms. Although these tools have provided many insights into brain functions (see Nicholson, 2006), they cannot replace genuine glass-box theories. The entities, states, and processes associated with cognitive mechanisms may never induce any direct perceptual experience as bacteria do when we watch them with a microscope. Even the most elaborated brain scan technology may not unravel these mechanisms. In fact, some have argued that functional neuroimaging has not yet contributed to an understanding of cognitive mechanisms (e.g. Coltheart, 2006), while others argue that this technique simply provides another dependent variable besides behavioural data to discriminate between competing psychological theories (Henson, 2005).

The thought experiment in this article was contrived to make this point obvious. Certainly, all branches of science increasingly exclude sense-perception (direct perception) as much as possible from playing the major role in the acquisition of observational evidence, and cognitive psychology is no exception here. Nevertheless neuroimaging data – like behavioural data (e.g. reaction time, difference limen, etc.) – can only be used to infer cognitive mechanisms and not to observe them directly (e.g. Hampton, Bossaerts, & O'Doherty, 2006; Poldrack, 2006; Sternberg, 2001). Although it seems impossible that neuroimaging data by themselves can prove or disprove the existence of a hypothesized cognitive mechanism or mental architecture, future glass-box theories may and should include these data to evaluate testable predictions derived from these theories. For example, promising theoretical approaches in this direction try to relate neural network models and neuroscience (e.g. Norman & O'Reilly, 2003) or apply formalized learning models to brain-imaging findings (e.g. Daw, O'Doherty, Dayan, Seymour, & Dolan, 2006; Forstmann *et al.*, 2008; see also the chapters by John P. O'Doherty and by Christian Büchel in this book).

Cognitive psychology needs glass-box theories because they are important for inferring cognitive mechanisms. Without such theories, cognitive psychology cannot leave behaviourism behind and proceed to a deep understanding of cognition. As explained above, the logical structure of these theories, however, is usually very complex, especially when these theories describe hidden mechanisms. This glass-box approach requires that one deduces testable predictions from a set of initial assumptions. It was argued that mathematics provides an important tool to build-up the inferential structure of a glass-box theory. Mathematics not only helps to establish this inferential structure but also avoids the trap that one incorrectly derives logically false conclusions from a model's basic assumptions. In addition, the deductive power of mathematics also helps to link psychological phenomena that are usually described and discussed in isolation. In fact, often a simple principle can account for several psychological low-level laws (e.g. Miller & Ulrich, 2003).

Acknowledgements

I am indebted to Volker Gadenne from whom I could learn much about the philosophy of science. I thank Jeff Miller for many suggestions and for reading the text with much deliberation. It was of great help to discuss the content of this article with Allen Osman and Hartmut Leuthold. Dominik Ulrich's effort in designing Figure 3.2 is highly appreciated. The Deutsche Forschungsgemeinschaft (UL 116/3) supported part of this work.

References

Adam, M. (2002). *Theoriebeladenheit und Objektivität: Zur Rolle von Beobachtungen in den Naturwissenschaften*. Frankfurt: Ontos Verlag.

Albert, D. (1968). Freies Reproduzieren von Wortreihen als stochastische Entleerung eins Speichers. *Zeitschrift für Experimentelle und Angewandte Psychologie, 15*, 564–581.

Bousfield, W. A. & Sedgewick, C. H. (1944). An analysis of sequences of restricted associative responses. *Journal of General Psychology, 30*, 149–165.

Bunge, M. (1967a). *Scientific Research I: The Search for System*. New York: Springer-Verlag.

Bunge, M. (1967b). *Scientific Research II: The Search for Truth*. New York: Springer-Verlag.

Coltheart, M. (2006). What has functional neuroimaging told us about the mind (so far)? *Cortex, 42*, 323–331.

Creelman, C. D. (1962). Human discrimination of auditory duration. *Journal of the Acoustical Society of America, 34*, 582–593.

Daw, N. D., O'Doherty, J. P., Dayan, P., Seymour, B., & Dolan, R. J. (2006). Cortical substrates for exploratory decisions in humans. *Nature, 441*, 876–879.

Forstmann, B. U., Dutilh, G., Brown, S., Neumann, J., von Cramon, D. Y., Ridderinkhof, K. R., & Wagenmakers, E.-J. (2008). Striatum and pre-SMA facilitate decision-making under time pressure. *Proceedings of the National Academy of Sciences, 105*, 17538–17542.

Gadenne, V. (2004). *Philosophie der Psychologie*. Hans Huber: Bern.

Goldstone, S. & Goldfarb, J. L. (1964). Auditory and visual time judgment. *Journal of General Psychology, 70*, 369–387.

Hacking, I. (1983). *Representing and Intervening*. Cambridge: Cambridge University Press.

Hampton, A. N., Bossaerts, P. & O'Doherthy, J. P. (2006). The role of the ventromedial prefrontal cortex in abstract state-based inference during decision making in humans. *The Journal of Neuroscience, 25*, 8360–8367.

Henson, R. (2005). What can functional neuroimaging tell the experimental psychologist? *The Quarterly Journal of Experimental Psychology, 58A*, 193–233.

Hogarth, R. M. (2001). *Educating Intuition*. Chicago, IL: The University of Chicago Press.

Kahneman, D., Slovic, P., & Tversky, A. (2005). *Judgement Under Uncertainty: Heuristics and Biases*. (21st printing). New York: Cambridge University Press.

Lewis, P. A. & Miall, R. C. (2003). Distinct systems for automatic and cognitively controlled time measurement: Evidence from neuroimaging. *Current Opinion in Neurobiology, 13*, 1–6.

Luce, R. D. (1993). *Sound and Hearing: A Conceptual Introduction*. Hillsdale, NJ: Lawrence Erlbaum.

MacCorquodale, K. & Meehl, P. E. (1948). On a distinction between hypothetical constructs and intervening variables. *Psychological Review, 55*, 95–107.

McGill, W. J. (1963). Stochastic latency mechanisms. In R. D. Luce, R. B. Bush, & E. Galanter (Eds), *Handbook of Mathematical Psychology*, (Vol. 1, pp. 309–360), New York: Wiley.

Miller, J. & Ulrich, R. (2003). Simple reaction time and statistical facilitation: A parallel grains model. *Cognitive Psychology, 46*, 101–151.

Nicholson, C. (2006). Thinking over fMRI and psychological science. *Observer (a publication of the Association for the Psychological Sciences), 19*, 21–27.

Norman, K. A. & O'Reilly, R. C. (2003). Modeling hippocampal and neocortical contributions to recognition memory: A complementary-learning-systems approach. *Psychological Review, 110*, 611–646.

Penney, T. B., Gibbon, J., & Meck, W. H. (2000). Differential effects of auditory and visual signals on clock speed and temporal memory. *Journal of Experimental Psychology: Human Perception and Performance, 26*, 1770–1787.

Poldrack, R. A. (2006). Can cognitive processes be inferred from neuroimaging data? *Trends in Cognitive Sciences, 10*, 59–63.

Raaijmakers, J. G. & Shiffrin, R. M. (1981). Search of associative memory. *Psychological Review, 88*, 93–134.

Raaijmakers, J. G. W. & Shiffrin, R. M. (2002). Models of memory. In H. Pashler & D. Medin (Eds), Stevens' *Handbook of Experimental Psychology*, (3rd Edn, Vol 2): *Memory and Cognitive Processes* (pp. 43–76). New York: John Wiley & Sons, Inc.

Rammsayer, T. H. & Ulrich, R. (2001). Counting models of temporal discrimination. *Psychonomic Bulletin & Review, 8*, 270–277.

Rammsayer, T. & Ulrich, R. (2005). No evidence for qualitative differences in the processing of short and long temporal intervals. *Acta Psychologica, 120*, 141–171.

Shapere, D. (1982). The concept of observation in science and philosophy. *Philosophy of Science, 49*, 485–525.

Skinner, B. F. (1950). Are theories of learning necessary? *Psychological Review, 57*, 193–216.

Sternberg, S. (2001). Separate modifiability, mental modules, and the use of pure composite measures to reveal them. *Acta Psychologica, 106*, 147–246.

Ulrich, R. & Dietz, K. (1985). The short-term storage as a buffer memory between long-term storage and the motor system: A simultaneous-processing model. *Journal of Mathematical Psychology, 29*, 243–270.

Ulrich, R., Nitschke, J., & Rammsayer, T. (2006). Crossmodal temporal discrimination: Assessing the predictions of a general pacemaker-counter model. *Perception & Psychophysics, 68*, 1140–1152.

Van Fraassen, B. C. (1980). *The Scientific Image*. Oxford: Claderndon Press.

Vorberg, D. & Ulrich, R. (1987). Random search with unequal search rates: Serial and parallel generalizations of McGill's model. *Journal of Mathematical Psychology, 31*, 1–23.

Wearden, J. H., Edwards, H., Fakhri, M., & Percival, A. (1998). Why "Sounds are jugded longer than lights": Application of a model of the internal clock in humans. *Quarterly Journal of Experimental Psychology, 51*B, 97–120.

Part 2

Learning and consolidation

Reinforcement learning mechanisms in the human brain: Insights from model-based fMRI

John P O'Doherty

Introduction

In order to survive, humans like other animals need in any given circumstance to be able to select those behaviours out of a range of possible behaviours that lead to the greatest probability of obtaining rewards or avoiding punishers. Such a capacity likely depends on the ability to make predictions about when and where rewards or punishers are going to occur, and to flexibly modify action selection in the light of such knowledge. In recent years, considerable interest has arisen in developing an understanding of the basic computations underlying such an ability. Reinforcement learning models are a class of algorithms originally derived from computer science, which have been found to have strong relevance for how real animals can learn to choose optimally in a stochastic environment (Sutton & Barto, 1998). In the present chapter we will review evidence for the applicability of reinforcement learning models to reward-learning and reward-based action selection in humans, with a particular emphasis on data derived from functional neuroimaging studies. We will begin by describing the basic mechanisms by which predictions of future reward as well as punishment can be learned, and their associated neural bases. Next we will consider the mechanisms underlying action selection for reward, as well as in learning to avoid punishers. We will also review instances where findings from functional neuroimaging studies are inconsistent with a simple reinforcement learning framework, and discuss the implications of these results for the development of a more complete theory of human choice.

Predicting future rewards or punishers

Prediction of an impending appetitive or aversive outcome can be studied through the phenomenon of classical or Pavlovian conditioning, whereby an arbitrary initially affectively neutral stimulus, termed the conditioned stimulus (CS) is repeatedly paired with another stimulus already endowed with appetitive or aversive affective value, usually termed the unconditioned stimulus (UCS). Over time the animal or human begins to develop affective responses to the CS, indicating that this stimulus has now taken on affective value to the organism by virtue of its predictive significance. Considerable progress has been made in identifying the brain regions involved in encoding predictions of future rewards or punishers. Single-unit recording studies in non-human primates and rodents have implicated neurons in a number of brain regions including the orbitofrontal cortex, lateral prefrontal cortex, amygdala, ventral, and dorsal striatum in responding following presentation of a cue predictive of subsequent rewarding or punishing consequences (Thorpe *et al.*, 1983; Schoenbaum *et al.*, 1998; Tremblay & Schultz, 1999; Paton *et al.*, 2006). Consistent with these findings, functional neuroimaging studies have also revealed activations in some of these areas during both appetitive and aversive Pavlovian conditioning in response to CS presentation (Buchel *et al.*, 1998; Gottfried *et al.*, 2002). For example, Gottfried *et al.* (2002) reported activity in both amygdala and orbitofrontal cortex following presentation of visual stimuli predictive of the subsequent delivery of both a pleasant and an unpleasant odour. Gottfried *et al.* (2003) aimed to investigate the nature of such predictive representations in order to establish whether such responses are related to the sensory properties of the unconditioned stimulus irrespective of its underlying reward value, or whether such responses are directly related to the reward value of the associated unconditioned stimulus. To address this, Gottfried *et al.* trained subjects to associate visual stimuli with one of two food odours: vanilla and peanut butter while being scanned with fMRI. Subjects were then subsequently removed from the scanner and fed to satiety on a food corresponding to one of the food odours in order to decrease the reward value of that odour, e.g. to decrease the value of the vanilla odour subjects were fed to satiety on vanilla ice-cream. Due to the selectivity of such a devaluation procedure, the value of the odour not eaten shows no such decrease, a phenomenon known as sensory-specific satiety (Rolls *et al.*, 1981). Following the devaluation procedure subjects were then placed back in the scanner and presented with the conditioned stimuli again in a further conditioning session. Neural responses to presentation of the CS paired with the devalued odour were found to decrease in orbitofrontal cortex and amygdala from before to after the satiation procedure, whereas no such decrease was evident for CS paired with the non-devalued odour. These results provide evidence that predictive representations related to presentation of a particular conditioned stimulus in amygdala and orbitofrontal cortex encode the value of the associated UCS and not merely its sensory properties. The above findings implicate a number of brain regions in encoding predictions of future rewarding or punishing consequences, when such predictions pertain to passive associations between stimuli and outcomes, without any action being required on behalf of the subject to bring such outcomes about. In a subsequent section we will consider the case where subjects' must actively make responses in order to obtain a reward or avoid a punisher and address whether in this context predictive representations are also present in the same brain regions.

Learning of predictive value representations

The finding of expected value signals in the brain raises the question of how such signals are learned in the first place. An influential theory from behavioural psychology put forward by Rescorla and Wagner suggests that learning of predictions are mediated by the degree of surprise engendered when an outcome is presented, or more precisely the difference between what is expected and what is received (Rescorla & Wagner, 1972; see Büchel this volume for a formalization of the R-W-model). Formally this is called a prediction error, which in the Rescorla-Wagner formulation can take on either positive or negative sign depending on whether an outcome is greater than expected (which would lead to a positive error signal), or less than expected (which would lead to a negative error). This prediction error is then used to update predictions associated with a particular stimulus or cue in the environment, so that if this cue always precedes say a reward (and hence is fully predictive of reward) eventually the expected value of the cue will converge to the value of the reward, at which point the prediction error is zero and no further learning will take place.

Initial evidence for prediction error signals in the brain emerged from the work of Wolfram Schultz and colleagues who observed such signals by recording from the phasic activity of dopamine neurons in awake behaving non-human primates undergoing simple Pavlovian or instrumental conditioning tasks with reward (Mirenowicz & Schultz, 1994; Schultz et al., 1997; Hollerman & Schultz, 1998; Schultz, 1998). The response profile of these neurons does not correspond to a simple Rescorla-Wagner rule but rather a real-time extension of this rule called temporal difference learning in which predictions of future reward are computed at each discrete time interval t within a trial, such that the error signal is generated by computing the difference in successive predictions (Schultz et al., 1997). This specific model provides a good approximation to the temporal profile of activity of these neurons during classical conditioning, in which the dopamine neurons first respond at the time of the UCS before learning is established but shift back in time within a trial to respond instead at the time of presentation of the cue once learning is established. In order to test for evidence of a temporal difference prediction error signal in the human brain, O'Doherty et al. (2003b) scanned human subjects while they underwent a classical conditioning paradigm in which associations were learned between arbitrary visual fractal stimuli and a pleasant sweet taste reward (glucose). One cue was followed most of the time by the taste reward, whereas another cue was followed most of the time by no reward. However in addition, subjects were exposed to low frequency 'error' trials in which the cue associated with reward was presented but the reward was omitted, and the cue associated with no reward was presented but a reward was unexpectedly delivered. The specific trial history that each subject experienced was next fed into a temporal difference model in order to generate a time-series which specified the model-predicted prediction error signal at three different time points in a trial from the time at which the CS is presented until the time at which the reward is delivered (three sessions later) (Figure 4.1A). This time-series was then convolved with a canonical haemodynamic response function and regressed against the fMRI data for each individual subject, in order to identify brain regions correlating with the model-predicted time-series. This analysis revealed significant correlations with the model-based predictions in a number of brain regions, most notably the ventral striatum (ventral putamen bilaterally) (Figure 4.1B) and orbitofrontal cortex, both prominent target regions of dopamine neurons 12 (Oades and Halliday, 1987). These results suggest that prediction error signals are present in the

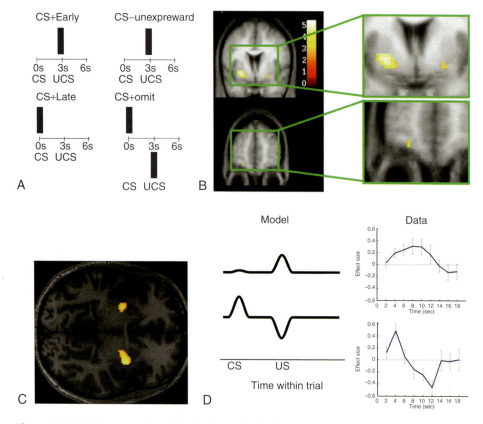

Figure 4.1 Prediction error signals in the human brain during appetitive and aversive learning. Illustration of model prediction error signals elicited in an experiment by O'Doherty *et al.* (2003) in which in one trial type (CS+) an arbitrary visual cue is associated 3 s later with delivery of a taste reward (1M glucose), and in another trial type (CS−) a different cue is followed by no taste. In addition, occasional 'surprise' trials occur in which the CS+ is presented but the reward is omitted (CS+omit), and the CS− is presented but a reward is unexpectedly delivered (CS− unexpreward). During CS+Early trials (early in training before learning is established) the PE signal should occur at the time of delivery of the reward, whereas by CS+late trials (late in training once learning is established) the signal should have switched to the time of presentation of the CS. On CS+omit trials a positive PE signal should occur at the time of presentation of the CS, but a negative PE signal should occur at the time the reward was expected (because the reward is omitted). CS−unexpreward trials should be associated with a positive signal at the time the reward is presented. Parts of human ventral striatum (top), and orbitofrontal cortex (bottom) showing a significant correlation with the temporal difference prediction error signal. Colour-bar depicts t-statistic of the group random effects statistics. Data from O'Doherty *et al.* (2003). Region of ventral striatum (bilaterally) correlating with temporal difference prediction errors elicited during second order conditioning with an aversive shock stimulus. From Seymour *et al.* (2004). Model-predicted prediction error signals on trials involving the unexpected presentation of the cue signaling pain (top left), and the unexpected omission of the cue signaling pain (bottom left), are shown alongside actual timecourses from these trials extracted from the ventral striatum (top right and bottom right). A very close correspondence between the model-predicted and actual BOLD responses can be seen after one takes into account the delay introduced by haemodynamic lag in the actual fMRI responses.

human brain during reward-learning, and that these signals conform to a response profile consistent with a specific computational model: temporal difference learning. The evidence discussed so far supports the presence of prediction error signals during learning involving appetitive or rewarding stimuli.

The next obvious question is whether such signals can be found to underlie learning about punishing as well as rewarding events. Evidence of a role for dopamine neurons in responding during aversive learning is mixed. Single-unit studies have generally failed to observe strong dopaminergic activity in response to aversive events (Schultz, 1998), and indeed it has been found that dopamine neurons may in fact inhibit responding during aversive stimulation such as tail pinch in rats (Ungless *et al.*, 2004). On the other hand, a number of studies measuring dopamine release in the striatum in rats have found evidence for increased dopamine levels during aversive as well as appetitive conditioning (Pezze & Feldon, 2004). However, as termination of an aversive stimulus can in itself be rewarding, the implications of these studies for understanding the role of dopamine in aversive learning are still debated. Irrespective of whether dopamine will turn out to play a role in aversive learning or not, existing evidence appears to rule out a role for phasic dopamine in encoding prediction errors for aversive events in the same way as appears to be the case during learning with rewards. This then raises the question of whether prediction error signals for aversive learning are present anywhere else in the brain, e.g. in the phasic activity of neurons carrying another neuromodulatory neurotransmitter? Although the suggestion that another neurotransmitter system such as serotonin may be involved in mediating aversive learning is intuitively and computationally appealing (Daw *et al.*, 2002), to date no direct evidence has emerged to support such a hypothesis.

In spite of this, neuroimaging studies have revealed strong evidence for the presence of prediction error signals in the human brain during aversive as well as appetitive learning. Seymour *et al.* (2004) scanned human subjects while they underwent a second-order conditioning paradigm in which the sequential presentation of two visual cues led to the subject receiving a mild but painful electric stimulation to the foot, whereas the sequential presentation of two other cues led to the subject obtaining a tickling but non painful electrical stimulation. On most trials the first cue signaling shock was followed by the second cue signaling shock and similarly for the stimuli signaling non-shock. However, on some rare trials in which the first cue presented signaled shock, the second cue to be presented unexpectedly signaled non-shock thereby inducing a negative prediction error. Similarly on occasional trials in which the first cue presented signaled non-shock, the second cue presented signaled shock, inducing a positive prediction error. A full temporal difference prediction error signal was then generated for each subject based on the trial-by-trial experience of that subject and correlated against the fMRI data. Significant correlations with TD prediction errors was found in ventral striatum bilaterally, in a region very close to that found to respond during prediction errors for reward (Figure 4.1D). These results demonstrate that prediction signals are also present in the brain during aversive conditioning, a finding that has been replicated a number of times subsequently (e.g. Seymour *et al.*, 2005). Given that such aversive signals in striatum are unlikely to depend on the afferent input of dopamine neurons, these findings also show that BOLD activity in ventral striatum should not be considered to be a pure reflection of the afferent input of dopamine neurons, an interpretation implicitly assumed in some of the reward imaging literature. Rather, activity in striatum is likely to also reflect the influence of a number of different neuromodulatory systems in addition to dopamine, input from other cortical and sub-cortical areas, as well as intrinsic computations within this region.

The studies discussed above demonstrate that prediction error signals are present during learning to predict both appetitive and aversive events, a finding consistent with the tenets of a prediction error based account of associative learning. However, merely demonstrating the presence of such signals in the striatum during learning does not establish whether such signals are causally related to learning or merely an epi-phenomenon. The first study aiming to uncover a causal link was that of Pessiglione and colleagues (2006) who manipulated systemic dopamine levels by delivering a dopamine agonist and antagonist while subjects were being scanned with fMRI during performance of a reward-learning task. Prediction error signals in striatum were boosted following administration of the dopaminergic agonist, and diminished following administration of the dopaminergic antagonist. Moreover, behavioural performance followed the changes in striatal activity, being increased following administration of the dopamine agonist and decreased following administration of the antagonist. These findings therefore support a causal link between prediction error activity in striatum and the degree of behavioural learning for reward.

Action selection for reward

While classical conditioning is a useful paradigm for studying the passive learning of reward predictions, to gain insight into the process by which humans can learn to perform actions in order to obtain reward it is necessary to turn to instrumental conditioning, which involves learning of stimulus–response or stimulus–response–outcome associations. It is here that reinforcement learning models become relevant. The basic idea behind most reinforcement learning models is that in order to choose optimally between different actions, an agent needs to maintain internal representations of the expected reward available on each action, and then subsequently choose the action with the highest expected value. Also central to these algorithms is the notion of a prediction error signal which is used to learn and update expected values for each action through experience, just as in the Rescorla-Wagner learning model for Pavlovian conditioning described earlier. In one such model – the actor/critic, action selection is conceived as involving two distinct components: a critic, which learns to predict future reward associated with particular states in the environment, and an actor which chooses specific actions in order to move the agent from state to state according to a learned policy (Barto, 1992, 1995). The critic encodes the value of particular states in the world and as such has the characteristics of a Pavlovian reward prediction signal described above. The actor stores a set of probabilities for each action in each state of the world, and chooses actions according to those probabilities. The goal of the model is to modify the policy stored in the actor such that over time, those actions associated with the highest predicted reward are selected more often. This is accomplished by means of the aforementioned prediction error signal that computes the difference in predicted reward as the agent moves from state to state. This signal is then used to update value predictions stored in the critic for each state, but also to update action probabilities stored in the actor such that if the agent moves to a state associated with greater reward (and thus generates a positive prediction error), then the probability of choosing that action in future is increased. Conversely, if the agent moves to a state associated with less reward, this generates a negative prediction error and the probability of choosing that action again is decreased.

Some computational neuroscientists have drawn analogies between the anatomy and connections of the basal ganglia, and possible neural architectures for implementing reinforcement learning models including the actor/critic. Houk et al. (1995) proposed that the actor and critic could be implemented within patch/striosome and matrix compartments distributed throughout the striatum. Montague et al. (1996) proposed that the ventral and dorsal striatum implemented the critic and actor respectively, on the grounds of extant knowledge of the putative functions of these structures at the time, derived primarily from animal lesion studies. In order to test these hypotheses, O'Doherty et al. (2004), scanned hungry human subjects with fMRI while they performed a simple instrumental conditioning task in which they were required to choose one of two actions leading to juice reward with either a high or low probability (Figure 4.2A). Neural responses corresponding to the generation of prediction error signals during performance of the instrumental task were compared to that elicited during a control Pavlovian task in which subjects experienced the same stimulus–reward contingencies but did not actively choose which action to select. This comparison was designed to isolate the actor, which was hypothesized to be engaged only in the instrumental task, from the critic, which was hypothesized to be engaged in both the instrumental and Pavlovian control tasks. Consistent with the proposal of a dorsal vs ventral actor/critic architecture, activity in dorsal striatum was found to be specifically correlated with prediction error signals when subjects were actively performing instrumental responses in order to obtain reward. By contrast ventral striatum was found to be active in both the instrumental and Pavlovian tasks (Figure 4.2B).

These results suggest a dorsal/ventral distinction within the striatum whereby ventral striatum is more concerned with Pavlovian or stimulus–outcome learning, while the dorsal striatum is more engaged during learning of stimulus–response or stimulus–response–outcome associations. However, it is important to note that the study was not designed to address whether learning of action values in the dorsal striatum is governed by state-value prediction errors generated from the critic, as implemented in the full actor/critic model. It is also plausible that action values within the dorsal striatum might be learned and updated directly as instantiated in other variants of reinforcement learning such as Q-learning or SARSA, in which action values are learned directly rather than being updated via prediction errors generated by the critic (Watkins & Dayan, 1992; Sutton & Barto, 1998). Indeed recent evidence from the single-unit recording of dopamine

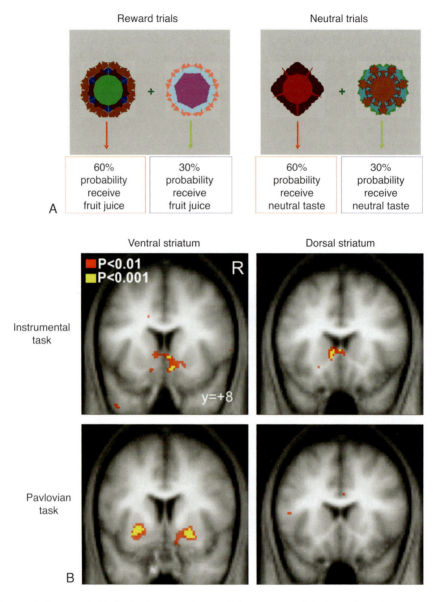

Figure 4.2 The actor/critic in the human striatum. (A) Instrumental choice task used by O'Doherty *et al.* (2004). On each trial of the reward condition subject chooses between two possible actions, one associated with a high probability of obtaining juice reward (60%), the other a low probability (30%). In a neutral condition subjects also choose between actions with similar probabilities but in this case they receive an affectively neutral outcome (tasteless solution). Prediction error responses during the reward condition of the instrumental choice task were compared to prediction error signals during a yoked Pavlovian control task. (B) Significant correlations with the reward prediction error signal generated by an actor/critic model were found in ventral striatum (ventral putamen extending into nucleus accumbens proper) in both the Pavlovian and instrumental tasks, suggesting that this region is involved in stimulus-outcome learning. By contrast a region of dorsal striatum (anteromedial caudate nucleus) was found to be correlated with prediction error signals only during the instrumental task, suggesting that this area is involved in stimulus-response or stimulus response outcome learning. Data from O'Doherty *et al.* (2004).

neurons supports the notion that these neurons may be involved in learning action-values directly as opposed to merely learning state values as would be predicted by the full actor/critic model (Morris *et al.*, 2006; Niv *et al.*, 2006). Nevertheless, the suggestion that human dorsal striatum is specifically involved under situations when subjects need to select actions in order to obtain reward has received support from a number of other fMRI studies, both model- and trial-based (Tricomi *et al.*, 2004; Haruno *et al.*, 2004).

Expected value of actions

This raises the question as to where in the brain expected values are represented during action learning for reward. A number of model-based fMRI studies have consistently implicated ventromedial prefrontal cortex in encoding the value of chosen actions. Kim *et al.* (2006) used a variant of the actor/critic algorithm to generate expected value signals as subjects made decisions between which of two possible actions to chose in order to obtain monetary reward, as well as in a different condition, to avoid losing money. In this study, different available actions were associated with distinct probabilities of either winning or losing money, such that in the reward condition one action was associated with a 60% probability of winning money, and the other action with only a 30% probability of winning. In order to maximize their cumulative reward, subjects should learn to choose the 60% probability action. In the avoidance condition, subjects were presented with a choice between the same probabilities, except in this context, 60% of the time after choosing one action they avoided losing money, whereas this only occurred 30% of the time after choosing the alternate action. In order to minimize their losses, subjects should learn to choose the action associated with the 60% probability of loss avoidance. Model-generated expected value signals for the action chosen were found to be correlated on a trial-by-trial basis with BOLD responses in bilateral orbitofrontal cortex and adjacent medial prefrontal cortex in both the reward and avoidance conditions, such that activity in these areas increased in proportion to the expected future reward associated with the specific action chosen (Figure 4.3A).

Similar results were obtained by Daw *et al.* (2006), who used a four armed bandit task in which 'points' (that would later be converted into money) were paid out on each bandit. However, unlike the studies described previously, in this case, the mean payoff available on each bandit drifted over time, such that no one bandit was consistently paying out more than the others, but at any one time some bandits paid out more than the others. As a consequence, subjects had to keep track of the mean payoffs available on each bandit over the course of the experiment, in order to work out which one paid out the most at any one moment. Model-predicted expected value signals specific to the action chosen were found to be correlated on a trial by trial basis with fMRI activity in ventromedial prefrontal cortex (Figure 4.3B). Taken together, these findings suggest that orbital and medial prefrontal cortex are involved in keeping track of the expected future reward associated with chosen actions, and that these areas show a response profile consistent with an expected value signal generated by reinforcement learning models.

So far we have considered evidence broadly supportive of reinforcement learning-based accounts of human decision-making. In the following section we will now discuss

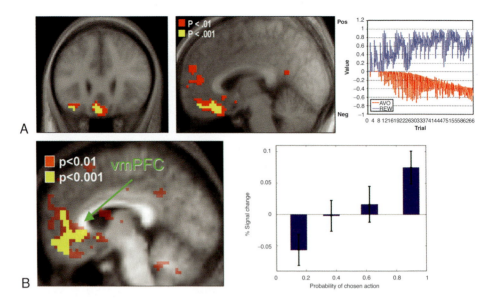

Figure 4.3 Expected value signals in ventromedial prefrontal cortex. (A) Regions of ventromedial prefrontal cortex (medial and central orbitofrontal cortex extending into medial prefrontal cortex) correlating with expected value signals generated by a variant of the actor/ critic model during an fMRI study of instrumental choice of reward and avoidance (left and middle panels). The model-predicted expected value signals are shown for one subject in the right panel for both the reward (blue) and avoidance (red) conditions. Data from Kim *et al.* (2006). (B) Similar regions of ventromedial prefrontal cortex correlating with model predicted expected value signals during performance of a four-armed bandit task with non-stationary reward distributions (left panel). BOLD signal changes in this region are shown plotted against model predictions (right panel), revealing an approximately linear relationship between expected value and BOLD signal changes in this region. Data from Daw *et al.* (2006).

learning situations and empirical findings that pose challenges for reinforcement learning-based accounts.

Challenges to reinforcement learning models of human choice

Avoidance learning

In avoidance learning, an animal or human learns to perform an action in order to avoid obtaining an aversive outcome. Unlike reward learning, avoidance learning is a form of instrumental conditioning not so easily accounted for by standard theories of reinforcement. The problem is that once an aversive outcome has been successfully avoided, the individual no longer experiences explicit reinforcement for their behaviour, and thus, behaviour appears to be maintained even in the absence of reinforcement (Solomon & Wynne, 1953). Yet according to reinforcement theory, such behaviour should rapidly extinguish. The fact that responding appears to be maintained even in extinction therefore runs counter to the basic assumptions of reinforcement learning theory. A parsimonious theoretical account of avoidance learning is to propose that successfully avoiding an aversive outcome in itself acts as a reward. Thus, avoidance behaviour is positively reinforced on each trial when the aversive outcome is avoided, just as receipt of reward reinforces behaviour during reward conditioning (Dickinson & Dearing, 1979; Gray, 1987). In this sense, avoidance of an aversive outcome could be considered to be an 'intrinsic reward,' with the same positive reinforcing properties as a real 'extrinsic' reward. A study by Kim *et al.*, mentioned previously was designed specifically to address this hypothesis. To briefly recapitulate: subjects were scanned while on each trial choosing from one of two actions in order to either win money or else avoid losing money. The fMRI data was then used to test whether successful avoidance of an aversive outcome recruited the same or different neural circuitry as that elicited by receipt of a reward itself. The rationale of the study was that should avoiding an aversive outcome act as a reward, then similar underlying neural circuitry should be recruited as that elicited during reward receipt. If, on the contrary, these two processes are found to engage completely distinct and non-overlapping neural circuitry, then this would suggest that avoidance and reward may depend on very distinct neural substrates, providing evidence against a reinforcement learning-based account of avoidance. Consistent with the former possibility, a part of the human brain previously implicated in responding to reward outcomes, the medial OFC, increased in activity following successful avoidance of the aversive outcome (Figure 4.4). Thus, these findings suggest that avoidance can after all be accommodated happily within the reinforcement learning framework. Notably, this study also provides a powerful example of where fMRI data can be used to provide insights into the psychological processes underlying a specific form of learning, that to date had been very difficult to address exclusively at the behavioural level.

Encoding abstract rules in a decision problem

A much more serious challenge to reinforcement learning theory comes from situations where a decision problem features higher order structure. Examples of such structure include the presence in a task of rules describing inter-dependencies between actions, rewards, and other exogenous variables such as time. Simple RL models assume the actions available in the world and the rewards that can be obtained from choice of those actions are independent from each other, such that in a given state, information gained about the rewards available from choice of one action provides no information about the rewards available from choice of another action. However, in many situations rules describing inter-dependencies between different actions do exist, and if subjects can exploit these rules, this will lead to greater reward than otherwise. One of the simplest examples of a decision task with such an abstract rule is probabilistic reversal learning (Cools *et al.*, 2002; O'Doherty *et al.*, 2003a). In this task, subjects can choose between one of two actions which give out monetary rewards or losses on a probabilistic basis, similar to the instrumental choice tasks outlined previously. However, in this case, at any one time, one of the actions pays out more reward than the other, such that if the subject continues to choose the high paying action they will obtain the greatest reward.

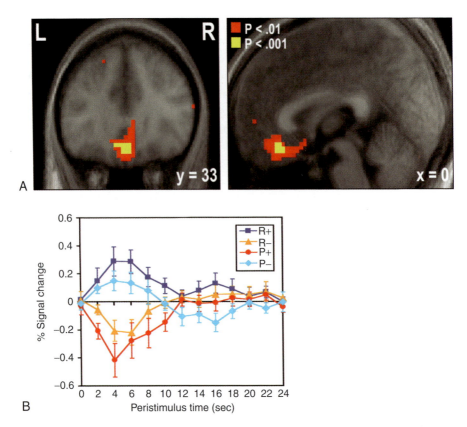

Figure 4.4 Avoidance of an aversive outcome recruits overlapping circuitry to receipt of reward (A) Medial OFC showing a significant increase in activity after avoidance of an aversive outcome as well as after obtaining reward. (B) Time-course plots of peak voxels in the OFC for four different outcomes: receipt of reward (R+), avoidance of an aversive outcome (P−), missed reward (R−), and receipt of an aversive outcome (P+). The plots are arranged such that time 0 corresponds to the point of outcome delivery. Data from Kim *et al.* (2006).

After a time the contingencies reverse, and the subject has to switch their choice of action in order to continue to maximize their reward. The structure in this task is the anti-correlation between the distributions of rewards available on the two actions: when one action is 'good' the other is 'bad' and vice-versa, as well as the rule that after a time the contingencies will reverse. A standard RL model could be used to learn such a task, but in this case the model would not incorporate the abstract rules in the reversal task but would instead simply learn about the values of the two actions independently.

However, what if a model were to incorporate such rules? In order to establish whether human subjects do use an abstract representation of the task structure in order to guide their choices, Hampton *et al.* (2006) scanned subjects with fMRI whilst they underwent probabilistic reversal learning. A computational model which incorporated the structure of the task was then constructed and fitted to both the behavioural and fMRI data. This structure-based model was implemented as a Hidden Markov model (HMM), where the hidden state to be estimated was the probability that on a given trial the 'correct' (or currently high reward value action) is being chosen. This model also incorporated the fact that the identity of the correct action would reverse from time to time. The structure-based model was found to provide a good fit to subjects' behaviour, and the signal derived from the model representing the probability that subjects were choosing the correct action (prior correct) was found to be significantly correlated at the time of action choice with fMRI activity in ventromedial prefrontal cortex (Figure 4.5A). The areas thus identified overlap markedly with those regions found to correlate with expected value derived from standard RL models outlined previously. This is perhaps not surprising as the prior correct signal from the HMM model is strongly co-linear with expected value signals derived from RL.

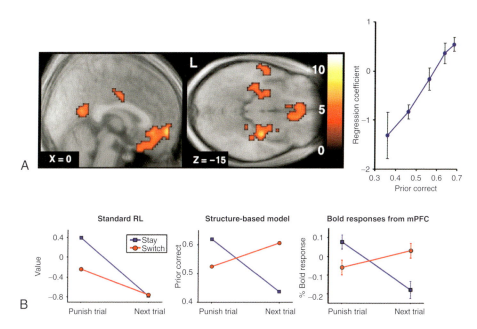

Figure 4.5 Expected value signals in ventromedial prefrontal cortex reflect abstract task structure. (A) Regions of ventromedial prefrontal cortex correlating with expected value signals while subjects performed a decision task with abstract structure: probabilistic reversal learning (left panel). Expected signals were generated by a model that incorporates the structure of the task. Plot of responses in this region against expected value signals reveal a strongly linear relationship. (B) Dissociating a model which incorporates the structure of the task (structure-based model) from standard RL models which do not incorporate the rules of the task. The predictions from standard RL and the structure-based model are plotted before and after switching action choice following a reversal, where the subject switches back to an action that was chosen previously (shown in left and middle panels in red). The structure-based model predicts that prior correct (which is co-linear with expected value) jumps up following a reversal, whereas the RL models predict no such increase. The actual BOLD signal in medial PFC shows a response profile consistent with the structure based model and not simple RL (right panel). Data from Hampton *et al.* (2006).

Model comparison: structure-based inference vs. standard RL

However, the key question is whether the model that incorporates the rules of the decision task can account *better* for subjects' behavioural and fMRI data than does standard RL, as this would provide evidence that human subjects *do* use knowledge of task structure in order to guide their choices as opposed to merely learning action values independently. In this study we therefore compared the goodness of fit of the HMM model to subjects' behavioural data to the fit achieved by a family of different RL models. The structure-based model was found to provide a significantly better fit to the behavioural data than did the best fitting RL model, even after adjusting for the number of free parameters in the model. Thus, even at the behavioural level, there is evidence to suggest that subjects are using knowledge of the structure of the reversal task in order to guide their choices.

In order to determine whether neural coding of expected values also reflected knowledge of this structure, we looked specifically at those times in the experiment when the predictions of the structure-based model and of the standard RL model would be maximally divergent. This happens to be immediately after subjects switch their choice of action. According to both RL and the structure-based model, subjects should switch their choice of action once they have a low expected value for that action, presumably after having received a string of non-rewarding outcomes after selecting that action on previous trials. Where the models diverge, is when subjects switch back to an action that they previously switched away from after a prior contingency reversal. According to standard RL, once subjects switch back to an action they should still have a low expected reward for that action because the last time they chose that action it had a low expected value (hence they switched away from it). However, according to the structure-based model, once subjects switch back to an action they previously switched away from, this time, they should have a high expected reward value, because they understand that the contingencies have reversed, and that therefore this action must now have a high reward value. Figure 4.5B shows the predictions of both the structure-based model and standard RL models alongside the actual signal at the time of choice extracted from the medial prefrontal cortex. As can be seen from this figure the actual fMRI data mirrors the predictions of the structure-based model, by showing that subjects' expectations of reward jumps up once they switch back to a previously chosen action following a reversal. In a further analysis, model-predictions from the structure-based model and standard RL model were both entered into a regression analysis against the fMRI data and the fit of both models to the fMRI data were directly compared. Once again, the structure-based model was found to provide a better fit to the fMRI data than the best-fitting RL model. These results suggest that subjects can take into account the abstract rules of a decision problem and that knowledge of such rules can modulate expected value signals in prefrontal cortex that in turn may be used to guide behavioural choice. This particular study provides an example of how fMRI data can be used to discriminate between competing computational models of cognitive function, by showing that neural signals are accounted better by one model than another. These findings therefore pose a significant challenge to simple reinforcement learning-based account of human choice. The implications of this challenge will be discussed in the final section of this chapter.

Exploration vs. Exploitation: A rewarding dilemma

Another important challenge to existing reinforcement learning models comes from a study by Daw *et al.* (2006) into the so-called exploration/exploitation dilemma, which emerges in any situation where multiple options are available to choose from, any of which could yield reward. The dilemma arises from the trade off between the need to explore each of the different actions in order to establish how much reward is paid out by each, and the desire to exploit the action which is currently known to have the highest reward. Clearly time spent exploring sub-optimal actions results in less reward being obtained, but at the same time it is necessary to explore in order to find potentially richer actions than the ones being pursued currently. A number of computational strategies have been proposed within the reinforcement learning framework to allow an agent to balance exploration and exploitation. The simplest method is the so-called epsilon greedy approach in which the action with the best predicted reward value is almost always chosen except for occasions which occur with probability ε, wherein an exploratory action is chosen. The soft-max approach involves putting the different action values through a sigmoidal function which essentially provides a 'soft threshold' so that the best action is usually selected, but sometimes a less good action is selected allowing that action to be explored. A more principled approach concerns estimating the uncertainty in the agents knowledge about the rewards available on each action and driving action selection to minimize uncertainty as well as to maximize reward. To address which of these mechanisms was being implemented in the human brain, Daw *et al.* looked for evidence of these different strategies while subjects performed a four armed bandit task (this task is described in more detail above). Remarkably, there was no evidence from the neuroimaging data to support the ε-greedy, soft-max or uncertainty-based accounts. Instead, a region of frontopolar cortex was found to become engaged on trials when subjects engaged in exploratory behaviour, defined as any trial in which subjects chose an action with a lower expected value than the best available action (Figure 4.6). Differential activity in this frontal region on exploratory compared to exploitative trials suggests a 'switching' account of exploratory behaviour whereby occasional exploratory actions are selected by engaging a prefrontal mechanism which switches off or wrests control from the default exploitative system, presumed to reside in ventromedial prefrontal cortex and striatum. The implications of this study are therefore, that existing computational strategies for addressing the exploration/exploitation dilemma may not account for how such a dilemma is actually resolved in the brain, providing another serious challenge to existing reinforcement learning models.

Implications toward a more complete theory of human choice

The findings described above show that reinforcement learning models have been remarkably successful in accounting for much of human behavioural and neural data during

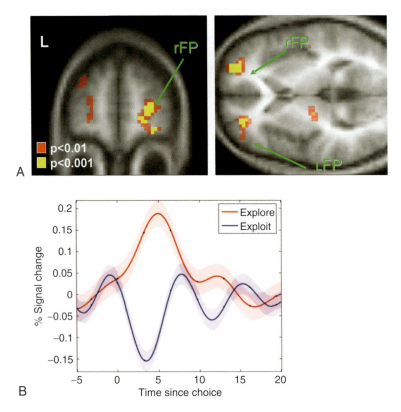

Figure 4.6 Exploration-related activity in frontopolar cortex. (A) Regions of left and right frontopolar cortex (lFP, rFP) showing significantly increased activation on exploratory compared with exploitative trials. Activation maps (yellow, P<0.001; red, P<0.01) are superimposed on a subject-averaged structural scan. (B) BOLD time courses averaged over exploratory (red line) and exploitative (blue line) decisions. Coloured fringes show error bars (representing s.e.m.). Data from Daw *et al.* (2006).

reward-learning and simple choice. However, simple versions of these models encounter difficulties in accounting for more complex aspects of choice behaviour such as under situations where a decision problem incorporates abstract rules or structure. Furthermore, existing computational approaches to the exploration/exploitation problem do not adequately account for neuroimaging results suggesting the presence of a 'switching' mechanism in frontal cortex related to exploratory behaviour. How can these findings be reconciled with reinforcement learning models? One possible approach is to consider distinct contributions of prefrontal and striatal systems to controlling behaviour. Whereas striatal circuitry may be involved in mediating simple reinforcement learning mechanisms such as those captured by the actor/critic or Q-learning, prefrontal cortex may instead be involved in learning about the structure or rules of the world, such as what features of the environment are relevant for the decision problem, and what the rules are for transiting from one state of the environment to another (Doya *et al.* 2002). In reinforcement learning this division of labour is often termed 'model-based reinforcement learning' – where the model-based part is concerned with building a model of the different states of the world, while the reinforcement learning part learns the values of these different states. This theory proposes that prefrontal and striatal systems co-operate as essentially one unified system that can produce adaptive reward-guided behaviour even in complex situations with higher order state transitions (Doya *et al.* 2002).

An alternative dual system hypothesis has been proposed by Daw *et al.* (2005), in the main to accommodate animal data suggesting the presence of two distinct mechanisms for controlling behaviour, a goal-directed system in which actions are selected with respect to the incentive value of goals, and a habit system in which actions are chosen based on learned stimulus-response associations without encoding the incentive value of the associated outcome (Balleine & Dickinson, 1998; for evidence in humans of goal-directed learning see Valentin *et al.*, 2007). The computational instantiation of this theory proposes that prefrontal cortex is involved in implementing a 'forward model' involving an on-line forward search through a decision tree, whereas striatum is involved in implementing simple or model-free reinforcement learning. According to this account, evidence from human imaging studies described here that activity in prefrontal cortex reflects the structure of the decision problem could be indicative of the operation of this 'model-based' forward system.

Future studies will be needed to resolve these two competing but related hypotheses. One way to address this would be to determine whether reinforcement learning-related activity in prefrontal cortex and striatum are dissociable from each other as would be predicted from the Daw *et al.* account, such that prefrontal activity would reflect learning about the structure of the decision problem while striatum would show only simple RL signals that do not reflect such structure. Alternatively should neural activity in both striatum and prefrontal cortex be found to reflect learning with higher order structure – this would provide evidence in support of the former proposal.

Conclusions

In this chapter we have reviewed evidence from functional neuroimaging demonstrating the applicability of reinforcement learning models and extensions of these models toward understanding the basic mechanisms underlying value-dependent learning in humans. We have also provided a number of examples where data from functional neuroimaging has been used as a means to discriminate between competing models of cognitive function, even when such models cannot be adequately discriminated on the basis of behavioural data alone. This provides support for the contention that at least within the field of reward-learning, functional neuroimaging provides a powerful tool with which to advance computational theories of psychological and neural function.

Acknowledgements

JOD is supported by a Searle Scholarship. The author would like to thank Nathaniel Daw, Peter Dayan, Ray Dolan, and Ben Seymour at UCL, and Peter Bossaerts, Alan Hampton, Hackjin Kim, and Vivian Valentin at Caltech, who were major collaborators on the work discussed here.

References

Balleine, B. W. & Dickinson, A. (1998). Goal-directed instrumental action: contingency and incentive learning and their cortical substrates. *Neuropharmacology*, *37*, 407–419.

Barto, A. G. (1992). Reinforcement learning and adaptive critic methods. In: D. A. White & D. A. Sofge (Eds), *Handbook of Intelligent Control: Neural, Fuzzy, and Adaptive Approaches*, pp. 469–491. New York: Van Norstrand Reinhold.

Barto, A. G. (1995). Adaptive critics and the basal ganglia. In: J. C. Houk, J. L. Davis, & B. G. Beiser (Eds), Models of Information Processing in the Basal Ganglia, pp. 215–232. Cambridge, MA: MIT Press.

Buchel, C., Morris, J., Dolan, R. J., & Friston, K. J. (1998). Brain systems mediating aversive conditioning: an event-related fMRI study. *Neuron*, *20*, 947–957.

Cools, R., Clark, L., Owen, A. M., & Robbins, T. W. (2002). Defining the neural mechanisms of probabilistic reversal learning using event-related functional magnetic resonance imaging. *Journal of Neuroscience*, *22*, 4563–4567.

Daw, N. D., Kakade, S., & Dayan, P. (2002). Opponent interactions between serotonin and dopamine. *Neural Networks*, *15*, 603–616.

Daw, N. D., Niv, Y., & Dayan, P. (2005). Uncertainty-based competition between prefrontal and dorsolateral striatal systems for behavioral control. *Nature Neuroscience*, *8*, 1704–1711.

Daw, N. D., O'Doherty, J. P., Dayan, P., Seymour, B., & Dolan, R. J. (2006). Cortical substrates for exploratory decisions in humans. *Nature*, *441*, 876–879.

Dickinson, A., & Dearing, M. (1979). Appetitive-aversive interactions and inhibitory processes. In: A. Dickinson & R. Boakes (Eds), *Mechanisms of Learning and Motivation*, pp. 203–231. Hillsdale, NJ: Erlbaum.

Doya, K., Samejima, K., Katagiri, K., & Kawato, M. (2002). Multiple model-based reinforcement learning. *Neural Computation*, *14*, 1347–1369.

Gottfried, J. A., O'Doherty, J., & Dolan, R. J. (2002). Appetitive and aversive olfactory learning in humans studied using event-related functional magnetic resonance imaging. *Journal of Neuroscience*, *22*, 10829–10837.

Gottfried, J. A., O'Doherty, J., & Dolan, R. J. (2003). Encoding predictive reward value in human amygdala and orbitofrontal cortex. *Science*, *301*, 1104–1107.

Gray, J. A. (1987). *The Psychology of Fear and Stress*. Cambridge: Cambridge University Press.

Hampton, A. N., Bossaerts, P., & O'Doherty, J. P. (2006). The role of the ventromedial prefrontal cortex in abstract state-based inference during decision making in humans. *Journal of Neuroscience*, *26*, 8360–8367.

Haruno, M., Kuroda, T., Doya, K., Toyama, K., Kimura, M., Samejima, K., Imamizu, H., & Kawato, M. (2004). A neural correlate of reward-based behavioral learning in caudate nucleus: a functional magnetic resonance imaging study of a stochastic decision task. *Journal of Neuroscience*, *24*, 1660–1665.

Hollerman, J. R., & Schultz, W. (1998). Dopamine neurons report an error in the temporal prediction of reward during learning. *Nature Neuroscience*, *1*, 304–309.

Houk, J. C., Adams, J. L., & Barto, A. G. (1995). A model of how the basal ganglia generate and use neural signals that predict reinforcement. In: J. C. Houk, J. L. Davis, & B. G. Beiser (Eds), *Models of Information Processing in the Basal Ganglia*, pp. 249–270. Cambridge: MIT Press.

Kim, H., Shimojo, S., & O'Doherty, J. P. (2006). Is avoiding an aversive outcome rewarding? Neural substrates of avoidance learning in the human brain. *PLoS Biology*, *4*, e233.

McClure, S. M., Berns, G. S., & Montague, P. R. (2003). Temporal prediction errors in a passive learning task activate human striatum. *Neuron*, *38*, 339–346.

Mirenowicz, J., & Schultz, W. (1994). Importance of unpredictability for reward responses in primate dopamine neurons. *Journal of Neurophysiology*, *72*, 1024–1027.

Montague, P. R., Dayan, P., & Sejnowski, T. J. (1996). A framework for mesencephalic dopamine systems based on predictive Hebbian learning. *Journal of Neuroscience*, *16*, 1936–1947.

Morris, G., Nevet, A., Arkadir, D., Vaadia, E., & Bergman, H. (2006). Midbrain dopamine neurons encode decisions for future action. *Nature Neuroscience, 9,* 1057–1063.

Niv, Y., Daw, N. D., & Dayan, P. (2006). Choice values. *Nature Neuroscience, 9,* 987–988.

Oades, R. D., & Halliday, G. M. (1987). Ventral tegmental (A10) system: Neurobiology. 1. Anatomy and connectivity. *Brain Res, 434,* 117–165.

O'Doherty, J., Critchley, H., Deichmann, R., & Dolan, R. J. (2003a). Dissociating valence of outcome from behavioral control in human orbital and ventral prefrontal cortices. *Journal of Neuroscience, 23,* 7931–7939.

O'Doherty, J., Dayan, P., Friston, K., Critchley, H., & Dolan, R. J. (2003b). Temporal difference models and reward-related learning in the human brain. *Neuron, 38,* 329–337.

O'Doherty, J., Dayan, P., Schultz, J., Deichmann, R., Friston, K., & Dolan, R. J. (2004). Dissociable roles of ventral and dorsal striatum in instrumental conditioning. *Science, 304,* 452–454.

Paton, J. J., Belova, M. A., Morrison, S. E., Salzman, C. D. (2006). The primate amygdala represents the positive and negative value of visual stimuli during learning. *Nature, 439,* 865–870.

Pessiglione, M., Seymour, B., Flandin, G., Dolan, R. J., & Frith, C. D. (2006). Dopamine-dependent prediction errors underpin reward-seeking behaviour in humans. *Nature, 442,* 1042–1045.

Pezze, M. A., & Feldon, J. (2004). Mesolimbic dopaminergic pathways in fear conditioning. *Progress in Neurobiology, 74,* 301–320.

Rescorla, R. A., & Wagner, A. R. (1972). A theory of Pavlovian conditioning: variations in the effectiveness of reinforcement and nonreinforcement. In: A. H. Black & W. F. Prakasy (Eds), *Classical Conditioning II: Current Research and Theory,* pp. 64–99. New York: Appleton Crofts.

Rolls, B. J., Rolls, E. T., Rowe, E. A., & Sweeney, K. (1981). Sensory specific satiety in man. *Physiology & Behavior, 27,* 137–142.

Schoenbaum, G., Chiba, A. A., & Gallagher, M. (1998). Orbitofrontal cortex and basolateral amygdala encode expected outcomes during learning. *Nature Neuroscience, 1,* 155–159.

Schultz, W. (1998). Predictive reward signal of dopamine neurons. *Journal of Neurophysiology, 80,* 1–27.

Schultz, W., Dayan, P., & Montague, P. R. (1997). A neural substrate of prediction and reward. *Science, 275,* 1593–1599.

Seymour, B., O'Doherty, J. P., Koltzenburg, M., Wiech, K., Frackowiak, R., Friston, K., & Dolan, R. (2005). Opponent appetitive-aversive neural processes underlie predictive learning of pain relief. *Nature Neuroscience, 8,* 1234–1240.

Seymour, B., O'Doherty, J. P., Dayan, P., Koltzenburg, M., Jones, A. K., Dolan, R. J., Friston, K. J., & Frackowiak, R. S. (2004). Temporal difference models describe higher-order learning in humans. *Nature, 429,* 664–667.

Solomon, R., & Wynne, L. (1953). Traumatic avoidance learning: Acquisition in normal dogs. *Psychological Monographs, 67,* 1–19.

Sutton, R. S., & Barto, A. G. (1998). *Reinforcement Learning.* Cambridge, MA: MIT Press.

Thorpe, S. J., Rolls, E. T., & Maddison, S. (1983). The orbitofrontal cortex: neuronal activity in the behaving monkey. *Experimental Brain Research, 49,* 93–115.

Tremblay, L., & Schultz, W. (1999). Relative reward preference in primate orbitofrontal cortex. *Nature, 398,* 704–708.

Tricomi, E. M., Delgado, M. R., & Fiez, J. A. (2004). Modulation of caudate activity by action contingency. *Neuron, 41*(2), 281–92.

Ungless, M. A., Magill, P. J., & Bolam, J. P. (2004). Uniform inhibition of dopamine neurons in the ventral tegmental area by aversive stimuli. *Science, 303,* 2040–2042.

Valentin, V. V., Dickinson, A., & O'Doherty, J. P. (2007). Determining the neural substrates of goal-directed learning in the human brain. *Journal of Neuroscience, 27,* 4019–4026.

Watkins, C. J., & Dayan, P. (1992). Q-learning. *Machine Learning, 8,* 279–292.

Chapter 5

Cognitive models in learning and reward processing

Christian Büchel

Introduction

The main topic of this chapter is how cognitive models relate to imaging neuroscience or more directly, if and how fMRI can assist in testing hypothesis about cognitive models. The first part will revisit the concept of cognitive theories and more precisely specify at what level fMRI might be valuable in this context. Two examples will then be presented in which (i) fMRI data from a learning experiment is analyzed in the context of a cognitive model, which helped to understand the underlying mechanisms and (ii) an example in which fMRI data was analyzed in the context of a model, but was able to refute or refine thinking about how that model is implemented in the brain. The latter example is especially important as the field has been faced with the criticism that strong predictions (e.g. through strong cognitive theories) have often biased the interpretation of the data towards an existing theory.

Cognitive models

Usually cognitive models are based on previous, mainly behavioural, data, and these models can be construed as a concept around a previous observation. If useful, this concept allows abstraction; so that the theory extends beyond the observations it is based on. Importantly, this allows making predictions based on the cognitive model or theory. These predictions are then testable by new experiments and three consequences might emerge (i) the theory is fully supported by the new data, (ii) the data does not support the theory, and (iii) the data partially supports the theory. In the latter case, the theory or model is usually extended adding new degrees of freedom at the cost of parsimony. This should be kept in mind, as introducing more and more free parameters to a model can easily account for a wealth of data; however, often these additional parameters lead to difficulties in interpreting the model.

Predictions for neuroimaging data based on a cognitive model or theory can be of two sorts: They can be spatial i.e. suggesting where a certain cognitive function is implemented in the brain or they can be temporal, i.e. making predictions about how a system responds to a certain constellation of stimuli in a given context. Previously, the only way to test spatial predictions of cognitive models was the classical neuropsychological lesion approach. In this framework, a patient with a certain lesion who had a certain cognitive deficit was studied to relate the lesion to the cognitive deficit. Predictions about the response patterns of the cognitive systems were mainly based on behavioural studies using reaction times or accuracy as the dependent variables.

With the advent of new neuroimaging techniques a new tool was introduced that is in principle capable of testing spatial and temporal predictions made by cognitive models. However, in contrary to the lesion approach, neuroimaging is a correlative technique and thus the signal change in a certain brain area does not necessarily prove that this region is essential for the task. It could well be an unspecific co-activation. However, in combination with a transient lesion techniques like transcranial magnetic stimulation (TMS) this disadvantage can be circumvented. For instance, the activation of the occipital cortex in blind volunteers as identified by functional neuroimaging (Sadato et al., 1996; Büchel, 1998; Büchel et al., 1998a; Röder et al., 1997) could have been an unspecific effect. Yet a TMS study was able to show a decrease in tactile reading performance in blind volunteers by disrupting processes in the occipital cortex, thereby directly showing the functional relevance of occipital areas for tactile processing in the blind (Cohen et al., 1997).

Before entering the discourse of how functional neuroimaging can inform cognitive theories, it is worth to revisit the theoretical background of how models can influence the interpretation of data and how data can shape cognitive models in general. A formal framework on how to combine data with a model is the Bayesian approach.

In essence Bayes' theorem tells how to update or revise beliefs (i.e. theories) in light of new evidence (i.e. data). Bayesian inference can be regarded as the prototypical scientific method because updating probabilities through Bayesian inference requires initial beliefs or models to start with and then to collect new data, and then to change the original theory according to the new information. Often the a priori knowledge about a model or more precisely about model parameters enters the framework as priors or prior distributions, i.e. in the Gaussian case says something about their mean and distribution around that mean. The data enters the system in the form of a likelihood.

The result of this process is the posterior distribution that can be considered as a compromise between the data and the prior information available. If the prior distribution is very narrow, i.e. there are strong a priori beliefs about a certain parameter and the data is very noisy the result is heavily influenced by the prior information, i.e. the model. In the opposite case where there is only weak a priori knowledge, i.e. the prior distribution is rather flat, the posterior distribution is mainly influenced by the data. Importantly this framework allows an adaptive control of the reliability of a priori information to enter the system translating this framework feasible for the interplay of cognitive models and neurophysiology: one can consider a cognitive model as a prior that enters the system, which will then be combined with the data, i.e. the likelihood. However, apart from the immediate appeal, this procedure can also be dangerous. In cases in which the cognitive model is overemphasized, i.e. using a very narrow prior one might bias the interpretation of the information towards the initial model.

The remainder of this chapter will comprise two empirical parts: in the first part data from an emotional learning paradigm with variable contingencies is used to illustrate the usefulness of a cognitive model in interpreting experimental data. In the second part, a somewhat opponent viewpoint is presented namely, a case in which the data was actually able to overrule a prior hypothesis based on a cognitive or microeconomic theory. It should be noted that both examples do not employ a formal Bayesian framework. However, it is noteworthy that the interpretation of the data is performed in a Bayesian sense, i.e. the models used in both data sets can be considered as priors (in the mind set of the experimenter) and that the conclusions that are drawn (posterior probability) are a function of the data and the model (i.e. prior).

Emotional learning with variable contingencies

In classical conditioning an organism is required to learn the association between a neutral stimulus (conditioned stimulus: CS) and an innately meaningful stimulus (unconditioned stimulus: UCS). Usually the innately meaningful (UCS) is behaviourally relevant (i.e. food reward, electric shock, or pain). Through repetitive presentation of the conditioned stimulus together with the unconditioned stimulus, the conditioned stimulus will eventually itself evoke an unconditioned response. This associative pattern emerges rather quickly if the conditioned stimulus is always followed by the unconditioned stimulus, i.e. employing a 100% reinforcement scheme. However, in the real world the situation is often more complicated and contingencies are less predictable and also tend to vary over time. What an organism has learned today might not be correct in two weeks time, calling for an adaptive mechanism that can readjust according to new evidence.

A crucial question in the context of classical conditioning is: 'which structures are responsible for establishing the link between the CS and the UCS'? Rodent (Quirk *et al.*, 1997) and human functional neuroimaging studies (Büchel *et al.*, 1998b; LaBar *et al.*, 1998) have revealed a pivotal role of the amygdala in this context. Importantly, the amygdala activation was strongest in the beginning, when the CS–UCS pairing was novel, and then decreased over time as the contingency was learnt by the organism. These studies used a fixed reinforcement scheme and were therefore not in a position to reveal the mechanism for the pairing of CS and UCS beyond the initial learning.

These initial studies were the motivation to investigate how different brain systems support the adaptation to variable contingencies in a classical conditioning task. In this task two neutral pictures were chosen as the conditioned stimuli (a face and house) and an aversive heat pain stimulus was used as the UCS (Glascher & Buchel, 2005). Faces and houses were used because they have clear and easily dissociable cortical representations in the occipito-temporal cortex (Kanwisher *et al.*, 1997; Epstein & Kanwisher, 1998). Initially, both the face and the house were reinforced with a UCS in 50% of all presentations. After some time, the reinforcement contingency for the face was increased to 100% and with a slight delay the reinforcement contingency for the house was also increased to 100%. In the following trials, these contingencies were slowly changed following a noisy sine and cosine. (Figure 5.1).

The initial hypothesis for this experiment comprised the notion that according to current reinforcement, the activation in cortical and subcortical areas will vary. The obvious question following this initial hypothesis is 'how precisely does the activity change'.

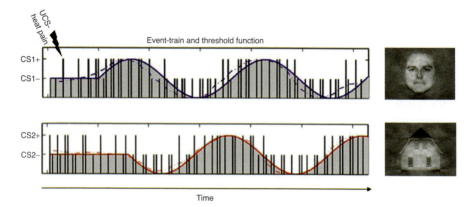

Figure 5.1 Variable contingencies in an aversive classical conditioning paradigm. Each 'stick' denotes the presentation of a CS, either a face (top) or house (bottom). Long sticks denote reinforced trials, i.e. are followed by the UCS (heat pain). After an initial period of 50% partial reinforcement, reinforcement is increased to 100% (top) or decreased to 0% (bottom) and then continues to vary according to a sinusoidal pattern (blue and red curve). Both reinforcement schemes were phase shifted with ¼ cycle, to render them uncorrelated. The dashed line visualizes the fit of the event with the idealized contingency curve.

For example, the signal could change rather quickly reflecting the change in contingency immediately, yet it is also possible that cortical or subcortical areas integrate information over a longer time period and therefore adjust their activity rather slowly. In addition, different brain areas could exhibit different time-courses of activation.

Conceptually, these different time-courses could be associated with the learning rate, a parameter that is common to many reinforcement learning algorithms. One such algorithm or model is that of Rescorla and Wagner initially devised to explain classical conditioning (Rescorla & Wagner, 1972a). The Rescorla-Wagner (RW) model has proven useful in the past to describe simple trial-based reinforcement learning. In this model a prediction is generated and then compared to the outcome once it is available.

The RW model allows the estimation of constantly updated outcome predictions. According to the RW model, the predicted outcome V_t is estimated as follows:

$$V_t = p_{t-1} \times u_t \tag{1}$$
$$\delta_t = (R_t - V_t)$$
$$p_t = p_{t-1} + \varepsilon \delta_t \times u_t$$

where V_t indicates the predicted outcome of trial t; u_t indicates the conditioned stimulus (CS) type at trial t and can be either 1 or 0 depending on the particular CS type presented at trial t; R_t indicates the actual outcome of trial t (shock or no shock); p_t indicates the change in prediction at trial t due to the prediction error δ_t at trial t ($R_t - V_t$); and ε indicates the learning parameter that controls the influence of the prediction error on the update of the prediction (Dayan & Abbott, 2001; Glascher & Buchel, 2005). If the prediction is correct, δ_t will be zero and no change will occur, if the actual outcome is smaller than the predicted outcome δ_t will be negative and the expectation will be reduced, otherwise δ_t will be positive and the expectation will be increased.

This outcome is compared against the initial prediction. If the prediction differs from the outcome the prediction for subsequent trials will be adjusted so that eventually the prediction matches the outcome. This adjustment of subsequent prediction is governed by the constant ε. If ε is zero the system does not update its predictions and therefore the system cannot learn. If ε is large, the current prediction error will heavily influence the prediction for the next trial, i.e. learning is instantaneous. By the recursive nature of the Rescorla Wagner model the constant epsilon can be seen as a rate constant that determines how fast the system can adapt and how strongly it considers past evidence (Figure 5.2).

In the case of variable contingencies ε is crucial to determine how flexible the system is i.e. how quickly it can adapt to new circumstances. This was the basis for the experimental hypothesis of the neuroimaging study. The research question was whether different brain structures are governed by different dynamics and therefore their signal could be best described by different values of ε. Considering the interpretation of ε as a variable that determines how strongly a system considers past evidence, we hypothesized that signal changes in classical learning related areas like the medial temporal lobe including the hippocampus and the amygdala would be best described by a low ε emphasizing their role in

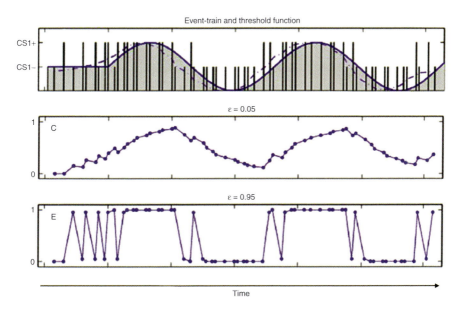

Figure 5.2 Different learning coefficients ε determine the prediction in a Rescorla-Wagner model in classical conditioning with variable contingencies. (Top) Each 'stick' denotes the presentation of a CS. Long sticks denote trials (CS+) that are followed by the UCS (heat pain). A low ε leads to slowly adapting predictions (middle), whereas a high ε leads to rapidly changing predictions (bottom). The difference can best be seen in the initial phase of 50% partial reinforcement. The predictions for a low ε slowly increase; the predictions based on a high ε wildly oscillate. The dashed line visualizes the fit of the event with the idealized contingency curve.

learning and memory. In contrast to learning and memory-related areas it was hypothe-sized that 'perceptual areas' like the fusiform face area or the parahippocampal place area would be best characterized by high values of ε allowing for instantaneous adaptation.

Figure 5.3 shows the result of this study. The fMRI time course in the fusiform face area was best explained by a regressor that was based on a RW model with a high epsilon. In contrast, fMRI signal in the right amygdala was best explained by a regressor based on a Rescorla Wagner model with a low epsilon.

In summary, this experiment is an example for how a cognitive theory like the Rescorla Wagner model can provide a framework for the analysis of fMRI data in a learning con-text. In addition to simple behavioural studies, in which a single learning rate ε can be estimated, the investigation of activation patterns in the whole brain using fMRI allowed us to further subdivide different brain areas by their ability to integrate information over different periods of time. This temporal distinction allowed to make inferences about whether a certain area is involved in 'storing' information as this is inversely linked to the learning parameter ε.

Applying the concepts of formal learning theory to guessing tasks

In the pervious section, the prediction error has briefly been introduced as a crucial signal for updating adaptive behaviour in the context of reinforcement learning. To recapitu-late, the prediction error represents the difference between the predicted and the actual outcome. In contrast to a learning task, in guessing tasks in which the outcome is probabilistic and the probabilities are graphically depicted (e.g. tossing a coin suggests 50% gain probability in a fair game) nothing can be learned that could improve subsequent performance. Therefore, a prediction error signal is not necessary for adapting

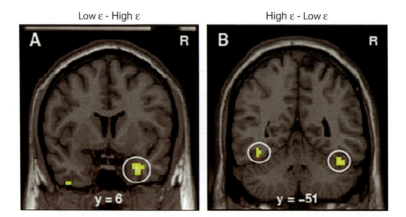

Figure 5.3 Coronal sections of T1 weighted MRIs highlighting activations related to different learning parameters ε. The predictions generated by a Rescorla-Wagner model with low ε best described activation in the amygdala and hippocampus (left). In contrast the activation in the fusiform face area was best predicted by a Rescorla-Wagner model using a high ε.

behaviour. Nevertheless, it is still possible that a prediction error signal is generated as suggested by previous studies (Knutson *et al.*, 2001).

If one starts from the Rescorla Wagner model (Rescorla & Wagner, 1972b) as described above (Eq. 1) some simplifications can be made to readily apply this framework to guessing paradigms. As there is nothing to be learnt, the recursive nature of the equation can be dropped. Therefore, the equation can be reduced to predictions and prediction errors without a dynamic updating component.

$$V = p \qquad\qquad (2)$$
$$\delta = (R - V)$$

where V indicates the predicted outcome; p indicates the prediction for that trial type; R indicates the actual outcome; note that V is kept constant and is not influenced by the prediction error   which is simply the difference between outcome R and the prediction V.

The crucial question is: 'which signal constitutes the prediction and how is it generated'. In guessing games with monetary rewards, the amount and probability of the possible reward could form the ingredients of this prediction. However, before coming back to this question an experiment is described that was used to investigate this research question.

In this study healthy volunteers performed repeated guesses to obtain monetary rewards. They were exposed to a visual stimulus showing the back side of eight playing cards. A certain amount of money (1€ coin or a 5€ note) could be placed on either a single card or on the corners of four cards (Figure 5.4, top left). Letting volunteers gamble for a single or 5€ allowed the manipulation of expected reward magnitude. Letting volunteers place their bets on a single or four cards allowed the manipulation of reward probability. After volunteers have placed their bets, an anticipation phase of four seconds followed. After this four second period all eight cards were flipped and the position of the red ace was visible. If this card touched the bet, the volunteer had gained the amount of money if not he had lost the money. In experimental terms this can be seen as a 2 x 2 x 2 factorial design with the factors reward magnitude (1 or 5€) reward probability (low or high) and outcome (gain or loss). Although the graphically depicted probability was 1/8 for one card and 1/2 for four cards, the actual probabilities used in the experiment were set to 26% and 66%. As the major goal of this study was to identify a possible 'prediction signal', emphasis was put on the anticipation phase. In a first step it was examined whether reward magnitude and reward probability are represented through neural activity changes in the human brain during reward anticipation. As shown by previous primate studies (Fiorillo *et al.*, 2003; Tobler *et al.*, 2005), dopaminergic midbrain neurons projecting to the ventral striatum were a possible candidate structure for the representation of predictions. These nonhuman primate studies by the group of W. Schultz have shown that during the anticipation of rewards dopaminergic midbrain neurons projecting to the ventral striatum express probability and magnitude of possible rewards by their firing rate.

Testing for main effect of reward magnitude in the described guessing paradigm revealed higher BOLD signals for 5€ trials compared to 1€ trials in the ventral striatum. In addition a similar region also showed increased bold signal for more likely rewards

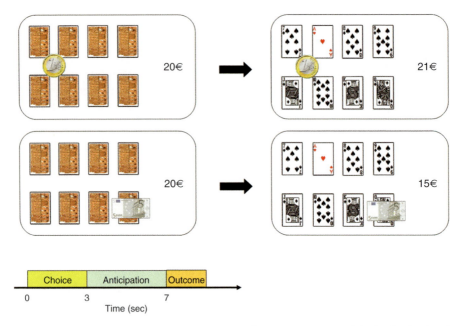

Figure 5.4 Task layout. Each guessing trial began with the presentation of the backside of eight playing cards. Initially, volunteers had to place money on individual playing cards. In some trials, money could be placed on the corners of four adjacent cards (top left), in others on a single card only (bottom left). This manipulation allowed us to control reward probability. 4.2 seconds after placing the bet, the cards were flipped (right). Seven of eight cards were black, the remaining one was a red ace. If the red ace was selected (top right), the volunteer gained the amount of money, and otherwise lost the money (bottom right).

(i.e. a main effect of probability) (Figure 5.5). This finding is in agreement with non-human primate data showing a modulation of firing rate of dopaminergic midbrain neurons related to expected reward magnitude (Tobler *et al.*, 2005) and probability (Fiorillo *et al.*, 2003). After establishing a representation of the ventral striatum for reward magnitude and probability the next step would be to establish a combined measure that could represent a value prediction.

Consider you are offered a choice of two simple games: You could either gamble for 10€ with a gain probability of 60% or alternatively you could gamble for 100€ with a gain probability of 50%. Considering these two options, most volunteers would chose option two, namely gamble for 100€ with a gain probability of 50%. But why? Early microeconomic theory going back to Blaise Pascal was interested in how people make decisions. Pascal and Pierre de Fermat had the idea that the product of expected reward magnitude and probability (the so-called expected value; EV) determines choice behaviour. Applied to the two gambling alternatives clearly shows that the preferred gamble of 100€ at 50% has the higher EV (50) as compared to the alternative (EV 6). Expected value could therefore be the code for a prediction in the simplified framework presented in equation 2. For completeness, it should be noted that although EV can explain choice behaviour in many circumstances, it fails to do so in many cases for instance when

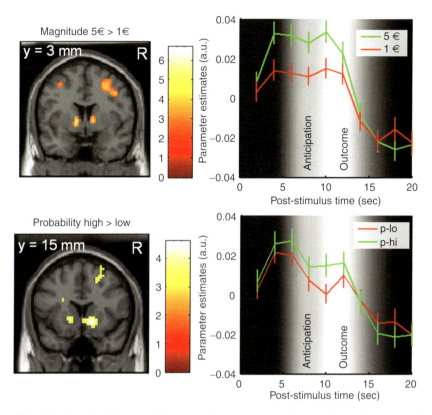

Figure 5.5 Activation during the anticipation of monetary rewards at P<0.001 (uncorrected) and voxel time-courses. The gray plateau from about 6–10 s is related to the BOLD response elicited by reward anticipation. (top) Main effect of magnitude showing stronger BOLD signal changes for trials with € 5.00 as opposed to € 1.00 in bilateral ventral striatum. (bottom) Main effect of probability showing stronger BOLD signal changes for trials with high reward probability in bilateral ventral striatum.

probabilities are either very low or high. Therefore, the field of behavioural economics has developed more elaborate models to universally account for human choice behaviour under risk and under uncertainty (Kahneman & Tversky, 1979).

To follow the lead that EV is the prediction signal, expected value was estimated for all four possible trial types. For example, gain related expected value of 5€ high probability trials was estimated as

$$EV_{gain} = 0.66 \cdot 5 \tag{3}$$

And the loss related part as

$$EV_{loss} = 0.34 \cdot -5 \tag{4}$$

Leading to a total EV of

$$EV_{total} = EV_{gain} + EV_{loss} = 0.66 \cdot 5 + 0.34 \cdot -5 = 1.60 \tag{5}$$

In contrast, low probability 5€ trials result in a negative expected value, because the likelihood of loss was higher than that of gain:

$$EV_{total} = EV_{gain} + EV_{loss} = 0.26 \cdot 5 + 0.74 \cdot -5 = -2.4 \tag{6}$$

Expected values for 1€ trials show a similar pattern (Figure 5.6A).

Based on the observed main effect of magnitude and probability, the ventral striatum was also considered a candidate region for the representation of EV. Although the signal time-courses in the ventral striatum (Figure 5.6B) were very similar to the prediction in Figure 5.6A, a major difference was observed. As predicted by EV, 5€ high probability trials lead to the greatest signal change. In addition, signal changes during anticipation for 1€ trials were significantly lower. So far, this pattern was in accordance with the notion of this area coding expected value. However, inspecting the bold response to 5€ low probability trials revealed a signal amplitude between 1€ trials and 5€ high probability trials. However, according to expected value, the signal for this trial type should be lowest. To confirm this finding, an additional independent sample comprising 24 volunteers was investigated, confirming the initial pattern. Revisiting the composition of EV offered a crucial hint. What if the ventral striatum sometimes also labelled as part of the 'reward system' of the brain, simply does not consider loss as an

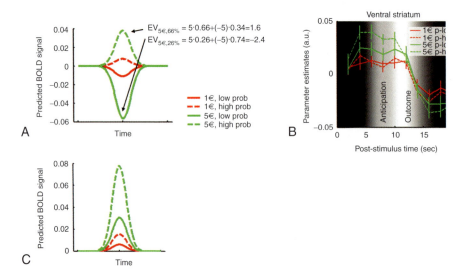

Figure 5.6 Expected values and signal changes in the ventral striatum. The actual values (A, C) are convolved with a Gaussian for a better visual comparison with BOLD responses. Total expected value (EV) is shown in (A). (B) fMRI signal change in the ventral striatum plotted separately for all four different trial types. During anticipation, the pattern is similar to the spredictions from the EV model (a). However, BOLD signal changes for 5 €, low probability trials are in between 1 € trials and the 5 €, high probability trials. This is in contradistinction to the model of EV (A). Comparing the ventral striatal time-course (B) with gain-related EV (C) i.e. without considering losses, the neuronal signal matches the model predictions.

option, i.e. is maximally optimistic? To investigate this, only the gain related part of expected value was considered (Eq. 3). With this modification the theoretical predictions of EV matched the observed signal in the ventral striatum (Figure 5.6C). Thus our data supports the notion that not total expected value (EV), but only gain related EV(EV+) is represented in the ventral striatum and reflects a possible 'prediction' against which outcomes are then compared. In agreement with this observation, a recent primate study (Bayer & Glimcher, 2005) and a with Parkinson's disease (PD) patients (Frank *et al.*, 2004) have suggested the possibility that gain-related predictions and the associated prediction errors might be expressed in the ventral striatum. In the primate study, dopamine spike rates in the postreward interval seemed to only encode positive reward prediction errors and dopamine was therefore attributed to the positive reward prediction error term of reinforcement learning models (Bayer & Glimcher, 2005). In PD patients, who have a dopaminergic deficit in the midbrain, better learning for the avoidance of choices that lead to negative outcomes as compared to learning from positive outcomes was observed. This bias was reversed by dopamine agonists (Bayer & Glimcher, 2005). Importantly, this example shows that an initial model that was used to predict the data was substantially modified by the data itself. In this particular instance, this was possible by a high signal-to-noise-ratio and the possibility to validate the data using an independent sample.

Conclusions

This chapter has shown two possibilities of how empirical data from functional neuroimaging can interact with cognitive models. In the first example, a cognitive model was helpful to interpret learning data using a learning parameter of the Rescorla-Wagner model. In addition to behavioural data in which only a single parameter could be applied, this approach allowed to identify cortical and subcortical structures showing different learning rates. In contrast, the second example showed that fMRI data that was not in agreement with an existing model was useful in modifying the model. However, this was only possible, because the data was unambiguous and an additional sample for cross validation was available. In other cases, in which only a single sample is available, this approach is more difficult, because if the data does not fit the assumed model, this could either mean that the sensitivity of the measurement technique is insufficient or indeed, the model is not correct.

   Although the models employed in this chapter did not enter the experimental framework in a formal Bayesian sense, the interpretation of the results, not only in these experiments but most experiments using explicit models, is performed in a similar way. In analogy to a formal Bayesian approach, the model can be considered the prior probability (in the mind of the experimenter), whereas the data enters the likelihood. Importantly, Bayesian inference is performed by the experimenter who takes his initial beliefs (priors) into account when interpreting the data. In this case, the prior is determined by the beliefs of the experimenter, i.e. a narrow prior for a firm and well-established model, and a flat prior for a more speculative model.

References

Bayer, H. M. & Glimcher, P. W. (2005). Midbrain Dopamine Neurons Encode a Quantitative Reward Prediction Error Signal. *Neuron, 47,* 129–141.

Büchel, C. (1998). Functional neuroimaging studies of Braille reading: cross-modal reorganization and its implications. *Brain, 121,* 1193–1194.

Büchel, C., Price, C., & Friston, K. (1998a). A multimodal language region in the ventral visual pathway. *Nature, 394,* 274–277.

Büchel, C., Morris, J., Dolan, R. J., & Friston, K. J. (1998b). Brain systems mediating aversive conditioning: an event-related fMRI study. *Neuron, 20,* 947–957.

Cohen, L. G., Celnik, P., Pascual-Leone, A., Corwell, B., Falz, L., Dambrosia, J., Honda, M., Sadato, N., Gerloff, C., Catala, M. D., & Hallett, M. (1997). Functional relevance of cross-modal plasticity in blind humans. *Nature, 389,* 180–183.

Dayan, P. & Abbott, L. F. (2001). *Theoretical Neuroscience.* Cambridge, MA: MIT Press.

Epstein, R. & Kanwisher, N. (1998). Acortical representation of the local visual environment. *Nature, 392,* 598–601.

Fiorillo, C. D., Tobler, P. N., & Schultz, W. (2003). Discrete coding of reward probability and uncertainty by dopamine neurons. *Science, 299,* 1898–1902.

Frank, M. J., Seeberger, L. C., & O'Reilly, R. C. (2004). By carrot or by stick: cognitive reinforcement learning in parkinsonism. *Science, 306,* 1940–1943.

Glascher, J. & Buchel, C. (2005). Formal learning theory dissociates brain regions with different temporal integration. *Neuron, 47,* 295–306.

Kahneman, D. & Tversky, A. (1979). Prospect theory: an analysis of decision under risk. *Econometrica, 4,* 263–291.

Kanwisher, N., McDermott, J., & Chun, M. M. (1997). The fusiform face area: A module in human extrastriate cortex specialized for face perception. *Journal of Neuroscience, 17,* 4302–4311.

Knutson, B., Adams, C. M., Fong, G. W., & Hommer, D. (2001). Anticipation of increasing monetary reward selectively recruits nucleus accumbens. *Journal of Neuroscience, 21,* RC159.

LaBar, K. S., Gatenby, J. C., Gore, J. C., LeDoux, J. E., & Phelps, E. A. (1998). Human amygdala activation during conditioned fear acquisition and extinction: a mixed-trial fMRI study. *Neuron, 20,* 937–945.

Quirk, G. J., Armony, J. L., & LeDoux, J. E. (1997). Fear conditioning enhances different temporal components of tone-evoked spike trains in auditory cortex and lateral amygdala. *Neuron, 19,* 613–624.

Rescorla, R. A. & Wagner, A. R. (1972a). A theory of Pavlovian conditioning: variations in the effectiveness of reinforcement and non reinforcement. In: A. H. Black & W. F. Prakasy (Eds), *Classical Conditioning II,* pp. 64–99. New York: Appleton-Century-Croft.

Rescorla, R. A. & Wagner, A. R. (1972b). A theory of Pavlovian conditioning: variations in the effectiveness of reinforcement and non-reinforcement. In: A. H. Black & W. F. Prakasy (Eds), *Classical conditioning II,* pp. 64–99. New York: Appleton-Century-Croft.

Röder, B., Rösler, F., & Hennighausen, E. (1997). Different cortical activation patterns in blind and sighted humans during encoding and transformation of haptic images. *Psychophysiology, 34,* 292–307.

Sadato, N., Pascual-Leone, A., Grafman, J., Ibanez, V., Deiber, M.-P., Dold, G., & Hallett, M. (1996). Activation of the primary visual cortex by Braille reading in blind subjects. *Nature, 380,* 526–528.

Tobler, P. N., Fiorillo, C. D., & Schultz, W. (2005). Adaptive coding of reward value by dopamine neurons. *Science, 307,* 1642–1645.

Chapter 6

Neuroimaging and interactive memory systems

Dara G. Ghahremani and Russell A. Poldrack

Introduction

The view of separate brain systems supporting different memory functions has gained wide support in the last few decades. The primary focus of researchers has been on dissociable memory functions supported by the medial temporal lobe (MTL) structures, including the hippocampus, from systems supported by other cortical and subcortical structures, such as the basal ganglia. While the MTL is thought to comprise the declarative memory system, supporting acquisition of flexibly accessible knowledge, the basal ganglia comprise procedural or non-declarative memory systems that underlie habit learning, a gradual acquisition of behavioural tendencies (Knowlton, Mangels, & Squire, 1996; Packard, Hirsh, & White, 1989). The focus on these two systems has arisen in large part due to dissociations in memory performance observed in neuropsychological and non-human animal studies. In general, patients with damage to the MTL or related structures (e.g. amnesics, Korsakoff's syndrome) tend to have poor declarative memory while those with damage to the basal ganglia (e.g. Parkinson's Disease, Huntington's Disease) have trouble with non-declarative learning. Such dissociations have pointed to the existence of biologically and psychologically distinct memory systems. More recently, neuroimaging techniques have allowed researchers to examine the relationship between these memory systems in humans. The availability of simultaneous recordings of the human brain offered by neuroimaging techniques has also informed neurocomputational theories of memory systems. The goal of this chapter is to review the neuropsychological and non-human animal findings and discuss ways in which neuroimaging research has advanced our understanding of memory systems in the human brain. In particular, we illustrate how neuroimaging has gone beyond confirming previous work outlining the important structures involved multiple memory systems to refining our understanding of how and when they are invoked.

Human neuropsychological evidence for multiple memory systems

Neuropsychological studies have offered important directions in identifying key brain structures involved in memory systems. While patients with focal damage to a particular brain region show deficits in performing certain memory tasks but not others, an inference can be made about the type of memory supported by structures within the damaged region. Perhaps the clearest example of this is that of patient HM who had his medial temporal lobes (MTL) surgically removed (Cohen & Squire, 1980; Scoville & Milner, 1957). As with most amnesics, the operation resulted in HM showing remarkable impairment in his ability to consciously remember material he had been exposed to after his operation (anterograde amnesia). However, he was not impaired on all types of memory tasks. In particular, he showed a dissociation in performance on tasks that assess two different types of memory – one that encompasses conscious recollection (*declarative memory*) or episodic memory (memory for spatio-temporally specific contexts) and another that does not require conscious memory access and is observed by experience-induced changes in performance (*non-declarative* or *procedural memory*). While HM had great difficulty with explicit memory tasks that assess declarative memory (e.g. recalling words from a previously studied list or recognizing pictures from a prior exposure), he showed normal performance on implicit memory tasks that assess non-declarative or procedural memory (e.g. completing word stems with words from a previously viewed list or more rapidly performing a task, such as picture categorization, on previously viewed items than for new items). Thus, studies on HM and many subsequent studies on amnesics have led to a major discovery in cognitive neuroscience – that structures within the medial temporal lobe crucially support declarative memory.

Neuropsychological studies of patients with basal ganglia disorders, such as Parkinson's Disease (PD), have highlighted the basal ganglia as encompassing another major memory system. While amnesic patients often show performance that is equivalent to controls on non-declarative tasks, PD patients who have compromised functioning of the striatum typically show worse performance on several of these tasks relative to healthy control participants (e.g. Knowlton *et al.*, 1996). Some of the most definitive studies come from observations of PD patients while performing the probabilistic classification learning task (PCT), a task introduced by Knowlton, Squire, and Gluck (1994). In this task, based on previous work by Gluck and Bower (1988), participants must learn to classify visual stimuli into one of two categories based on trial-by-trial feedback. This feedback is probabilistic, such that participants cannot rely on simply remembering the outcome from the previous encounter with each stimulus (i.e. cannot rely on episodic memory retrieval); rather, they must integrate information over many trials to form a representation of the optimal stimulus-response associations. In a common version of this task, known as the 'weather prediction' task, the participant is instructed to predict the weather based on a set of geometric features presented on four individual cards, which are presented in all possible combinations (Figure 6.1). Knowlton *et al.* (1996) demonstrated a double dissociation between classification learning and declarative memory: amnesic patients show normal PCT-learning but impaired declarative memory, while PD patients show the opposite pattern. The deficit for PCT learning in PD patients has been replicated by Shohamy *et al.* (2004), and a parallel deficit in Huntington's Disease patients was observed by Knowlton *et al.* (1996). Thus, it appears that different forms of damage to the basal ganglia lead to a similar deficit in PCT learning.

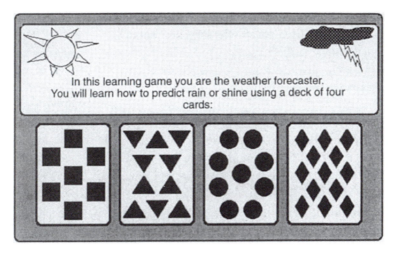

Figure 6.1 Cues presented to participants in the weather prediction task, a probabilistic classification learnig task used by Knowlton *et al.* (1996). One to four cards appeared on the screen during each trial. The participants were required to predict sun shine or rain based on these cues.

Support from non-human animal studies for interactive multiple memory systems

Non-human animal studies (e.g. rodent studies) have used lesion techniques, pharmacological manipulations, and neuronal recording techniques to examine the interactivity of multiple memory systems. One of the most striking results comes from inter-cerebral drug infusion studies in rodents that involve temporarily inactivating specific brain regions using local anesthetics (e.g. lidocaine) (e.g. Packard & McGaugh, 1996). These studies suggest that multiple memory systems are invoked at different time scales during learning. In these experiments, rats must travel down the arms of a 'plus-maze' in search of food. During a training phase, they start from the 'south' arm of the maze and learn to find the food located in the 'west' arm. During probe trials the rats are placed at the opposite starting point ('north' arm). A left turn (the correct response when starting from the south arm during training trials) is interpreted as an expression of 'response' memory while a right turn suggests expression of 'place' memory. When a probe trial appears early in training, the rat expresses place memory, but when probed after many trials of training, it expresses response memory. This behavioral difference at different times during learning is linked with dissociations between the MTL and basal ganglia strctures. Early learning is supported by MTL structures while later learning is supported by basal ganglia structures. Inactivation of the hippocampus just prior to the initial probe trial impairs expression of place learning, whereas inactivation of the caudate prior to the second probe not only impairs expression of response learning but, interestingly, elicits expression of place learning. Packard (1999) showed that infusion of glutamate into these structures (thus non-selectively activating them) resulted in a similar trade-off between memory systems. These studies suggest that while multiple memory systems may encode similar information, they may be differentially engaged during the expression of memory depending on the stage of training.

Non-human animal studies have also alluded to how memory systems may compete or interfere with each other. Evidence for competitive interference between systems comes from studies showing *enhanced* performance in rats with lesions in the hippocampus or caudate-putaman. In the 'win-stay' radial maze task in which rats must visit various spatial locations twice within a session, the hippocampal spatial memory system may interfere with the rat revisiting a location where it had already found and consumed the food. Hippocampal lesioned rats are not impeded by their prior spatial experience and are better able to learn this task (McDonald & White, 1993; Packard *et al.*, 1989). Conversely, lesions of the caudate-putamen facilitate performance on a spatial discrimination task ('Y-maze' task) in which performance may be impeded by interference from response learning strategies. Taken together, these findings point to possible ways in which memory systems may interfere, and possibly compete, with one another to serve task goals.

Human neuroimaging studies of memory systems

Non-human animal studies of memory systems have provided a basis on which to think more deeply about human memory systems in terms of their interaction, but fundamental differences between species (such as language, a significant mediator of mnemonic processes) limit the inferences that can be made about human memory based on these studies. While human patient studies have been informative in determining major components of memory systems, they are limited in several ways. For one, lesions are rarely restricted to distinct brain structures and often involve gross damage to several areas. In addition, given what we know about the redundancy (and competitive interference) between memory systems in animal studies, human lesion studies offer little insight into how intact memory systems interact to give rise to memory performance. In this regard, neuroimaging techniques, such as Positron Emission Tomography (PET) or functional MRI (fMRI), provide an advantage in allowing researchers to measure activity in multiple brain areas simultaneously while experiment participants perform various memory tasks.

Neuroimaging studies of healthy populations

Human fMRI studies have shed light on the dynamics of interaction between memory systems in the normal, healthy brain. In an early blocked-design fMRI study of the PCT, a comparison of PCT and baseline task (a task equating the perceptual-motor demands of the PCT) blocks showed deactivation of MTL over the course of learning, suggesting less reliance on MTL across time (Poldrack, Prabhakaran, Seger, & Gabrieli, 1999). In a follow-up event-related fMRI study, Poldrack *et al.* (2001) showed the relationship between MTL and basal ganglia structures during the course of learning. Specifically, an inverse relationship was found between the two structures with MTL showing greater activation than the caudate nucleus early in learning while the reverse was found later in learning. Moreover, an inverse correlation was found between these two brain structures across individuals suggesting individual differences in the way participants perform the task (presumably, either relying more on their declarative or non-declarative memory systems).

The study also found differential reliance either on the MTL or caudate depending on whether the task emphasized use of declarative or non-declarative memory (i.e. via paired-associate learning or feedback-based learning, respectively).

In an fMRI study that aimed to dissociate contributions of separate memory systems to learning, Foerde, Knowlton, and Poldrack (2006) showed that PCT learning is supported by different brain systems depending on the task demands. During learning, participants performed the PCT either with full attention (single-task) or while distracted with a secondary task (dual-task). After training participants were given a probe memory test in which they responded without receiving feedback. While performance during acquisition and the probe test did not differ between the single- and dual-task conditions, a striking dissociation was found when correlating probe performance with brain activation. Probe performance on items learned during the single-task condition was correlated with hippocampal activity whereas striatal activity correlated with performance on items learned during dual-task conditions. Moreover, in a separate test of their declarative knowledge, participants showed better performance on single-task items than dual-task items, suggesting greater reliance on their declarative memory system during single-task learning conditions, affording increased ability to flexibly apply knowledge gained during these conditions.

Importantly, this study shows that equivalent learning performance can be supported by different memory systems depending on task demands, and confirms the notion that knowledge flexibility depends on the type of memory system invoked during acquisition. It also suggests that competition between memory systems may be more observable during the expresion of knowledge gained during learning than during the acquisition period. Moreover, it highlights the unique role of neuroimaging techniques in revealing the involvement of these different systems during learning.

Neuroimaging studies of patient populations

Neuroimaging studies have also revealed the extent to which patients with lesions rely on uninjured brain systems as a means of compensating for their injuries. In an fMRI study of early stage PD patients performing the PCT, patients showed greater MTL activation than controls despite exhibiting equivalent performance (Moody, Bookheimer, Vanek, & Knowlton, 2004) suggesting that they invoked MTL-dependent strategies to perform this typically striatum-dependent task. Similarly, Voermans et al. (2004) examined learning of a virtual maze in patients with Huntington's disease and normal controls. Whereas control subjects engaged the caudate nucleus during learning, the patients exhibited less activity in the caudate and increased activity in the hippocampus. Both of these findings suggest that the hippocampal memory system may compensate for deficits in striatal learning mechanisms.

Neuroimaging studies of motor and skill learning

Neuroimaging studies of motor and perceptual skill learning have also found a negative relationship between MTL and basal ganglia (Jenkins et al., 1994; Poldrack & Gabrieli, 2001) similar to that found in the PCT studies mentioned above. These studies found greater activity in the striatum (putamen and caudate, respectively) accompanied by decreased activity in the MTL during learning. Another PET imaging study comparing performance on a planning task (the Tower of London) in PD patients and controls showed differential activation in the caudate and hippocampus despite equal behavioural performance between the two groups (Dagher, Owen, Boecker, & Brooks, 2001). Not surprisingly, PD patients showed weaker activation in caudate regions than controls; however, they also showed greater hippocampal activation relative to controls, suggesting invocation of MTL-dependent strategies to perform the task. Further evidence of an inverse relationship between the two memory systems comes from a neuroimaging study of rule-learning that found decreases in hippocampal activation along with increased activation in the caudate head as learning progressed (Seger & Cincotta, 2006).

Neuroimaging studies and models of learning

Neuroimaging and patient studies of the PCT both show that the presence of feedback may modulate the involvement of different memory systems in learning. Poldrack *et al.* (2001) showed that feedback-based PCT learning elicits greater striatal activation than non-feedback-based learning (observational learning). Moreover MTL signal increased when feedback was not present during learning. This fMRI study inspired a follow-up study on PD patients. Shohamy *et al.* (2004) showed that, while PD patients' performance on the PCT without feedback was equivalent to controls, they were severely impaired at learning the same information through feedback-based learning.

Neuroimaging studies have further implicated the basal ganglia in processing of feedback. Aron *et al.* (2004) performed an event-related fMRI study of a PCT in which stimulus, delay, and feedback events were modeled and examined separately. An examination of the feedback events revealed robust activation in the striatum and midbrain (putatively the dopaminergic substantia nigra and ventral tegmental area). Another fMRI study of the PCT by Ghahremani and Poldrack (2007) that used a modified version of the weather prediction task aimed to determine the influence of feedback type on the ventral striatum (VS), a major target of midbrain dopamine neurons, by providing either informational feedback alone (the category of 'rain' or 'sunshine') or feedback in the form of monetary reward reinforcers (e.g. gain of $1 for correct performance, loss of $.50 for incorrect performance) (Figure 6.2). This study found greater activation for positive versus negative feedback in the VS for both types of feedback (Figure 6.3). Moreover, the VS showed a larger response for monetary rewards than positive information-only feedback, consistent with many studies showing sensitivity of the VS to primary (e.g. food) and secondary (e.g. money) rewards (see O'Doherty, 2004; Schultz, 2000 for reviews). These neuroimaging results confirm an important role for the striatum and the dopaminergic system in the processing of feedback for non-declarative memory.

The midbrain dopamine system has been interpreted in non-human animal neurophysiology studies as providing an important error signal for learning, known as 'prediction error' (Schultz, 2002). A prediction error signal is the mismatch between expected and actual reward outcomes. Several neuroimaging studies have shown correlations

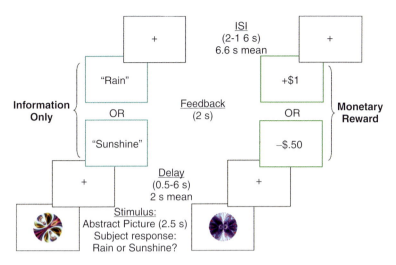

Figure 6.2 Schematic event sequence during a single trial of the simplified version of the weather prediction task used by Ghahremani and Poldrack (2007) in which either money or outcome information alone was presented as feedback. ISI – inter-stimulus interval.

between ventral striatum activity and computed prediction error signals in the context of classical (McClure, Berns, & Montague, 2003; O'Doherty *et al.*, 2003) and instrumental (O'Doherty, 2004; Tanaka *et al.*, 2004) conditioning, involving primary or conditioned rewards. Participants in the standard PCT only receive feedback in the form of information without such types of rewards. Rodriguez *et al.* (2006) aimed to determine whether striatal regions associated with feedback in the fMRI PCT study of Aron *et al.* (2004) showed prediction error signals similar to studies in which primary or conditioned rewards were offered. Using a Rescorla-Wagner model of reinforcement learning (Rescorla & Wagner, 1972), they showed strong correlations between ventral striatum/ nucleus accumbens activation and prediction error signals. These results suggest that the circuitry involved in reward learning may be more generally involved in a mechanism that supports the non-declarative basal ganglia-based memory system.

Neuroimaging evidence for memory system interaction

Although the notion of interactions between memory systems has been discussed by many non-human animal and neuroimaging studies, few studies provide evidence for a mechanism that mediates this interaction. Given that there is weak evidence for direct anatomical connections from striatum to MTL (*cf.*, Poldrack & Packard, 2003), it is likely that other brain regions play a role in mediating activity between the two regions. To determine potential causal relationships between the MTL, striatum, and other brain regions, including areas within the prefrontal cortex (PFC), Poldrack and Rodriguez (2003) performed an effective connectivity analysis on the fMRI data of the PCT of Poldrack *et al.* (2001) using path analysis. Path analysis uses the covariance between regions to test models of causal influence between those regions (Bollen, 1989).

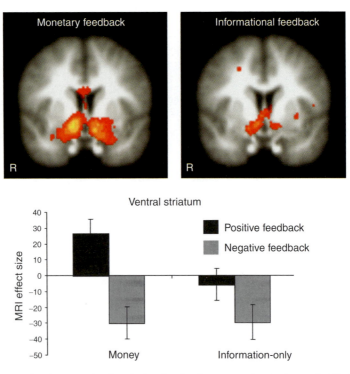

Figure 6.3 Ventral striatum activation during feedback presentation in the probabilistic classification learning fMRI study of Ghahremani and Poldrack (2007). The top panel shows statistical maps for the contrasts of positive versus negative feedback presented in the form of money (left) and outcome information-alone (right) (coronal slices at y=6, MNI coordinates; thresholded at Z<2.3, cluster-corrected at p<0.05). The bottom panel shows the MRI effect size of ventral striatum activation during the two forms of feedback presented.

Depending on how well the model fits the data, one can claim that the path coefficients are indices of causal influence between variables (Bollen, 1989; Pearl, 2000). Results from this analysis indicated that the anterior cingulate acts as a mediating region between the MTL and the striatum. Poldrack and Rodriguez (2004) postulated that this PFC mediation may be facilitated by neuromodulatory systems, emphasizing the dopaminergic system in particular. The results of Voermans *et al.* (2004) are also consistent with the role of the PFC in modulating the interaction between striatum and hippocampus. They employed an effective connectivity analysis known as a psychophysiological interaction analysis (Friston *et al.*, 1997) which examines how connectivity between regions is modulated by experimental conditions. Voermans *et al.* (2004) found that both the hippocampus and regions in the superior frontal and anterior cingulate cortex showed increased interaction with the caudate in patients with compromised basal ganglia function versus controls. These results are also consistent with other work suggesting that the anterior cingulate may be generally involved in exerting control by affecting the engagement of other brain regions (Kerns *et al.*, 2004).

Conclusion

Neuroimaging techniques have further advanced our understanding of multiple memory systems in the human brain by affording examination of activity in multiple brain regions recorded simultaneously over time. This ability has allowed memory researchers to pursue questions about memory systems and their interaction that could not be directly addressed with experiments on brain damaged patients, such as amnesics and PD patients. Not only has neuroimaging confirmed the notion of distinct brain structures corresponding to different psychological categories of memory (i.e. declarative/non-declarative); it has also offered insights into the interaction of these regions. For instance, the inverse relationship between MTL and basal ganglia structures found in several studies sheds light on the dynamics between these two systems over the time course of learning, and several studies in controls and patients suggest that the balance of activity between the two systems can be shifted depending on the learning strategies used. Moreover, neuroimaging has allowed the ability to separately examine different components of learning trials (e.g. stimulus/response and feedback presentations). This has helped to differentiate components of the learning process that seem to be supported by separate memory systems (e.g. feedback processing subserved by the striatum and dopaminergic systems). In addition, connectivity analyses of fMRI data have suggested that memory system interactions may rely upon mediation by regions outside the MTL and basal ganglia. Such analyses can guide further neuroimaging and patient studies to more precisely determine how other brain regions, such as those within prefrontal cortex, serve to modulate memory system interaction. Furthermore, as a complement to neuroimaging techniques, more sophisticated behavioural paradigms that manipulate shifts in learning strategies could offer a sharper picture of when and how memory systems interact.

Over all, the introduction of advanced neuroimaging techniques in the fields of psychology and neuroscience has expanded progress in human memory systems research, approaching questions which were not previously addressable. We expect the great potential of this method to continue inspiring new achievements in our understanding of how memory systems function and interact.

Acknowledgements

This work was supported by grants from the Whitehall Foundation and National Science Foundation (BCS-0223843) to RP.

References

Aron, A. R., Shohamy, D., Clark, J., Myers, C., Gluck, M. A., & Poldrack, R. A. (2004). Human midbrain sensitivity to cognitive feedback and uncertainty during classification learning. *Journal of Neurophysiology*, 92(2), 1144–1152.

Bollen, K. A. (1989). *Structural Equations with Latent Variables*. New York: Wiley.

Cohen, N. J. & Squire, L. R. (1980). Preserved learning and retention of pattern-analyzing skill in amnesia: dissociation of knowing how and knowing that. *Science*, 210(4466), 207–210.

Dagher, A., Owen, A. M., Boecker, H., & Brooks, D. J. (2001). The role of the striatum and hippocampus in planning: a PET activation study in Parkinson's disease. *Brain*, *124*(Pt 5), 1020–1032.

Foerde, K., Knowlton, B. J., & Poldrack, R. A. (2006). Modulation of competing memory systems by distraction. *Proceedings of the National Academy of Sciences of the United States of America*, *103*(31), 11778–11783.

Friston, K. J., Buechel, C., Fink, G. R., Morris, J., Rolls, E., & Dolan, R. J. (1997). Psychophysiological and modulatory interactions in neuroimaging. *Neuroimage*, *6*(3), 218–229.

Ghahremani, D. G. & Poldrack, R. A. (2007). Comparing high- and low-incentive rewards as feedback in probabilistic classification learning: an fMRI study. *Society for Neuroscience Abstracts, 773.8.*

Gluck, M. A. & Bower, G. H. (1988). Evaluating an adaptive network model of human learning. *Journal of Memory and Language*, *27*, 166–195.

Gluck, M. A. & Bower, G. H. (1988). From conditioning to category learning: an adaptive network model. *Journal of Experimental Psychology. General*, *117*(3), 227–247.

Jenkins, I. H., Brooks, D. J., Nixon, P. D., Frackowiak, R. S., & Passingham, R. E. (1994). Motor sequence learning: a study with positron emission tomography. *Journal of Neuroscience*, *14*(6), 3775–3790.

Kerns, J. G., Cohen, J. D., MacDonald, A. W., 3rd, Cho, R. Y., Stenger, V. A., & Carter, C. S. (2004). Anterior cingulate conflict monitoring and adjustments in control. *Science*, *303*(5660), 1023–1026.

Knowlton, B. J., Mangels, J. A., & Squire, L. R. (1996). A neostriatal habit learning system in humans. *Science*, *273*(5280), 1399–1402.

Knowlton, B. J., Squire, L. R., & Gluck, M. A. (1994). Probabilistic classification learning in amnesia. *Learning & Memory*, *1*(2), 106–120.

Knowlton, B. J., Squire, L. R., Paulsen, J. S., Swerdlow, N. R., Swenson, M., & Butters, N. (1996). Dissociations within nondeclarative memory in Huntington's disease. *Neuropsychology*, *10*, 538–548.

McClure, S. M., Berns, G. S., & Montague, P. R. (2003). Temporal prediction errors in a passive learning task activate human striatum. *Neuron*, *38*(2), 339–346.

McDonald, R. J. & White, N. M. (1993). A triple dissociation of memory systems: hippocampus, amygdala, and dorsal striatum. *Behavioral Neuroscience*, *107*(1), 3–22.

Moody, T. D., Bookheimer, S. Y., Vanek, Z., & Knowlton, B. J. (2004). An implicit learning task activates medial temporal lobe in patients with Parkinson's disease. *Behavioral Neuroscience*, *118*(2), 438–442.

O'Doherty, J. P. (2004). Reward representations and reward-related learning in the human brain: insights from neuroimaging. *Current Opinion in Neurobiology*, *14*(6), 769–776.

O'Doherty, J. P., Dayan, P., Friston, K., Critchley, H., & Dolan, R. J. (2003). Temporal difference models and reward-related learning in the human brain. *Neuron*, *38*(2), 329–337.

Packard, M. G. (1999). Glutamate infused posttraining into the hippocampus or caudate-putamen differentially strengthens place and response learning. *Proceedings of the National Academy of Sciences of the United States of America*, *96*(22), 12881–12886.

Packard, M. G., Hirsh, R., & White, N. M. (1989). Differential effects of fornix and caudate nucleus lesions on two radial maze tasks: evidence for multiple memory systems. *Journal of Neuroscience*, *9*(5), 1465–1472.

Packard, M. G. & McGaugh, J. L. (1996). Inactivation of hippocampus or caudate nucleus with lidocaine differentially affects expression of place and response learning. *Neurobiology of Learning and Memory*, *65*(1), 65–72.

Pearl, J. (2000). *Causality: Models, Reasoning, and Inference*. Cambridge, UK and New York: Cambridge University Press.

Poldrack, R. A., Clark, J., Pare-Blagoev, E. J., Shohamy, D., Creso Moyano, J., Myers, C., *et al.* (2001). Interactive memory systems in the human brain. *Nature, 414*(6863), 546–550.

Poldrack, R. A. & Gabrieli, J. D. (2001). Characterizing the neural mechanisms of skill learning and repetition priming: evidence from mirror reading. *Brain, 124*(Pt 1), 67–82.

Poldrack, R. A. & Packard, M. G. (2003). Competition among multiple memory systems: converging evidence from animal and human brain studies. *Neuropsychologia, 41*(3), 245–251.

Poldrack, R. A., Prabhakaran, V., Seger, C. A., & Gabrieli, J. D. (1999). Striatal activation during acquisition of a cognitive skill. *Neuropsychology, 13*(4), 564–574.

Poldrack, R. A. & Rodriguez, P. (2004). How do memory systems interact? Evidence from human classification learning. *Neurobiology of Learning and Memory, 82*(3), 324–332.

Rescorla, R. A. & Wagner, A. R. (1972). A theory of Pavlovian conditioning: variations in the effectiveness of reinforcement and nonreinforcement. In A. H. Black & W. F. Prokasy (Eds), *Classical Conditioning II: Current Research and Theory* (pp. 64–99). New York: Appleton Century Crofts.

Rodriguez, P. F., Aron, A. R., & Poldrack, R. A. (2006). Ventral-striatal/nucleus-accumbens sensitivity to prediction errors during classification learning. *Human Brain Mapping, 27*(4), 306–313.

Schultz, W. (2000). Multiple reward signals in the brain. *Nature Reviews. Neuroscience, 1*(3), 199–207.

Schultz, W. (2002). Getting formal with dopamine and reward. *Neuron, 36*(2), 241–263.

Scoville, W. B. & Milner, B. (1957). Loss of recent memory after bilateral hippocampal lesions. *Journal of Nneurology, Neurosurgery, and Psychiatry, 20*(1), 11–21.

Seger, C. A. & Cincotta, C. M. (2006). Dynamics of frontal, striatal, and hippocampal systems during rule learning. *Cerebral Cortex, 16*(11), 1546–1555.

Shohamy, D., Myers, C. E., Grossman, S., Sage, J., Gluck, M. A., & Poldrack, R. A. (2004). Cortico-striatal contributions to feedback-based learning: converging data from neuroimaging and neuropsychology. *Brain, 127*(Pt 4), 851–859.

Tanaka, S. C., Doya, K., Okada, G., Ueda, K., Okamoto, Y., & Yamawaki, S. (2004). Prediction of immediate and future rewards differentially recruits cortico-basal ganglia loops. *Nature Neuroscience, 7*(8), 887–893.

Voermans, N. C., Petersson, K. M., Daudey, L., Weber, B., Van Spaendonck, K. P., Kremer, H. P., *et al.* (2004). Interaction between the human hippocampus and the caudate nucleus during route recognition. *Neuron, 43*(3), 427–435.

Chapter 7

Contributions of functional neuroimaging to theories of category learning

Paul J. Reber

Introduction

A question occasionally levied of researchers in functional imaging is 'what have your methods shown that we did not already know based on another experimental technique?' This is a fair question as a good number of early functional neuroimaging studies had an initial goal of validating the technique and thus often confirmed hypotheses about functional neuroanatomy (e.g. that the medial temporal lobe is critical for memory formation). Functional neuroimaging and in particular, functional magnetic resonance imaging (fMRI), has grown in popularity and use significantly over the past decade. As experimental design and data analysis techniques have become more sophisticated, two types of answers to the basic 'what have we learned?' question have been presented. One is to provide a better connection to neuroscience for cognitive processes. For example, experimental cognitive psychology shows the existence of the phenomenon of visual object priming and fMRI with similar paradigms finds that it is closely connected with changes in evoked activity in extrastriate visual cortex. In this way, neuroimaging has added anatomical localization to the phenomenon as part of the data for a theory of priming to incorporate. A second type of answer comes from attempts to use the data that can be obtained with fMRI to disambiguate between competing cognitive theories. Our ongoing research has been using fMRI to provide evidence in support of a specific theory of the cognitive representations that support visual category learning. In this approach, localization of changes in neural activity is not the end-goal of the fMRI study, but a data-point aimed at deciding between theories of categorization that may be difficult or impossible to separate purely by behavioural measures.

Category learning

Judging the category membership of a novel object is a fundamental cognitive component operation that contributes to object perception, semantic memory retrieval, reasoning, and problem solving. There are a number of methods by which category membership can be determined. When confronted with a novel, small, furry, four-legged animal, and attempting to determine whether it is a cat or a dog, one can explicitly search for characteristic features (cat's whiskers, wagging tail) and apply a category rule to the features to decide membership. Another possibility is to compare the novel animal to cats and dogs previously seen and identify which group is most similar. A third approach conjectures the idea of maintaining the representation of a prototypical cat and dog reflecting the most common features of the category and using these for comparison. A fourth possibility is that no explicit retrieval of rules, prior examples or a prototype occurs but that object-related processing within the visual system determines the object's category as part of visual identification.

A distinction between this last method of categorization and the preceding three is the lack of reference to information about explicit memory for previously seen examples of a category. Acquisition of conscious, declarative memory for facts, events, and rules depends materially on the medial temporal lobe (MTL). However, several studies have suggested that there appear to be additional, nondeclarative memory systems that support category learning for some tasks (e.g. Knowlton & Squire, 1993). These studies indicate that brain regions outside the MTL, areas that participant in memory without awareness, may play an important role in some sorts of category learning. These dissociations do not tell us what types of learning or representation are going on in nondeclarative category memory.

While memory systems theory proposes different neural substrates for different types of categorization, a significant challenge in developing theories of categorization is a general problem of indeterminacy between cognitive models. We can experimentally control the stimuli used to drive category learning, the stimuli used to assess category knowledge and measure the responses made by participants. However, it is possible that this may not be enough to disambiguate between competing models of category learning and knowledge.

As an example, Figure 7.1 gives two common types of category learning hypotheses, a prototype model and an exemplar model, applied to learning a category of dot patterns (as in Posner & Keele, 1969). The leftmost column shows the experimentally controlled elements: the study patterns, test pattern, and labels the processing stages. Both example theories are based on an initial encoding/learning process during which the study stimuli are used to develop an internal representation. For the Prototype model, the internal representation captures the 'gist' or underlying commonality of the category. Exemplar models represent knowledge by storage of the previously seen exemplars. When test stimuli are encountered, the Prototype model conjectures that they are compared to the abstracted prototype and if the match is sufficiently similar, the stimulus is endorsed as a category member. In the Exemplar model, test stimuli are compared to all the stored examples and an average similarity is calculated. If this average similarity meets the response criterion, it is endorsed as a category member. But which of these hypotheses correctly describes human cognitive processes? Determining this is complicated by a serious disambiguation problem for some versions of these hypotheses. In particular, if the encoding process for the Prototype theory is based on a linear combination of stimulus features to create the gist representation and the test process for the Exemplar theory is

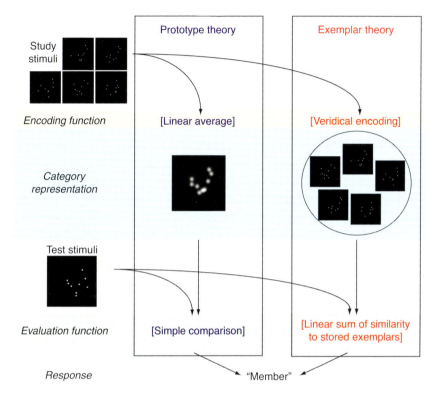

Figure 7.1 Schematic of two theories of category learning. The Prototype theory is based on creating a prototype representation from studied items that reflects the central tendency, linearly calculated from the positions of the stimulus elements (dots). The Exemplar theory stores veridical traces of the seen exemplars. At Test, the Prototype theory compares the test item to the learned prototype to judge membership while the Exemplar theory compares the test item to all stored exemplars via a linear similarity metric. Because linear operations are commutative (the order of operations does not matter) both theories are guaranteed to make identical predictions about the category membership response. These theories are difficult or impossible to decide between without additional information about the internal representational state that exists after learning'.

based on linear weighting of similarity across features to decide membership (as in Figure 7.1), then the theories are fundamentally indistinguishable based solely on categorization response behaviour. Since linear operations are commutative (i.e. it does not matter what order they are effected), predictions from this Prototype theory will be identical to an Exemplar theory that uses a comparison process that matches the information processing in the encoding process of the Prototype theory (and vice versa).

Distinguishing between these hypotheses requires making additional assumptions, such as inferring that the encoding process should be more cognitively demanding than the retrieval process for the Prototype theory and the reverse should be try for the Exemplar theory. However, this type of information processing assumption depends on an accurate model of the cognitive demands these processes require in the brain and the validity of these assumptions may be unclear. For example, the calculation of a gist representation appears complex (in Prototype theories), but may be accomplished very efficiently by an attractor-based neural network. The rapid comparison of a test stimulus to a large number of stored exemplars (in Exemplar theories) would likewise appear to be computationally intensive, but may be a fast process when implemented in a parallel distributed system via pattern completion.

Another approach to resolving the theoretical positions is based on attempting to incorporate a wider range of data beyond basic categorization responses. The representation hypothesized by the Exemplar theory contains veridical memory traces of the prior stimuli. These traces could therefore be used not just in categorization judgements, but also to support recognition memory judgements about prior experience with specific test stimuli. Similarity effects in recognition memory have been used to suggest that cognitive processing with recognition memory representations appears to share functionality with categorization processing. Evidence that a common set of representations is used to support both categorization and recognition judgements is therefore evidence for Exemplar theory.

Neuropsychology

The theory that a single common set of representations supports both recognition and categorization judgements appears to be inconsistent with findings of dissociations between recognition memory and category learning (Knowlton & Squire, 1993; Knowlton, Squire, & Gluck, 1994; Knowlton, Ramus, & Squire, 1992). Knowlton & Squire (1993) provided the first clear demonstration of this dissociation was with the dot-pattern classification task (Posner & Keele, 1969) used as an example in Figure 7.1. Patients who had neurological damage to the MTL and severely impaired declarative memory exhibited category learning at the same rate as age-matched healthy controls in an experimental incidental learning situation. All participants were shown 40 dot patterns drawn from a category defined by a central prototype without any instruction to learn the category. After a short delay of 5 minutes, enough to remove the availability of the stimuli from working memory and require dependence on long-term memory, participants were instructed that they would be given a categorization task with novel stimuli. For each new dot pattern, they were asked to indicate whether they thought it was a member of the same category seen prior to the delay. Both amnesic patients and matched controls performed reliably better than chance and at similar levels. In contrast, when a similar procedure was used to lead up to a recognition test, the amnesic patients were significantly impaired at recognizing dot patterns seen before the delay. Knowlton & Squire (1993) interpreted this result as indicating that the acquisition of representations supporting future categorization judgements was spared in the amnesic patients while acquisition of representations supporting future recognition judgements was impaired (due to the patients' MTL damage). This result suggested that the two types of representations are separately stored in the brain.

Single dissociations with neuropsychological patients are not always thoroughly convincing. An important concept was described by Shanks & St. John (1994) termed the 'sensitivity criterion'. The concern they raised was that some implicit learning tasks might happen to be differentially sensitive to low levels of knowledge (or degraded knowledge) than explicit memory tasks such as recognition memory. If the cognitive processing required by an implicit learning task happened to function such that a little knowledge goes a long way towards performance, it could theoretically be possible to observe an apparent dissociation even if a common set of representations were involved. Nosofsky & Zaki (1998) presented a computational account of categorization and recognition with dot patterns that shows how exactly this could happen for the dot-pattern categorization task.

In their model, a common set of representations is acquired by both patients and healthy controls. The patients' representations are degraded due to their memory disorder such that they are less precise. Loss of precision has differing effects on categorization and recognition. Because categorization is entirely based on similarity of the test item being evaluated to the category representations, loss of precision in representation does not significantly affect performance. However, since a recognition judgement requires a precise assessment of whether a specific item has been seen before (i.e. similarity effects make the task harder, not easier), the patients' performance would be significantly impaired compared to controls.

This model, like other sensitivity-based theories, predicts that whenever above chance performance is observed by memory-impaired patients on an implicit task, there should be some trace of explicit memory for the material (although the patients are impaired). Squire & Knowlton (1995) examined the performance of the severely amnesic patient E.P. on the dot-pattern category learning task and found that he exhibited normal category learning with no evidence at all of any explicit (recognition) memory for the stimuli. This finding provides the strongest possible form of a single dissociation between intact and impaired memory processes. However, even this result may not be entirely convincing. Palmeri & Flannery (1999) 'simulated' a disorder of memory by simply not presenting the training stimuli and found that healthy college students were able to perform better than chance on a dot-pattern categorization test, but not a recognition test (in theory, the participants were able to extract information about the category by comparison to other test times during the test itself). This result cast doubt on the strength of the above-chance performance of amnesic patients in this task. In addition, the complete absence of recognition memory for dot-patterns observed in Squire & Knowlton (1995) depends on a null result obtained in a single patient.

The theoretical debate over the representations acquired in the dot-pattern categorization task provides an illustrative example of the difficulty of resolving a question that depends fundamentally on the content of representations that cannot be directly observed. The basic neuropsychological dissociation of Knowlton & Squire (1993) suggests separate representations supporting category knowledge and recognition memory. However, those data do not directly disconfirm the alternate theory proposed by Nosofsky & Zaki (1998). The situation is analogous to the problem of discriminating between Prototype and Exemplar models: two very different theories of knowledge make predictions consistent with the available data. In the absence of a double dissociation, (which has not been observed between recognition and categorization), neuropsychological research may be unable to clearly discriminate between the two competing theoretical perspectives.

Functional neuroimaging

The advent of functional neuroimaging of cognitive processing has provided another method to examine the representations that support categorization processes in order to disambiguate between competing theories of category learning. The ability to assess the neural correlates of processes and representations with functional magnetic resonance imaging (fMRI) can provide evidence tying knowledge to specific neural systems. This additional data can constrain theoretical interpretation and resolve the intractable ambiguity faced by pure experimental and neuropsychological studies.

Data about brain function collected with fMRI is inherently correlational in nature. In isolation, functional neuroimaging data cannot identify the specific neural basis of a cognitive function, nor is the imaging resolution sufficient to uncover the specific neural representations. However, this additional source of data, in conjunction with existing experimental and neuropsychological data, allows for construction of a coherent theoretical account that brings converging evidence together from each technique. It is the convergence of neuroscience and information processing methods facilitated by fMRI that best demonstrates how theories of cognition are informed by functional neuroimaging.

A series of studies of the neural correlates of category learning in the dot pattern categorization task will be reviewed. Based on these findings, a specific hypothesis about the nature of implicit category learning within the visual system is presented. This hypothesis attempts to incorporate information about the memory systems and general organization of the brain to account for a broad range of data from different techniques.

Dot pattern categorization

The dot pattern categorization task introduced by Posner & Keele (1969) involves exposing participants to set of simple images of dot patterns, typically nine white dots on a black background, and observing incidental category learning. The category of dot patterns is defined by an underlying prototype pattern and all stimuli used in the experimental session for study and test are distortions of this underlying prototype created by jittering the dots into new positions (see Figure 7.2). In a version of the paradigm that has been used extensively in neuropsychological and neuroimaging studies, the patterns are shown to the participants one at a time with instructions to simply 'indicate the center dot in the pattern'. No mention of the category is made, so any learning is incidental. This is the task that Knowlton & Squire (1993; Squire & Knowlton, 1995) used in their finding that memory-disordered patients learned the underlying category at a normal rate, although they are significantly impaired at recognizing this kind of stimuli. A key claim of this hypothesis is that there are separate representations of the memories of dot-patterns that support recognition memory and categorization judgements. The alternate hypothesis,

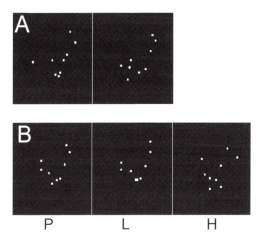

P   L   H

Figure 7.2 (A) Study items used during incidental learning of a dot pattern category. Study items are novel distortions created from an unseen prototype that defines the category. (B) Test items used to assess category knowledge. P is the underlying prototype that defines the category; L is a 'low distortion' category member which is very similar to the prototype; H is a 'high distortion' category member.

best embodied by the model of Nosofsky & Zaki (1998), was that there is a single store of memory that is degraded in memory-disordered patients and that these degraded representations can support category judgements but not recognition. The first functional neuroimaging study of this task, (Reber, Stark, & Squire, 1998a) aimed to identify neural correlates of the representation that supports dot pattern categorization.

The prior hypotheses about the neural correlates of category representations can be partly derived from neuropsychological studies. Damage to the MTL causes memory impairments for recognition and recall. Thus, the MTL would be a likely candidate for knowledge-associated activity under the single-system hypothesis. However, no strong prior hypothesis predicted where activity would be observed under the multiple memory systems hypothesis, only that it would be a brain region that operated independently from the MTL. A challenge to using neuroimaging to test the competing hypotheses is that the lack of observed activity differences in a brain region (e.g. the MTL) cannot be used to draw a strong inference that this region is uninvolved in the task being studied. fMRI depends critically on contrasts between tasks or conditions and the failure to find differential activity in the task of interest can be due to accidental activity in the control task or high levels of chronic baseline activity in the region.

To identify neural activity associated with the category representation, Reber, Stark, and Squire (1998a) examined activity evoked by dot-pattern stimuli after category learning. Participants learned the category in the traditional incidental manner of observation of stimuli derived from an unseen prototype. After learning, participants performed a categorization test in which the stimuli were arranged into blocks of mostly categorical patterns or mostly non-categorical patterns. Differences in activity during these two types of blocks should reflect differential involvement of the category representations, with greater contributions of category knowledge occurring during the blocks of mostly categorical patterns. The key finding (Figure 7.3A) was a reduction in activity in early visual cortex for stimuli in the learned category. The direction of change in activity was unanticipated, but similar to observations of reduced activity for previously seen stimuli in visual priming tasks (Schacter & Buckner, 1998). This effect appears to reflect fluent processing for stimuli within the learned category (e.g. less effortful and activity evoking) and is dubbed the Categorical Fluency Effect (CFE).This finding supports the multiple systems model of category learning and suggests that incidental category learning in this case is supported by non-declarative memory operating within visual cortex. However, this initial result was not definitive for several reasons. First, the non-categorical stimuli were randomly generated patterns, leaving open the possibility demonstrated by Palmeri and Flannery (1999) that participants were differentially processing the categorical stimuli during the test (e.g. the within-item similarity of the categorical patterns was producing the CFE). Second, the lack of observed activity within the MTL cannot be used to rule out the possibility that declarative memory for the dot patterns was affecting performance.

A second study (Reber, Stark, & Squire, 1998b) addressed these concerns by replicating the CFE using non-categorical stimuli that were drawn from an unseen category (but having the same within-category similarity during the test) and also introducing a similar recognition task for cross-group comparison. This study replicated the CFE (Figure 7.3B) during the categorization test and additionally observed a very different pattern of activity for old and new items during recognition. During recognition, no evidence of reduced activity in visual cortex for previously seen dot patterns was observed, even when ROI-driven methods were used to investigate small changes (Figure 7.3C). The dissociation in neural activity between categorization and recognition is similar to the dissociations between priming and recognition memory seen in fMRI (Donaldson, Petersen, & Buckner, 2001).

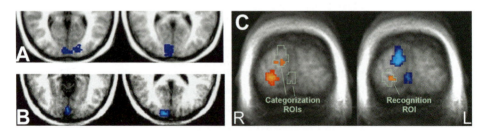

Figure 7.3 (A) fMRI results from Reber, Stark & Squire (1998a) showing the reduction in evoked posterior occipital activity that occurred after incidental learning of a category of dot patterns, the Categorical Fluency Effect. (B) Replication of this result in Reber, Stark, and Squire (1998b). (C) Comparison of posterior activity evoked during recognition and categorization of dot patterns. Regions of activity activated by the other task are shown outlined in green with a low-threshold analysis of evoked activity used to provide the best estimate of the direction of activity. For Recognition, red reflects greater activity for old than new stimuli. For categorization, blue reflects greater activity for category non-members than category members.

The second study strengthened the hypothesis that visual cortex is materially involved in representing knowledge of the dot pattern categories and that these representations do not participate in recognition memory. They raised a further question of why the CFE or some similar response does not occur during recognition if the category learning process is supposed to be incidental and automatic. If top-down processes can affect category-specific activity in the visual cortex, this raises the possibility that the differential task demands of making recognition and categorization judgements may be affecting the observed pattern of evoked neural activity. Neither of the first two studies attempted to characterize the whole network of brain regions that participate in these two types of judgements.

A third study (Reber, Buxton, & Wong, 2002) examined activity during both categorization and recognition judgements in contrast with a common control task (counting and judging odd/even number of dots). These contrasts identified a wider network of active brain regions involving prefrontal, parietal, and occipital cortical areas with different subregions active in the two tasks (Figure 7.4A,B). The more direct double-subtraction (areas where the recognition – counting difference was larger than the categorization – counting difference) identified greater activity for recognition in the medial temporal

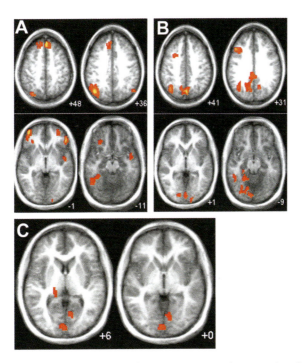

Figure 7.4 (A) Greater activity for category judgements compared to counting dots from Reber *et al*. (2002). (B) Greater activity for recognition judgements compared to counting dots. (C) Comparison of recognition and categorization activity by reference to the common control task. Red regions indicate greater activity for recognition judgements compared to categorization judgements.

lobe and posterior visual cortex (Figure 4C). These differences are consistent with Reber, Stark, and Squire (1998b) since the absence of a CFE during recognition would lead to generally higher activity in posterior visual cortex. In addition, this study provided the first evidence that the MTL was selectively involved in recognition of dot patterns. All three studies support the idea of differential involvement of occipital cortex in incidental category learning and declarative memory and the MTL supporting recognition memory. Cross-task comparisons between recognition and categorization cannot independently rule out the possibility of high-level task demands between these two tasks were affecting the pattern of evoked activity. A fourth study capitalized on the fact that the multiple category learning systems hypothesis does not require that all categorization depend only on the visual cortex. Healthy participants, who can use their long-term declarative memory to retrieve information about prior examples in order to consciously reason about category membership have multiple methods for accomplishing category learning.

In Reber *et al.* (2003), two groups of participants learned dot-pattern categories using different instructions. One group learned via the traditional incidental training, but a second group was told explicitly that the study items all came from the same category and they should attempt to learn it. The first group once again exhibited the CFE. The second group did not exhibit the CFE, showed greater activity for category members in several brain regions and using ROI analysis techniques were found to have elevated activity in the MTL for category members (Figure 7.5). A single system model of category learning cannot easily account for these results. If a common set of representations supports both recognition and categorization, certainly different categorization strategies should rely on common representations and produce generally similar neural correlates. Across this series of studies, functional neuroimaging of the hidden representations that support categorization judgements provided consistent support for the hypothesis that a separate system exists for category learning that does not depend on the MTL. The double dissociations observed in neuroimaging studies provide stronger evidence in support of multiple systems than the single dissociations observed in neuropsychology have.

In addition to reinforcing the hypothesis that multiple category learning systems function in the brain, the activity pattern reflected in the CFE also supports a specific hypothesis about how implicit dot-pattern category learning occurs. This type of learning appears to depend on changes within sensory, visual cortex such that after learning, future processing of category members is more efficient. This mechanism appears to reflect a rational type of plasticity for the visual system to maintain, the ability to re-wire to facilitate the processing of categories of previously seen objects. However, important questions can be raised as to the plausibility of this hypothesis since it depends on fairly rapid plasticity within adult sensory cortex. This type of plasticity would need to be maintained without interfering with established basic visual processing. In addition, a mechanism by which the fluency effect can contribute to categorization but not affect recognition will need to be identified. The fMRI results cannot rule out the possibility that the CFE reflects a correlate of the categorization process that depends on an area that has not yet been observed to exhibit differential activity. Because of its fundamentally correlational nature, fMRI will likely be most effective for generating new specific hypotheses about cognitive

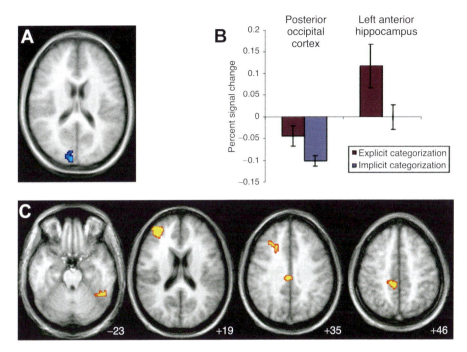

Figure 7.5 Comparison of evoked activity for incidental and explicit category learning of dot patterns from Reber *et al.* (2003). (A) Replication of the CFE. (B) ROI analysis showing greater activity in the MTL during explicit category judgements with less of a CFE effect occurring in visual cortex. (C) Regions of increased activity for category members following explicit category learning (compared with non-categorical patterns).

neuroscience processes. As demonstrated here, exploring these new hypotheses will often provide ideas about how to bridge systems and cellular neuroscience with cognitive processes and functions.

For the case of dot-pattern categorization, functional neuroimaging has advanced the basic theory by providing evidence in support of multiple category learning systems that could not be obtained through neuropsychological or experimental studies alone. In parallel with this series of studies, a separate line of research has been examining a different dissociation within category learning systems by contrasting the roles of the MTL and the basal ganglia (particularly, the caudate nucleus).

The role of the caudate in category learning

A second neuropsychological dissociation between category learning and explicit memory was reported by Knowlton, Squire, and Gluck (1994). In this task, which is known as the 'weather prediction' task based on the cover story, participants gradually learn a probabilistic classification scheme where four arbitrary cues (cards with geometric shapes) are used to predict a binary outcome (rainy or sunny weather). The task is learned via trial and error with feedback given after every outcome prediction. With practice, participants become able to make above-chance predictions although they may not be able to describe the relationships between the cues and outcomes. Knowlton, Squire, and Gluck (1994) found that amnesic patients exhibited normal initial learning of this task although they were impaired on explicit memory for elements of the task.

This initial single dissociation was followed up in a second study (Knowlton, Mangels, & Squire, 1996) that found the opposite dissociation in patients with Parkinson's disease. These patients exhibited impaired category learning although their explicit memory for the task elements was normal. This double dissociation strongly implies that separate brain regions support this kind of category learning and explicit memory. Further, the category learning appears to depend on the intact function of the basal ganglia, which is disordered in Parkinson's Disease (PD).

However, even this double dissociation is not completely convincing independent of other evidence due to details of task performance. The performance of amnesic patients was only similar to controls over the first 50 trials of training. Over the next 150 trials, healthy participants out-performed the amnesic patients. This result suggests that the intact MTL contributed to the healthy controls' performance after the initial 50-trial learning period. It is therefore somewhat curious that the patients with PD, who have intact MTL function would not exhibit more effective learning by relying on the MTL. Further complications emerged from a failure to replicate intact learning by amnesic patients (Hopkins *et al.*, 2004) and by a report of intact early category learning by PD patients who appeared to rely on the MTL (Moody *et al.*, 2004). An alternate hypothesis that the task requires an ongoing interaction between the MTL and basal ganglia cannot easily be ruled out.

A functional neuroimaging study of the probabilistic classification task provided additional evidence for two competing memory systems to be involved. Poldrack *et al.* (2001) used fMRI to observe the neural correlates of performing the probabilistic classification task and a control task that used similar stimuli that required explicit learning of associations. Increased activity in the basal ganglia (specifically the caudate) was associated with performing probabilistic classification as had been seen previously (Poldrack *et al.*, 1999). In contrast, increased activity in the MTL was associated with the explicitly learned paired-associate task. This study found that increased activity in one system was associated with a tendency for the other system to be de-activated below the resting baseline. This may reflect competition between the two systems, or may reflect a different mode of operation in the de-activated system (e.g. a sparse pattern of neural firing might produce less activity in fMRI even when that activity is still critical to task performance). Whether competition can be confidently concluded, the observed double dissociation reinforces the hypothesis that separate memory systems in the basal ganglia and MTL appear to support category representations and explicit memory for this task as well.

In parallel with research on the probabilistic classification task, a series of experiments examining category learning in tasks where the stimuli can be described in a simple two-dimensional space led to the development of the COVIS model (Ashby *et al.*, 1998). The Competition between Verbal and Implicit Systems model hypothesized that learning conscious, rule-based categories depends on the prefrontal cortex but that a separate system of implicit category learning relies on connections between posterior caudate

regions and extra-striate visual cortex. Like the hypotheses about dot-pattern and probabilistic classification, this model is based on the idea that separate representations exist
reflecting knowledge that can support category judgements for implicit and explicit tasks.
The two types of category learning hypothesized to depend on separate neural systems are
typically termed Rule-Based (RB) and Information-Integration (II) (Fig. 6A,B). RB categorization is hypothesized to depend on conscious knowledge and testing verbalizeable
rules. II categorization is hypothesized to depend on implicit feedback-driven integration
of information about the stimulus dimensions and the category label.Like probabilistic
classification, II learning is hypothesized to depend materially on the basal ganglia. RB
learning depends on several neural structures including prefrontal cortical regions supporting working memory, hypothesis testing, and response selection. In addition, RB
categorization depends on explicit memory representations supported by the MTL
(Ashby & Valentin, 2007). The proposed dissociation in the neural representation of the
information that contributes to these two kinds of categorization goes against single-
system models of recognition and categorization proposed in some exemplar theories.
The RB/II distinction proposes two different types of category representations, one that

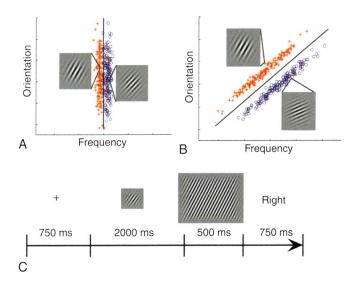

Figure 7.6 (A) Diagrammatic representation of an RB category structure. Stimuli are sine wave
gratings each represented in a 2-dimenstional space based on the frequency of light/dark
oscillations and the orientation of the pattern (from vertical to horizontal). The category shown
shows a red (left) category of lower-frequency stimuli separate from a blue (right) category of
higher-frequency stimuli. The rule that defines the two categories is therefore based solely on
frequency relative to the boundary. (B) Diagrammatic representation of an II category
structure. Distinguishing between the two categories requires integrating information about
both frequency and orientation. (C) Structure of the category learning procedure. Each trial
contains a stimulus presented for 2000ms during which time the participant makes a judgement
about the category membership. This is followed by a mask and feedback about the accuracy of
the category response.

depends on the MTL and one that does not. It differs from the model of categorization that emerged from the dot-pattern studies in that the implicit category learning process depends on the basal ganglia rather than changes within sensory cortex.

Evidence for the distinction between RB and II categorization comes from a series of experimental studies that have identified behavioural dissociations between the two types of category learning. In particular, two functional dissociations have been identified for RB and II category learning. Maddox et al. (2003) compared the effect of delaying feedback by 2.5s during category learning for RB and II categorization. This manipulation was found to selectively impair II categorization. The theoretical basis of this finding is that II categorization depends on close temporal association between the stimulus to be categorized, the label to be associated and feedback as to whether the label given was correct. In contrast, RB is hypothesized to depend partly on working memory (WM) and therefore information about stimuli, label, and response can be maintained over delays of several seconds in order to support learning.

While the involvement of WM in RB categorization allows this type of learning to be insensitive to feedback-delay, RB learning has been shown to be sensitive to secondary tasks that imposed a WM load concurrent with category learning (Waldron & Ashby, 2001; Maddox & Ashby, 2004; Zeithamova & Maddox, 2006). In each of these studies, the concurrent WM load affected RB categorization more than II categorization. The double dissociation created by the manipulations of delay and WM load strongly implies separate cognitive processes supporting RB and II category learning that have different operating characteristics.

The basis of the theory of separate RB and II category learning systems is grounded in ideas about the cognitive neuroscience of category learning. Testing these theories has proven challenging with neuropsychological studies of patient populations for several reasons. First, the RB system is hypothesized to depend on prefrontal cortex for WM maintenance, the MTL, and also the anterior basal ganglia to provide information about feedback supporting hypothesis testing. Thus patients with PD or other etiologies that produce dysfunction in the basal ganglia will not necessarily show dissociations between RB and II category learning (Ashby et al., 2003; Filoteo et al., 2005). Task complexity as represented by the number of relevant stimulus dimensions is important in these studies (Filoteo et al., 2005). In addition, a chronic challenge is that with these simple two-dimensional categorization tasks, whenever one system is damaged, the other system is capable of exhibiting at least partial learning of the task, making a strong double dissociation difficult to observe. Functional neuroimaging provides an excellent tool for doing exactly this and both reinforcing the dissociation between types of category learning and generating hypothesis about specific mechanisms of learning.

In Nomura et al. (2007), two groups of participants learned a simple two-dimensional categorization task structured to support either RB or II category learning. The categories to be learned were constructed to produce roughly similar levels of category learning over 320 trials of training (Figure 7.6). On each trial, a circular patch of a sine-wave grating was shown and participants tried to identify which of two categories it belonged to. After responding, the stimulus was masked and then feedback was given as to whether the response was correct. Participants performed this task over four 11-minute runs (80 trials per run) while whole-brain fMRI data were collected. The key contrast was between activity evoked on correct and incorrect responses in order to identify success-correlated neural activity.

Success-correlated activity was observed in a number of brain regions, notably including the MTL during RB category learning, and in the posterior caudate during II category learning. Using a technique of aligning targeted neuroanatomical structures (ROI-AL; Stark & Okada, 2003), a double dissociation was observed with significantly larger success-related differences in the MTL during RB than II and significantly larger success-related differences in the caudate during II than RB (Figure 7.7). The dissociation observed with fMRI reinforces the behavioural dissociation across studies (Maddox *et al.*, 2003; Waldron & Ashby, 2001) in support of the hypothesis that there are two distinct systems for learning RB and II categorizations. While recognition memory was not directly assessed, this result further argues against single-representation system models that hypothesize a common set of memories being the basis for all categorization and recognition processes. As evidence mounts for multiple knowledge stores from different paradigms, it appears that it will be more productive to pursue research into the operating characteristics and processing constraints of these different systems from a multiple

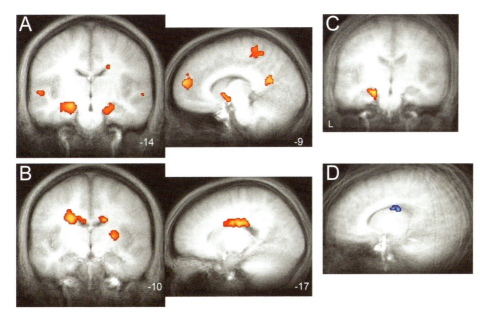

Figure 7.7 Success-correlated activity for (A) RB and (B) II categorization as found in Nomura *et al.* (2007). Red indicates greater activity for correct than incorrect responses. Notably, during RB categorization increased activity is observed bilaterally in the MTL for correct responses. In contrast, during II increased activity is observed in the posterior caudate during successful responses. A direct comparison of success-correlated activity obtained via ROI analysis is shown in (C) RB>II, and (D) II>RB. Red regions indicate a greater difference for successful than unsuccessful categorization during RB categorization. Blue indicates a greater difference during II categorization.

category learning systems approach. The localization of key contributions to the MTL and caudate also provides candidate hypotheses about the cognitive operation of the RB and II systems. The involvement of the MTL in successful RB suggests that explicit recollection plays a critical role. A likely candidate for this would be to memorize a reference stimulus at or near the boundary between the two candidates. Judging category membership would then require retrieving the boundary item and comparing a test stimulus to it along the key dimension. Performing this contrast (and maintaining knowledge of the relevant dimension) would likely depend heavily on WM and spatial attention processes.

Hypotheses about the operation of the II category learning system can be derived from information about the neurophysiological properties of the cortico-striatal loops that appear to be critically involved in successful II categorization. Three key properties of these circuits have been proposed to be relevant for category learning. First, the basal ganglia provides a dopamine-dependent reward signal that is necessary for feedback-driven learning (Wickens, 1990; Smiley et al., 1994). Second, there is a many-to-one convergence of projections from extrastriate cortex onto individual spiny neurons (Wilson, 1995). This would support information compression needed for a small number of spiny neurons in the caudate to influence a greater number of cortical neurons and this type of information compression would naturally tend to create categorical representations (because the smaller number of neurons would be insufficient to represent the individual details of a large number of representations). Third, the connections from cortex onto the spiny neurons is returned to the same region (Middleton & Strick, 2000) which would allow the learning supported by feedback to be reflected in the development of representations in the cortex with its greater representational capacity. These properties suggest that II category learning is likely to result in prototype-style representations where clusters of stimuli become captured by a central tendency (e.g. the Striatal Pattern Classifier model of Ashby & Waldron, 1999).

As with the example of studies of dot-pattern categorization, functional neuroimaging of RB and II category learning provided evidence aimed at a core theoretical debate about the nature of the underlying representations. Data obtained using fMRI supports models based on multiple category learning systems in each of the three tasks reviewed here. In each case, functional neuroimaging provides evidence of dissociable processes and/or representations between an implicit form of category learning and explicit memory processes that can support both recognition and conscious category learning.

Conclusions

Within the domain of human category learning, functional neuroimaging has been able to advance the core theory by establishing dissociations that were difficult or impossible to observe with other techniques. Multiple and single system theories primarily differ in the number and form of the cognitive and neural representations used and do not always clearly differ in specific predictions about behaviour. Techniques based solely on assessing behaviour to infer the underlying process depend on inferences about those unseen elements to support specific approaches. As in the first example presented here, comparing categorization based on prototypes and exemplars, observations based only on input and output may be incapable of distinguishing between competing theories. Additional assumptions are necessary and where these assumptions can be connected to neuroanatomical structures with known functions, functional neuroimaging can provide a method for disambiguating between competing frameworks.

A key idea for exemplar models of categorization is that the exemplars that support category judgements may also be part of the declarative memory system (i.e. they can also be consciously recognized). The neuropsychological dissociation reported by Knowlton and Squire (1993) suggested that category learning does not depend on declarative memory, but this single dissociation was shown to be unconvincing by the computational approach of Nosofsky & Zaki (1998). The modeling work did not rule out the multiple systems hypothesis, but showed that the neuropsychological dissociation did not necessarily rule out a single-system hypothesis. However, these competing hypotheses make quite different predictions about what should be observed with functional neuroimaging. The multiple systems hypothesis predicts that there should be dissociable activity patterns for implicit category learning and declarative memory (either recognition or explicit category learning) whereas the single-system hypothesis predicts common activity patterns likely involving the MTL. A series of fMRI experiments examining category-specific activity during dot-pattern categorization found that incidental category learning was dissociable from recognition memory (Reber *et al.*, 1998b, 2002) and explicit category learning (Reber *et al.*, 2003). The observed dissociation argues strongly in favour of a multiple systems theory of category learning.

Further evidence for multiple categorization systems comes from studies of probabilistic classification (e.g. Poldrack *et al.*, 2001) and comparisons of RB and II category learning (e.g. Nomura *et al.*, 2007). In these paradigms, evidence for a dissociation between types of learning was observed in patient groups (e.g. Knowlton *et al.*, 1996) or through different experimental manipulations (Maddox *et al.*, 2003). In both cases fMRI studies reinforced the dissociation between types of learning. Learning that required explicit memory or conscious discovery and use of rules was associated with activity in the MTL. Implicit category learning was associated with activity in the basal ganglia. As with the studies of dot-pattern categorization, the dissociation supports the theory of multiple memory systems supporting category learning.

The localization of neural correlates associated with implicit category learning also facilitates the development of specific theories of the operation of category learning outside of the MTL. The studies implicate different regions and therefore suggest different neurobiological mechanisms supporting different types of implicit category learning. Incidental learning of dot-pattern categories has been consistently associated with changes in activity in visual sensory cortex suggesting a rewiring of perceptual processing to facilitate identification of category members. Implicit learning of II categories and probabilistic classification has been associated with the basal ganglia. The neurophysiological properties of cortico-striatal loops may be important for understanding the operating characteristics of this form of category learning.

The hypotheses about the core underlying processes and learning mechanisms that emerge from these studies make behavioural predictions that can be tested in further experimental work. For example, based on the localization of activity changes in early visual cortex, we have begun to examine the retinotopic specificity of dot-pattern category learning (Kim et al., 2003). In addition the consistent observation of a reduction in evoked activity for the learned category led to an initial study of perceptual processing speed with these stimuli (Huang et al., 2005). The correlational nature of fMRI means that localization of changes should be seen only as a candidate hypothesis for identifying mechanisms, since the possibility of additional unobserved changes cannot be ruled out. The CFE in posterior visual cortex is certainly correlated with categorization, but whether it is causally related to making successful categorization judgements or a consequence of processes occurring elsewhere cannot be established definitively with neuroimaging. Hypotheses connected to the implicated neural systems can use properties like retinotopic organization (in visual cortex) or the need to have temporally contingent reward signals (in the posterior basal ganglia; Maddox et al., 2003) in experimental design.

The ability of functional neuroimaging to bridge from cognitive hypotheses to systems neuroscience to the neurobiological properties of cells within the system is an important strength of the method. Cognitive hypotheses about the processes between stimulus perception and response have had to conjecture what types of information processing occurs in the neural systems of the brain. Functional neuroimaging permits observation of correlates of those information processing elements. Experimental design aimed at observing a dissociation can disambiguate between competing hypotheses. Observations of activity patterns can generate novel hypotheses about specific processes and mechanisms. Both types of design have moved forward the theoretical development of the systems of category learning in the brain using cognitive designs, fMRI observations of system-level activity, and known neurophyiological properties to conjecture specific mechanisms.

Acknowledgements

Thanks to Larry Squire and Craig Stark for their collaborative effort on the dot pattern categorization work, Emi Nomura for her lead role in the RB and II categorization with Todd Maddox and Vince Filoteo, and to the NU Cognitive Brain Mapping Group, especially Todd Parrish, Darren Gitelman, and Marsel Mesulam. The research reviewed here was supported by NIH R01 MH58748 and an McDonnell Foundation award to support 'Interdisciplinary Collaborative Consortium on the Cognitive Neuroscience of Category Learning'.

References

Ashby, F. G., Alfonso-Reese, L. A., Turken, A. U., & Waldron, E. M. (1998). A neuropsychological theory of multiple systems in category learning. *Psychological Review, 105*, 442–481.

Ashby, F. G., Noble, S., Filoteo, J. V., Waldron, E. M., & Ell, S. W. (2003). Category learning deficits in Parkinson's disease. *Neuropsychology, 17*, 115–124.

Ashby, F. G. & Valentin, V. V. (2007). Computational cognitive neuroscience: Building and testing biologically plausible computational models of neuroscience, neuroimaging, and behavioral data. In Statistical and Process Models for Cognitive Neuroscine and Aging, Eds. M. J. Wegner, C. Shuster, Mahwah, NJ, US: Lawrence Erlbaum Associates. pp. 15–58.

Ashby, F. G. & Waldron, E. M. (1999). On the nature of implicit categorization. *Psychonomic Bulletin & Review, 6*, 363–378.

Donaldson, D. I., Petersen, S. E., & Buckner, R. L. (2001). Dissociating memory retrieval processes using fMRI: evidence that priming does not support recognition memory. *Neuron, 31*, 1047–1059.

Filoteo, J. V., Maddox, W. T., Salmon, D. P., & Song, D. D. (2005). Information-integration category learning in patients with striatal dysfunction. *Neuropsychology, 19*, 212–222.

Hopkins, R. O, Myers, C. E, Shohamy, D., Grossman, S., & Gluck, M. A. (2004). Impaired probabilistic category learning in hypoxic subjects with hippocampal damage. *Neuropsychologia, 42*, 524–535.

Huang, V. & Reber, P. J. (2005). Observing fluency in visual category learning behavior. *Soc for Neuroscience Abs.*, Vol 31.

Kim, G. -Y. & Reber, P. J. (2003). Retinotopic specificity in dot pattern categorization. Cognitive Neuroscience Society 10th Annual meeting. NewYork: Cognitive Neuroscience Society.

Knowlton, B. J., Mangels, J. A., & Squire, L. R. (1996). A neostriatal habit learning system in humans. *Science, 273*, 1399–1402.

Knowlton, B. J., Ramus, S. J., & Squire, L. R. (1992). Intact artificial grammar learning in amnesia: Dissociation of category-level knowledge and explicit memory for specific instances. *Psychological Science, 3*, 172–179.

Knowlton, B. J. & Squire, L. R. (1993). The learning of categories: parallel brain systems for item memory and category knowledge. *Science, 262*, 1747–1749.

Knowlton, B. J., Squire, L. R., & Gluck, M. A. (1994). Probabilistic classification learning in amnesia. *Learning & Memory, 1*, 106–120.

Maddox, W. T. & Ashby, F. G. (2004). Dissociating explicit and procedural-learning based systems of perceptual category learning. *Behavioral Processes, 66*, 309–332.

Maddox, W. T., Ashby, F. G., & Bohil, C. J. (2003). Delayed feedback effects on rule-based and information-integration category learning. *Journal of Experimental Psychology: Learning, Memory & Cognition, 29*, 650–662.

Middleton, F. A. & Strick, P. L. (2000). Basal ganglia and cerebellar loops: motor and cognitive circuits. *Brain Research: Brain Research Reviews, 31*, 236–250.

Moody, T. D. Bookhemier, S. Y. Vanek, Z., & Knowlton, B. J. (2004). An implicit learning task activates medial temporal lobe in patients with Parkinson's disease. *Behavioral Neuroscience, 118*, 438–442.

Nomura, E. M., Maddox, W. T., Filoteo, J. V., Ing, A. D., Gitelman, D. R., Parrish, T. B., Mesulam, M. M., & Reber, P. J. (2007). Neural correlates of rule-based and information-integration visual category learning. *Cerebral Cortex, 17*, 37–43.

Nosofsky R. & Zaki S. (1998). Dissociations between categorization and recognition in amnesic and normal individuals: An exemplar-based interpretation. *Psychological Science, 9*, 247–255.

Palmeri, T. J. & Flanery, M. A. (1999). Learning about categories in the absence of training: Profound amnesia and the relationship between perceptual categorization and recognition memory. *Psychological Science, 10*, 526–530.

Poldrack, R. A., Prabhakaran, V., Seger, C. A., & Gabrieli, J. D. (1999). Striatal activation during acquisition of a cognitive skill. *Neuropsychology, 13*, 564–574.

Poldrack, R. A., Clark, J., Pare-Blagoev, E. J., Shohamy, D., Creso-Moyano, J., Myers, C. E., & Gluck, M. A. (2001). Interactive memory systems in the brain. *Nature, 414*, 546–550.

Posner, M. I. & Keele, S. W. (1968). On the genesis of abstract ideas. *Journal of Experimental Psychology, 77*, 353–363.

Reber, P. J, Gitelman, D. R., Parrish, T. B., & Mesulam, M.-M. (2003). Dissociating explicit and implicit category knowledge with fMRI. *Journal of Cognitive Neuroscience, 15,* 574–685.

Reber, P. J., Stark, C. E. L., & Squire, L. R. (1998a). Cortical areas supporting category learning identified using functional magnetic resonance imaging. *Proceedings of the National Academy of Sciences, USA, 95,* 747–750.

Reber, P. J., Stark, C. E. L., & Squire, L. R. (1998b). Contrasting cortical activity associated with declarative and nondeclarative memory. *Learning & Memory, 5,* 420–428.

Reber, P. J., Wong, E. C., & Buxton, R. B. (2002). Comparing the brain areas supporting nondeclarative categorization and recognition memory. *Cognitive Brain Research, 14,* 245–257.

Schacter, D. L. & Buckner, R. L. (1998). Priming and the brain. *Neuron, 20,* 185–195.

Shanks, D. R. & St. John, M. F. (1994). Characteristics of dissociable human learning systems. *Behavioral and Brain Sciences, 17,* 367–447.

Smiley, J. F., Levey, A. I., Ciliax, B. J., & Goldman-Rakic, P. S. (1994). D1 dopamine receptor immunoreactivity in human and monkey cerebral cortex: predominant and extrasynaptic localization in dendritic spines. *Proceedings of the National Academy of Sciences, USA, 91,* 5720–5724.

Squire, L. R. & Knowlton, B. J. (1995). Learning about categories in the absence of memory. *Proceedings of the National Academy of Sciences, USA, 92,* 12470–12474.

Stark, C. E. L. & Okada, Y. (2003). Making memories without trying: medial temporal lobe activity associated with incidental memory formation during recognition. *Journal of Neuroscience, 23,* 6748–6753.

Waldron, E. M. & Ashby, F. G. (2001). The effects of concurrent task interference on category learning: evidence for multiple category learning systems. *Psychonomic Bulletin & Review, 8,* 168–176.

Wickens, J. (1990). Striatal dopamine in motor activation and reward-mediated learning: steps towards a unifying model. *Journal of Neural Transmission, General Section, 80,* 9–31.

Wilson, C. (1995). *The Contribution of Cortical Neurons to the Firing Pattern of Striatal Spiny Neurons.* Cambridge, MA: Bradford

Zeithamova, D. & Maddox, W. T. (2006). Dual-task interference in perceptual category learning. *Memory & Cognition, 34,* 387–398.

Chapter 8

Declarative memory consolidation

Guillén Fernández and Indira Tendolkar

Introduction

Memory consolidation cannot be defined easily in a strict sense, because researchers from widely different fields in psychology and neuroscience are using this term very broadly for all operations taking place after initial memory formation that lead to long-term memory traces. There are certain dimensions along which memory consolidation can be refined more stringently. One dimension describes the level of observation. Thus, one can distinguish molecular and cellular aspects of consolidation summarized by the term 'synaptic consolidation' on one end of this dimension from system-level aspects of memory consolidation ('system consolidation') at the other end (for review Dudai, 2004). At the cellular level, consolidation is thought to enable long-term changes in synaptic efficacy and thus neural cell communication; a process requiring protein synthesis and leading to structural changes of neurons and their synapses (for review Kandel, 2001). Consolidation at the system level in contrast describes network changes by which large-scale representations of recent and remote memories differ. Here, we will focus on operations underlying the latter one, system level consolidation and their outcomes.

   Another dimension along which memory consolidation can be more readily specified is the kind of memory stabilized. Memory consolidation for declarative and non-declarative forms of memory seems to be based on fundamentally different neural operations, at least at the system level (Walker & Stickgold, 2005; Ellenbogen *et al.*, 2006). This book chapter focuses on declarative memory consolidation at the human brain system level and recent advances in characterizing the neural underpinnings of this fundamental mnemonic operation.

   The transition from labile to more stable forms of memory is called consolidation ('Konsolidierung') since the seminal work of Müller and Pilzecker (1900). They performed a large series of experiments based on one principal study-test design that was influenced by the work of Ebbinghaus (1885), but nevertheless truly innovative at that time. Subjects had to memorize lists of pairs of nonsense syllables at study and to recall one syllable of the pair when cued by the other one at test. They found reduced recall rates for a first study list when a second list was presented shortly after the first one, indicating that the memory of the first list was still in a labile state. In contrast, they did not find this memory impairing effect when they extended the interval between the two study lists and thus, they concluded that the memory traces of the first lists got already consolidated and were thus less vulnerable to disruption. However, Müller and Pilzecker observed this time-depended disruption of original learning only with very short intervals of a few minutes (e.g. six minutes). Thus, though their work introduced the term and principal idea of memory consolidation, they actually did not really provide the initial empirical basis for the consolidation theory but rather the interference theory, explaining retroactive inhibition. Nevertheless, the work by Müller and Pilzecker stimulated memory consolidation research in three directions, one investigating the nature and duration of retrograde amnesia in brain damaged patients, one testing the vulnerability of memories to electroconvulsive therapy, and another probing the effect of sleep on forgetting curves. We will try to give a short overview of these three lines of research below.

Initial empirical evidence

The idea that newly acquired memories are vulnerable was rapidly used to explain retrograde amnesia in patients. Burnham (1903) described two patients with retrograde amnesia induced by traumatic life events in one case and an epileptic seizure in the other case and explained this finding with the fact that memories acquired shortly before the incident were never completely organized. Although this and other early reports linked retrograde amnesia to a transition from labile to stabile memory traces, the close link between a specified organic brain lesion and retrograde amnesia was not introduced until the seminal work of Scoville and Milner (1957). Brenda Milner assessed carefully the amnesia of patient H.M. induced by the removal of the medial temporal lobe bilaterally for the treatment of drug resistant epilepsy (Scoville & Milner, 1957). This study provided the fundament for the present day view on system-level consolidation of declarative memories as a process by which a recent memory becomes gradually independent of the hippocampus, and cortical regions become increasingly engaged. Numerous following studies on patients with amnesia based on temporal lobe damage suggest that the temporal extend of the retrograde aspect of their amnesia is correlated with the anatomical extend of their damage. Patients with lesions limited to the hippocampus show a temporally limited retrograde amnesia of a few years while patients with more extended lesions of the medial temporal lobes have extended and ungraded amnesias covering several years or even decades (for a review on this topic: Squire et al., 2004). However, there is currently an ongoing debate (Moscovitch et al., 2005) whether certain types of declarative memories never get hippocampally independent and others get almost instantaneously independent of the hippocampus when new memories can easily be integrated in an already existing knowledge network or schema (Tse et al., 2007). The retrieval of vivid autobiographical memories might stay hippocampally dependent. On the other hand, memories might naturally become detached from their original temporo-spatial context with time and thus they might elicit less vivid recolective experiences as recent memories do. Regardless, of this reduction in vividness patients with retrograde amnesia have the preserved ability to access their remote past in a flexible way as shown by several case reports (e.g. Teng & Squire, 1999).

Investigating the temporal gradient of retrograde amnesia induced by electroconvulsive shocks as treatment of mental illnesses or in experimental settings with animals was important in estimating experimentally the time course of memory consolidation. The first studies were done in experimental animals (e.g. mice) by Duncan (1949) who revealed a temporally graded retrograde amnesia, but as in the behavioural studies by Müller and Pilzecker with a rather short gradient. Electroconvulsive shocks caused retrograde memory impairments only up to 15 minutes after learning. However, retrospective studies in humans estimated a much longer retrograde effect of electroconvulsive treatment on declarative memory. Depressed patients given a series of electroconvulsive shocks for relief of their disease exhibited a temporal gradient of retrograde amnesia. Memories acquired up to three years prior to the treatment were impaired, while more remote memories were not affected (Squire et al., 1975). This result provided initial experimental evidence for a rather long-lasting process of consolidation in humans, at least when assessed retrospectively.

The role of sleep in cognition has fascinated experimentalists and philosophers since the early days of science (Aristotle 350 B.C.E). In modern science, the non-linearity of the forgetting curve, as initially assessed experimentally by Ebbinghaus (1885), prompted Jenkins and Dallenbach (1924) to investigate the role of sleep on memory retention. They tested their subjects with the same nonsense syllables as Ebbinghaus did, but they manipulated in addition to the duration of the study-test interval the way the subjects spend this time. The subject who slept between the study phase and the retrieval test showed less forgetting with a forgetting curve that stayed almost stable after the initial dip. A finding that was interpreted as evidence for how sleep stabilizes recently acquired memory traces. However, this kind of correlational evidence cannot cleanly distinguish between an active process of memory stabilization from a passive effect of sleep by reducing retroactive interference during wakefulness. Only recently, a more causative relationship between sleep and memory consolidation has been confirmed. Actually, there appears a specific contribution of the deep sleep stages, so-called slow-wave sleep, to declarative memory formation (e.g. Plihal & Born, 1999; Tucker et al., 2006). These sleep stages are electrophysiologically characterized by slow EEG oscillations (< 1 Hz) and the induction of such slow oscillation-like field potential, in contrast to faster (5 Hz) ones by transcranial electrical stimulation during a period of emerging slow wave sleep, enhances the retention of declarative memories (Marshall et al., 2006). Thus, this elegant study provides initial evidence for an active role of slow oscillations of field potentials as they occur during slow wave sleep in declarative memory consolidation. In sum, there is ample evidence supporting the conclusion that slow wave sleep plays an active role in declarative memory consolidation.

Evidence from animal studies

The reports mentioned above and other studies probing declarative memory consolidation in healthy human subjects and brain-damaged patients are complemented by several lines of research using experimental animals. Lesion studies have been used to determine the time course of memory consolidation prospectively and to determine brain regions that are critically important for recent and remote memory retrieval. The identification of critical brain regions and their dissociation between recent and remote memory retrieval has also been explored by a series of studies assessing memory retrieval-related brain activity in rodents using mapping methods which measure either regional metabolism by way of (14C)2-deoxglucose uptake or expression of activity-regulated genes like c-fos. Finally, electrophysiologists have discovered potentially a direct correlate of active consolidation processes by revealing task-specific replay pattern during periods of rest or sleep that followed certain learning tasks.

Neuropsychological studies of brain damaged patients identifying a temporally graded retrograde amnesia have proven the time-limited role of the hippocampus and related structures in the medial temporal lobe in memory retrieval. However, these retrospective studies are limited in their explanatory power when estimating the time course of this hippocampal-neocortical transfer, because remote memories are usually retrieved and thus re-encoded often since their initial acquisition. Thus, Zola-Morgan and Squire studied retrograde amnesia prospectively in monkeys to make a proper estimation for the time-course of declarative memory consolidation at the brain system level (1990). The monkeys included in that study were trained to discriminate 100 pairs of objects beginning 16, 12, 8, 4, and 2 weeks before both hippocampi were removed (20 different pairs at each time period). Two weeks after surgery, memory was assessed by presenting each of the 100 object pairs again for a single-choice trial. Normal monkeys exhibited forgetting; that is, they remembered recently learned objects better than objects learned many weeks earlier. Monkeys whose hippocampi were removed were severely impaired at remembering recently learned objects (2 and 4 weeks), but they remembered objects learned 12 weeks ago as well as normal monkeys did and significantly better than they remembered objects learned more recently. These results show that the hippocampus is required for memory retrieval for only a limited period of time after learning. After about 8 to 12 weeks, its role in memory retrieval diminishes, and a more permanent memory gradually develops independently of the hippocampus, probably in neocortex.

Turning away from the lesion approach and towards an activation approach, also in experimental animals, confirmed the decline in hippocampal contributions to memory retrieval and identified a medial prefrontal region as involved in remote memory retrieval. Bontempi and colleagues (1999) showed with autoradiography using (14C)2-deoxyglucose uptake in rats that recall of spatial information acquired five days before testing (i.e. recent condition) was associated with a hippocampal activity increase in contrast to the retrieval of information acquired 25 days before testing (remote condition). Testing the opposite contrast (i.e. remote versus recent retrieval) revealed activity increases in the ventromedial prefrontal cortex and the temporal neocortex. This finding, which was replicated and extended several times, confirms a hippocampal-neocortical transfer within a rather short time frame of 20 days. This time frame appears much shorter than the temporal gradient of retrograde amnesia in retrospective studies in humans based either on brain damages patients or patients receiving electroconvulsive treatment. Moreover, this finding revealed for the first time a special role of the ventromedial prefrontal cortex in remote memory retrieval, a result that has not been predicted based on human data before. However, the critical role of this brain region in remote memory retrieval has been confirmed by focused brain lesion studies. Takehara and coworkers (2003) damaged either the hippocampus or the medial prefrontal cortex of rats at various time intervals after establishing trace eye-blink conditioning. They choose trace eye-blink conditioning to clarify such reorganization, because hippocampal damage produces temporally graded retrograde amnesia. When ablated one day after learning, the hippocampal lesion group of rats exhibited a severe impairment in their conditioned response, whereas the medial prefrontal lesion group showed only a slight decline. With an increase in interval between learning and ablation, the effect of the hippocampal lesion diminished and that of the medial prefrontal lesion increased. Thus, when ablated four weeks after learning, the hippocampal lesion group exhibited normal performance, but the medial prefrontal lesion group failed to retain the conditioned response. In other words Takehara and his coworkers revealed a clear double dissociation. While hippocampal ablation leads to retrieval impairments of recent but not remote memories, medial prefrontal ablation leads to retrieval impairments of remote but not recent memories. Thus, these results provide strong evidence that consolidation is accompanied by the transfer of critical binding nodes from the hippocampus to the ventromedial prefrontal cortex. A finding that got subsequently confirmed also in human subjects (Takashima *et al.*, 2006) and that might prompt a revision of the classical view on system level consolidation, because it assumes a neocortical pointer or integrator that succeeded the hippocampus (Frankland & Bontempi, 2005, see below).

As already shortly described, neuropsychological studies of brain-damaged patients and studies with experimental animals implementing either the lesion approach or an activation approach identified the hippocampal-neocortical transfer during declarative memory consolidation, but they did not reveal the mechanism by which this transfer is accomplished. Marr (1971) was the first who proposed a model of hippocampal-neocortical transfer integrating sleep as a critical feature. He suggested that sleep would provide a suitable period for this transfer, because it would mitigate interference due to continuous input during wakefulness. Moreover, he proposed rehearsal trials occurring during sleep that strengthen initially hippocampal-neocortical connections and finally inter-neocortical connections enabling memory retrieval independent of the hippocampus. An electrophysiological mechanism that potentially underlies this initial idea of Marr has been later identified by Wilson and McNaughton (1994). They simultaneously recoded from a large number of single hippocampal neurons during three specific behaviours: a spatial exploration phase and a pre- as well as post behaviour sleep phase. When firing activity of pairs of neurons within these ensembles was highly correlated in the exploration phase, this correlation was also enhanced during subsequent sleep, but low during preceding sleep. In contrast, firing patterns that were uncorrelated during behaviour remained uncorrelated in the subsequent sleep period. This specific sleep reactivation was particular prominent during slow-wave sleep. Subsequently, Skaggs and McNaughton (1996) showed that this reactivation pattern contains information about the temporal order of firing patterns observed during pre-sleep behaviour, probably with time-compression. These pioneering studies and numerous studies performed thereafter also recording simultaneously from neocortical and hippocampal cells (e.g. Ji & Wilson, 2007) showed post-learning replay, which might be neural correlate of active consolidation, but the link between these replay patterns and the behavioural outcome of consolidations has not been established stringently.

Human imaging work

Predictions

The work summarized so far allows one to outline a list of predictions for functional neuroimaging studies probing declarative memory consolidation. (1) The hippocampal activation associated with declarative memory retrieval should get weaker with consolidation. (2) This process should be an active process linked to slow-wave sleep and not a passive time dependent effect. (3) Neocortical, most likely medial prefrontal activation associated with declarative memory retrieval should get stronger with consolidation. (4) Brain activity during slow-wave sleep should be associated to brain activity during pre-sleep behaviour as a correlate of replay.

Retrospective studies

Lesion studies in brain-damaged patients have shown that the medial temporal lobe with the hippocampus at its core is, in contrast to recent memory retrieval, not necessary for remote memory retrieval. As outlined above, this finding paved the way for the consolidation theory at the human brain system level. To confirm this putative transfer of memory traces or binding nodes from the hippocampus to the neocortex in healthy subjects, researchers have rapidly used functional neuroimaging to compare brain activity associated with recent and remote memory retrieval. Initially, all studies took a retrospective approach by presenting subjects with information from earlier phases of their lives compared to recent information of an equal type usually during a recognition memory test. Mostly, this remote information was gathered from autobiographical memory, because it mimics best what can be tested in patients with retrograde amnesia. Additionally, remote memories were tested with retrieving general knowledge (e.g. famous persons, events, etc.) from an earlier life phase of subjects.

Somehow counterintuitive to the lesion data available, the vast majority of imaging studies testing autobiographical memory retrieval did not reveal a temporal gradient of hippocampal contributions or at least a reduced hippocampal activation associated with remote as compared to recent memory retrieval (Maguire et al., 2001; Ryan et al., 2001; Maguire & Frith, 2003; Addis et al., 2004; Gilboa et al., 2004; Piolino et al., 2004; Rekkas & Constable, 2005; Steinvorth et al., 2006; Viard et al., 2007). At first sight, these findings seem to contradict the 'classical' consolidation theory and support the multiple-trace theory, which proposes that retrieval of vivid episodic memories remain hippocampally dependant (Moscovitch *et al.*, 2005). This theory dissociates personal semantic memories which are based in the neocortex from 'true' autobiographical memories that are more relying on an episodic, vivid component, whereby only the latter ones may engage the medial temporal lobes and the hippocampus in particular. However, the discrepancy between lesion and imaging literature may simply reflect the principal difference between these two methods, the lesion method identifies brain regions that are essential for a certain task and functional imaging identifies brain regions that are engaged in such a task. In other words, in healthy subjects the medial temporal lobe might always participate in vivid autobiographical memory retrieval, but this participation is not essential for retrieval of consolidated neocortical memory traces. Moreover, most of these studies used a block rather than an event-related design making it impossible to distinguish transient event-related effects (such as the remoteness of each memory) from state-related changes in activity unrelated to the processing of specific stimuli but which are tonically maintained across a block of trials (Otten *et al.*, 2002).

In addition to these issues, there is an ongoing debate of how to assess autobiographical memories. Typically, weeks prior to scanning, subjects get interviewed in a semi-structured manner to acquire information forming the base for individual stimuli of different remoteness and associated to either general semantic knowledge or personal events (Nadel *et al.*, 2000). However, due to reactivation in such pre-scan interviews and throughout lifetime, the true remoteness of autobiographical memories may be questionable and hence any hippocampal involvement may be related to recollection of the pre-scan interview or other occasions. Nevertheless, some studies have accounted for that by interviewing close family members (Piolino *et al.*, 2004; Viard *et al.*, 2007) and still found an increase of hippocampal activity, making it less likely that the experimental reactivation is indeed contaminating remote memories with new, recent episodic memories of the interview. However, these studies did not exclude event memories that had become semanticized (Moscovitch *et al.*, 1999; Rosenbaum *et al.*, 2001).

Yet, a few studies found evidence for a decrease of hippocampal activation as a function of remoteness as predicted by the consolidation theory (Niki & Luo, 2002; Piefke *et al.*, 2003). Both studies had a blocked design and required subjects to recollect remote and recent episodes upon cueing and not simply recognize information they had encountered before. However, particularly the instruction Piefke and colleagues used (i.e. 'Please remember the events and situations of your personal life history specified in the displayed sentences as vividly and emotionally as possible') in their study resembled very much the one, which was used by Viard and colleagues and which resulted in an increase of hippocampal activity. Maguire and Frith (2003) used a parametric event-related random-effects design in a large group of subjects of young and old age to overcome some of the limitations of previous neuroimaging studies and found that activity in the right hippocampus declined with the remoteness of the material, though left hippocampal activation did not change. The authors suggested that it is important to take into account the lateral asymmetry when trying to understand the hippocampal involvement in remote memory.

Another commonly applied method in retrospective studies of remote memory retrieval is to measure neural activity related to recognition of pictures of people who were famous in particular periods (Haist *et al.*, 2001; Bernard *et al.*, 2004; Douville *et al*, 2005). For example, Haist and colleagues (2001 presented faces of celebrities from six decades (1940s to 1990s) in a blocked design to elderly subjects. They found decreased activation in the right anterior medial temporal lobe with increasing remoteness of their stimuli, supporting a time-limited role of this brain region in remote memory retrieval. In contrast to the results obtained in this blocked design, Bernard and colleagues (2004) found by applying an event-related design a hippocampal activation involved in successful recognition of faces of famous people independent of remoteness. In a related study, Douville and colleagues (2005 replicated this result when using names of famous people as stimuli. Moreover, the right anterior hippocampal/parahippocampal region showed a difference in activity whereby recent famous names produced the largest activity, foils the lowest, and remote famous names were in between. Again, it is not obvious why, apart from methodological issues such as blocked design opposed to event-related design, similar experimental set-ups produce such contradictory results. Moreover, it is difficult to interpret the data in the concept of consolidation of episodic memories since the retrieval of famous faces or names reflects mainly semantic memory, unless self-referent instructions are given that demand to recollect personal memories associated with these names. However, this was not done in any of the above mentioned studies.

In sum, imaging studies testing memory consolidation retrospectively do not provide a coherent pattern of results regarding the involvement of the hippocampus in remote memory retrieval. The studies probing remote memory retrieval in the autobiographic domain show often but not always hippocampal participation independently of remoteness. However, taking the principal difference between imaging and lesion studies into account; these studies can not falsify the consolidation theory, stating that the hippocampus is not essential for remote memory retrieval. Moreover, the retrospective approach has fundamental limitations in the sense that remoteness is graded on a very coarse scale on which recent memories often span periods of five or even ten years, and memories used as stimuli are those which are usually retrieved often until recently during normal life and/or in a prescan interview and thus they represent always quite recent memories, just with a longer history than truly recent memories.

Prospective studies

To have a better experimental control of remoteness, several laboratories have started to implement prospective designs in imaging studies. Here, subjects study different sets of stimuli at different time points prior to the test session in the scanner. Thus, remoteness can be manipulated within the experiment and all items are encoded equally. Certainly, these studies have to operate for practical reasons on an entirely different time scale than retrospective studies; but a time scale of up to several weeks is possible in line with prospective studies observing system-level consolidation in experimental animals or sleep studies in humans (see above). Although the prospective approach allows much more control of stimulus remoteness than a retrospective design, it has also particular limitations that have to be kept in mind. In particular, the contrast between remote and recent memory retrieval in prospective studies is typically confounded either by difference in task difficulty/memory performance in studies in which encoding was equated or by differences in encoding in studies in which memory performance was equated by some kind of study manipulation. Nevertheless prospective study designs are particularly useful to investigate the change in neural activity as a function of the time course of consolidation. The principle idea in this kind of studies is that declarative memory formation is performed in a standardized experimental setting. Consequently retrieval of this information is tested, whereby delay of retrieval reflects consolidation. By these means, brain activity associated to correctly retrieved information can be compared that has been either acquired recently or remotely within the experimental set-up. Moreover, the experimental setting allows studying the effects of different sleep phases (as outlined before) on the brain activation.

The first of these prospective fMRI studies was conducted by Stark and Squire (2000), who compared neural activity in the medial temporal lobe between three separate recognition memory experiments with different study-test intervals that ranged from 30 minutes to one week. They found an increase in activity for correctly recognized items, which was most prominent in the posterior aspect of the hippocampus and which was independent of the duration of the study-test delay. Given the timing of retrospective testing, the authors concluded that the interval of one week was possibly too short to observe any changes in MTL activity related to declarative memory consolidation. However, this study has been done in the early days of event-related fMRI with rather small numbers of subjects and other methodological limitations potentially causing limited power to detect the time effect, particularly since more recent prospective studies were indeed able to find differences even within a couple of days (Orban *et al.*, 2006; Takashima *et al.*, 2006).

Orban and colleagues (2006 combined for the first time in an imaging study on declarative memory consolidation the prospective design with a sleep manipulation. They used a memory task requiring the retrieval of spatial navigational information and brain activity was probed immediately after learning and three days later. Importantly, subjects were either allowed to have regular sleep in the first night after initial learning or they were totally sleep-deprived in this night. Hippocampal activity decreased from immediate to remote retrieval independent of the factor of sleep. Moreover, subjects that were allowed to sleep showed a significantly increased striatal activity after three days compared to sleep-deprived subjects. The first finding might be in line with the consolidation theory and shows a potential effect of consolidation within a relatively short time scale of three days. The later finding is in line with studies showing a smooth transition between hippocampal and striatal contributions to navigational memory retrieval, shown by extended training or in cases with damage to the basal ganglia already after short training (Iaria *et al.*, 2003; Hartley *et al.*, 2003; Voermans *et al.*, 2004). The authors concluded that sleep supports the transfer from a hippocampal system to a striatal system. However, this conclusion is based on a comparison between subjects who slept and were sleep-deprived. Hence, sleep-deprivation might in fact mediate active processes disturbing memory so that it remains difficult to generalize these sleep-related findings and interpret the data in terms of sleep effects on consolidation.

Takashima and colleagues (2006 were not only able to support the rapid hippocampal-neocortical transfer as a function of consolidation but also to show the effect of slow-wave sleep on that. Here, declarative memory consolidations was assessed over the time course of three months and correlated with the duration of slow-wave sleep during a nap, which subjects took after an initial study session on the first day. Subjects initially memorized a large set of photographs of natural landscapes. Subsequently, memory for four different subsets of these stimuli was probed four times within three months on day 1, 2, 30, and 90. During each session, a recognition memory test was performed on these remote items that were intermixed with recent items (i.e, memorized just prior to scanning) and new items. Behaviourally, Takashima and colleagues found a positive across subject correlation between the duration of slow-wave sleep and memory performance for items memorized prior to but not after the nap. This selective correlation confirms once more the specific association between slow wave sleep and declarative memory consolidation and it substantiates the idea that the consolidation process itself may cause the hippocampal trace decay rather than a passive time-dependant process associated with forgetting. Brain activity related to stimuli correctly recognized with high confidence was assessed across time. A progressively decreasing hippocampal activation for correctly and confidentially recognized remote items was found next to an increasing anterior ventral medial prefrontal activation for correctly and confidentially recognized remote items (Figure 8.1). Moreover, the reduction in hippocampal activity related to remote memory retrieval on the first day correlated across subjects with the duration of slow wave sleep, indicating that the behavioural effect of consolidation is indeed associated with a reduced hippocampal involvement.

Gilboa and colleagues (2004 argued that the vividness of retrieved information is critical for the hippocampal activation. Hence, the decrease of hippocampal activity may be related to a less vivid memory over time. While this is certainly a possibility, which, however, does not contradict the notion that consolidation goes along with reduced hippocampal contributions to memory retrieval, Takashima and colleagues argued against this possibility, because they used only trials associated with confident hits and the largest hippocampal activity decrease occurred on day one across the nap and between day one and two despite improving or at least stable memory performance. The progressive ventro-medial prefrontal activity increase with progressive remoteness represents the first human data confirming the data obtained in rodents (Bontempi et al., 1999; Takehara et al., 2003). This brain region is most likely not the place where item related memory traces are stored, but this region might serve as a binding node for or pointer towards distributed representations in posterior brain regions and thus, it may support a similar function for remote memory retrieval as the hippocampus for recent memory retrieval.

Though the data of Takashima and colleagues (2006 are in line with the classical consolidation model, in which memories get hippocampally independent, the results of Bosshardt and colleagues presented in two consecutive papers show evidence that might speak against this conclusion and that might be in favour of the multiple trace theory.

In an initial study Bosshardt and colleagues investigated subjects during retrieval of word pairs, they had learned one day or 10 minutes before (Bosshardt *et al.*, 2005a). The authors varied the level of associations and used the Remember/Know paradigm (Tulving 1985) to probe those trials that are more likely to engage episodic memory retrieval and thus the hippocampus (Eldridge *et al.*, 2000). Most critically, Bosshardt and colleagues used for the encoding of the remote pairs a sentence generation task and for the recent pairs a semantic relatedness task to equate performance levels at retrieval between the two conditions, but performance was actually better for remote than recent items. Thus, the increase of left hippocampal activity for remote over recent trials may also be related to the differences in the amount of encoding and the actually differences in retrieval, because they used a blocked design and hence they could not probe selectively retrieval related activity as it has been possible in event-related designs as used by Takashima and colleagues.

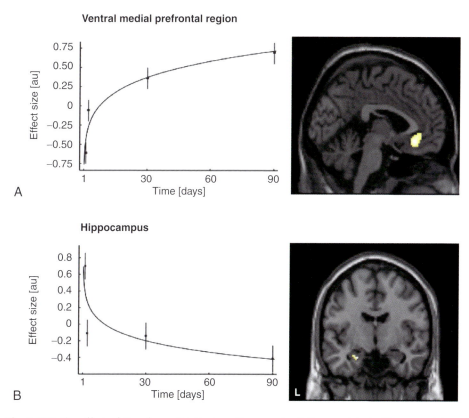

Figure 8.1 The effect of time (consolidation) on the neural activity associated with successful and confident memory retrieval (time by condition interaction). Only two brain regions were found by Takashima and coworkers (2006) that either increased or decreased systematically their activity over the course of 90 days: (A) A ventral medial prefrontal region showed an increase in activity related to confident remote hits over time. (B) In contrast, the hippocampus showed a decline in activity. Maps are thresholded at p<0.05, corrected. Note that the power law function was fitted to the observations for descriptive purposes only. (Reprinted with permission).

In a second experiment, Bosshardt and colleagues extended their design and compared retrieval-related brain activity at day one and one month after study phase (Bosshardt *et al.*, 2005b). In that experiment, the learning runs were increased for half of the stimuli. By these means, the authors sought to disentangle the factors of remoteness and memory performance. Moreover, subjects were separated into a group of good learners and a group of poor learners whereby activity for remote and recent information was only compared within the group of good learners. Their retrieval-related hippocampal and neocortical activity increased from the day to the month lag. This increase was observed both when retrieval performance was matched between the day and the month lag and when the learning procedure for information retrieved at the day and the month lag was matched. Hence, this study appears in stark contrast to the above-outlined predictions of the consolidation theory, because the pattern of results suggests that retrieval of remote memory does not get independent of the hippocampus. Contrary, this study seems to support the multiple trace theory (Moscovitch *et al.*, 2005).

Studies on replay

While all imaging studies reviewed so far investigated the effect of consolidation on brain activity related to memory retrieval a few recent studies probed nocturnal replay, the putative correlate of active consolidation (Peigneux *et al.*, 2004; Rasch *et al.*, 2007). In the first of these studies, Peigneux and colleagues measured regional cerebral blood flow with positron emission tomography while subjects performed a navigational memory task, slept in the scanner after intensively performing that navigational memory task, and slept in the scanner without prior training. The navigational memory task resulted in robust activation of the hippocampus. Activity in the same area was found again and selectively during slow wave sleep in the night following the navigational memory task only, but not during the control night. Moreover, hippocampal activity during slow wave sleep correlated positively with the improvement in memory performance across the night. Thus, this study provided initial evidence for slow wave sleep specific replay activity in humans. More recently Rasch and colleagues (2007) used an elegant study design to probe replay activity more specifically related to a particular memory acquired prior to sleep. In that study subjects learned a series of object locations while exposed to a particular smell in the evening before sleep. One day later, memory for object locations was enhanced when that smell was re-applied during slow wave sleep in between. This finding was specific for the smell, the kind of memory (declarative), the conjunction between smell and memory task during encoding, and the sleep stage during which the smell was applied. Moreover, Rasch and colleagues (2007 showed that the re-exposure of the specific smell applied at study during slow wave sleep but not other sleep stages was associated with a hippocampal activity increase revealing that this particular memory is replayed in the hippocampus during slow wave sleep. This finding clearly shows that indeed memory reactivation during slow wave sleep causes memory consolidation – the first time that such a mechanistic account for declarative memory consolidations has been identified. Taken together, these studies provide compelling evidence for the idea that replay during slow wave sleep is causative for consolidation of specific declarative memories.

In a related study, Peigneux and colleagues (2006 pursued the endeavour to probe post-learning replay associated with consolidation to the wake state. They used again a navigational memory task thought to be hippocampus-dependant and an implicit motor sequence learning task, which rather relies on motor and premotor areas as well as striatum and cerebellum. Functional MRI was conducted during an auditory oddball task before and after participants conducted either the navigational or the procedural learning task outside the scanner. After spatial learning, activity during the oddball task increased in brain regions associated with spatial learning. Likewise, immediately after the procedural learning, increased activity was seen in a distributed set of cortical and subcortical regions commonly associated with the motor sequence learning task used. These results indicate that learned information is already processed during the first hours of post-training wakefulness even when subjects simultaneously perform an unrelated cognitive task. Though slow wave sleep appears to play a prominent role in declarative memory consolidation, post-encoding processes of memory consolidation seem to be initiated immediately and do occur during both sleep and wakefulness.

Conclusions

The functional imaging literature reviewed here seems to confirm most predictions outlined above and based on human lesion data, experimental animal research, and theoretical work. There are clearly conflicting results regarding the question whether hippocampal activation associated with remote and recent declarative memory retrieval differ. Data derived from brain-damaged patients and experimental animals led to the prediction that remote memories can be retrieved independently from the hippocampus. This prediction has been confirmed by retrospective and prospective imaging studies, but several imaging studies did not find reduced hippocampal activation for remote as opposed to recent memory retrieval. Given the heterogeneity of study designs, this partial discrepancy cannot be easily explained by a specific (set of) design feature(s). To date the most parsimonious explanation for the fact that several imaging studies probing the outcome of declarative memory consolidation found at least as much hippocampal activity for remote as for recent memory retrieval lies in the conceptual difference between the lesion and the imaging approach. It might just be the case that under certain, yet unknown circumstance the hippocampus does participate in remote memory retrieval although its participation is not critical as shown by numerous neuropsychological studies of patients with bilateral hippocampal damage. The second prediction mentioned above that declarative memory consolidation is an active process linked to slow-wave sleep has been univocally confirmed by several behavioural and imaging studies by now. Initial evidence has been provided verifying the hypothesis that neocortical, most likely medial prefrontal areas are involved in remote declarative memory retrieval. Finally, recent imaging studies have provided a unique view on active processes underlying declarative memory consolidation by assessing hippocampal activity during slow-wave sleep associated to brain activity during pre-sleep behaviour as a correlate of replay.

Functional neuroimaging of declarative memory consolidation is yet in an embryonic state as a field of research and thus some conflicting results are to be expected. Regardless of these conflicts, however, most predictions made by the consolidation theory based on human lesion and experimental animal data have been well confirmed already – for the first time in healthy humans. Thus, it is the first time that phenomena underlying consolidation like replay or the consequences thereof can now be assessed in healthy humans. In this way neuroimaging studies provide information about interacting brain regions and thus it confirms and refines hypothesis derived from the consolidation theory at the brain system level. Despite this translational success, functional neuroimaging has not yet provided fundamentally new insights into how consolidation transfers recent memories into a more stable form. However, more current work has established a set of powerful experimental designs that can prospectively investigate ongoing consolidation (Peigneux *et al.*, 2004; Rasch *et al.*, 2007) and the consequence of this fundamental mnemonic operation (Takashima *et al.*, 2006) in great detail. In other words, these experimental approaches provide the arena for gaining fundamentally new insights in declarative memory consolidation at the human brain system level.

References

Addis, D. R., Moscovitch, M., Crawley, A. P., & McAndrews, M. P. (2004). Recollective qualities modulate hippocampal activation during autobiographical memory retrieval. *Hippocampus, 14*(6), 752–762.

Aristotle. (350 B.C.E) On sleep and sleeplessness (translated by J. I. Beare published in Ross, W. D. (Ed.) (1930). The works of Aristotle (vol. 3). Oxford: Clarendon Press)

Bernard, F. A., Bullmore, E. T., Graham, K. S., Thompson, S. A., Hodges, J. R., & Fletcher, P. C. (2004). The hippocampal region is involved in successful recognition of both remote and recent famous faces. *Neuroimage, 22*(4), 1704–1714.

Bontempi, B., Laurent-Demir, C., Destrade, C., & Jaffard, R. (1999). Time-dependent reorganization of brain circuitry underlying long-term memory storage. *Nature, 400*(6745), 671–675.

Bosshardt, S., Schmidt, C. F., Jaermann, T., Degonda, N., Boesiger, P., Nitsch, R. M., Hock, C., & Henke, K. (2005a). Effects of memory consolidation on human hippocampal activity during retrieval. *Cortex, 41*(4), 486–498.

Bosshardt, S., Degonda, N., Schmidt, C. F., Boesiger, P., Nitsch, R. M., Hock, C., & Henke, K. (2005b). One month of human memory consolidation enhances retrieval-related hippocampal activity. *Hippocampus, 15*(8), 1026–1040.

Burnham, W. H. (1904). Retroactive amnesia: Illustrative cases and a tentative explanation. *American Journal of Psychology, 14*, 382–396.

Douville, K., Woodard, J. L., Seidenberg, M., Miller, S. K., Leveroni, C. L., Nielson, K. A., Franczak, M., Antuono, P., & Rao, S. M. (2005). Medial temporal lobe activity for recognition of recent and remote famous names: an event-related fMRI study. *Neuropsychologia, 43*(5), 693–703.

Dudai, Y. (2004). The neurobiology of consolidations, or, how stable is the engram? *Annual Review of Psychology, 55*, 51–86.

Duncan, C. P. (1949). The retroactive effect of electroshock on learning. *Journal of Comparative and Physiological Psychology, 42*, 32–44.

Ebbinghaus, H. (1885). *Über das Gedächtnis*. Leipzig: Duncker & Humboldt.

Eldridge, L. L., Knowlton, B. J., Furmanski, C. S., Bookheimer, S. Y., & Engel, S. A. (2000). Remembering episodes: a selective role for the hippocampus during retrieval. *Nature Neuroscience*, *3*(11), 1149–1152.

Ellenbogen, J. M., Payne, J. D., & Stickgold, R. (2006). The role of sleep in declarative memory consolidation: passive, permissive, active or none? *Current Opinion in Neurobiology*, *16*(6), 716–722.

Ebbinghaus, H. (1885). Über das Gedächtnis [On memory]. Reprint: (1966) Amsterdam, Netherlands: E. J. Bonset.

Frankland, P. W. & Bontempi, B. (2005). The organization of recent and remote memories. *Nature reviews. Neuroscience*, *6*(2), 119–130.

Gilboa, A., Winocur, G., Grady, C. L., Hevenor, S. J., & Moscovitch, M. (2004). Remembering our past: functional neuroanatomy of recollection of recent and very remote personal events. *Cerebral Cortex*, *14*(11), 1214–1225.

Haist, F., Bowden Gore, J., & Mao, H. (2001). Consolidation of human memory over decades revealed by functional magnetic resonance imaging. *Nature Neuroscience*, *4*(11), 1139–1145.

Hartley, T., Maguire, E. A., Spiers, H. J., & Burgess, N. (2003). The well-worn route and the path less traveled: distinct neural bases of route following and wayfinding in humans. *Neuron*, *37*(5), 877–888.

Iaria, G., Petrides, M., Dagher, A., Pike, B., & Bohbot, V. D. (2003). Cognitive strategies dependent on the hippocampus and caudate nucleus in human navigation: variability and change with practice. *Journal of Neuroscience*, *23*(13), 5945–5952.

Jenkins, J. G. & Dallenbach, K. M. (1924). Obliviscence during sleep and waking. *American Journal of Psychology*, *35*, 605–612.

Ji, D. & Wilson, M. A. (2007). Coordinated memory replay in the visual cortex and hippocampus during sleep. *Nature Neuroscience*, *10*(1), 100–107.

Kandel, E. R. (2001). The molecular biology of memory storage: a dialogue between genes and synapses. *Science*, *294*(5544), 1030–1038.

Maguire, E. A., Henson, R. N., Mummery, C. J., & Frith, C. D. (2001). Activity in prefrontal cortex, not hippocampus, varies parametrically with the increasing remoteness of memories. *Neuroreport*, *12*(3), 441–444.

Maguire, E. A. & Frith, C. D. (2003). Lateral asymmetry in the hippocampal response to the remoteness of autobiographical memories. *Journal of Neuroscience*, *23*(12), 5302–5307.

Marr, D. (1971). Simple memory: a theory for archicortex. *Philos Trans R Soc Lond B Biol Sci*, *262*(841), 23–81.

Marshall, L., Helgadottir, H., Molle, M., & Born, J. (2006). Boosting slow oscillations during sleep potentiates memory. *Nature*, *444*(7119), 610–613.

Moscovitch, M., Yaschyshyn, T., Ziegler, M., & Nadel, L. (1999). Remote episodic memory and retrograde amnesia: was Endel Tulving right all along? In: E. Tulving (Ed.), *Memory, Consciousness, and the Brain: The Tallinn Conference* (pp. 331–345). New York: Psychology.

Moscovitch, M., Rosenbaum, R. S., Gilboa, A., Addis, D. R., Westmacott, R., Grady, C., McAndrews, M. P., Levine, B., Black, S., Winocur, G., & Nadel, L. (2005). Functional neuroanatomy of remote episodic, semantic and spatial memory: a unified account based on multiple trace theory. *Journal of Anatomy*, *207*(1), 35–66.

Müller, G. E. & Pilzecker, A. (1900). Experimentelle Beiträge zur Lehre vom Gedächtnis. *Z Psychol* (*Ergänzungsband 1*), 1–288.

Nadel, L., Samsonovich, A., Ryan, L., & Moscovitch, M. (2000). Multiple trace theory of human memory: computational, neuroimaging, and neuropsychological results. *Hippocampus*, *10*(4), 352–368.

Niki, K. & Luo, J. (2002). An fMRI study on the time-limited role of the medial temporal lobe in long-term topographic autobiographic memory. *Journal of Cognitive Neuroscience*, *14*(3), 500–507.

Orban, P., Rauchs, G., Balteau, E., Degueldre, C., Luxen, A., Maquet, P., & Peigneux, P. (2006). Sleep after spatial learning promotes covert reorganization of brain activity. *Proceedings of the National Academy of Sciences of the United States of America, 103*(18), 7124–7129.

Otten, L. J., Henson, R. N., & Rugg, M. D. (2002). State-related and item-related neural correlates of successful memory encoding. *Nature Neuroscience, 5*(12), 1339–1344.

Peigneux, P., Laureys, S., Fuchs, S., Collette, F., Perrin, F., Reggers, J., Phillips, C., Degueldre, C., Del Fiore, G., Aerts, J., Luxen, A., & Maquet, P. (2004). Are spatial memories strengthened in the human hippocampus during slow wave sleep? *Neuron, 44*(3), 535–545.

Peigneux, P., Orban, P., Balteau, E., Degueldre, C., Luxen, A., Laureys, S., & Maquet, P. (2006). Offline persistence of memory-related cerebral activity during active wakefulness. *PLoS Biology, 4*(4), e100.

Piefke, M., Weiss, P. H., Zilles, K., Markowitsch, H. J., & Fink, G. R. (2003). Differential remoteness and emotional tone modulate the neural correlates of autobiographical memory. *Brain, 126*(Pt 3), 650–668.

Piolino, P., Giffard-Quillon, G., Desgranges, B., Chetelat, G., Baron, J. C., & Eustache, F. (2004). Re-experiencing old memories via hippocampus: a PET study of autobiographical memory. *Neuroimage, 22*(3), 1371–1383.

Plihal, W. & Born, J. (1999). Effects of early and late nocturnal sleep on priming and spatial memory. *Psychophysiology, 36*(5), 571–582.

Rasch, B., Büchel, C., Gais, S., & Born, J. (2007). Odor cues during slow-wave sleep prompt declarative memory consolidation. *Science, 315*(5817), 1426–1429.

Rekkas, P. V. & Constable, R. T. (2005). Evidence that autobiographic memory retrieval does not become independent of the hippocampus: an fMRI study contrasting very recent with remote events. *Journal of Cognitive Neuroscience, 17*(12), 1950–1961.

Rosenbaum, R. S., Winocur, G., & Moscovitch, M. (2001). New views on old memories: re-evaluating the role of the hippocampal complex. *Behavioural Brain Research, 127*(1,2), 183–197.

Rosenbaum, R. S., Ziegler, M., Winocur, G., Grady, C. L., & Moscovitch, M. (2004). "I have often walked down this street before": fMRI studies on the hippocampus and other structures during mental navigation of an old environment. *Hippocampus, 14*(7), 826–835.

Ryan, L., Nadel, L., Keil, K., Putnam, K., Schnyer, D., Trouard, T., & Moscovitch, M. (2001). Hippocampal complex and retrieval of recent and very remote autobiographical memories: evidence from functional magnetic resonance imaging in neurologically intact people. *Hippocampus, 11*(6), 707–714.

Scoville, W. B. & Milner, B. (1957). Loss of recent memory after bilateral hippocampal lesions. *Journal of Neurology, Neurosurgery, and Psychiatry, 20*(1), 11–21.

Skaggs, W. E. & McNaughton, B. L. (1996). Replay of neuronal firing sequences in rat hippocampus during sleep following spatial experience. *Science, 271*(5257), 1870–1873.

Squire, L. R., Slater, P. C., & Chace, P. M. (1975). Retrograde amnesia: temporal gradient in very long term memory following electroconvulsive therapy. *Science, 187*(4171), 77–79.

Squire, L. R., Stark, C. E., & Clark, R. E. (2004). The medial temporal lobe. *Annual Review of Neuroscience, 27*, 279–306.

Stark, C. E. & Squire, L. R. (2000). fMRI activity in the medial temporal lobe during recognition memory as a function of study-test interval. *Hippocampus, 10*(3), 329–337.

Steinvorth, S., Corkin, S., & Halgren, E. (2006). Ecphory of autobiographical memories: an fMRI study of recent and remote memory retrieval. *Neuroimage, 30*(1), 285–298.

Takashima, A., Petersson, K. M., Rutters, F., Tendolkar, I., Jensen, O., Zwarts, M. J., McNaughton, B. L., & Fernández, G. (2006). Declarative memory consolidation in humans: a prospective functional magnetic resonance imaging study. *Proceedings of the National Academy of Sciences of the United States of America, 103*(3), 756–761.

Takehara, K., Kawahara, S., & Kirino, Y. (2003). Time-dependent reorganization of the brain components underlying memory retention in trace eye blink conditioning. *Journal of Neuroscience*, *23*(30), 9897–9905.

Teng, E. & Squire, L. R. (1999). Memory for places learned long ago is intact after hippocampal damage. *Nature*, *400*(6745), 675–677.

Tse, D., Langston, R. F., Kakeyama, M., Bethus, I., Spooner, P. A., Wood, E. R., Witter, M. P., & Morris, R. G. (2007). Schemas and memory consolidation. *Science*, *316*(5821), 76–82.

Tucker, M. A., Hirota, Y., Wamsley, E. J., Lau, H., Chaklader, A., & Fishbein, W. (2006). A daytime nap containing solely non-REM sleep enhances declarative but not procedural memory. *Neurobiology of learning and memory*, *86*(2), 241–247.

Tulving, E. (1985). Memory and consciousness. *Canadian Journal of Psychology*, *26*, 1–12.

Tulving, E., Schacter, D. L., McLachlan, D. R., & Moscovitch, M. (1988). Priming of semantic autobiographical knowledge: a case study of retrograde amnesia. *Brain and Cognition*, *8*(1), 3–20.

Viard, A., Piolino, P., Desgranges, B., Chetelat, G., Lebreton, K., Landeau, B., Young, A., De La Sayette, V., & Eustache, F. (2007). Hippocampal activation for autobiographical memories over the entire lifetime in healthy aged subjects: an fMRI study. *Cerebral Cortex*, *17*, 2453–2467.

Voermans, N. C., Petersson, K. M., Daudey, L., Weber, B., Van Spaendonck, K. P., Kremer, H. P., & Fernández, G. (2004). Interaction between the human hippocampus and the caudate nucleus during route recognition. *Neuron*, *43*(3), 427–435.

Walker, M. P. & Stickgold, R. (2005). It's practice, with sleep, that makes perfect: implications of sleep-dependent learning and plasticity for skill performance. *Clinics in Sports Medicine*, *24*(2), 301–317.

Wilson, M. A. & McNaughton, B. L. (1994). Reactivation of hippocampal ensemble memories during sleep. *Science*, *265*(5172), 676–679.

Zola-Morgan, S. M. & Squire, L. R. (1990). The primate hippocampal formation: evidence for a time-limited role in memory storage. *Science*, *250*(4978), 288–290.

Chapter 9

On the intimate relationship between neurobiology and function in the theoretical analysis of human learning and memory

Alan Richardson-Klavehn, Zara M. Bergström, Elena Magno, Gerasimos Markopoulos, Catherine M. Sweeney-Reed, and Maria Wimber

Introduction

In writing the current chapter, we set ourselves the task of achieving a balanced perspective on the relationship between functional (information-processing) and neurobiological approaches to the understanding of human learning and memory, in view of recent controversies concerning the compatibility and relative usefulness of these approaches. We argue that neurobiological information, including information from functional neuroimaging, is essential in informing functional theory, but that functional theory is in turn essential to increasing the specificity of theorizing concerning how representations and processes of learning and memory relate to their neurobiological substrates (see also Shallice, 2003). First, however, we define the scope of the chapter, and note the important medical and societal applications of neuroimaging research on learning and memory.

Commonality of theoretical and methodological issues across the fields of learning and of memory

The current section of this volume has reviewed the neuroimaging of learning, focussing on research using functional magnetic resonance (haemodynamic) imaging. Here we use the term neuroimaging more broadly to cover both haemodynamic and electrophysiological investigations, given the increasing spatial resolution of electrophysiological data (e.g. from magnetoencephalography, MEG), combined with advances in visualizing spatiotemporal patterns in such data (e.g. Düzel et al., 2003; Lobaugh, West, & McIntosh, 2001; McIntosh & Lobaugh, 2004; Sweeney-Reed & Nasuto, 2007), and the increasing tendency to combine haemodynamic and electrophysiological data, with an accompanying increase of knowledge about the relationships between the two kinds of signals in relation to learning and memory (e.g. Fiebach, Gruber, & Supp, 2005; Düzel, Richardson-Klavehn et al., 2005;

Schott, Richardson-Klavehn *et al.*, 2006; see also Logothetis & Wandell, 2004). Ultimately, both kinds of methods index the activity of large assemblies of nerve cells.

The distinction between neuroimaging research on learning and on memory, as embodied in the organisation of this volume, is also to some extent artificial. In his classic work *Principles of Learning and Memory* (1976), Robert G. Crowder had the following to say concerning the definitions of learning and of memory (pp. 3–4):

> Formulating a definition of *learning* is an instructive exercise, pondering the various inclusions and exclusions that must be added to any straightforward statement, but for the present purposes we may simply describe it as a change in the organism that occurs at a particular time as a function of experience. (Experience, of course, may also produce many other changes that are not learning.) The change in the brain that constitutes learning corresponds to what gets entered into memory. However, this change, learning, cannot be observed directly and therefore some indirect performance test must be used to infer that learning has occurred. The basic form of such a test is a comparison of performance that could reflect the learning experience with control performance, in which the critical experience is missing. Learning is inferred from a difference as a function of the experience. To recapitulate…the acquisition process (learning) may only be studied through performance in a memory test (retention plus retrieval)…The term "memory" is used for both the product of learning and the process of retention and retrieval.

Crowder's analysis raises some interesting issues, given the changes in theoretical focus and research methods in the science of learning and memory after 1976 (for brief histories see Bower, 2000; Squire, 2004; Squire & Kandel, 1999; Tulving, 2001). Firstly, it points out that a focus on learning, rather than defining a conceptually distinct research area, represents a focus on experimental *paradigms* of learning and memory that examine gradual acquisition and retention of information across multiple experiences, in contrast to the episodic memory paradigms reviewed elsewhere in this volume, which typically focus on the acquisition and retention of information from single experiences. The area of memory consolidation reviewed by Fernández and Tendolkar (this volume) is a good case in point, in that the theoretical concern is to explain how memory records of individual episodes are transformed over time, and/or with repeated retrieval, to become stable and relatively immune to forgetting, or to become context-independent semantic representations (e.g. Moscovitch *et al.*, 2005).

In this context, it is also interesting to note that Crowder's description of how learning is measured (i.e. by reference to a no-learning control condition) reads remarkably like a definition of repetition priming (i.e. the facilitation of cognitive processing with repetition), an expression of learning and memory on which research subsequently burgeoned (e.g. Henson, 2003; Richardson-Klavehn & Bjork, 1988; Roediger & McDermott, 1993; Schacter & Buckner, 1998; Schacter, Wig, & Stevens, 2007; Tulving & Schacter, 1990; Wiggs & Martin, 1998). The typical focus of repetition priming paradigms is on the impact of single episodes on later cognitive performance, measured by contrast with a control (baseline) condition in which such a relevant episode has not occurred, and it is known that some information that can be regarded as episodic, such as information about the original presentation modality and some other aspects of the presentation context, is retained and influences the later expression of repetition priming (e.g. Jacoby, 1983a; Richardson-Klavehn & Gardiner, 1996; Richardson-Klavehn, Clarke, & Gardiner, 1999;

Roediger & Srinivas, 1993). These paradigms, therefore, explicitly bridge the study of learning and memory (see also Kirsner, Speelman, & Schofield, 1993, for an explicit analysis of the similarities between priming and skill acquisition). Not surprisingly, therefore, current theoretical issues in the areas of learning and of memory have considerable commonality, notably the persistent cross-paradigmatic issue of the extent to which heterogeneity in mental representations and/or processes is necessary to account for different manifestations of learning and memory (i.e. the abstractionist vs. non-abstractionist debate, or the issue of unitary vs. multiple learning and memory systems; see Richardson-Klavehn & Bjork, 1988; see also Poldrack & Foerde, 2008; Squire, 2004). This debate can be traced to the 17th–18th century debate between the empiricist philosophers John Locke and George Berkeley over the necessity of postulating a distinct class of abstract ideas in addition to specific ideas in order to explain mental function (with the term 'ideas' in both cases referring to kinds of mental representation). Here Locke was the precursor of abstractionist or multiple systems perspectives, and Berkeley was the precursor of non-abstractionist or unitary perspectives (although Locke's position has precedents in Descartes and Aristotle).

Secondly, it is interesting to consider Crowder's (1976) statement that 'this change, learning, cannot be observed directly' (p. 3) in the light of the flood of subsequent information about the neural basis of learning and memory, some of which is reviewed in the current volume. Major advances have been made in understanding the brain changes responsible for learning and memory at the neuronal, neurotransmitter, molecular, and genetic levels (for accessible introductions see Le Doux, 2002; Linden, 2007; Rose, 1993; Squire & Kandel, 1999; see also Kandel, 2001). But brain-activity measurements are not direct measures of these brain changes, and thus Crowder's statement remains essentially true, at least regarding the results of research with living humans. Despite intensive work that might link these two levels of scientific enquiry (e.g. Buzsáki, 1996; Buzsáki & Draguhn, 2004; Hasselmo & McClelland, 1999; Laughlin & Sejnowski, 2003; Paulsen & Sejnowski, 2000; Sejnowski & Paulsen, 2006; Varela et al., 2001), bridging the gap remains an awesome task (but see Schott, Seidenbecher et al., 2006, for an example of recent neuroimaging work that begins to bridge this gap).

Critical applications of neuroimaging of learning and memory

One major theme of the current volume is to counter sceptical arguments regarding the value of brain-imaging methods in informing functional psychological theories of learning and memory, and all of the chapters in the current section of this volume provide examples of the use of neuroimaging to discriminate theories or models at the functional level. Whether or not these specific uses are convincing, and whatever one's general position on the issue of whether neuroimaging data can in principle discriminate between functional theories (e.g. Coltheart, 2006a; Henson, 2005, 2006a; Poldrack, 2006; Rugg, this volume) – and in particular on whether they can elucidate the ever-contentious issue regarding unitary vs. multiple learning and memory systems – understanding the brain basis of learning and memory is critical to understanding and possibly remediating pathological changes in learning and memory, which are of ever-increasing societal importance. For example, neuroimaging can potentially make an important contribution by revealing differences in learning and memory-related brain activity between 'at risk' individuals for Alzheimer and other forms of dementia, and those individuals not at risk, which might not yet be observable in behaviour as measured by neuropsychological tests, thus allowing effective targeting of new generations of preventative drugs (e.g. Cummings, Doody, & Clark, 2007; Mosconi *et al.*, 2007; Reimann, 2007; Stam *et al.*, 2003). In this context, as reviewed in part by Fernández and Tendolkar (this volume), neuroimaging might provide an important scientific window on 'cognitively silent' (Craik, 2002; see also Tulving, 2001), but clinically critical, learning and memory processes such as memory formation and consolidation. Furthermore, as Ghahremani and Poldrack (this volume) and Reber (this volume) illustrate, neuroimaging research can point to differences in the strategies used by patients (e.g. Parkinson dementia patients) and normal control participants, or older and younger participants, to solve learning and memory tasks, even when the groups are not behaviourally distinguishable on the particular tasks chosen. This information could, once again, prove of considerable clinical and therapeutic relevance. Neuroimaging of reinforcement learning, as reviewed by Büchel (this volume) and O'Doherty (this volume), could potentially inform understanding and treatment of addictive and obsessive–compulsive conditions in which inappropriate stimulus–reward and/or stimulus–avoidance associations have been acquired (e.g. Murray *et al.*, 2008; Remijnse *et al.*, 2006). We believe that experimental cognitive psychologists should be proud (*cf.* Page, 2006) that their theoretical and methodological expertise plays a key role in such societally important applications of neuroimaging research, which 'promise to revolutionize medical research and practice in neurology and psychiatry' (Squire & Kandel, 1999, p. 214), regardless of whether such research feeds back to inform functional theories of learning and memory (see also Henson, 2005).

Chapter overview

In the remainder of this chapter, we (1) comment from an evolutionary neurobiological perspective on the role of knowledge about the brain in elucidating functional theories of learning and memory, (2) present two examples that seem to us to illustrate in a telling way the theoretical value of measuring brain activity in relation to understanding learning and memory function, (3) comment on some of the theoretical and methodological issues facing attempts to distinguish unitary and multiple systems accounts of learning and memory, and (4) comment on some current issues in the use of dissociations to separate learning and memory functions.

Could neurobiology ever inform functional theories of learning and memory?

The debate between advocates (e.g. Henson, 2005, 2006a, 2006b; Poldrack, 2006; Rugg, this volume) and critics (e.g. Coltheart, 2004, 2006a, 2006b; Harley, 2004a, 2004b; Page, 2006) of neuroimaging as a tool to inform cognitive theory has been carried out at two levels. One is the *in principle* level: i.e. could information about the brain, including information from neuroimaging, *ever* inform or constrain functional theories? At this level the critical view (e.g. Coltheart, 2004; 2006a; Harley, 2004a, 2004b; Page, 2006; Uttal, 2001; Van Orden & Kloos, 2003; Van Orden & Paap, 1997; Van Orden, Pennington, & Stone, 2001) questions the relevance of function to brain-activity inferences (e.g. Henson, 2005, 2006a), and brain-activity to function inferences (Henson, 2005; Poldrack, 2006), and the fundamental assumption of some degree of systematic function-to-brain-activity mapping that underlies both kinds of inference (Henson, 2005, 2006a, 2006b; Poldrack, 2006; Shallice, 2003), as well as the relevance of other neurobiological data. The other is the *in practice* level: i.e. are there examples of neuroimaging data, or for that matter behavioural or neuropsychological data, ever discriminating conclusively between functional theories? The latter debate has been conducted via arguments concerning specific theories and datasets, and appears to have reached bedrock over an issue that Coltheart (2006b, p. 425) terms 'Henson's Gambit'. That is, the argument that neuroimaging data have not yet conclusively discriminated between functional theories might be sacrificially conceded by neuroimaging researchers, but this concession exposes their critics to the rejoinder that behavioural data and purely functional theories of cognition have not produced any scientific consensus either. In this latter respect, a reasonable compromise (Henson, 2005, 2006b) is to accept that no single dataset will provide conclusive confirmation or disconfirmation of a specific theory, and that science proceeds rather via a Darwinian process of natural selection, whereby successful theories, or classes of theories that make generally similar predictions (e.g. J. A. Anderson & Hinton, 1981; J. R. Anderson, 1978, 1985; J. R. Anderson & Lebiere, 2003; Chomsky, 1980), gradually emerge from large bodies of research (e.g. Baddeley, 2003; Coltheart & Davies, 2003).

Here, however, along with Henson (2006b), we are more concerned with the *in principle* issue in relation to theories of learning and memory. That is, we are concerned with the critical view that the hardware (or rather 'wetware') implementation of learning and memory processes in the brain is simply irrelevant to their functional explanation by psychological theory (e.g. Coltheart, 2004, 2006a; Harley, 2004a, 2004b; Morton, 1984; Page, 2006; Putnam, 1975). The response that we are, as neuroimaging scientists, interested in the entire mind/brain entities that underlie learning and memory is a reasonable one (e.g. Buchsbaum & D'Esposito, this volume; see also Squire, 2004; Squire & Kandel, 1999; Tulving, 2000), and is consistent with the important clinical and therapeutic applications mentioned in the Introduction, but will no doubt be less than satisfying to dyed-in-the-wool advocates of the functional information-processing approach to cognition.

At a general level, the *in principle* critiques of neurobiological approaches to cognition (e.g. Coltheart, 2004, 2006a; Harley, 2004a, 2004b; Page, 2006) often rely on a strong adherence to functionalism as a philosophical theory about the mind and its relationship to the brain (e.g. Putnam, 1975). This doctrine was in the modern era stimulated by the development of the Turing machine and the digital computer, but traces its roots to Aristotle, who 'solved' the mind/body problem by distinguishing between form (soul) and the substance having that form (body). Thus, according to functionalist doctrine, an understanding of form and function (mind) does not require an understanding of substance (brain). Given developments in thought about the mind since the original formulations of functionalism, such adherence to functionalism on the part of cognitive theorists raises highly complex and contentious general arguments regarding the value of functionalist, connectionist, and dynamical systems views of the mind and brain, and how these are interrelated (for an introduction see Bechtel & Abrahamsen, 2002; see also Churchland, 2002; Henson, 2005, 2006b; Mainzer, 2007).

Pending developments in that area, however, there is already some reason to believe that a strong functionalist perspective may not be efficient from a scientific point of view in achieving a general understanding of human learning and memory (see also Bechtel, 2002; Henson, 2005, 2006a, 2006b; Rugg, this volume). This problem is, after all, a difficult and complex one, many critical aspects of which still resist a comprehensive understanding after over a century of scientific research. An evolutionary neurobiological perspective suggests that our sophisticated learning and memory functions evolved as part and parcel of the evolution of our complex nervous system (e.g. Churchland, 2002; Jerison, 1973; Hakeem et al., 2005; Hart, Hart, & Pinter-Wollman, 2008; Klein et al., 2002; Laughlin & Sejnowski, 2003; Linden, 2007; Mainzer, 2007; Oakley, 1983; Roth & Dicke, 2005; Roth & Wulliman, 2001; Schenker, Desgouttes, & Semendeferi, 2005; Sejnowski & Paulsen, 2006; Sherry & Schacter, 1987; Squire, 2004; Striedter, 2005; Tulving, 1983, 1985, 2000; Velichkovsky, 2002). Given current knowledge about the brain, one might then already take issue with the strong functionalist claim that 'A system with as many degrees of freedom as the brain can imitate to within the accuracy relevant to psychological theory any structure one can hope to describe' (Putnam, 1975, p. 302). The fact that this statement is rather optimistic is indicated by the elementary example that the neurons of the brain, given their known timing properties, would be incapable of implementing a serial search process through the thousands of face representations stored in memory in order to identify a particular face, while producing behavioural reaction times for face identification on the order of hundreds of milliseconds (Henson, 2005). Similar considerations apply to word identification (e.g. Cohen et al., 2000; Nobre, Allison, & McCarthy, 1994). These simple examples illustrate that 'though psychological theories can be phrased purely in algorithmic terms – representations, processes, mappings, transforms – without reference to brain regions or neurons, this does not mean that they are not ultimately constrained by such implementational details' (Henson, 2005, p. 224; see this article also for a discussion, in relation to brain function, of logical and causal relationships between Marr's (1982) levels of explanation).

Moreover, consideration of other fundamental characteristics of our learning and memory capabilities – including both notable strengths and weaknesses – suggests that they may be intimately connected with the nature of the wetware of the nervous system, and may represent an optimal solution for intelligent adaptive behaviour within the constraints of this wetware (e.g. J. R. Anderson & Milson, 1989; J. R. Anderson & Schooler, 2000; J. R. Anderson & Labiere, 2003; Bjork, 1989; Bjork & Bjork, 1992; Klein et al., 2002; Laughlin & Sejnowski, 2003; Richardson-Klavehn & Bjork, 2002; Sejnowski, 1981; Sejnowski & Paulsen, 2006; Sherry & Schacter, 1987). The amazing strengths include the successful acquisition and retention of vast quantities of information, with no known limit to the amount of information that can be stored across a lifetime, and the ability to generalize across widely varying inputs, such as in the learning of categories, concepts, and rules (e.g. Richardson-Klavehn & Bjork, 2002; see also Ghahremani & Poldrack, this volume; Reber, this volume); the equally impressive weaknesses include forgetting, interference, memory distortions and illusions, and decline of certain learning and memory functions with normal ageing (e.g. Richardson-Klavehn & Bjork, 2002; Schacter, 2001). Furthermore, retrieving information from memory, which occurs at just about every (waking) moment, is not a simple readout process, but dynamically changes the state of memory, enhancing the future accessibility of the retrieved information, and sometimes simultaneously impairing the retrievability of other information (i.e. the well-documented phenomenon of *retrieval-induced forgetting*; M.C. Anderson, Bjork, & Bjork, 1994; M. C. Anderson & Spellman, 1995; Bjork & Bjork, 1992; for reviews see M. C. Anderson & Levy, 2007; Levy & M. C. Anderson, 2002; Norman, Newman, & Detre, 2007). These considerations suggest that human learning and memory, in general character, have very little in common with the information storage and retrieval systems of digital computers, and that it is not surprising that the once popular functionalist-inspired computer metaphor for learning and memory achieved only limited theoretical success. Most fundamentally, it does not provide a natural explanation for the *dynamic* and *constructive* properties of our learning and memory capabilities (Richardson-Klavehn & Bjork, 2002; see also our discussion of retrieval inhibition in the next main section of this chapter).

The parallel-distributed-processing (connectionist) approach to learning and memory, which developed as an alternative to the computer metaphor (e.g. J. A. Anderson & Hinton, 1981; Hasselmo & McClelland, 1999; McClelland, 2000; McClelland & Rogers, 2003; Sejnowski, 1981), viewed information processing as being more similar in general character to that of an analogue radio than to that of a digital computer: Its fundamental task is reliable discrimination of signals, by which is meant significant or interpretable patterns of activity, from noise generated by the comparative unreliability across space and time of the individual elements of the wetware (i.e. nerve cells or assemblies thereof), which unreliability contrasts markedly with the reliability across space and time of the basic hardware elements of the digital computer (Laughlin & Sejnowski, 2003; but see also Sejnowski & Paulsen, 2006, for qualification). Whatever the successes and failures of the connectionist approach with regard to specific models (e.g. McClelland, 2000; McClelland & Goddard, 1996; McClelland, McNaughton, & O'Reilly, 1995; McClelland & Rogers, 2003; see also J. R. Anderson & Labiere, 2003) – and whatever the ultimate implications of these models for the philosophical issues concerning functionalism (e.g. Bechtel & Abrahamsen, 2002) – these models *as a class* provided important insights regarding how some of the dynamic and constructive properties of human learning and memory, both the strengths and the weaknesses, might emerge naturally from the basic character of the wetware, and provided solutions to various conundrums that arose from the computer metaphor. These include the spatial metaphor for storage (e.g. Roediger, 1980), which implausibly tends to imply serial memory search processes, and can result in the circular assumption that we know what we are seeking from memory and where it is stored before we retrieve it. Connectionist models show explicitly how multiple memory records can be searched simultaneously, and by doing so naturally incorporate a retrieval principle which we have called *selective resonance* (Richardson-Klavehn & Bjork, 2002; see also Eysenck, 1979; Fisher & Craik, 1977; Lockhart, 2002; Nairne, 2002; Ratcliff, 1978). That is, in order for successful retrieval of specific information to occur, stimuli (cues) in the retrieval environment must not only cause sympathetic resonance in relevant memory records (i.e. the *encoding specificity principle*, and accompanying *general abstract processing system framework*; e.g. Tulving, 1983, 2001), but must also fail to cause sympathetic resonance (or *homophony*; Semon, 1923) in irrelevant memory records (i.e. the *cue-overload principle*; e.g. Watkins & Watkins, 1975; see also Nairne, 2002).

More generally, connectionist models incorporate the notion of memory as a 'filter' between inputs and outputs (e.g. Sejnowski, 1981), which does away with the implausible notion that learning (encoding) involves copying features of stimuli into memory (i.e. memory traces are no more likely to be copies of the information they represent than are perceptual representations), and makes it possible to see how learning and memory capabilities may have evolved hand in hand with perceptual capabilities (e.g. J. A. Anderson & Hinton, 1981; Sejnowski & Paulsen, 2006; but see also Craik, 2002; Tulving, 2001, for further discussion of the relationship between perception and memory). They also raise fruitful questions about the level of analysis that may need to be invoked in theories of learning and memory to provide explanations, rather than simply redescriptions, of certain fundamental processes, such as interference and forgetting, a comprehensive theory of which has proved elusive (e.g. Crowder, 1976; see also M. C. Anderson, 2003). Explaining such dynamic properties requires an understanding of how memory representations interact with each other during encoding, storage, and retrieval, which ultimately may require a lower level of theoretical analysis than that employed in traditional information-processing approaches (e.g. J. A. Anderson & Hinton, 1981). These conclusions about insights from the connectionist approach follow whether or not one believes that this approach will ultimately assist in bridging the massive gap between our knowledge of learning and memory at the functional and brain-systems levels and at the cellular and molecular levels (e.g. Kandel, 2001; Squire & Kandel, 1999). We note, nevertheless, that the study of oscillations and interareal oscillatory synchrony in electrophysiological data, combined with connectionist modelling of such phenomena, appears to have considerable promise in bridging these levels (e.g. Buzsáki, 1996; Buzsáki & Draguhn, 2004; Düzel, Richardson-Klavehn et al., 2005; Hasselmo & McCelland, 1999; Laughlin & Sejnowski, 2003; Paulsen & Sejnowski, 2000; Sejnowski & Paulsen, 2006; Varela et al., 2001; see also the first part of the next main section of this chapter).

In summary, learning and memory appears to provide a particularly good example of the shortcomings of a purely functionalist scientific approach. From an evolutionary neurobiological perspective – and with a concurrent appreciation of the dynamic and constructive properties of learning and memory – it seems reasonable to argue that scientific understanding of the functioning of the wetware at the appropriate level or levels of description is likely to go hand in hand with scientific understanding of the functional properties of our learning and memory capabilities, and one might argue that the experience of the last hundred years or so has already taught us this lesson. If so, neuroimaging (defined broadly, as in the Introduction, to include both haemodynamic and electrophysiological techniques) clearly has a critical role to play, along with other neurobiological methods. We next consider two examples where neuroimaging research appears to have provided important information concerning human learning and memory function that could not easily have been provided by other methods, such as neuropsychological or purely behavioural research.

Observing the 'unobservable'

Imaging learning 1: Encoding processes

Here we return to Crowder's (1976) observation, noted in the Introduction, that the changes in the human brain that constitute learning cannot be observed directly. In relation to this observation, a particular theme running through this volume as a whole is that neuroimaging methods may provide 'windows on the mind' that cannot be provided by behavioural data or by introspection or self-report measures. Craik (2002; see also Tulving, 2001), for example, draws attention to the possibility that critical learning and memory encoding processes may be 'cognitively silent' (p. 315). Here he means that, although encoding involves laying down a record of ongoing psychological and presumably neural processing activity (e.g. Kolers & Roediger, 1984; Roediger, Weldon, & Challis, 1989), establishing that record in the brain may require additional neural encoding or consolidation processes that are not easily amenable to behavioural or introspective observation, as testified by the performance of amnesic patients (e.g. with medial temporal lobe damage), whose ongoing information processing can be similar to that of normal people, but who simply cannot lay down a record of that processing that is of sufficient quality to support later conscious recollection (e.g. Mayes, 2000). These putative cognitively silent encoding processes seem to qualify as functionally relevant.

A particular contribution of neuroimaging research on learning and memory has been to begin to provide a window on such processes, via paradigms in which brain activity during encoding, or during a learning phase in which encoded information is practised (or sometimes, avoided; see the next subsection of this chapter), is separated on the basis of the later memory fate of the information. Such research has already provided striking findings that could not easily be provided by purely behavioural research. For example, it has been possible to separate encoding processes associated with later conscious recollection of the encoding episode from encoding processes associated with later perceptual-lexical repetition priming (Düzel, Richardson-Klavehn et al., 2005; Schott, Richardson-Klavehn et al., 2006; Schott, Richardson-Klavehn et al., 2002), both in space and time. In haemodynamic measurements (Schott, Richardson-Klavehn et al., 2006; see also Paller et al., this volume) the typical encoding-related (including hippocampal) activations appear to be specific for later conscious recollection and not priming, whereas activity predicting later priming occurs in ventral visual stream areas implicated in stimulus identification that are very similar (as revealed by inclusive masking analysis) to the areas that show priming-related deactivations at retrieval (Schott, Henson, Richardson-Klavehn *et al.*, 2005; for a review, see Schacter *et al.*, 2007).

Strikingly, some encoding processes associated with later priming have been found, via electrophysiological (MEG) measurements, to occur during the early time window of stimulus identification itself (within 250 ms after stimulus presentation), and have been source-localized to similar ventral visual stream areas as implicated by the fMRI data (Düzel *et al.*, 2005). Some of these electrophysiological activity differences, such as changes in the synchrony patterns of alpha (~10 Hz) oscillations across ventral visual stream areas, also occur prior to stimulus presentation, suggesting a critical role of top-down attentional control in facilitating Hebbian learning (for explanation, see McClelland, 2000; Paulsen & Sejnowski, 2000; Squire & Kandel, 1999) in stimulus identification networks, by inducing more coordinated and systematic responding to stimulus features (thus reducing 'noise' in the system). Such pre-stimulus brain-activity differences also counter explanations in terms of item-selection artefacts. Counterintuitive aspects of these findings, namely that priming is predicted by reduced rather than increased haemo-dynamic responses in ventral visual stream areas (Schott, Richardson-Klavehn *et al.*, 2006), as well as reductions in the amplitude of beta and gamma (> 20 Hz) oscillations source-localized to similar ventral visual stream areas with MEG (Düzel *et al.*, 2005), have suggested new hypotheses concerning differences between processes underlying priming at encoding and retrieval (Schott, Richardson-Klavehn *et al.*, 2006), which would not have been entertained on the basis of behavioural data alone, and which provide a basis for more specific tests for similarities and differences between the properties of encoding processes for priming and for conscious recollection. More generally, the electrophysio-logical findings regarding encoding processes for priming and for conscious recollection (Düzel *et al.*, 2005; Schott *et al.*, 2002) point up the value of a multimodal imaging approach in which the time (and increasing spatial) resolution of electrophysiological data complements the spatial resolution of haemodynamic data.

At a theoretical level the results appear relevant to non-abstractionist views of percep-tual-lexical priming as depending on memory traces for the same whole prior processing episodes that support conscious recollection (e.g. Jacoby, 1983a, 1983b), because, at least at face value, one might then only expect neural dissociations between priming and conscious recollection at retrieval, but not at encoding. The apparent role of the medial temporal lobe in encoding selectively for later conscious recollection, and the apparent instantiation of both encoding and retrieval processes for priming within stimulus iden-tification areas, with the encoding processes occurring in part during the time window of stimulus identification itself, both appear to create difficulties for this position, as well as some other unitary approaches. At very least, they provide challenging data for unitary learning and memory theorists to explain (see Baddeley, 2003, and our discussions of memory systems and of dissociation data in the next two main sections of this chapter). On the other hand, the results appear to fit in well with multiple systems views that attribute perceptual-lexical priming to the operation of encapsulated perceptual representation systems (e.g. Tulving & Schacter, 1990).

A critical caveat is that memory-related activity changes localized to particular brain regions (e.g. in the case of priming, the ventral visual stream) do not necessarily indicate that these regions are themselves storage sites for the relevant memory records. Addressing this problem represents a general challenge for neuroimaging research on learning and memory, and again points up the huge gap between knowledge at the functional and brain systems levels, and at the cellular and molecular levels, at least in humans (e.g. Kandel, 2001; Squire & Kandel, 1999). In the current context, it might be argued that the connectivity changes in the brain responsible for priming occur 'upstream' of the regions identified by Düzel et al. (2005) and Schott, Richardson-Klavehn et al. (2006), but that priming-related encoding activity was apparent in stimulus identification regions owing to the nature of the back-averaging procedure (i.e. because priming, at retrieval, depends on perceptual-lexical information). The relevant memory records might, therefore, encode a larger constellation of information, but exert their influence at retrieval via these 'modular' stimulus identification regions (e.g. Sherry & Schacter, 1987). Strangely (cf. Coltheart, 2006a; Harley, 2004a, 2004b; Page, 2006), consideration of this issue suggests that localizing learning-and-memory-related connectivity changes to particular anatomical structures or networks may turn out to be crucial in discriminating between functional theories of learning and memory (see also Humphreys & Price, 2001). That is, knowledge concerning the anatomy and functional role of particular brain regions, in addition to that currently provided by neuroimaging in humans, is important (see also Rugg, this volume).

Other recent electrophysiological findings have indicated that pre-stimulus brain-activity state is also critical for encoding processes that later support conscious recollection (e.g. Otten et al., 2006; Guderian, Schott, Richardson-Klavehn, & Düzel, under review; Düzel & Guderian, this volume). The spatial resolution of MEG data has allowed localization of some aspects of this pre-stimulus brain activity, as well as post-stimulus item-related brain activity, to the medial temporal lobe (Guderian et al., under review; Düzel & Guderian, this volume). Of particular interest here is the finding that a medial temporal lobe oscillatory brain state in the theta (~4 to ~7 Hz) frequency range predicts successful memory formation independent of the cognitive level of processing (deep vs. shallow) engaged during study of the to-be-remembered information. The latter findings may begin to provide a window on the cognitively silent and processing-independent encoding process for later conscious recollection hypothesized by Craik (2002) and Tulving (2001), and suggest, contrary to some assertions (Coltheart, 2006a), that neuroimaging research may well be able to distinguish aspects of memory encoding relating to ongoing cognitive processing from more specifically episodic-memory-related aspects of encoding. As a further example of this separation, Schott, Fenker, Zierhut, Heinze, Düzel, and Richardson-Klavehn (under review) have used psychophysiological interactions analysis of fMRI data (Friston et al., 1997) to demonstrate strikingly different connectivity patterns between hippocampus and neocortical regions during successful encoding under deep compared with under shallow study processing (see also Schott et al., 2002, for electrophysiological data showing a spatiotemporal dissociation between level of processing and episodic encoding success).

Imaging learning 2: Processes and consequences of retrieval avoidance

A further telling illustration of the value of neuroimaging data in illuminating mental processes is provided by research on *retrieval inhibition* (e.g. M. C. Anderson & Levy, 2007; M. C. Anderson & Spellman, 1995; Bjork, 1989). Here the theoretical concern is with dynamic processes that control interference from irrelevant, out-of-date, or otherwise undesirable (e.g. negative emotional) memories. As an aside, in reference to the discussion of the general character of human learning and memory in the previous main section of this chapter, it is worth noting that such inhibitory mechanisms would never have been suggested by the functionalist computer metaphor for learning and memory; rather, the need to consider such mechanisms arises from the natural susceptibility of our learning and memory processes to interference, which may be an intrinsic property of our highly parallel wetware architecture, and the fact that individual memories do not seem to be stored in discrete packets or locations but rather as patterns across distributed networks (e.g. J. A. Anderson & Hinton, 1981; Hasselmo & McClelland, 1999; Laughlin & Sejnowski, 2003; McClelland, 2000; McClelland & Goddard, 1996; McClelland *et al.*, 1995; Paulsen & Sejnowski, 2000; Squire & Kandel, 1999), as discussed in the previous main section of this chapter. Moreover, the notion of retrieval inhibition at the functional level is directly inspired by the well-known occurrence of inhibitory processes at the neurobiological level. One paradigm employed to study such inhibitory memory control processes involves asking participants, through repeated training, to learn to *avoid* retrieving previously learned information in the presence of cues that would normally remind them of that information. Under some circumstances, such avoidance in the presence of reminders can lead to that information later being less retrievable than it otherwise would be owing to the normal forgetting processes that are correlated with the passage of time (e.g. M. C. Anderson & Green, 2001; M. C. Anderson *et al.*, 2004).

What mental processes happen at the very time that experimental participants are learning to avoid retrieval that are responsible for the later forgetting fate of the avoided material? Because retrieval is being stopped during the avoidance training, there is no adequate behavioural index at the time of that training, and devising subjective (introspective) indices of whether, and how, retrieval has been avoided involves one in a mire of scientific problems. Instead, neuroimaging findings have begun to provide answers. Avoiding retrieval in the presence of reminders results in haemodynamic response increases in a number of brain regions implicated in cognitive control, including dorsolateral prefrontal cortex, ventrolateral prefrontal cortex, frontopolar cortex, and anterior cingulate cortex (M. C. Anderson *et al.*, 2004; Depue, Curran, & Banich, 2007). In contrast, haemodynamic activity in medial temporal lobe and visual representational regions is reduced (M. C. Anderson *et al.*, 2004; Depue *et al.*, 2007). The magnitude of the event-related-potential (ERP) correlate of recollection (e.g. Rugg, this volume) obtained from electroencephalography (EEG), a late left parietal voltage positivity, is also reduced during retrieval avoidance (Bergström, Velmans, de Fockert, & Richardson-Klavehn, 2007). These findings collectively indicate successful reduction of recollection via cognitive control, at the time at which avoidance of retrieval actually occurs. Indeed, Bergström *et al.* (2007) showed that recollection of previously successfully learned material can be reduced to the point where there is little difference in retrieval-related ERPs between avoiding retrieval of material previously successfully learned and attempting retrieval of material previously not successfully learned.

Such neuroimaging findings have also begun to provide a resolution of the issue of why avoiding retrieval in the presence of reminders sometimes produces later forgetting (e.g. M. C. Anderson & Green, 2001; M. C. Anderson *et al.*, 2004) and why it sometimes does not (e.g. Bergström *et al.*, 2007; Bulevich *et al.*, 2006; Hertel & Calcaterra, 2005). Critical here are the questions of what strategies participants employ to avoid retrieval, and of whether the later forgetting, if it occurs, is inhibitory (i.e. reflects suppression of the memory representation itself) or whether it reflects non-inhibitory mechanisms such as interference from competing memories. Avoiding retrieval might involve substituting alternative thoughts for the avoided memory (Hertel & Calcaterra, 2005), which would produce competing (interfering) memories at retrieval, rather than inhibiting the representation of the avoided memory itself. Bergström, de Fockert, and Richardson-Klavehn (under review) examined this issue by asking one randomly assigned group of participants to avoid retrieval by substituting alternative thoughts in the presence of reminders (thought substitution group), and another randomly assigned group to avoid retrieval by simply focusing on the reminder itself and keeping the to-be-avoided memory out of consciousness without substituting an alternative thought (thought suppression group). EEG was recorded during this training phase and, in the absence of behavioural or self-report measures of retrieval avoidance, provided a critical index of whether these different instructions actually created any difference at all in the strategies used by participants to avoid retrieval. That is, the null hypothesis that the avoidance strategies of the groups were identical despite different instructions predicts no difference in brain activity between the groups as indexed by ERPs time-locked to the presentation of the reminders during avoidance training. As it turned out, however, this null hypothesis of no difference in brain activity was clearly rejected, providing an example of the value of the kind of process-to-brain-activity inference, or forward inference, described by Henson (2005, 2006a, 2006b; see also Rugg, this volume).

Critically, the different retrieval avoidance strategies, as created by the avoidance-instruction manipulation and as indexed by the ERP data, also led to different later behavioural forgetting consequences. As shown in Figure 9.1 (top left panel), the thought substitution group later only showed forgetting when retrieval was cued with the same reminder as used during avoidance training, but not with a new reminder not used during training, suggesting that competing memories had been associated with the reminder used during avoidance training, creating later interference. In striking contrast, the thought suppression group showed forgetting with both previously used and new reminders, suggesting that the representations of the avoided memories themselves had been inhibited (see M. C. Anderson & Green, 2001; M. C. Anderson *et al.*, 2004).

Bergström *et al.* also used brain-activity-to-function inference, or reverse inference (Henson, 2005, 2006a; Poldrack, 2006; Rugg, this volume), to draw more specific conclusions about

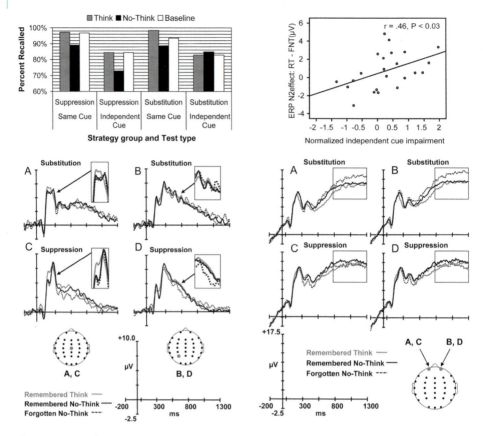

Figure 9.1 Data from Z. M. Bergström, J. de Fockert, and A. Richardson-Klavehn (under review). Top left panel: Final cued recall. Same-cue test: Word recall cued with the same associate cue used during the initial study phase. Independent-cue test: Word recall cued with a novel associate cue not used previously in the experiment. Think condition: Words that were recalled during the Think/No-Think training phase intervening between the study phase and the final test, in response to the associate cue used at study. No-Think condition: Words whose recall was avoided during the intervening Think/No-Think training phase, in the presence of the associate cue used at study. Baseline condition: Words initially studied but not cued in the intervening Think/No-Think training phase. Both thought suppression and thought substitution groups showed significant final recall impairment for No-Think items compared to Baseline items on the same-cue test, but only the thought suppression group showed a significant final recall impairment for No-Think items on the independent-cue test. Top right panel: Across-participants brain-behaviour correlation in the thought suppression group between the N2-like ERP effect recorded during the Think/No-Think training phase (average voltage difference between subsequently remembered Think items and subsequently forgotten No-Think items from 180 to 225 ms across the parietal sites P3, PZ, and P4) and the amount of subsequent inhibitory forgetting (normalized difference between Baseline and No-Think items) on the final independent-cue recall test. Bottom panels: ERPs recorded during the Think/No-Think training phase intervening between the study phase and the final cued recall tests. Data for No-Think items are separated by later forgetting fate on the final cued recall tests. The head-plots schematically depict the electrode locations, and the boxes within the figures emphasize the portions of the waveforms that are of principal interest. Bottom left panel: Grand average ERPs in the substitution group (A & B) and the suppression group (C & D) at the vertex (CZ; A & C) and at a left parietal site (P3; B & D). Bottom right panel: Grand average ERPs in the substitution group (A & B) and the suppression group (C & D) at left (A & C) and right (B & D) frontopolar sites.

the nature of the different strategies during avoidance training that led to these different types of later forgetting. The grand average ERP data are shown in the bottom two panels of Figure 9.1. An N2-like ERP effect related to strategy for avoiding retrieval (because it was similar for avoided material subsequently remembered and subsequently forgotten) was twice as large in the thought suppression group as in the thought substitution group (see Figure 9.1, bottom left panel), and the size of this N2-like strategy effect predicted the amount of subsequent inhibitory (i.e. cue-independent) forgetting of the avoided material across participants in the thought suppression group ($r = 0.46$, $p < .03$; Figure 9.1, top right panel). This N2-like strategy effect has spatial and temporal similarities with the N2 effects observed during stopping of overt motor acts (e.g. Kopp, Rist, & Mattler, 1996; Van Veen & Carter, 2002), although it emerged earlier and was somewhat smaller in magnitude than many motor-stopping N2 effects. Moreover, only the thought suppression group showed a reduction in the late left parietal ERP positivity related to conscious recollection (Bergström *et al.*, 2007; Rugg, this volume) for avoided material that was subsequently forgotten (see Figure 9.1, bottom left panel). Finally, the non-inhibitory forgetting in the thought substitution group was predicted by a right frontal slow shift during avoidance training (see Figure 9.1, bottom right panel) that resembles a frontal slow-shift that has been associated with selection among competing memories (Johansson *et al.*, 2006). These behavioural and ERP findings complement previous haemodynamic evidence linking stopping of overt actions and stopping of memory retrieval (e.g. M. C. Anderson *et al.*, 2004; see also Levy & M. C. Anderson, 2002), and provide further scientific evidence for voluntary memory suppression as proposed by Freud (1915/1957). Whether or not these particular theoretical interpretations stand the test of time, the findings just described illustrate more generally the considerable value of brain-activity measurements in learning paradigms in which measurements of overt behaviour are not feasible.

On the meaning of the term 'memory system': function, space, and content

Questions concerning the ability of neuroimaging research to elucidate cognitive theory are brought into sharp focus by the continued lively debate over whether learning and memory is a unitary entity, or whether there is heterogeneity in memory systems, as is assumed, e.g. by Ghahremani and Poldrack (this volume; see also Poldrack & Foerde, 2008) and Reber (this volume). Those who argue that the available behavioural, neuropsychological, and neuroimaging evidence fails to conclusively reject a unitary view of memory (see also Rajah & McIntosh, 2005) have used three connected strategies (e.g. Berry, Henson, & Shanks, 2006; Berry, Shanks, & Henson, 2006, 2008; Kinder & Shanks, 2001, 2003; Ostergaard & Jernigan, 1993; Newell, Lagnado, & Shanks, 2007; Plaut, 1995, 2003; Speekenbrink, Channon, & Shanks, 2008). The first is to question the existing evidence of dissociations between different memory measures, a substantial proportion of which, in the learning and memory area, consists of single dissociations (i.e. cases where a variable, such as a comparison of patients and control participants, or a comparison of one study condition with another, influences performance on one memory test but not another), on the basis that the null hypothesis has been accepted for one of the tests, which could simply reflect a lack of statistical power (and indeed power is often low in small sample neuropsychological studies; see Ostergaard & Jernigan, 1993; Dunn, 2003). The second is to show with new data that such dissociations are not replicable, i.e. that one memory test simply shows a larger effect of the relevant variable than the other memory test. The third is to show formally that a unitary learning and memory model can simulate some of the dissociations that do exist (e.g. greater deficits of brain-damaged patients on one learning and memory test compared with another, and sometimes double dissociations across patient groups and tests). Finally, some memory systems theorists have themselves argued that the neuropsychological evidence does not allow unambiguous conclusions because the memory measures compared have often been insufficiently matched, either at encoding, retrieval, or both (Ryan & Cohen, 2003; see also Reingold, 2003).

A furthermore general criticism of the multiple-memory-systems approach is that the functional characteristics of the putative differentiable memory systems are poorly specified (e.g. Weldon, 1999). Systems theorists have responded by arguing that their approach naturally accounts for a wider range of behavioural, neuropsychological, and neuroimaging data than do unitary approaches, and that unitary approaches, especially modelling approaches, often introduce 'unnatural' assumptions or devices in order to account for neuropsychological data, especially double dissociations (e.g. Poldrack & Foerde, 2008). Another kind of response is that the memory-systems approach is a pretheoretical orientation (i.e. a philosophy of doing science), thus questioning the relevance of all the concerns just reviewed (e.g. Tulving, 2000, 2001). Under this perspective, the psychology of learning and memory is simply redefined as being concerned with the relevant mind/ brain systems and how they interact to influence behaviour (e.g. Buchsbaum & D'Esposito, this volume; Tulving, 2001; see also Kim & Baxter, 2001; Kesner & Rogers, 2004; Mizumori *et al.*, 2004; Squire, 2004; Squire & Kandel, 1999).

We suspect we are not alone in finding neither of these kinds of response fully satisfying. The former kind of response, that the memory systems approach naturally accounts for a wider range of data than unitary approaches, invites the rejoinder that any theory incorporating more constructs is bound to account for a wider range of data (e.g. Richardson-Klavehn & Bjork, 1988), especially if the constructs are not well specified (e.g. J. R. Anderson, 1978, 1985; Weldon, 1999). The latter, more philosophical, kind of response demonstrates that the memory-systems debate is a microcosm of the more general debates concerning functionalism and the cognition/brain relationship discussed in the second main section of this chapter. Extending the argument that we made there, we see no reason why it should not be possible to develop theories that are in tune with or inspired by neurobiology, while also providing detailed specifications of functional properties that would satisfy experimental psychologists in the functional information-processing tradition (e.g. as argued by J. A. Anderson & Hinton, 1981; see also Shallice, 2003).

In considering the implications of attempting such a theoretical synthesis, it is worth referring back to a statement of the scientific task from an information-processing perspective: 'Any general theory of memory must specify at least four things: how information is represented, the type of information that is stored and retrieved, the nature of the storage and retrieval operations, and the format of the store' (Murdock, 1982, p. 610). This statement, when applied to the multiple-memory-systems issue, suggests a multiplicity of aspects in which the hypothetical memory systems might differ with respect to their functional properties alone, and calls for a precise specification from multiple systems theorists of what the functional differences are. There is, additionally, the dimension of *spatiality*, under the reasonable assumption that learning and memory processes are instantiated in the brain. Sherry and Schacter (1987) clearly had such issues in mind when they provided one of the most detailed analyses to date of the meaning of the claim that there are multiple memory systems. Here, they speak of information-processing modules, as postulated by Fodor (1983), such as might be involved in perceptual and language processing:

> One possibility is that all modules output to a common memory system and gain access to this information via a common retrieval mechanism. This is a relatively clear case of a unitary memory system…A second possibility is that each module has its own memory system but that each of these module-specific memories operates according to the same rules. We would not call this state of affairs multiple memory systems either…There is a third possibility, however, that each module has its own acquisition, retention, and retrieval processes and that the rules of operation of these processes differ across modules. According to our usage of the term, only here do we find multiple memory systems (p. 441).

In terms of their analysis, it is apparent that the characteristics of the hypothesized memory systems still await considerable clarification some 20 years later: It remains to be demonstrated that there are spatially separated memory systems in the brain that, functionally, obey completely different rules of operation. For example, the same formally described encoding, storage, and/or retrieval process(es) could conceivably be instantiated at different locations in the brain (Henson, 2005; Richardson-Klavehn, 1986; Sherry & Schacter, 1987) or could operate on different informational content, which in many cases, owing to the known content-specialisation of certain brain regions, would be expected to be accompanied by spatial differences in the brain (Sherry & Schacter, 1987; Khader & Rösler, this volume, Rugg, this volume). Indeed, the reality of such possibilities is pointed up by the data presented by Büchel (this volume), which suggest that learning-related brain-activity changes described by a Rescorla-Wagner feedback-processing rule are instantiated in amygdala/hippocampus and in fusiform face area, albeit with different learning-rate parameter values for the former and latter areas.

As another example, owing to the wetware properties of the brain, selective-resonance-like processes (e.g. J. A. Anderson & Hinton, 1981; Eysenck, 1979; Nairne, 2002; Ratcliff, 1978; Richardson-Klavehn & Bjork, 2002) might play a role in many different forms of memory retrieval, that may be instantiated in different anatomical structures or different brain networks. The notion that memory encoding processes involve laying down a record of ongoing cognitive processing activity at the time of encoding (e.g. Kolers &

Roediger, 1984; Roediger *et al.*, 1989), whether, e.g., for verbal information, pictorial information, or whether processing is shallow or deep, suggests again that formally similar encoding processes might be instantiated at different anatomical locations or in different brain networks. Furthermore, the notion that encoding of new information is intimately related to retrieval of pre-existing information, as pointed up by the levels-of-processing approach to human learning and memory (e.g. Craik, 2002; Richardson-Klavehn & Bjork, 2002; Richardson-Klavehn, Gardiner, & Ramponi, 2002; see also Squire, 2007), suggests that selective-resonance-like processes may be involved in some aspects of encoding processes as well as retrieval processes (but see also Tulving, 2001). As a final example, recent research has suggested that the phenomenon of retrieval induced forgetting – the dynamic functional property whereby retrieval of particular information causes forgetting of other information (see the second and third main sections of this chapter) – may cut across widely different manifestations of memory, such as memory for episodic information, and memory for lexical and semantic information (e.g. Bäuml, 2002; Johnson & M. C. Anderson, 2004; Levy *et al.*, 2007; Norman *et al.*, 2007), thus prompting a search for the common functional mechanisms involved (e.g. Norman *et al.*, 2007; see also Rajah & McIntosh, 2005).

This discussion suggests that the theoretical enterprise is a highly complex one, one conception of which is that we must specify a point in a four (or more) dimensional space in which the formal properties of encoding, storage, and retrieval processes can be either homogeneous or heterogeneous, with a further dimension being whether these processes are instantiated in the same or different anatomical locations or by different functional-anatomical networks (Henson, 2005; Richardson-Klavehn, 1986; Sherry & Schacter, 1987; Weldon, 1999). The situation becomes even more complex when one considers that encoding, storage, and retrieval processes may not simply be formally homogeneous vs. heterogeneous, but rather might share some functional components (e.g. selective resonance properties, dynamic forgetting processes, etc.), while differing in other critical aspects (e.g. decision and monitoring processes) at other levels of theoretical description (e.g. J. A. Anderson & Hinton, 1981; Henson, 2005).[1]

The *components of processing* point of view put forward as a resolution of the unitary vs. multiple systems debate captures some of these points regarding the complexity of the enterprise, by arguing that some processes are common to different manifestations of learning and memory, and others different across these manifestations (e.g. Roediger,

---

[1] The analysis presented here assumes for the sake of argument that theoretical decisions about encoding processes, memory representations, and retrieval processes could at some level of analysis be orthogonal. This orthogonality likely does not hold even at the level of traditional information-processing theory (Palmer, 1978; J. R. Anderson, 1978). Retrieval processes, e.g., to some extent specify the structure of their representational inputs (J. R. Anderson, 1978). Further, in connectionist approaches, there are strong connections between certain theoretical assumptions regarding encoding, storage, and retrieval processes (e.g., J. A. Anderson & Hinton, 1981; McClelland, 2000). The point of the analysis is simply to make clear that multiple-memory-systems theories should be able to specify more precisely how encoding processes, storage processes, and retrieval processes differ or do not differ across hypothetical memory systems.

Buckner, & McDermott, 1999; Ramponi, Richardson-Klavehn, & Gardiner, 2004, 2007; see also Chater, 2003; Moscovitch, 1994, 2000). These complexity issues are also addressed in a more general way by Henson (2005) in relation to neuroimaging, in his discussion of different possible function-to-brain-structure mappings at different levels of theoretical description (see also Rugg, this volume). In the context of all these complexities, the view of unitary learning and memory theorists – that on the basis of parsimony one should not reject unitary models until there is a need to do so on the basis of falsifying evidence – does appear to have some considerable force (e.g. Berry *et al.*, 2008; see also Brown & Lamberts, 2003). A model-testing approach in which additional well-specified theoretical constructs are only added when there is an absolute need to do so in order to fit the data would be one approach to achieving the requisite level of theoretical specificity (e.g. Berry *et al.*, 2008; Brown & Lamberts, 2003; Coltheart & Davies, 2003; see also McClelland, 2000; McClelland & Goddard, 1996; and McClelland *et al.*, 1995 for this type of approach to solving the problem of catastrophic interference in connectionist networks).

We address the issue of whether extant data already require the rejection of unitary functional models in the next main section of this chapter. Here we note that a particular problem that may emerge when heterogeneity of representations and/or processes is incorporated into more formal models is that models may cease to be identifiably different owing to the number of free parameters – at least when they are tested only against behavioural data (e.g. J. R. Anderson, 1978, 1985). In this situation, analysis of how such models, or classes of models, might be realized in the structures and networks of the brain may play an increasingly critical role in theory development (e.g. J. R. Anderson & Lebiere, 2003; Squire, 2004). As Rugg (this volume) points out, if characterizations of particular neural structures are available on an independent basis (e.g. anatomical characterizations of internal structure, and of connectivity with other structures), which suggest that these structures are constrained to implement formally different computational processes, and do not just differ in the informational content of their processing, and if these structures also turn out to be differentially involved in different, dissociable, manifestations of learning and memory, it might be possible to make theoretical progress at both functional and neural levels. In short, knowledge about the brain is of critical importance (Rugg, this volume).

More generally, an approach based on the evolution of our functional neuroanatomy would suggest that it is likely that different brain systems have evolved at different times to deal with retention of different types (e.g. procedural learning and priming vs. conscious recollection of personal episodes), and that these may have some different functional properties (e.g. McClelland, 2000; McClelland & Goddard, 1996; McClelland *et al.*, 1995; Sherry & Schacter, 1987; Tulving, 1983, 2000), but that some functional properties may have been conserved across these systems, as suggested by the components-of-processing perspective just discussed (e.g. Roediger *et al.*, 1999; see also McClelland, 2000; McClelland & Goddard, 1996; McClelland *et al.*, 1995). The prospect of an interplay of this evolutionary neurobiological perspective with the functional model-testing perspective (e.g. Berry *et al.*, 2008; Brown & Lamberts, 2003; Coltheart &

Davies, 2003) in the context of neuroimaging and neuropsychological data is an exciting one, and we suspect that the impact of such a theoretical synthesis will be that the unitary versus multiple-memory-systems debate will dissolve in the face of theories that are not only better specified but also more encompassing. The scientific task, however, remains formidable. We next consider some empirical strategies for progressing with that task.

Dissociations in context

The critical importance of reversed associations

The concept of *dissociation* between different memory measures (e.g. Richardson-Klavehn & Bjork, 1988) has become central to modern learning and memory research, including neuroimaging research (e.g. Henson, 2005; 2006a, 2006b; Ghahremani & Poldrack, this volume; Reber, this volume; Rugg, this volume). There has been much debate about whether behavioural, neuropsychological, and neuroimaging dissociations are able to provide conclusive evidence for or against particular functional theories (e.g. Baddeley, 2003; Brown & Lamberts, 2003; Bullinaria & Chater, 1995; Coltheart & Davis, 2003; Chater, 2003; Dunn, 2003; Dunn & Kirsner, 2003; Humphreys & Price, 2001; Juola, 2003; McCloskey, 2003; Olton, 1989; Plaut, 1995, 2003; Reingold, 2003; Ryan & Cohen, 2003; Shallice, 1988, 2003; Van Orden & Kloos, 2003; Van Orden *et al.*, 2001; see also the citations in regard to the memory systems debate in the previous main section of this chapter).[2]

Clear progress appears to have been made with the introduction of the concept of *reversed association* (e.g. Dunn, 2003; Dunn & Kirsner, 1988), which means, at a behavioural level, that when Test 1 and Test 2 show both a double dissociation (i.e. a crossover interaction or negative association) and a parallel effect (i.e. a positive association) within the same experiment, it is impossible to construct a monotonic function relating the efficiency of a single cognitive process (or resource; see Shallice, 1988, 2003) to performance in the two tests. Either pattern taken on its own would admit such a monotonic function. That is, the crossover interaction can be explained by assuming that process efficiency is monotonically positively related to performance in Test 1 and monotonically negatively related to performance in Test 2, and the parallel effect can be explained by assuming that

---

[2] Here we do not discuss more general claims that dissociation data can never address the issue of homogeneity versus heterogeneity of higher mental representations and/or processes (e.g., Uttal, 2001; Van Orden & Kloos, 2003; Van Orden & Paap, 1997; Van Orden *et al.*, 2001), which rely on questioning the assumption of pure insertion that underlies the dissociation approach in behavioural, neuropsychological and neuroimaging research and the assumption of some degree of systematicity in function-to-brain-structure and function-to-brain-activity mapping in neuropsychological and neuroimaging research. Such claims would appear to make scientific investigation using conventional experimental methods impossible. By contrast, conventional experimental investigation of complex dynamical systems appears to be eminently possible, as illustrated by successes in the physical and biological sciences. For further discussion see Bechtel (2002), Henson (2005, 2006a, 2006b) and Poldrack (2006).

process efficiency is monotonically positively related to performance in both tests. One cannot, however, have it both ways unless one violates the fundamental assumption of monotonicity of measurement, and thus when a statistically significant reversed association occurs, it appears that one must reject a single-process model.[3]

Henson (2005, 2006a) extends this logic to the demonstration of qualitative rather than quantitative differences in brain activity between different experimental conditions during the use of function-to-brain-activity (forward) inference for haemodynamic imaging, whereby the activity in two different brain regions is treated as analogous to behaviour in two different tests. A contrast between two experimental conditions that are hypothesized to differ in a particular functional aspect must yield a crossover interaction (i.e. a negative relationship) between activity in the two different brain regions; in the same experiment, both brain regions must display an increase in activity (i.e. a positive relationship) as a function of an experimental contrast (such as the contrast of each experimental condition against a fixation baseline). This pattern makes it less likely that activity in the two regions is simply inversely related as a function of the efficiency of a unitary functional process (e.g. via reciprocal inhibitory connections between the two regions). This approach appears to have considerable promise, especially when the two brain regions involved might be expected to implement different functions based on independent neural, especially neuroanatomical, evidence regarding internal structure, and connectivity (e.g. Humphreys & Price, 2001; Rugg, this volume; see also the previous main section of this chapter).

Here we note additionally that the theoretical value of reversed associations for learning and memory research – as we believe is also the case for simple dissociations or simple associations (see the next subsection) – depends very much on the *context* in which they occur (i.e. the particular variables that produce the dissociation and association, and their relation to theory). Our argument departs from the observation that the occurrence of a reversed association, while providing useful information from a measurement point of view (e.g. Dunn, 2003), does not in and of itself give information about the nature of the two cognitive processes that it necessitates. Such inferences must be made within the context of the particular experiment, dependent on the particular variables studied and their theoretical motivation (see also Henson, 2005, 2006a; Rugg, this volume; Shallice, 1988; Tulving, 1985). One can, e.g. think of behavioural reversed associations that are trivial theoretically. Suppose, e.g. that there are two patient groups who display a double dissociation. That is, Patient Group A is impaired on Memory Test 1 but not on Memory Test 2, compared its matched normal control group. Group B is impaired on Memory Test 2 but not on Memory Test 1, again compared to its matched normal control group. Now suppose that one half of each patient group, and one half of each of the control groups, is visually impaired, or has an impairment in motor responding, which impairs

---

[3] Here we gloss over the possibility that monotonicity might be violated in some cases, as, e.g., in the case of the Yerkes-Dodson law, which postulates an inverted U-shaped function relating arousal to performance. With regard to learning and memory processes, monotonicity appears to be a reasonable working assumption.

performance on both Memory Test 1 and Memory Test 2 for these halves of all four groups compared with the other halves of all four groups. The double dissociation pattern is therefore reproduced at two different levels of overall test performance, and this parallel effect (positive association) superimposed on the double dissociation (negative association) thus constitutes a reversed association. That result would tell us that performances in the tests are not always monotonically negatively correlated with each other, and not always monotonically positively correlated with each other, which of course is valuable measurement information (e.g. Dunn, 2003). But, from a theoretical viewpoint, such a pattern would tell us almost nothing, because the processes producing the parallel effect are too far removed (cognitively too far 'upstream' or 'downstream') from the memory processes of interest in regard to the double dissociation. We use the term *cognitive closeness* to describe the theoretical relationship between the variables that produce the double dissociation and the parallel effect, which needs to obtain in order to make the reversed association theoretically informative.

Similar arguments concerning cognitive closeness appear to apply to the learning and memory processes producing the double dissociations which are a necessary precondition for observing reversed associations. The criticism that unitary learning and memory modeling approaches resort to 'unnatural' devices in order to account for neuropsychological double dissociations (Poldrack & Foerde, 2008) can be reinterpreted as the criticism that the hypothetical processes producing one 'half' of the double dissociation are not cognitively close enough to those producing the other 'half' of the double dissociation to be theoretically convincing (e.g. one half of the dissociation may be produced by memory processes within these models, the other half by perceptual processes; see, e.g. Kinder & Shanks, 2001, 2003).

Our argument concerning cognitive closeness can be extended to neuroimaging reversed associations. Henson's (2005, 2006a) reversed association requirement for demonstrating a qualitative difference in brain activity appears, on consideration, to be necessary but not sufficient to ground theoretical claims of multiple learning and memory processes. For example, two brain regions could be reciprocally interconnected as a function of a single learning and memory process, thus producing a double dissociation in a comparison of two experimental conditions, but these two brain regions could both be activated in the same direction by input from visual or auditory identification regions in comparison with a fixation baseline – which might occur if the two memory-related brain regions both receive input from sensory-perceptual areas via independent parallel connections – thus producing the required reversed association. One might, therefore, introduce the additional requirement that the experimental or participant variables producing the neuroimaging reversed association are both variables that, under the null hypothesis of a single learning and memory process, would lead to a positive relationship between activity in the two regions, or to a negative relationship between activity in the two regions, but not to both positive and negative relationships. That is, in the terms introduced here, the variable producing the association across regions must be cognitively close to the variable producing the double dissociation across regions.

The requirement to ground claims of multiple learning and memory processes on theoretically informative reversed associations is an ambitious one, and it largely remains to be seen to what extent reversed associations can be demonstrated, especially in neuroimaging research, in which the relevant comparisons and statistical analyses have as yet rarely been reported (Henson, 2005, 2006a). It also largely remains to be seen how this approach can be applied to the activity of networks of brain regions (Henson, 2006a), and to electrophysiological data (Mecklinger & Jäger, this volume; Paller *et al.*, this volume; Rugg, this volume). There might also be limitations to the underlying working assumption that regional brain activity is monotonically related to cognitive process (or resource) efficiency and/or to behavioural performance (e.g. Henson, 2005, 2006a; Shallice, 2003; see also our Footnote 3). The empirical strategy of seeking reversed associations, however, appears particularly relevant to recent hypotheses that multiple memory systems in the brain compete to influence behaviour (e.g. Kim & Baxter, 2001; Kesner & Rogers, 2004; Mizumori *et al.*, 2004; see also Ghahremani & Poldrack, this volume; Poldrack & Foerde, 2008; Reber, this volume), because such views might predict inverse relationships between activity in the competing brain systems, which prima facie might be consistent with multiple brain systems implementing a unitary psychological function. A particular challenge in this respect is incorporating sufficient experimental conditions within the time constraints of neuroimaging experiments in order to be able to demonstrate theoretically informative reversed associations.

Theoretically informative reversed associations in research using purely behavioural dependent measures are also as yet uncommon in the literature, but some such data patterns have already been observed (see also Dunn & Kirsner, 1988). Richardson-Klavehn *et al.* (1999), e.g. showed such a reversed association by contrasting intentional and incidental word-stem completion tests that differed only in that, in the former test, participants were instructed to try to complete stems with previously studied words, and in the latter test, participants were instructed to complete stems with the first words coming to mind. The word-stem test cues corresponded to both studied and non-studied words, and the constitution of the test list in terms of stimuli and sequence was identical across groups. Prior to this test, words were studied under three conditions. Participants either generated words from incomplete sentences together with the first letter of each of the target words, which virtually guaranteed successful generation, and said the target words aloud (Generate condition), read visually presented target words and made a judgment as to the pleasantness of each word's meaning (Read-Semantic condition), or read visually presented target words and counted the number of syllables that each word contained (Read-Phonemic condition). Study condition was manipulated within subjects within each test group, with a counterbalanced order, and the order of the cues corresponding to the three types of studied words within the test list, as well as of the cues corresponding to non-studied words, was randomized.

The results are shown in Figure 9.2, in which priming in the incidental test group (i.e. the likelihood of producing target words in the incidental test for stems corresponding to studied words minus the corresponding likelihood for stems corresponding to non-studied target

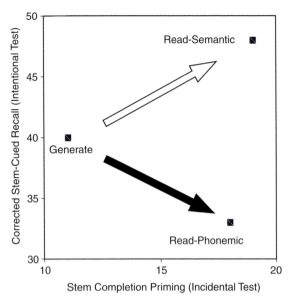

Figure 9.2 A reversed association between memory tests presenting identical word-stem retrieval cues, and differing only in instructions to the two participant groups (data from Table 1 of A. Richardson-Klavehn, A. J. B. Clarke, & J. M. Gardiner (1999), *Consciousness and Cognition, 8*, 271–284). Percentage stem-cued recall, corrected for baseline guessing, in the intentional test group is plotted against percentage priming in the incidental test group (following Dunn & Kirsner, 1988). Study condition (Generate, Read-Phonemic, Read-Semantic) was manipulated within subjects within each test group. The positive association between the tests is indicated by the unfilled arrow; the negative association between the tests is indicated by the filled arrow. All differences between study conditions within each test were statistically significant, except for the difference in priming between the Read-Semantic (19%) and Read-Phonemic conditions (18%) in the incidental test. Furthermore, significant priming was observed compared to the non-studied baseline in all study conditions in the incidental test, and stem-cued recall was significantly above the guessing baseline in all study conditions in the intentional test. The same reversed association pattern occurs when data uncorrected for baseline performance are plotted (because the baseline correction amounts to subtracting a constant value for non-studied items from the values for studied items within each test), and when test performance in the Generate condition is not conditionalized on successful generation at study (conditionalized data are shown).

words) is plotted against corrected cued recall in the intentional test group (i.e. the likelihood of responding with studied target words minus the likelihood of guessing with non-studied target words). This way of depicting the data was advocated by Dunn and Kirsner (1988). The critical data pattern for current purposes is that the Generate condition produced better performance than the Read-Phonemic condition in the intentional test, but worse performance than the Read-Phonemic condition in the incidental test (i.e. a double dissociation or negative association indicated by the filled arrow in Figure 9 .2), and that the Read-Semantic condition produced better performance than the Generate condition in both tests (i.e. a parallel effect or positive association indicated by the unfilled arrow in Figure 9.2). It therefore appears impossible to construct a monotonically positive or a monotonically negative function relating the efficiency of a single memory process to performance in the two tests, even though they presented identical physical retrieval cues and differed only in the instructions to participants (*cf.* Ryan & Cohen, 2003). The experiment also fulfils the cognitive closeness requirement that the processes engaged by the study conditions were relevant to memory in a theoretically interesting way (see also Richardson-Klavehn, Lee, Joubran, & Bjork, 1994, for a further example of a theoretically interesting, but less clear-cut, reversed association, between perceptual identification priming and recognition memory). From a formal standpoint, these results appear to present a serious challenge to single-system theories postulating that priming and intentional test performance depend on the same underlying memory representations (e.g. Berry, Henson *et al.*, 2006; Berry, Shanks *et al.*, 2006, 2008), because it is by no means clear how different means of access to the same representations would cause the ordinal rearrangement of the means of some study conditions, but not others, as a function only of a manipulation of test instructions.

Why did the data pattern displayed in Figure 9.2 occur? Our theoretical interpretation is that the intentional test engaged controlled retrieval, which benefits from prior processing of semantic information, thus producing advantages for the Generate and Read-Semantic study conditions over the Read-Phonemic condition in that test. By contrast, priming in the incidental test was relatively insensitive to prior processing of semantic information (as indicated by the very similar priming for the Read-Semantic and Read-Phonemic conditions), but rather benefited from match in sensory modality between study and test, thus producing priming advantages for the Read-Semantic and Read-Phonemic conditions over the Generate condition in that test (although the generate condition did produce significant priming).[4]

The dissociations of the incidental test from the intentional test (see the next subsection for further discussion) also show that priming in the incidental test primarily reflected involuntary or unintentional memory retrieval, given that the tests had identical physical retrieval cues, and differed only in instructions (by the logic of the *retrieval intentionality criterion*; Schacter, Bowers, & Booker, 1989; see also Richardson-Klavehn & Gardiner, 1998). Critically, however, the modality-match effect was also evident in the intentional test, as evidenced by the advantage of the Read-Semantic over the Generate condition in that test. The conclusion is that performance in the intentional test reflected a mix of controlled retrieval and stimulus-driven automatic retrieval or priming (see also Richardson-Klavehn & Gardiner, 1996; Richardson-Klavehn *et al.*, 2002). The intentional

---

[4] In this particular experiment, the test cues (i.e., word stems) were always visually presented, raising the possible objection that the effect of study modality did not concern perceptual match between study and test stimuli, but rather an overall modality effect. Here it is important to note that other research using incidental auditory stem-completion tests has clearly established that modality effects relate to match between study and test stimuli, because such tests, in contrast to visual tests, show advantages for auditory over visual study presentation (e.g., Schacter & Church, 1992).

test participants were instructed not to guess, and their observed likelihood of guessing with unstudied target words was fairly low (11%). Thus, these data, along with other data (Craik, Moscovitch, & McDowd, 1994; Gardiner, Ramponi, & Richardson-Klavehn, 1999; Richardson-Klavehn et al., 2002; Richardson-Klavehn & Gardiner, 1996; Schott et al., 2005) suggest that conscious recollection of prior episodes can either reflect automatic stimulus-driven retrieval, or more controlled search-like retrieval (see also Moscovitch, 1994, 2000). This theoretical conclusion contrasts with two-process models that equate conscious recollection with controlled retrieval, and unconscious memory with automatic retrieval (e.g. Jacoby, 1998; Jacoby, Toth, & Yonelinas, 1993; for discussion see Richardson-Klavehn, Gardiner, & Java, 1996; Richardson-Klavehn et al., 2002; Schott et al., 2005).

The more general implication of the reversed association that we have just described is that seeking associations as well as dissociations between learning and memory measures within the same experiment can contribute to the goal of specifying which processes are common to, versus different across, the different measures, as suggested by the components-of-processing approach discussed in the previous main section of this chapter (e.g. Roediger et al., 1999). Such an empirical strategy should therefore be central to progressing beyond the unitary vs. multiple-memory-systems arguments discussed there. With respect to neuroimaging, such a strategy would begin to specify which processes are common across learning-and-memory-related brain regions or networks, and which are different across regions or networks, and at which level in the functional hierarchy these similarities and differences occur (e.g. J. A. Anderson & Hinton, 1981; Henson, 2005). We pursue the implications of these arguments in the next subsection.

Broader theoretical implications of conjunctions of dissociations and associations

Crossed double dissociations (i.e. double dissociations as a function of a single experimental manipulation; see Dunn & Kirsner, 1988) between priming and intentional test performance, such as the one just described, are quite common in the literature, but have typically been reported in isolation rather than in conjunction with parallel effects (e.g. Jacoby, 1983a; Winnick & Daniel, 1970; for reviews, see Richardson-Klavehn & Bjork, 1988; Roediger & McDermott, 1993). Using Dunn and Kirsner's (1988) logic, it would be possible, in principle, to explain such dissociations by arguing that priming is negatively related to the efficiency of a single learning and memory process, and that intentional test performance is positively related to that same process (or the converse). To our knowledge, however, such a view has never actually been advanced with regard to these data patterns. Furthermore, we know of no reports suggesting that priming and intentional test performance are negatively correlated across participants and/or items, and there are a number of memory-relevant experimental variables, such as level of item-specific attention at encoding, that can produce parallel effects on priming and intentional test performance (e.g. Richardson-Klavehn & Bjork, 1988; Stone, Ladd, & Gabrieli, 2000; Stone et al., 1998; Turk-Browne, Yi, & Chun, 2006; Vuilleumier et al., 2005).

Single-system models of priming and intentional test performance also generally predict either parallel effects or imperfect single dissociations, in which a variable influences intentional test performance much more strongly than it influences priming (e.g. Berry, Henson *et al.*, 2006; Berry, Shanks *et al.*, 2006, 2008; Kinder & Shanks, 2001, 2003; see also Bullinaria & Chater, 1995). Against this general background context, the reported crossed double dissociations have more force than they have a right to from a purely formal point of view, and, along with the reversed association described in the previous subsection, also appear to represent a challenge to the view that priming and intentional test performance depend on common memory representations (see, e.g. Berry *et al.*, 2008). That is, the theoretical and empirical context in which the crossed double dissociations have been observed is once again critical (see also Baddeley, 2003; Chater, 2003; McCloskey, 2003).

A further point arising from this discussion of reversed associations is that single dissociations and parallel effects across learning and memory measures also can have considerable theoretical value in the appropriate theoretical and measurement context (see also Tulving, 1985, who argued that certain views of the relationship between memory systems – such as 'embeddedness' – predict only single dissociations, and not double dissociations). Single dissociations, in which a variable influences intentional test performance and not priming, might reflect the lower reliability of the priming measures, which reflects the involvement of more non-episodic-memory-related cognitive processes in typical priming measures than in typical intentional test measures (e.g. Buchner & Brandt, 2003), and means that power to detect effects of some variables on priming measures may often be low. This point is especially well taken in regard to neuropsychological group studies of priming, where the power to detect priming deficits in the patient group has sometimes been so small that the patients would have needed to show negative priming in order for a statistically significant priming deficit to be observed (Ostergaard & Jernigan, 1993; see also Dunn, 2003).

However, there have also been instances in which null effects on priming have occurred in conjunction with considerable power. One such instance concerns the effect of level of processing at study on later performance in word-stem completion. Given that the appropriate shallow and deep study tasks are used (whereby the shallow study task must engage lexical processing; see Richardson-Klavehn & Gardiner, 1998), power to detect very small effects of level of processing has approached unity, but no effect of level of processing has been detected (Richardson-Klavehn & Gardiner, 1996, 1998; Richardson-Klavehn *et al.*, 1999; see the latter article for a meta-analysis). Consistent with these data, there has been no sign of sensitivity to level of processing at study in the brain-activity predictors of later priming as measured with MEG and EEG (Düzel *et al.*, 2005; Schott *et al.*, 2002). Corresponding intentional word-stem completion tests in all cases showed substantial effects of level of study processing, even when baseline (non-studied item) performance was equated with those in the incidental tests, thus ruling out possible differences in response bias (e.g. Reingold, 2003) across tests (Richardson-Klavehn & Gardiner, 1996, 1998; Richardson-Klavehn *et al.*, 2002). Because external cues were identical across tests, with only the instructions differing, these results suggest that the presence or absence of level-of-processing effects on priming in incidental word-stem completion tests can act as a rather sensitive behavioural marker for the presence or absence of contamination of the incidental test by controlled retrieval strategies.

With regard to parallel effects (associations) across memory tests, the reversed association logic points up the theoretical value of observing such effects in conjunction with dissociations within the same experiment. For example, Richardson-Klavehn and Gardiner (1998) used such a pattern to show that a very low-level graphemic encoding task produced a deficit in word-stem completion priming, in comparison with another shallow (phonemic) encoding task and with a deep encoding task that could not be attributed to contamination of the incidental test by voluntary retrieval strategies. This result helped to resolve a long-standing controversy over when level-of-processing effects on priming occur (e.g. Brown & Mitchell, 1994), and to establish the level of representation (perceptual-lexical) at which priming in the word-stem completion test occurs (see also Ramponi et al., 2007, for similar evidence regarding the impact of low-level graphemic study tasks on conceptual priming). Ramponi et al. (2004) used the same logic to examine deficits in conceptual priming and conceptually cued recall in older participants, and showed that older participants, in comparison with younger participants, display preserved conceptual priming when the stimuli employed (in this case word-pairs) have established pre-experimental representations, but simultaneously show impaired conceptual priming with stimuli that have less well-established pre-experimental representations. In matched conceptually cued recall tests, older participants were impaired relative to younger participants with both kinds of stimuli. Thus again, there was a combination of a dissociation (i.e. an age effect on cued recall but not on conceptual priming for stimuli with established representations), and a parallel effect (an age effect on cued recall and on conceptual priming for stimuli with less well established representations). Because cues corresponding to the different types of stimuli were randomly intermixed in the test list, this pattern ruled out a significant role of contamination of the incidental test by voluntary or controlled retrieval strategies in the younger participants. In complementary experiments with younger participants only, Ramponi et al. (2007) showed that conceptual priming for stimuli with less well established representations is influenced by level of study processing (phonemic vs. semantic), whereas conceptual priming for stimuli with well established representations is little so influenced. Again, matched conceptually cued recall tests showed level-of-processing effects for both kinds of stimuli, producing a combination of parallel effect and dissociation that makes it difficult to attribute the parallel effect to contamination of the incidental test of conceptual priming by voluntary or controlled retrieval. From a measurement point of view (e.g. Dunn, 2003), such conjunctive data patterns (i.e. dissociation plus association) also make it difficult to attribute the absence of level-of-processing effects on priming under some conditions to lack of statistical power, because such effects do occur in other conditions within the same experiments.

Our substantive theoretical interpretation of these data patterns (Ramponi et al., 2004, 2007; see also Gardiner, Richardson-Klavehn et al., 2001) is that conceptual priming and cued recall of stimuli with less well established representations require an intra-stimulus strengthening process at study that is less likely to occur for older participants and shallower levels of study processing. By contrast, conceptual priming of established representations can occur without this strengthening process both in older participants and at shallower levels of study processing. In addition, conceptually cued recall, unlike conceptual priming, involves binding items to their episodic context at study, which is less likely to occur for older participants and shallower levels of processing, thus explaining age and level-of-processing effects on conceptually cued recall for both established and less well established representations. In short, the intra-stimulus strengthening process is important for both conceptual priming and conceptually cued recall tests, whereas the episodic binding process is important mainly for the conceptually cued recall test. These results illustrate again that, in general, the experimental strategy of producing parallel effects in the context of dissociations can establish component processes that are common to, versus different across, different learning and memory tests (e.g. Roediger *et al.*, 1999), and thus assists in going beyond the unitary vs. multiple systems arguments discussed in the previous main section of this chapter. In the light of Henson's (2005, 2006a) analyses of the resolving power of dissociations in haemodynamic neuroimaging, such an empirical strategy might also be of value for future neuroimaging research.

Dissociation evidence: Interim summary

Formal measurement issues are clearly critical in the cautious theoretical interpretation of dissociations and, in these terms, the concept of reversed association (Dunn & Kirsner, 1988) appears to be a considerable advance for the interpretation of behavioural, neuropsychological, and neuroimaging data. The theoretical force of such reversed associations, however, as with the component dissociations and associations that go to produce reversed associations, remains dependent on the theoretical context and the particular variables under consideration (see also Baddeley, 2003; Chater, 2003; McCloskey, 2003; Shallice, 1988). Similar arguments regarding dissociations in neuroimaging data and their theoretical and neuroanatomical context have been made by Henson (2005, 2006a) and Rugg (this volume), but we have additionally suggested that the notion of cognitive closeness of the experimental variables to the hypothetical learning and memory process or processes is critical to the theoretical resolution of behavioural and neuroimaging reversed associations. Furthermore, given appropriate statistical and experimental checks (*cf.* Dunn, 2003; Ostergaard & Jernigan, 1993), we believe that single dissociations can still be of considerable theoretical value when observed in conjunction with associations (see also Chater, 2003; Tulving, 1985). That is, the central insight offered by Dunn and Kirsner (1988) – that dissociations between measures are of most theoretical value when they occur in the context of associations between measures – has a broad range of applicability in neuroimaging, neuropsychological, and purely behavioural research.

Conclusions

As a complement to the chapters on learning in the current section of this volume, we have here attempted to present a general view of learning and memory as a dynamic and constructive capability, the psychological understanding of which is likely to require understanding of the brain, both structural and functional, and at many different levels. Critical debate of the issues involved in relating neuroimaging dissociations and other kinds of dissociation data to cognitive theory in recent years have revealed important principles that can be used to improve the theoretical resolution of future neuroimaging, neuropsychological, and purely behavioural research on learning and memory. Contrary to recent suggestions that the neurobiological level of analysis may replace the psycho-logical level, we have argued here that further developments in the specificity of cogni-tive-level theories, and in understanding how the representation and processing components of these specific theories relate to brain function and anatomy, are critical to progressing beyond the long-standing debate regarding unitary versus multiple learning and memory systems, as well as other theoretical debates in the area of learning and memory (see also Shallice, 2003). Greater communication and collaboration between researchers studying learning and memory at the level of cognitive theories and models, and those with a neurobiological orientation, appears to us, therefore, to be essential for scientific progress.

Acknowledgements

The order of the last five authors is alphabetical. Preparation of this chapter was sup-ported by grants from the Alexander von Humboldt Foundation (Stiftung) and the German Science Foundation (Deutsche Forschungsgemeinschaft: Grants RI1847 and SFB779TPA7), and by the Federal State of Sachsen-Anhalt, Germany, and we thank these organizations. We thank Chris Berry, Rik Henson, Frank Rösler, and David Shanks for discussion and comments on a previous version of this chapter. Any errors, inconsisten-cies, and omissions that remain are of course ours alone. The first author also thanks Edite Grinberga for support and encouragement during the research and writing of this chapter.

References

Anderson, J. A. & Hinton, G. E. (1981). Models of information processing in the brain. In G. E. Hinton & J. A. Anderson (Eds), *Parallel Models of Associative Memory* (pp. 9–48). Hillsdale, NJ: Erlbaum.

Anderson, J. R. (1978). Arguments concerning representations for mental imagery. *Psychological Review, 85*, 249–277.

Anderson, J. R. (1985). Ebbinghaus's century. *Journal of Experimental Psychology: Learning, Memory, and Cognition, 11*, 436–438.

Anderson, J. R. & Lebiere, C. (2003). The Newell test for a theory of cognition. *Behavioural and Brain Sciences, 26*, 587–601.

Anderson, J. R. & Milson, R. (1989). Human memory: An adaptive perspective. *Psychological Review, 96*, 703–719.

Anderson, J. R. & Schooler, L. J. (2000). The adaptive nature of memory. In E. Tulving & F. I. M. Craik (Eds), *Oxford Handbook of Memory* (pp. 557–570). New York: Oxford University Press.

Anderson, M. C. (2003). Rethinking interference theory: Executive control and the mechanisms of forgetting. *Journal of Memory and Language*, *49*, 415–445.

Anderson, M. C., Bjork, R. A., and Bjork, E. L. (1994). Remembering can cause forgetting: Retrieval dynamics in long-term memory. *Journal of Experimental Psychology: Learning, Memory and Cognition*, *20*, 1063–1087.

Anderson, M. C. & Green, C. (2001). Suppressing unwanted memories by executive control. *Nature*, *410*, 366–369.

Anderson, M. C. & Levy, B. J. (2007). Theoretical issues in inhibition: Insights from research on human memory. In D. S. Gorfein & C. M. MacLeod (Eds), *Inhibition in Cognition* (pp. 81–102). Washington, DC: American Psychological Association.

Anderson, M. C., Ochsner, K. N., Kuhl, B., Cooper, J., Robertson, E., Gabrieli, S. W., Glover, G. H., & Gabrieli, J. D. (2004). Neural systems underlying the suppression of unwanted memories. *Science*, *303*, 232–235.

Anderson, M. C. & Spellman, B. A. (1995). On the status of inhibitory mechanisms in cognition: Memory retrieval as a model case. *Psychological Review*, *102*, 68–100.

Baddeley, A. D. (2003). Double dissociations: Not magic, but still useful. *Cortex*, *39*, 139–131.

Bäuml, K. -H. (2002). Semantic generation can cause episodic forgetting. *Psychological Science*, *13*, 356–360.

Bechtel, W. (2002). Decomposing the mind-brain: A long-term pursuit. *Brain and Mind*, *3*, 229–242.

Bechtel, W. & Abrahamsen, A. (2002). *Connectionism and the Mind: Parallel Processing, Dynamics, and Evolution in Networks* (2nd Edn). Oxford, UK: Blackwell.

Bergström, Z. M., Velmans, M., de Fockert, J., & Richardson-Klavehn, A. (2007). ERP evidence for successful voluntary avoidance of conscious recollection. *Brain Research*, *1151*, 119–133.

Bergström, Z. M., de Fockert, J., & Richardson-Klavehn, A. (under review). *ERP and behavioural evidence for direct suppression of unwanted memories.*

Berry, C. J., Henson, R. N. A., & Shanks, D. R. (2006). On the relationship between repetition priming and recognition memory: Insights from a computational model. *Journal of Memory and Language*, *55*, 515–533.

Berry, C. J., Shanks, D. R., & Henson, R. N. A. (2006). On the status of unconscious memory: Merikle and Reingold (1991) revisited. *Journal of Experimental Psychology: Learning, Memory, and Cognition*, *32*, 925–935.

Berry, C. J., Shanks, D. R., & Henson, R. N. A. (2008). A single-system account of the relationship between priming, recognition, and fluency. *Journal of Experimental Psychology: Learning, Memory, and Cognition, 34*, 97–111.

Bjork, R. A. (1989). Retrieval inhibition as an adaptive mechanism in human memory. In H. L. Roediger III & F. I. M. Craik (Eds), *Varieties of Memory and Consciousness: Essays in Honor of Endel Tulving* (pp. 309–330). Hillsdale, NJ: Erlbaum.

Bjork, R. A. & Bjork, E. L. (1992). A new theory of disuse and an old theory of stimulus fluctuation. In A. F. Healy, S. M. Kosslyn, & R. M. Shiffrin (Eds), *Essays in Honor of William K. Estes* (Vol. 2, pp. 35–67). Hillsdale, NJ: Erlbaum.

Bower, G. H. (2000). A brief history of memory research. In F. I. M. Craik and E. Tulving (Eds.), *Oxford Handbook of Memory* (pp. 3–32). New York: Oxford University Press.

Brown, A. S. & Mitchell, D. B. (1994). A revaluation of semantic versus nonsemantic processing in implicit memory. *Memory and Cognition*, *22*, 533–541.

Brown, G. D. A. & Lamberts, K. (2003). Double dissociations, models, and serial position curves. *Cortex*, *39*, 148–152.

Buchner, A. & Brandt, M. (2003). Further evidence for systematic reliability differences between explicit and implicit memory tests. *Quarterly Journal of Experimental Psychology*, *56*A, 193–209.

Bulevich, J. B., Roediger, H. L. III, Balota, D. A., & Butler, A. C. (2006). Failures to find suppression of episodic memories in the think/no-think paradigm. *Memory and Cognition, 34*, 1569–1577.

Bullinaria, J. A. & Chater, N. (1995). Connectionist modelling: Implications for cognitive neuropsychology. *Language and Cognitive Processes, 10*, 227–264.

Buzsáki, G. (1996). The hippocampo-neocortical dialogue. *Cerebral Cortex, 6*, 81–92.

Buzsáki, G. & Draguhn, A. (2004). Neuronal oscillations in cortical networks. *Science, 304*, 1926–1929.

Chater, N. (2003). How much can we learn from double dissociations?. *Cortex, 39*, 167–169.

Chomsky, N. (1980). *Rules and Representations.* New York: Columbia University Press.

Churchland, P. S. (2002). *Brain-wise: Studies in Neurophilosophy.* Cambridge, MA: MIT Press.

Cohen, L., Dehaene, S., Naccache, L., Lehéricy, S., Dehaene-Lambertz, G., Hénaff, M. A., & Michel, F. (2000). The visual word form area: Spatial and temporal characterization of an initial stage of reading in normal subjects and posterior split-brain patients. *Brain, 123*, 291–307.

Coltheart, M. (2004). Brain imaging, connectionism, and cognitive neuropsychology. *Cognitive Neuropsychology, 21*, 21–25.

Coltheart, M. (2006a). What has functional neuroimaging told us about the mind (so far)? *Cortex, 42*, 323–331.

Coltheart, M. (2006b). Perhaps functional neuroimaging has not told us anything about the mind (so far). *Cortex, 42*, 422–427.

Coltheart, M. & Davies, M. (2003). Inference and explanation in cognitive neuropsychology. *Cortex, 39*, 188–191.

Craik, F. I. M. (2002). Levels of processing: Past, present…and future? *Memory, 10*, 305–318.

Craik, F. I. M., Moscovitch, M., & McDowd, J. M. (1994). Contribution of surface and conceptual information to performance on implicit and explicit memory tasks. *Journal of Experimental Psychology: Learning, Memory and Cognition, 20*, 864–875.

Crowder, R. G. (1976). *Principles of Learning and Memory.* Hillsdale, NJ: Erlbaum.

Cummings, J. L., Doody, R., & Clark, C. (2007). Disease-modifying therapies for Alzheimer disease: Challenges to early intervention. *Neurology, 69*, 1622–1634.

Depue, B. E., Curran, T., & Banich M. T. (2007). Prefrontal regions orchestrate suppression of emotional memories via a two-phase process. *Science, 317*, 215–219.

Dunn, J. C. (2003). The elusive dissociation. *Cortex, 39*, 177–179.

Dunn, J. C. & Kirsner, K. (1988). Discovering functionally independent mental processes: The principle of reversed association. *Psychological Review, 95*, 91–101.

Dunn, J. C. & Kirsner, K. (2003). What can we infer from double dissociations? *Cortex, 39*, 1–7.

Düzel, E., Habib, R., Schott, B., Schoenfeld, A., Lobaugh, N., McIntosh, A. R., Scholz, M., & Heinze, H.-J. (2003). A multivariate, spatiotemporal analysis of electromagnetic time-frequency data of recognition memory. *Neuroimage, 18*, 185–197.

Düzel, E., Richardson-Klavehn, A., Neufang, M., Schott, B. H., Scholz, M., & Heinze, H.-J. (2005). Early, partly anticipatory, neural oscillations during identification set the stage for priming. *NeuroImage, 25*, 690–700.

Eysenck, M. W. (1979). Depth, elaboration, and distinctiveness. In L. S. Cermak & F. I. M. Craik (Eds), *Levels of Processing in Human Memory* (pp. 89–118). Hillsdale, NJ: Erlbaum.

Fiebach, C. J., Gruber, T., & Supp. G. G. (2005). Neuronal mechanisms of repetition priming in occipitotemporal cortex: Spatiotemporal evidence from functional magnetic resonance imaging and electroencephalography. *Journal of Neuroscience, 25*, 3414–3422.

Fisher, R. P. & Craik, F. I. M. (1977). The interaction between encoding and retrieval operations in cued recall. *Journal of Experimental Psychology: Human Learning and Memory, 3*, 701–711.

Fodor, J. A. (1983). *The Modularity of Mind.* Cambridge, MA: Bradford.

Friston, K. J., Büchel, C., Fink, G. R., Morris, J., Rolls, E., & Dolan, R. J. (1997). Psychophysiological and modulatory interactions in neuroimaging. *Neuroimage*, 6, 218–229.

Freud, S. (1915/1957). Repression (Trans. J. Strachey). In J. Strachey (Ed.), *The Standard Edition of the Complete Psychological Works of Sigmund Freud* (pp. 146–158). London, UK: Hogarth.

Gardiner, J. M., Ramponi, C., & Richardson-Klavehn, A. (1999). Response deadline and subjective awareness in recognition memory. *Consciousness and Cognition*, 8, 484–496.

Gardiner, J. M., Richardson-Klavehn, A., Ramponi, C., & Brooks, B. M. (2001). Involuntary level-of-processing effects in perceptual and conceptual priming. In M. Naveh-Benjamin, M. Moscovitch, & H. L. Roediger III (Eds), *Perspectives on Human Memory and Cognitive Aging: Essays in Honor of Fergus Craik* (pp. 71–82). New York: Psychology Press.

Guderian, S., Schott, B. H., Richardson-Klavehn, A., & Düzel, E. (under review). *Medial temporal theta state before an event predicts episodic encoding success in humans.*

Hakeem, A. Y., Hof, P. R., Sherwood, C. C., Switzer, R. C. III, Rasmussen, L. E. L., & Allman, J. M. (2005). Brain of the African elephant (loxodonta africana): Neuroanatomy from functional resonance images. *The Anatomical Record*, 287A, 1117–1127.

Harley, T. A. (2004a). Does cognitive neuropsychology have a future? *Cognitive Neuropsychology*, 21, 2–16.

Harley, T. A. (2004b). Promises, promises. *Cognitive Neuropsychology*, 21, 51–56.

Hart, B. L., Hart, L. A., & Pinter-Wollman, N. (2008). Large brains and cognition: Where do elephants fit in? *Neuroscience and Biobehavioral Reviews*, 32, 86–98.

Hasselmo, M. E. & McClelland, J. L. (1999). Neural models of memory. *Current Opinion in Neurobiology*, 9, 184–188.

Henson, R. N. A. (2003). Neuroimaging studies of priming. *Progress in Neurobiology*, 70, 53–81.

Henson, R. N. A. (2005). What can functional neuroimaging tell the experimental psychologist? *Quarterly Journal of Experimental Psychology*, 58A, 193–233.

Henson, R. N. A. (2006a). Forward inference using functional neuroimaging: Dissociations versus associations. *Trends in Cognitive Sciences*, 10, 64–69.

Henson, R. N. A. (2006b). What has (neuro)psychology told us about the mind (so far)? A reply to Coltheart (2006). *Cortex*, 42, 387–392.

Hertel, P. T. & Calcaterra, G. (2005). Intentional forgetting benefits from thought substitution. *Psychonomic Bulletin and Review*, 12, 484–489.

Humphreys, G. W. & Price, C. J. (2001). Cognitive neuropsychology and functional brain imaging: Implications for functional and neuroanatomical models of cognition. *Acta Psychologica (Amsterdam)*, 107, 119–153.

Jacoby L. L. (1983a). Remembering the data: Analyzing interactive processes in reading. *Journal of Verbal Learning and Verbal Behavior*, 22, 485–508.

Jacoby, L. L. (1983b). Perceptual enhancement: Persistent effects of an experience. *Journal of Experimental Psychology: Learning, Memory, and Cognition, 9*, 21–38.

Jacoby, L. L. (1998). Invariance in automatic influences of memory: Toward a user's guide for the process-dissociation procedure. *Journal of Experimental Psychology: Learning, Memory, and Cognition, 24*, 3–26.

Jacoby, L. L., Toth, J. P., & Yonelinas, A. P. (1993). Separating conscious and unconscious influences of memory: Measuring recollection. *Journal of Experimental Psychology: General, 122*, 139–154.

Jerison, H. (1973). *Evolution of the Brain and Intelligence.* New York: Academic Press.

Johansson, M., Aslan, A., Bäuml, K. H., Gabel, A., & Mecklinger, A. (2006). When remembering causes forgetting: Electrophysiological correlates of retrieval-induced forgetting. *Cerebral Cortex, 17*, 1135–1141.

Johnson, S. K. & Anderson, M. C. (2004) The role of inhibitory control in forgetting semantic knowledge. *Psychological Science, 15*, 448–453.

Juola, P. (2003). One word, one module? *Cortex, 39*, 135–137.

Kandel, E. R. (2001). The molecular biology of memory storage: A dialogue between genes and synapses. *Science, 294*, 1030–1038.

Kesner, R. P. & Rogers, J. (2004). An analysis of independence and interactions of brain substrates that subserve multiple attributes, memory systems, and underlying processes. *Neurobiology of Learning and Memory, 82*, 199–215.

Kim, J. J. & Baxter, M. G. (2001). Multiple brain-memory systems: The whole does not equal the sum of its parts. *Trends in Neurosciences, 24*, 324–330.

Kinder, A. & Shanks, D. R. (2001). Amnesia and the declarative/procedural distinction: A recurrent network model of classification, recognition, and repetition priming. *Journal of Cognitive Neuroscience, 13*, 648–669.

Kinder, A. & Shanks, D. R. (2003). Neuropsychological dissociations between priming and recognition: A single-system connectionist account. *Psychological Review, 110*, 728–744.

Kirsner, K., Speelman, C. P., & Schofield, P. (1993). Implicit memory and skill acquisition: Is synthesis possible? In M. E. J. Masson & P. Graf (Eds), *Implicit Memory: New Directions in Cognition, Development, and Neuropsychology* (pp. 119–140). Hillsdale, NJ: Erlbaum.

Klein, S. B., Cosmides, L., Tooby, J., & Chance, S. (2002). Decisions and the evolution of multiple memory systems: Multiple systems, multiple functions. *Psychological Review, 109*, 306–329.

Kolers, P. A. and Roediger, H. L. III (1984). Procedures of mind. *Journal of Verbal Learning and Verbal Behavior, 23*, 425–449.

Kopp, B., Rist, F., & Mattler, U. (1996). N200 in the flanker task as a neurobehavioral tool for investigating executive control. *Psychophysiology, 33*, 282–294.

Laughlin, S. B. & Sejnowski, T. J. (2003). Communication in neural networks. *Science, 301*, 1870–1874.

Le Doux, J. (2002). *Synaptic Self*. New York: Penguin.

Levy, B. J. & Anderson, M. C. (2002). Inhibitory processes and the control of memory retrieval. *Trends in Cognitive Sciences, 6*, 299–305.

Levy, B. J., McVeigh, M. D., Marful, A., & Anderson, M. C. (2007). Inhibiting your native language: The role of retrieval-induced forgetting during second-language acquisition. *Psychological Science, 18*, 29–34.

Linden, D. J. (2007). *The Accidental Mind: How Brain Evolution has Given Us Love, Memory, Dreams, and God*. Cambridge, MA: Harvard University Press.

Lobaugh, N. J., West, R., & McIntosh, A. R. (2001). Spatiotemporal analysis of experimental differences in event-related potential data with partial least squares. *Psychophysiology, 38*, 517–530.

Lockhart, R. S. (2002). Levels of processing, transfer-appropriate processing, and the concept of robust encoding. *Memory, 10*, 397–403.

Logothetis, N. K. & Wandell, B. A. (2004). Interpreting the BOLD signal. *Annual Review of Physiology, 66*, 735–769.

Mainzer, K. (2007). The emergence of mind and brain: An evolutionary, computational, and philosophical approach. *Progress in Brain Research, 168*, 115–132.

Marr, D. (1982). *Vision: A Computational Investigation into the Human Representation and Processing of Visual Information*. San Francisco, CA: W. H. Freeman.

Mayes, A. (2000). Selective memory disorders. In E. Tulving & F. I. M. Craik (Eds), *Oxford Handbook of Memory* (pp. 427–440). New York: Oxford University Press.

McClelland, J. L. (2000). Connectionist models of memory. In E. Tulving & F. I. M. Craik (Eds), *Oxford Handbook of Memory* (pp. 583–596). New York: Oxford University Press.

McClelland, J. L. & Goddard, N. H. (1996). Considerations arising from a complementary learning systems perspective on hippocampus and neocortex. *Hippocampus, 6*, 654–665.

McClelland, J. L., McNaughton, B. L., & O'Reilly, R. C. (1995). Why there are complementary learning systems in the hippocampus and neocortex: Insights from the successes and failures of connectionist models of learning and memory. *Psychological Review, 102*, 419–457.

McClelland, J. L. & Rogers, T. T. (2003). The parallel distributed processing approach to semantic cognition. *Nature Reviews Neuroscience, 4*, 310–322.

McCloskey, M. (2003). Beyond task dissociation logic: A richer conception of cognitive neuropsychology. *Cortex, 39*, 196–202.

McIntosh, A. R. & Lobaugh, N. J. (2004). Partial least squares analysis of neuroimaging data: Applications and advances. *Neuroimage, 23, Supplement 1*, S250–S263.

Mizumori, S. J. Y., Yeshenko, O., Gill, K. M., & Davis, D. M. (2004). Parallel processing across neural systems: Implications for a multiple memory system hypothesis. *Neurobiology of Learning and Memory, 82*, 278–298.

Morton, J. (1984). Brain-based and non-brain-based models of language. In D. Caplan, A. R. Lecours, & A. Smith (Eds), *Biological Perspectives on Language* (pp. 40–64). Cambridge, MA: MIT Press.

Mosconi, L., Brys, M., Glodzik-Sobanska, L., de Santi, S., Rusinek, H., & de Leon, M. J. (2007). Early detection of Alzheimer's disease using neuroimaging. *Experimental Gerontology, 42*, 129–138.

Moscovitch, M. (1994). Memory and working-with-memory: Evaluation of a component process model and comparison with other models. In D. L. Schacter & E. Tulving (Eds), *Memory Systems of 1994* (pp. 269–310). Cambridge, MA: MIT Press.

Moscovitch, M. (2000). Theories of memory and consciousness. In E. Tulving & F. I. M. Craik (Eds), *Oxford Handbook of Memory* (pp. 609–626). New York: Oxford University Press.

Moscovitch, M., Rosenbaum, R. S., Gilboa, A., Addis, D. R., Westmacott, R., Grady, C., McAndrews, M. P., Levine, B., Black, S., Winocur, G., & Nadel, L. (2005). Functional neuroanatomy of remote episodic, semantic and spatial memory: A unified account based on multiple trace theory. *Journal of Anatomy, 207*, 35–66.

Murdock, B. B. (1982). A theory for the storage and retrieval of item and associative information. *Psychological Review, 89*, 609–626.

Murray, G. K., Corlett, P. R., Clark, L., Pessiglione, M., Blackwell, A. D., Honey, G., Jones, P. B., Bullmore, E. T., Robbins, T. W., & Fletcher, P. C. (2008). Substantia nigra/ventral tegmental reward prediction error in psychosis. *Molecular Psychiatry, 13*, 267–276.

Nairne, J. S. (2002). The myth of the encoding-retrieval match. *Memory, 10*, 389–395.

Newell, B. R., Lagnado, D. A., & Shanks, D. R. (2007). Challenging the role of implicit processes in probabilistic category learning. *Psychonomic Bulletin & Review, 14*, 505–511.

Nobre, A. C., Allison, T., & McCarthy, G. (1994). Word recognition in the human inferior temporal lobe. *Nature, 372*, 260–263.

Norman, K. A. Newman, E. L., & Detre, G. (2007). A neural network model of retrieval-induced forgetting. *Psychological Review, 114*, 887–953.

Oakley, D. A. (1983). The varieties of memory: A phylogenetic approach. In A. R. Mayes (Ed.), *Memory in Humans and Animals* (pp. 20–82). Wokingham, UK: Van Nostrand Reinhold.

Olton, D. S. (1989). Inferring psychological dissociations from experimental dissociations: The temporal context of episodic memory. In H. L. Roediger & F. I. M. Craik (Eds), *Varieties of Memory and Consciousness: Essays in Honor of Endel Tulving* (pp. 161–178). Hillsdale, NJ: Erlbaum.

Ostergaard, A. L. & Jernigan, T. L. (1993). Are word priming and explicit memory mediated by different brain structures? In M. E. J. Masson & P. Graf (Eds), *Implicit Memory: New Directions in Cognition, Development, and Neuropsychology* (pp. 327–350). Hillsdale, NJ: Erlbaum.

Otten, L. J., Quayle, A. H., Akram, S., Ditewig, T. A., & Rugg, M. D. (2006). Brain activity before an event predicts later recollection. *Nature Neuroscience, 9*, 489–491.

Page, M. P. A. (2006). What can't functional neuroimaging tell the cognitive psychologist? *Cortex, 42*, 428–443.

Palmer, S. E. (1978). Fundamental aspects of cognitive representation. In E. Rosch & B. B. Lloyd (Eds), *Cognition and Categorization* (pp. 259–303). Hillsdale, NJ: Erlbaum.

Paulsen, O. & Sejnowski, T. J. (2000). Natural patterns of activity and long-term synaptic plasticity. *Current Opinion in Neurobiology, 10*, 172–179.

Plaut, D. C. (1995). Double dissociations without modularity: Evidence from connectionist neuropsychology. *Journal of Clinical and Experimental Neuropsychology, 17*, 291–321.

Plaut, D. C. (2003). Interpreting double dissociations in connectionist networks. *Cortex, 39*, 138–141.

Poldrack, R. A. (2006). Can cognitive processes be inferred from neuroimaging data? *Trends in Cognitive Sciences, 10*, 59–63.

Poldrack, R. A. & Foerde, K. (2008). Category learning and the multiple memory systems debate. *Neuroscience and Biobehavioral Reviews, 32*, 197–205.

Putnam, H. (1975). Philosophy and our mental life. In H. Putnam (Ed.), *Mind, Language, and Reality: Philosophical Papers Volume 2* (pp. 291–303). New York: Cambridge University Press.

Rajah, M. N. & McIntosh, A. R. (2005). Overlap in the functional neural systems involved in semantic and episodic memory retrieval. *Journal of Cognitive Neuroscience, 17*, 470–482.

Ramponi, C., Richardson-Klavehn, A., & Gardiner, J. M. (2004). Level of processing and age affect involuntary conceptual priming of weak but not strong associates. *Experimental Psychology, 51*, 159–164.

Ramponi, C., Richardson-Klavehn, A., & Gardiner, J. M. (2007). Component processes of conceptual priming and associative cued recall: The roles of preexisting representation and depth of processing. *Journal of Experimental Psychology: Learning, Memory, and Cognition, 33*, 843–862.

Ratcliff, R. (1978). A theory of memory retrieval. *Psychological Review, 85*, 59–108.

Reimann, E. M. (2007). Linking brain imaging and genomics in the study of Alzheimer's disease and aging. *Annals of the New York Academy of Sciences, 1097*, 94–113.

Reingold, E. M. (2003). Interpreting dissociations: The issue of task comparability. *Cortex, 39*, 174–176.

Remijnse, P. L., Nielen, M. M., van Balkom, A. J., Cath, D. C., van Oppen, P., Uylings, H. B., & Veltman, D. J. (2006). Reduced orbitofrontal-striatal activity on a reversal learning task in obsessive-compulsive disorder. *Archives of General Psychiatry, 63*, 1225–1236.

Richardson-Klavehn, A. (1986). *Theories of Retrieval and the Episodic-Semantic Distinction.* Thesis submitted to the University of California, Los Angeles, in partial fulfilment of the requirements of the PhD degree.

Richardson-Klavehn, A. & Bjork, R. A. (1988). Measures of memory. *Annual Review of Psychology, 39*, 475–543.

Richardson-Klavehn, A. & Bjork, R. A. (2002). Memory, long-term. In L. Nadel (Ed.), *Encyclopedia of Cognitive Science* (Vol. 2, pp. 1096–1105). London, UK: Nature Publishing Group.

Richardson-Klavehn, A., Clarke, A. J. B., & Gardiner, J. M. (1999). Conjoint dissociations reveal involuntary "perceptual" priming from generating at study. *Consciousness and Cognition, 8*, 271–284.

Richardson-Klavehn, A. & Gardiner, J. M. (1996). Cross-modality priming reflects conscious memory, but not voluntary memory. *Psychonomic Bulletin and Review, 3*, 238–244.

Richardson-Klavehn, A. & Gardiner, J. M. (1998). Depth-of-processing effects on priming in word-stem completion: Tests of the voluntary-contamination, lexical processing, and conceptual processing hypotheses. *Journal of Experimental Psychology: Learning Memory and Cognition, 24*, 593–609.

Richardson-Klavehn, A., Gardiner, J. M., & Java, R. I. (1996). Memory: Task dissociations, process dissociations and dissociations of consciousness. In G. Underwood (Ed.), *Implicit Cognition* (pp. 85–158). Oxford, UK: Oxford University Press.

Richardson-Klavehn, A., Gardiner, J. M., & Ramponi, C. (2002). Level of processing and the process-dissociation procedure: Elusiveness of null effects on estimates of automatic retrieval. *Memory*, *10*, 349–364.

Richardson-Klavehn, A., Lee, M. G., Joubran, R., & Bjork, R. A. (1994). Intention and awareness in perceptual identification priming. *Memory and Cognition*, *22*, 293–312.

Roediger, H. L. III. (1980). Memory metaphors in cognitive psychology. *Memory and Cognition*, *8*, 231–246.

Roediger, H. L. III, Buckner, R. L., & McDermott, K. B. (1999). Components of processing. In J. K. Foster & M. Jelicic (Eds), *Memory: Systems, Process, or Function?* (pp. 31–65). Oxford, UK: Oxford University Press.

Roediger, H. L. III. & McDermott, K. B. (1993). Implicit memory in normal human subjects. In F. Boller & J. Grafman (Eds), *Handbook of Neuropsychology* (Vol. 8, pp. 63–131). Amsterdam, Netherlands: Elsevier.

Roediger, H. L. III., Weldon, M. S., & Challis, B. H. (1989). Explaining dissociations between implicit and explicit measures of retention: A processing account. In H. L. Roediger & F. I. M. Craik (Eds), *Varieties of Memory and Consciousness: Essays in Honor of Endel Tulving* (pp. 67–84). Hillsdale, NJ: Erlbaum.

Roediger, H. L. III. & Srinivas, K. (1993). Specificity of operations in perceptual priming. In M. E. J. Masson & P. Graf (Eds), *Implicit Memory: New Directions in Cognition, Development, and Neuropsychology* (pp. 17–48). Hillsdale, NJ: Erlbaum.

Rose, S. (1993). The M*aking of Memory: From Molecules to Mind*. London: Bantam Press.

Roth, G. & Dicke, U. (2005). Evolution of the brain and intelligence. *Trends in Cognitive Sciences*, *9*, 250–257.

Roth, G. & Wulliman, M. F. (Eds), (2001). *Brain Evolution and Cognition*. New York: Wiley.

Ryan, J. D. & Cohen, N. J. (2003). Evaluating the neuropsychological dissociation evidence for multiple memory systems. *Cognitive, Affective, and Behavioral Neuroscience*, *3*, 168–185.

Schacter, D. L. (2001). *The Seven Sins of Memory*. Boston, MA: Houghton Mifflin.

Schacter, D. L., Bowers, J., & Booker, J. (1989). Intention, awareness, and implicit memory: The retrieval intentionality criterion. In S. Lewandowsky, J. C. Dunn, & K. Kirsner (Eds), *Implicit Memory: Theoretical Issues* (pp. 47–65). Hillsdale, NJ: Erlbaum.

Schacter, D. L. & Buckner, R. L. (1998). Priming and the brain. *Neuron*, *20*, 185–195.

Schacter, D. L. & Church, B. A. (1992). Auditory priming: Implicit and explicit memory for words and voices. *Journal of Experimental Psychology: Learning, Memory, and Cognition*, *18*, 915–930.

Schacter, D. L., Wig, G. S., & Stevens, W. D. (2007). Reductions in cortical activity during priming. *Current Opinion in Neurobiology*, *17*, 171–176.

Schenker, N. M., Desgouttes, A. M., & Semendeferi, K. (2005). Neural connectivity and the cortical substrates of cognition in hominoids. *Journal of Human Evolution*, *49*, 547–569.

Schott, B. H., Fenker, D. B., Zierhut, K., Heinze, H.-J., Düzel, E., & Richardson-Klavehn, A. (under review). *Task-dependent increases in cortico-hippocampal functional connectivity during successful episodic memory formation*.

Schott, B. H., Henson, R. N., Richardson-Klavehn, A., Becker, C., Thoma, V., Heinze, H.-J., & Düzel, E. (2005). Redefining implicit and explicit memory: The functional neuroanatomy of priming, remembering, and control of retrieval. *Proceedings of the National Academy of Sciences USA*, *102*, 1257–1262.

Schott, B. H., Richardson-Klavehn, A., Heinze, H.-J., & Düzel, E. (2002). Perceptual priming versus explicit memory: Dissociable neural correlates at encoding. *Journal of Cognitive Neuroscience*, *14*, 578–592.

Schott, B. H., Richardson-Klavehn, A., Henson, R. N. A., Becker, C., Heinze, H.-J., & Düzel, E. (2006). Neuroanatomical dissociation of encoding processes related to priming and explicit memory *Journal of Neuroscience, 26,* 792–800.

Schott, B. H., Seidenbecher, C. I., Fenker, D. B., Lauer, C. J., Bunzeck, N., Bernstein, H.-G., Tischmeyer, W., Gundelfinger, E. D., Heinze, H.-J., & Düzel, E. (2006). The dopaminergic midbrain participates in human episodic memory formation: Evidence from genetic imaging. *Journal of Neuroscience, 26,* 1407–1417.

Sejnowski, T. J. (1981). Skeleton filters in the brain. In G. E. Hinton & J. A. Anderson (Eds), *Parallel Models of Associative Memory* (pp. 189–212). Hillsdale, NJ: Erlbaum.

Sejnowski, T. J. & Paulsen, O. (2006). Network oscillations: Emerging computational principles. *Journal of Neuroscience, 26,* 1673–1676.

Semon, R. (1923). *Mnemic Psychology* (Trans. B. Duffy). London, UK: Allen & Unwin.

Shallice, T. (1988). *From Neuropsychology to Mental Structure.* Cambridge, UK: Cambridge University Press.

Shallice, T. (2003). Functional imaging and neuropsychology findings: How can they be linked? *NeuroImage, 20,* Supplement 1, S146–S154.

Sherry, D. F. & Schacter, D. L. (1987). The evolution of multiple memory systems. *Psychological Review, 94,* 439–454.

Speekenbrink, M., Channon, S., & Shanks, D. R. (2008). Learning strategies in amnesia. *Neuroscience and Biobehavioral Reviews, 32,* 292–310.

Squire, L. R. (2004). Memory systems of the brain: A brief history and current perspective. *Neurobiology of Learning and Memory, 82,* 171–177.

Squire, L. R. (2007). Rapid consolidation. *Science, 316,* 57–58.

Squire, L. R. & Kandel, E. R. (1999). *Memory: From Mind to Molecules.* New York: Scientific American Library.

Stam, C., van der Made, Y., Pijnenburg, Y., & Scheltens, P. (2003). EEG synchronization in mild cognitive impairment and Alzheimer's disease. *Acta Neurologica Scandinavica, 108,* 90–96.

Stone, M., Ladd, S. L., & Gabrieli, J. D. E. (2000). The role of selective attention in perceptual and affective priming. *American Journal of Psychology, 113,* 341–358.

Stone, M., Ladd, S. L., Vaidya, C. J., & Gabrieli, J. D. E. (1998). Word-identification priming for ignored and attended words. *Consciousness and Cognition, 7,* 238–258.

Striedter, G. F. (2005). *Principles of Brain Evolution.* Sunderland, MA: Sinauer.

Sweeney-Reed, C. M., & Nasuto, S. J. (2007). A novel approach to detection of synchronisation in the EEG based on empirical mode decomposition. *Journal of Computational Neuroscience, 23,* 79–111.

Tulving, E. (1983). *Elements of Episodic Memory.* New York: Oxford University Press.

Tulving, E. (1985). On the classification problem in learning and memory. In L.-G. Nilsson & T. Archer (Eds), *Perspectives on Learning and Memory* (pp. 67–94). Hillsdale, NJ: Erlbaum.

Tulving, E. (2000). Concepts of memory. In E. Tulving & F. I. M. Craik (Eds), *Oxford Handbook of Memory* (pp. 33–43). New York: Oxford University Press.

Tulving, E. (2001). Does memory encoding exist? In M. Naveh-Benjamin, M. Moscovitch, & H. L. Roediger III (Eds), *Perspectives on Human Memory and Cognitive Aging: Essays in Honor of Fergus Craik* (pp. 6–27). New York: Psychology Press.

Tulving, E. & Schacter, D. L. (1990). Priming and human memory systems. *Science, 247,* 301–306.

Turk-Browne, N. B., Yi, D.-J., & Chun, M. M. (2006). Linking implicit and explicit memory: Common encoding factors and shared representations. *Neuron, 49,* 917–927.

Uttal, W. R. (2001). *The New Phrenology: The Limits of Localizing Cognitive Processes.* Cambridge, MA: MIT Press.

Van Orden, G. C. & Kloos, H. (2003). The module mistake. *Cortex, 39,* 164–166.

Van Orden, G. C. & Paap, K. R. (1997). Functional neuroimages fail to discover pieces of mind in parts of the brain. *Philosophy of Science Proceedings, 64,* S85–S94.

Van Orden, G. C., Pennington, B. F., & Stone, G. O. (2001). What do double dissociations prove? *Cognitive Science, 25,* 111–172.

Van Veen, V. & Carter, C. S. (2002). The timing of action-monitoring processes in the anterior cingulate cortex. *Journal of Cognitive Neuroscience, 14,* 593–602.

Varela, F., Lachaux, J.-P., Rodriguez, E., & Martinerie, J. (2001). The brainweb: Phase synchronization and large-scale integration. *Nature Reviews Neuroscience, 2,* 228–239.

Velichkovsky, B. M. (2002). Heterarchy of cognition: The depths and highs of a framework for memory research. *Memory, 10,* 405–419.

Vuilleumier, P., Schwartz, S., Duhoux, S., Dolan, R. J., & Driver, J. (2005). Selective attention modulates neural substrates of repetition priming and "implicit" visual memory: Suppressions and enhancements revealed by fMRI. *Journal of Cognitive Neuroscience, 17,* 1245–1260.

Watkins, O. C. & Watkins, M. J. (1975). Buildup of proactive inhibition as a cue-overload effect. *Journal of Experimental Psychology: Human Learning and Memory, 104,* 442–452.

Weldon, M. S. (1999). The memory chop-shop: Issues in the search for memory systems. In J. K. Foster & M. Jelicic (Eds), *Memory: Systems, Process, or Function?* (pp. 162–204). Oxford, UK: Oxford University Press.

Wiggs, C. L. & Martin, A. (1998). Properties and mechanisms of perceptual priming. *Current Opinion in Neurobiology, 8,* 227–233.

Winnick, W. A. & Daniel, S. A. (1970). Two kinds of response priming in tachistoscopic word recognition. *Journal of Experimental Psychology, 84,* 74–81.

Part 3

Working memory control processes and storage

Chapter 10

Toward characterizing the neural correlates of component processes of cognition

Matthew R. Johnson and Marcia K. Johnson

Introduction

Human cognition is a challenging area of inquiry. Ironically, the same intricacies of the mind that allow us to examine it also frustrate our progress; getting our thinking devices to understand their own mechanisms of operation sometimes feels like chasing one's shadow. The mind's flexibility requires many concepts to describe its many functions: For example, in the domain of memory, we use different terms for 'remembering' how to ride a bicycle and 'remembering' the events of the day the training wheels came off (procedural vs. declarative memory [Cohen & Squire, 1980]), or for remembering the phone number we just looked up (working memory [Baddeley, 1992; Baddeley & Hitch, 1974]) and our phone number from childhood (long-term memory). We categorize memory by its informational content (e.g. episodic vs. semantic memory [Tulving, 1983]), by the types of processes we think are engaged (e.g. familiarity vs. recollection [Atkinson & Juola, 1974; Jacoby & Dallas, 1981; Mandler, 1980; Tulving, 1985]; shallow vs. deep encoding [Craik & Lockhart, 1972]; or perceptual vs. reflective processing [Johnson & Hirst, 1991]), or by the brain regions that are involved (e.g. the medial temporal lobe vs. the basal ganglia [Poldrack & Packard, 2003; Poldrack & Rodriguez, 2004]).

Such broad categorizations of memory are not necessarily mutually exclusive; for instance, whether one is able to recollect a stimulus or merely recognize it as familiar may have something (but not everything) to do with whether it was initially encoded deeply or shallowly (see Yonelinas, 2002). In turn, such seemingly different subjective experiences as a feeling of familiarity or of more embellished recollection may involve partially overlapping brain structures. A closely related issue specific to process-oriented approaches is that key concepts may be complex and involve multiple sub-processes. For example, even simple working memory tasks require encoding, maintenance, updating, and selection processes. One such task sometimes used to operationalize the process of 'working memory' is the N-back task, which minimally requires one not only to perceive the features of a stimulus, construct an internal representation of it, and add that representation to an existing queue of N previously presented stimuli, but also to compare the first and last representations to decide if they are the same, recall the appropriate action to take, make a button press or other overt response, and remove the oldest representation from the queue. Furthermore, some of these sub-processes could easily be shared with a number of other cognitive tasks which may or may not be considered 'working memory' tasks *per se*. Also, as the complexity of a task grows, there is the increasing likelihood that different people will use different strategies (i.e. differing combinations or sequences of component processes) to perform the task (Johnson *et al.*, 2005). Thus, for multiple reasons, the greater the complexity of a task or a proposed cognitive process, the more difficult it may be to characterize. At the same time, general concepts used to characterize mental activity during complex tasks, e.g. 'working memory', 'executive function', and 'cognitive control' likely share some or many of the same underlying cognitive and neural components.

While general constructs such as working memory, executive function, and cognitive control focus attention on important domains and help organize findings, researchers also recognize the importance of unpacking these complex ideas into constituent elements (e.g. structures or processes): For example, the work of Baddeley and colleagues in characterizing the phonological loop, visuo-spatial sketchpad, and central executive subcomponents of working memory (Baddeley, 1984, 1996; Baddeley, Lewis, & Vallar, 1984; Baddeley & Lieberman, 1980; Salame & Baddeley, 1982) or the work of Cohen, Carter and others in dissociating elements of cognitive control, particularly the role of the anterior cingulate cortex (ACC) in detecting conflict (Botvinick, Nystrom, Fissell, Carter, & Cohen, 1999; Carter *et al.*, 1998; Kerns *et al.*, 2004; MacDonald, Cohen, Stenger, & Carter, 2000). In our lab, we have found it useful to adopt a component-process approach, using a model that defines a set of basic 'building blocks' of cognition that, when combined, could form the many more complex operations of which the mind is capable. Here, we first provide an overview of this model and then describe studies using neuroimaging to test and more completely characterize its component processes.

A component-process model: the MEM framework

The framework we have used to guide our investigation of the neural correlates of cognition is the Multiple-Entry, Modular (MEM) framework (Johnson, 1992; Johnson & Hirst, 1993; Johnson & Reeder, 1997). At different times, MEM has been discussed in the context of a 'memory' model (Johnson, 1992) or a model of 'cognition' more generally construed (Johnson & Reeder, 1997) because it is both: One of the core features of MEM is that each processing component is assumed to create memory records of its own processing. Thus, there is no distinction in MEM between components that store memory representations and those that perform ongoing information processing. Though this idea was initially articulated in a primarily cognitive context (Johnson, 1983; Kolers & Roediger, 1984), work in the neurosciences and in computational modeling has provided support for the idea that long-term storage of memory representations of a stimulus is mediated in cortex by changes in synaptic strength in the circuits that were initially used to perceive and/or think about that stimulus (McClelland, McNaughton, & O'Reilly, 1995; Mishkin, 1982; Miyashita, 1993; Squire & Alvarez, 1995).

In the MEM architecture (Figure 10.1), the most fundamental distinction is between components that serve Perceptual (P) versus Reflective (R) forms of processing (Johnson, 1983, 1997; Johnson & Hirst, 1993; Johnson & Reeder, 1997). These are organized into two perceptual subsystems (P-1 and P-2) shown in Figure 10.1C and two reflective subsystems (R-1 and R-2) shown in Figure 10.1B. Each of the four subsystems includes component processes. P-1 processes may be, in a sense, considered 'lower-level' versions of P-2 processes, and likewise R-1 processes may be considered 'lower-level' versions of R-2 processes. As represented by the vertical placement of the planes in Figures 10.1B and 1C, the subsystems reflect a hypothesized hierarchy related to their evolutionary history and the degree to which the processes in each generate an experience of conscious awareness or control: P-1 processes are associated the least with conscious awareness/control, followed by increasing awareness/control from P-2, R-1, and R-2 processes, respectively.

Low-level perceptual processes (P-1) include *locating* stimuli, *resolving* stimulus configurations (e.g. detecting edges), *tracking* stimuli, and *extracting* invariants from perceptual arrays (e.g. cues specifying the rapid expansion of features in the visual field that indicates a stimulus is coming toward you). Although, as noted above, we are generally

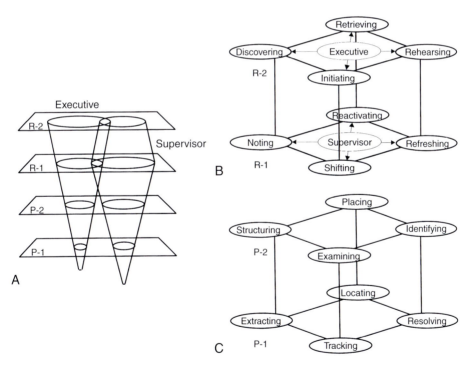

Figure 10.1 The MEM architecture. (A) Cones representing executive and supervisor agendas. The width of a cone as it passes through the R-2, R-1, P-2, and P-1 subsystems indicates the degree to which each type of agenda is involved with processing at these levels. (B) Eight reflective component processes associated with R-2 and R-1 levels of processing. (C) Eight perceptual component processes associated with P-2 and P-1 levels of processing.

unaware of the processing that occurs at the P-1 level, the learning that occurs within P-1 can allow us to improve in, for example, understanding an unfamiliar accent or catching a baseball. Higher-level perceptual processes (P-2) include *placing* objects in spatial relation to each other, *identifying* objects, *examining* or perceptually investigating stimuli (e.g. guided by perceptual schemas), and *structuring* or abstracting a pattern of organization from temporally extended stimuli (e.g. syntactic structure from language). These processes generate and allow us to learn about our phenomenal perceptual world of objects and events (e.g. that round objects roll and apples are often red and can be eaten).

The MEM reflective R-1 and R-2 subsystems propose processes that allow us to sustain, revive, organize, and manipulate information that may no longer be present in the immediate perceptual environment. R-1 component processes include *noting* relations among stimuli or thoughts, *shifting* attention, *refreshing* active information so that it is foregrounded relative to competing information, and *reactivating* information that is not currently active. The proposed component processes of R-2 are conceptually analogous to those in R-1, but are more deliberate (controlled). They include *discovering* (e.g. looking for relations), *initiating* (processes or sequences of processes), *rehearsing* (to keep information active), and *retrieving* (e.g. remembering via systematic self-cuing). Comparing *reactivating* versus *retrieving* illustrates the difference between R-1 and R-2 processes. One example of *reactivating* is when a memory record is (non-deliberately) activated by a partial match between ongoing reflection or perception and records of previous processing, for example, when a current thought or stimulus brings to mind relatively automatically the memory of a previous similar situation or stimulus. In contrast, an example of *retrieving* is when a person deliberately uses some strategy to systematically search their memory. For example, in trying to retrieve the name of a restaurant, one might try to think of people who would likely have told them about a restaurant (Baddeley, 1982; Reiser, 1986).

Importantly, though in MEM we refer to 'component processes', 'subsystems', or 'modules', a central tenet of the framework is that complex behaviours are constructed from flexibly recruited combinations and interactions of such components. MEM components should not be construed as 'modular' in the sense intended by Fodor (1983). MEM *agendas*, similar to the concepts of schemas, scripts, or plans (e.g. Miller, Galanter, & Pribram, 1960; Norman & Shallice, 1986; Stuss & Benson, 1986), coordinate and combine component processes to achieve one's goals (e.g. identify an object, recall a shopping list, plan one's weekend activities). Agendas may be specific or general, simple or complex, well-learned or newly formed; but in each case, an agenda constitutes a plan (e.g. representation of a goal) for cognition that includes one or more component subprocesses. In Figures 10.1A and 10.1B, *supervisor* refers to agendas that are predominantly active in subsystem R-1 and *executive* refers to those agendas predominantly active in subsystem R-2. Supervisor agendas tend to be simpler and more rote or schematized, whereas executive agendas are more complex, deliberate, and analytic. In both cases, agendas constitute the mechanisms of controlling cognition and monitoring outcomes.

Supervisor and executive agendas often invoke sequences of subprocesses that occur at multiple levels of processing. Hence, they are depicted as two cones in Figure 10.1A that pass through planes corresponding to the R-2, R-1, P-2, and P-1 subsystems. The width of each cone as it passes through a plane represents the degree to which executive or supervisor processes are presumed to recruit processes within that subsystem. Thus, although the primary domains of the supervisor and executive are subsystem R-1 and R-2, respectively, both supervisor and executive agendas are hypothesized to be able to influence, and draw upon, all four subsystems, although to different degrees. Importantly, supervisor and executive agendas are capable of influencing each other, as indicated by the overlap in the two reflective subsystems in Figure 10.1A. This feature of the MEM architecture provides a mechanism for self-reflection and other forms of complex cognition.

MEM is a mid-level model of cognition; MEM component subprocesses are not indivisible (in fact, see Johnson & Hirst, 1993; Johnson & Reeder, 1997 for discussions of ways in which some component processes might be further decomposed). Rather, MEM attempts to provide a general framework for reducing the vast space of human cognition to combinations of a relatively small and manageable number of components. (In this endeavour, we express the implicit hope that human cognition might follow a Pareto principle of sorts; i.e. fully describing a system as complex and flexible as the human mind could require a 'model' as complex as the system itself, but we can nevertheless aspire to create models that capture a large proportion of the mind's functions with a manageably small degree of complexity.) MEM also provides a means of organizing the results of investigations directed at more fine-grained levels of analysis than represented in MEM, namely by grouping finer subdivisions within a MEM component subprocess (e.g. within *rehearsing* or *identifying*). MEM is primarily a process-based model rather than a content-based one. Thus people are thought to be capable of performing operations like *tracking*, *identifying*, *reactivating*, etc., on a wide range of modalities of percepts and thoughts (e.g. auditory, pictorial, tactile, emotional, semantic). For example, one could further divide *identifying* into identifying based on visual information, identifying based on auditory information, etc.

MEM and neuroimaging

Just as conceptual psychological models like MEM can be informed by and help provide a context for investigating and understanding findings from neuropsychological studies of brain damaged patients (e.g. disrupted explicit memory and preserved acquisition of emotional associations, Johnson, Kim, & Risse, 1985), there should be a synergistic relation between such models and findings from neuroimaging. Research using neuroimaging has grown explosively since the early- to mid-1990s, and the knowledge base of replicable findings has grown to the point that we can begin to reason bidirectionally about the relationships between cognition and brain activity. Although there is some controversy over the productivity of the relation between cognitive psychology and neuroimaging (e.g. Uttal, 2001; but see Henson, 2005), the final judgement will rest on how much this partnership contributes to a cumulative science of mental function. The advantages and potential limitations of an additional source of new hypotheses and constraints in theorizing (i.e. neuroimaging evidence) are analogous to advantages and limitations following from procedures and traditions of other approaches (e.g. mathematical models; computer simulations). In any event, the challenges of using neuroimaging techniques such as functional magnetic resonance imaging (fMRI) to adduce evidence about theoretical constructs are not in principle greater or different than those of using cognitive/behavioural methods. Attempting to find the correspondence between cognitive operations and brain activity shares many problems with attempting to operationalize theoretical cognitive processes in cognitive-behavioural studies. Just as it is difficult to find a 'pure' behavioural index of a particular cognitive process, it is also difficult to relate tasks to activated brain regions or interactions between regions in a one-to-one manner. And, just as we can classify cognitive processes at different levels of abstraction, brain structures can also be classified at different levels (e.g. genes, molecules, cells, circuits, gyri, or cerebral hemispheres). In both domains the challenge is to find appropriate levels of abstraction that capture a maximal amount of variance in the observed data with a minimal amount of theoretical complexity. When the structure in question is large, it may be that different theoretical labels can describe similar amounts of variance, producing multiple models of roughly equal validity. For example, the idea that prefrontal cortex (PFC) is involved in cognitive control (Miller & Cohen, 2001) and the idea that PFC represents information in working memory (Courtney, 2004) may be equally apt accounts at a general level of description.

With resolutions typically on the order of a few millimeters, current functional neuroimaging methods afford a moderate degree of spatial discriminability, reliably localizing regions of maximal activity to a portion of a particular gyrus/sulcus, but not to a particular cell layer or cortical column. We began with the question of whether the mid-level spatial resolution afforded by fMRI would be appropriate for the mid-level 'conceptual resolution' of a cognitive model like MEM.

The refresh process

We have initially focused our neuroimaging studies on the component process of *refreshing*: the act of thinking of, or foregrounding, a representation of a thought or percept which was activated just a moment earlier and has not yet become inactive. We reasoned that if fMRI can provide a neural picture of this relatively simple process, we can then test hypotheses about other processes to assess whether distinct component processes as proposed in MEM could be dissociated neurally.

We also hypothesized that refreshing is likely to play a role in more complex constructs frequently discussed in the neuroimaging literature, especially working memory and executive function. This is because refreshing acts as both a basic maintenance process (i.e. refreshing a representation has the effect of prolonging its activation) as well as a manipulation process (i.e. by virtue of selecting or biasing one representation relative to others [Johnson et al., 2005; Raye, Johnson, Mitchell, Greene, & Johnson, 2007]). By characterizing the behavioural and neural correlates of refreshing, we hoped to shed further light on how refreshing contributes to more complex tasks, and perhaps explain in terms of shared component processes some of the common brain activity observed in neuroimaging studies of diverse tasks (e.g. Duncan & Owen, 2000).

Behavioural correlates of refreshing

In a behavioural study of the refresh process, Johnson and colleagues (Johnson, Reeder, Raye, & Mitchell, 2002) projected words onto a computer screen one at a time, and participants were instructed to read and say all words aloud as quickly as possible. Response times were recorded using a voice key apparatus. Some words were presented only once (*read* condition), some were followed immediately by the same word again (*repeat* condition), and some were followed immediately by a dot (•) that signaled participants to think of the just-previous word and say it aloud (*refresh* condition). A surprise recognition memory test for the words from the three conditions, randomly intermixed with new words, was administered a few minutes after the conclusion of the incidental encoding task.

Two effects of primary interest were observed. First, whereas participants were faster to say words in the *repeat* condition than in the *read* condition (consistent with repetition-priming effects [Tulving & Schacter, 1990]), they were slower to say words in the *refresh* condition than in the *repeat* and *read* conditions. Thus, a clear behavioural dissociation was observed between the R-1 process of *refreshing* and the P-2 process of *identifying* (the MEM perceptual subprocess most directly tested by the *read* and *repeat* conditions), given similar conceptual content. These results suggested that it could be possible to dissociate these processes neurally as well. It is important to recognize that, even in a task as simple as this, the *refresh* condition probably involved additional component processes in that participants had to *note* the dot and *initiate* a refresh. However, a control experiment revealed no difference between response times in the *read* condition and a condition in which participants were instructed merely to say 'dot' when the dot appeared, suggesting that the observed difference in response times between the *read* and *refresh* conditions was indeed primarily due to the process of refreshing word representations.

The second result of interest was greater recognition memory for words in the *refresh* condition than either the *repeat* or *read* conditions (and, as one would expect, greater memory for words in the *repeat* condition than in the *read* condition). This again demonstrates the dissociability of the refresh process from perceptual processes, and it is consistent with the MEM idea that separate (and thus potentially behaviourally distinguishable) memory records are created for information handled by each component subprocess. It is worth mentioning that later studies of the refresh process using different classes of stimuli sometimes show no advantage of *refresh* over *repeat* conditions for subsequent recognition memory (Johnson *et al.*, 2005). This suggests that people are better able to refresh some stimuli than others, or that during the recognition memory test, people draw upon memory records generated by different MEM component processes to varying degrees depending on the type of stimulus (e.g. perhaps people rely relatively more on R-1 and R-2 records when tested with word stimuli but relatively more on P-1 and P-2 records for pictures of people or abstract patterns).

Basic neural correlates of refreshing

Early fMRI investigations of the refresh process confirmed our initial hypothesis that it would be possible to distinguish relatively basic component subprocesses of cognition from one another via functional neuroimaging. Raye and colleagues (Raye, Johnson, Mitchell, Reeder, & Greene, 2002, Experiment 1) performed an event-related fMRI study with similar conditions to those described above in the behavioural study by Johnson and colleagues (2002). As shown in Figure 10.2A, there were three conditions (*read*, *repeat*, and *refresh*), randomly intermixed. In the *read* condition, the critical item was preceded by a different, novel word; in the *repeat* condition, the critical item was preceded by the same word; and in the *refresh* condition, a dot cued participants to think back to the just-presented word. The initial part of the hemodynamic activity should thus be comparable (reflect reading a word) in all conditions, and differences in haemodynamic activity between conditions should reflect differences in processing occurring during the second part of the trial, associated with reading a word for the first time, reading a word again, or refreshing a word.

Regions in which activity in the *refresh* condition was significantly greater than in both the *repeat* and *read* conditions included a region of left dorsolateral prefrontal cortex (DLPFC; middle frontal gyrus, Brodmann area 9; see Figure 10.2B) as well as two left parietal regions. The refresh-related DLPFC activity was of particular note due to that region's strong associations with working memory and general executive functioning, in which the refresh process is presumed to play a part. Raye and colleagues suggested that reported DLPFC activity in various working memory tasks (e.g. Cohen *et al.*, 1997; Petrides, Alivisatos, Meyer, & Evans, 1993; Smith & Jonides, 1999) may have been due, in part, to refresh-related activity. Experiments 2 and 3 reported by Raye *et al.* were control experiments intended to rule out alternative sources of the observed activity in DLPFC. Experiment 2 used a blocked design to verify that the observed activity was not due to task-switching (i.e. effects of performing different conditions from trial to trial). Experiment 3 demonstrated that refresh-related DLPFC activity was not due to the need to interpret a symbolic stimulus (i.e. the dot cue). Participants merely read or refreshed words silently, indicating that reflection is sufficient to identify refresh-related changes in neural activity without the need for an overt response.

Several subsequent fMRI studies of refreshing (Johnson, Mitchell, Raye, & Greene, 2004; Johnson, Raye, Mitchell, Greene, & Anderson, 2003; Johnson *et al.*, 2005) confirmed and extended the results found by Raye and colleagues (2002). For example, a study investigating age-related differences in refreshing using the same design identified the same refresh-related DLPFC region in a new sample of young adults (compare Johnson *et al.*, 2004, and Raye *et al.*, 2002). Johnson and colleagues (2003) identified somewhat different regions of left DLPFC associated with refreshing words, objects, and abstract patterns, suggesting that information type affects the part of DLPFC that is maximally activated by refreshing. Across studies with different types of stimuli (e.g. auditory and visual words, objects, abstract patterns, pictures of people, locations), refresh-related activity has consistently been observed in left lateral PFC, primarily distributed along the middle frontal gyrus (see Figure 10.2D). Refresh-related activity has also been seen, but less often, in right PFC. The exact location of left PFC activity and the presence and extent of right-hemisphere refresh activity may depend not only on the type of information refreshed but also on the other types of information being refreshed in the same study and the other types of operations being engaged (Johnson *et al.*, 2005).

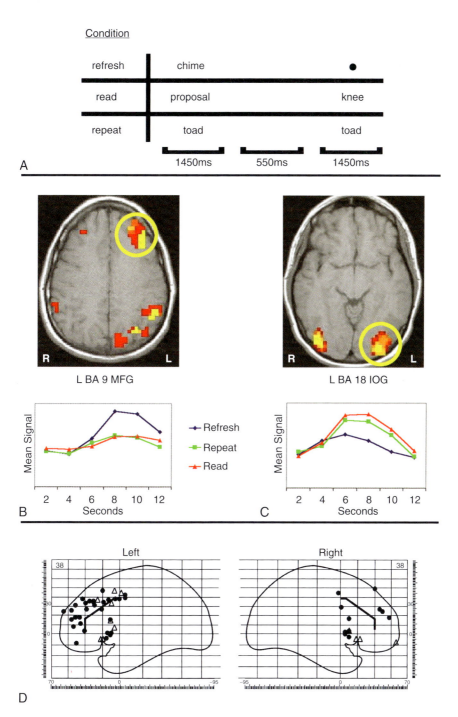

Figure 10.2 (A) Examples of the *refresh*, *read*, and *repeat* conditions used in Raye *et al.* (2002) and other studies. (B) Greater activity for refreshing than reading or re-reading word stimuli in left DLPFC. Adapted from Raye *et al.* (2002). (C) Greater activity for reading or re-reading word stimuli than refreshing in left occipital cortex. Adapted from Raye *et al.* (2002). (D) Maxima of refresh-related activity plotted for several studies. Circles indicate refreshing a single item, triangles indicate refreshing one of three items. Middle frontal gyrus is above the line, inferior frontal gyrus below. Adapted from Johnson *et al.* (2005). BA: Brodmann area, IOG: inferior occipital gyrus, MFG: middle frontal gyrus.

Distinguishing activity associated with different component reflective processes

It is important to compare the network of areas that are associated with refreshing to those associated with other reflective component processes, to more precisely identify which activation patterns are specific to the process of refreshing, which are specific to other component processes, and which are shared. Observing different patterns of activation between refresh and other reflective component processes would suggest that the observed refresh-related activity is specific to that process. Conversely, similar patterns of activation between refresh and other reflective processes could suggest that, as they are operationalized, either (a) refreshing and other component processes invoke a common component such as process *initiation* or (b) the two proposed component processes are not different, at least at the cognitive and neural levels of analysis afforded by the MEM framework and fMRI, respectively. Naturally, the comparison between refreshing and another component process could also yield a mixture of shared and distinct brain regions, or an outcome in which two processes might differ not in the areas activated but in the relative magnitude of activation in the same areas.

Johnson and colleagues (2003) compared the results of an fMRI experiment that included refreshing visually presented words and line drawings of objects (Experiment 1) with an experiment requiring participants to *note* (another R-1 process) whether or not a visually presented word or object was the same as one which had been presented previously (Experiment 2). The primary intent of analysing these two data sets together was to examine whether PFC activity appeared to be functionally organized around the type of component process invoked (i.e. *refreshing* versus *noting*), the type of information involved (e.g. words versus drawings), a combination of both organizational schemes, or neither (that is, some PFC areas might be flexibly recruited for multiple component processes and types of information, and thus not exhibit organization by either process or type or information). The results of Experiment 1 identified separate (but nearby) areas in left DLPFC for *refreshing* words versus drawings, whereas the results of Experiment 2 identified separate (but nearby) areas of right PFC that were activated for *noting* the repetition of words versus drawings. The fact that different regions were activated for different materials (holding operation constant within each experiment) supported a role of information type in the functional organization of PFC. Furthermore, a statistical comparison of the two experiments revealed an area of left DLPFC that was active for *refreshing* (across information type) but not for *noting*. Thus, the results of this study supported a functional organization of PFC both by type of information and type of process.

Other findings have also indicated that activity in different areas within left PFC may be differentially involved in refreshing versus other R-1 component processes. Johnson and colleagues (2005) presented the results of a meta-analysis that identified refresh-related areas of frontal cortex by pooling data across several studies, which allowed them to examine task-related activity both in regions that typically occur and in regions that may not have been significant in each study when analysed separately. Two areas of particular interest were a typical area of left DLPFC (middle frontal gyrus, Brodmann areas 9/6) similar to that reported by Raye and colleagues (2002) and a less frequently observed area of left anterior PFC (middle/superior frontal gyri, Brodmann areas 10/46). The DLPFC area showed greater variability in magnitude of activation across refresh studies compared to the anterior PFC area. This suggested that activity in the DLPFC area may reflect the nature of what is being represented whereas the anterior area may be serving a more general function such as process initiation. To test this hypothesis, Raye and colleagues (2007) performed an fMRI study in which brain activity in a *refresh* condition (as before, presentation of a word followed by a dot cuing participants to refresh the word) was compared to activation in an *act* condition (presentation of a word followed by a square cuing participants simply to press a button), and both were compared to a *read* condition (presentation of a word followed by another, different word).

Consistent with Raye and colleagues' (2007) hypothesis, an area of left DLPFC was more active for the *refresh* than the *act* condition (see Figure 10.3A).[1] This difference between the *refresh* and *act* conditions in left DLPFC is consistent with the hypothesis that this area is involved in foregrounding and/or maintaining a representation. In contrast, in a left anterior PFC area (superior frontal gyrus; Brodmann area 10, see Figure 10.3B) there was no difference in activity between the *refresh* and *act* conditions, although activity was greater in both than in the *read* condition, suggesting that left anterior PFC is associated with the component process of *initiating* rather than foregrounding a representation per se. Other investigators have emphasized the importance of DLPFC in selective attention, task management (e.g. maintaining a task context), or manipulation of information (e.g. D'Esposito, Postle, Ballard, & Lease, 1999; MacDonald *et al.*, 2000; Miller & Cohen, 2001; Petrides, 2000; Smith & Jonides, 1999). All of these proposed DLPFC functions involve foregrounding some information so that it has a competitive advantage (is more available) or confers a competitive advantage over (biases, e.g. Miller & Cohen, 2001) other information. We have proposed that refreshing is one mechanism by which such foregrounding occurs. It has also been suggested that anterior PFC (or frontopolar cortex), is involved in processing internally generated information (Christoff & Gabrieli, 2000), establishing 'task sets' (Passingham & Sakai, 2004), maintaining information about contexts and goals (Courtney, 2004), or monitoring and integrating subgoals (Braver & Bongiolatti, 2002). We have proposed that a common theme uniting these proposals is a shared demand for *initiating* (or *shifting* between) different agendas, or different active representations or stimulus features. In the case of studies contrasting refreshing with relatively automatic processes such as reading words, DLPFC may be sufficient. For more complex stimuli, or for negotiating between multiple non-automatic agendas (e.g. *refresh*, *act*), anterior PFC may be required.

A second experiment by Raye and colleagues (2007) compared *refreshing* to the R-2 process of *rehearsing*. For the *refresh* condition, a word was presented followed by the

---

[1]   In Figure 10.3A, in DLPFC, although there was less activity in the read than refresh condition, there was more activity in the read than act condition. In other studies, there was little activity in DLPFC in the read condition (compare Figure 10.3A with Figures 10.2B and 10.3C). This suggests that participants may have sometimes spontaneously refreshed in the read condition. One possibility is that such uncued refreshes are more likely to occur on read trials in some task contexts than others.

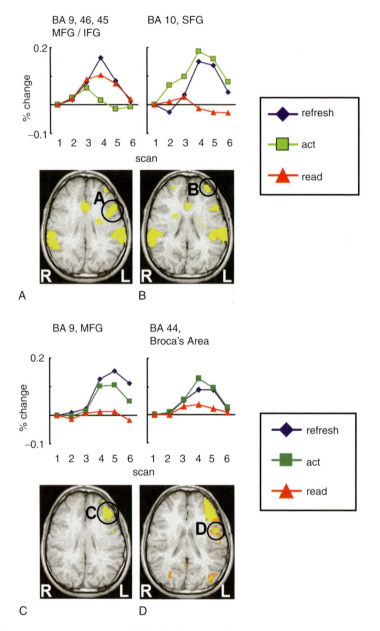

Figure 10.3 Data from Raye *et al*. (2007). (A) Greater activity for the *refresh* condition than the *act* condition in left DLPFC. (B) Similar activity for the *refresh* and *act* conditions in left anterior PFC. (C) Greater activity for the *refresh* condition than the *rehearse* condition in left DLPFC. (D) Greater activity for the *rehearse* condition than the *refresh* condition in Broca's area. All panels adapted from Raye *et al*. (2007). See text for details. BA: Brodmann area, IFG: inferior frontal gyrus, MFG: middle frontal gyrus, SFG: superior frontal gyrus.

letter 'V', cuing participants to refresh the visual aspect of the just-presented word. For the *rehearse* condition, a word was presented followed by the letter 'S', cuing participants to subvocally say the just-presented word twice. In the MEM framework, *rehearsing* is a distinct component R-2 process that is located just above the R-1 process of refreshing (see Figure 10.1B). This proximity indicates some similarity in function – in this case, both are mechanisms for keeping representations active. However, refreshing is a simpler, briefer, and relatively more automatic process, while rehearsing (for verbal information) typically involves more deliberate, subvocal repetition, often of multiple items, over several seconds. As distinct processes, *refreshing* and *rehearsing* should exhibit some differentiation in their neural signatures. Previous studies have located activity related to subvocal rehearsal in left ventrolateral prefrontal cortex (VLPFC) and have distinguished it from other (e.g. storage and executive) components of verbal working memory (Awh *et al.*, 1996; Chein & Fiez, 2001; Smith & Jonides, 1999), providing further support for the hypothesis that rehearse-related activity should be separable from refresh-related activity in left DLPFC. Of course, rehearsal studies typically involve several items, often presented visually and maintained (i.e. converted to a phonological code and cycled through repeatedly) over several seconds. Thus the contrast between thinking once briefly of the appearance of a just-seen stimulus, versus saying it twice subvocally, was intended to be a manipulation that would minimally engage a phonological loop but not result in substantial differences in 'time on task' between conditions.

Raye and colleagues (2007; Experiment 2) found two areas of interest that were more active in the *refresh* condition than the *rehearse* condition: an area of left DLPFC (middle frontal gyrus, Brodmann area 9) and an area bridging the precentral and middle frontal gyri (Brodmann area 6). These regions were also both identified as refresh-related areas in the meta-analysis by Johnson and colleagues (2005). A third area of interest was also found that was more active in the *rehearse* condition than the *refresh* condition. It was located in the inferior frontal gyrus (Brodmann area 44/6), including Broca's area. It is worth noting that both the refresh- and rehearse-related areas of interest, though most active in their preferred condition, also showed some activity in the non-preferred condition, although none of the areas showed appreciable activity during the *read* condition. Thus, although the *refresh* and *rehearse* conditions were neurally differentiable from each other, they appeared to show some degree of common activity as well. This is consistent with the MEM hypothesis that the more complex processes along the vertical edges of the cubes in Figure 10.1 (i.e. those closer to the top of the figure) might, through evolution, be variations of or elaborations upon the more rudimentary processes along the same edge (i.e. those closer to the bottom of the figure). That is, some overlap in brain regions subserving functionally and phylogenetically related processes would be consistent with this speculation.

Raye and colleagues (2007) also reported results of functional connectivity analyses. In Experiment 1, activity in the left anterior PFC region, which was equally active for both *refresh* and *act* trials and appeared to subserve the initiation of non-automatic actions, was more strongly correlated with activity in left DLPFC during *refresh* trials and more strongly with activity in left pre- and post-central gyri during *act* trials. These analyses illustrate a primary assumption of most neuroimaging research: cognitive processes are transactions among regions (e.g. Friston, 1994; Horwitz, 1994; McIntosh & Gonzalez-Lima, 1994). The results also illustrate a primary goal: that once a satisfactory mapping between brain regions and component processes is achieved, data on interactions between brain regions may generate or confirm hypotheses about the interactions between cognitive processes. Here, the correlation results suggest that during *refresh* trials, as a function of the cue, *initiating* (associated with left anterior PFC) plays a role in recruiting *refreshing* (associated with left DLPFC) or, during act trials, plays a role in recruiting a motor response (associated with motor/somatosensory areas in left pre- and post-central gyri). These results are consistent with the predictions of the MEM framework and demonstrate the ways in which different component processes may work together in different circumstances. Of course this account remains a hypothesis to be verified with further studies.

Refreshing as an executive function

The above sections have primarily focused on identifying the fundamental neural correlates of the refresh process, distinguishing it from other component cognitive processes, and elaborating on its role in reflective (e.g. working memory) functions that involve both the maintenance and the manipulation of representations. The neuroimaging work described thus far has primarily focused on the prefrontal correlates of refreshing, given the historically strong associations between PFC and the kinds of controlled, executive, and working memory functions that the proposed reflective processes in MEM support (e.g. Johnson & Reeder, 1997). For the purposes of the following discussion, we will group these working memory, cognitive control, and other reflective functions together under the general conceptual umbrella of 'executive function'.

Contemporary theories of PFC executive function (e.g. Miller & Cohen, 2001) suggest that the overarching purpose of the PFC is to direct thought (e.g. manipulate information) in the service of goals (or, in MEM terms, *agendas*) by sending signals to other areas of cortex that bias the flow of information and the patterns of neural activity in those areas. A related theory of working memory is that PFC helps to maintain active representations by modulating activity in the same posterior areas initially used in stimulus perception (Curtis & D'Esposito, 2003; Petrides, 1994; Ranganath & D'Esposito, 2005; Ruchkin, Grafman, Cameron, & Berndt, 2003). These views of executive function and working memory are consistent with the types of processes embodied in the MEM architecture's R-1 and R-2 level functions. If these theories are correct and if the *refresh* process is, as we believe, a basic component of executive function, we should not only find refresh-related activity in PFC but also evidence that refreshing can modulate activity in areas of cortex outside of PFC.

While we have previously reported refresh-related activity in areas beyond PFC, e.g. parietal cortex and precuneus (e.g. Raye *et al.*, 2002, 2007), these regions were not our primary focus. Recently, to more completely characterize the neural substrates of the refresh process and provide further evidence for refreshing as an executive function,

M. R. Johnson and colleagues (M. R. Johnson, Mitchell, Raye, D'Esposito, & Johnson, 2007) conducted an fMRI study to determine whether refreshing a visual stimulus could modulate activity in posterior regions of cortex thought to primarily support visual perception (i.e. P-1 and P-2 processing). There were four conditions of primary interest, two *refresh* conditions and two *repeat* conditions. In all four conditions, participants initially saw a screen containing two pictures side-by-side; one picture was always of a face and the other of a scene. After a brief, 500 msec delay, in the *Repeat_S* and *Repeat_F* conditions, the scene (face) stimulus was shown a second time; in the *Refresh_S* condition, a dot appeared where the scene stimulus had been, cuing participants to refresh (think back to, visualize) the scene picture; and in the *Refresh_F* condition, a dot appeared where the face stimulus had been, cuing participants to refresh the face picture.

In this study, we also administered a localizer task in order to locate areas of posterior cortex that selectively responded more to either faces or scenes (relative to the other stimulus class) during perception. A priori regions of interest (ROIs) included the parahippocampal place area (PPA; Epstein & Kanwisher, 1998) and fusiform face area (FFA; Kanwisher, McDermott, & Chun, 1997), which were identified bilaterally for each participant. Additional ROIs identified in a group-level analysis included areas of bilateral precuneus, bilateral middle occipital gyrus, and bilateral retrosplenial cortex, all of which responded more during perception of scenes than during perception of faces, and an area of right inferior occipital gyrus, which responded more during perception of faces than during perception of scenes. After these areas were identified, their activity during the main refresh task was assessed to see if it was modulated by which representation was refreshed, that is, by comparing activity in the *Refresh_S* and *Refresh_F* conditions. We also compared activity in these regions between *refresh* and *repeat* trials to examine the relative influences of reflective and perceptual processing, respectively, on activity in posterior perceptual regions.

Refresh-related activity was observed in areas of both DLPFC and anterior PFC, replicating prior work and suggesting that participants were indeed performing the refresh task similar to previous studies. Modulatory effects (i.e. differential activity) from refreshing faces vs. scenes were observed in bilateral PPA (see Figure 10.4A), bilateral retrosplenial cortex, left middle occipital gyrus, and left precuneus (activity in the *Refresh_S* condition was greater than in the *Refresh_F* condition), and in right FFA and right inferior occipital gyrus (activity in the *Refresh_F* condition was greater than in the *Refresh_S* condition). Importantly, the *Refresh_S* and *Refresh_F* conditions contained identical perceptual input (an initial screen containing one face and one scene, followed by a second screen showing only a dot) with the only difference being whether the dot indicated that participants should refresh the face or the scene. Thus, these results indicate that a brief, basic act of reflection (e.g. refreshing a face or a scene) is sufficient to induce modulatory activity in posterior regions of cortex that activate preferentially to that type of information during perception.

In addition, we (M. R. Johnson *et al.*, 2007) compared the overall activation difference for *repeat* conditions minus *refresh* conditions (i.e. perceptual activity minus reflective activity) in the four scene-selective ROIs (PPA, retrosplenial cortex, precuneus, and

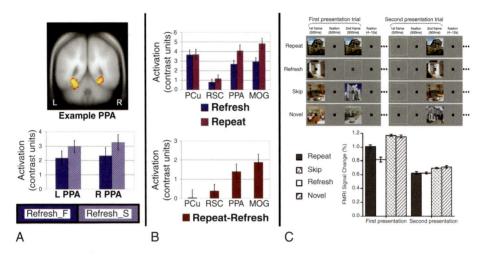

Figure 10.4 (A) Evidence of modulatory refresh effects in bilateral PPA. Adapted from M. R. Johnson *et al.* (2007). (B) A gradient for reflection versus perception, with little difference between *refresh* and *repeat* conditions in more anterior/superior scene-selective areas and significantly more activity for *repeat* than *refresh* conditions in more posterior/inferior areas. Adapted from M. R. Johnson *et al.* (2007). (C) Task description and data from right PPA, adapted from Yi et al. (2008). Refreshing and repeating scene stimuli produced similar degrees of repetition attenuation at a second presentation compared to stimuli that had been seen only once (*skip* condition). See text for details. MOG: middle occipital gyrus, PCu: precuneus, PPA: parahippocampal place area, RSC: retrosplenial cortex.

middle occipital gyrus). An anatomical gradient of relative responsiveness to reflection and perception was found, with the most anterior and superior area (precuneus) showing essentially no difference between *refresh* and *repeat* activity, and areas located more posteriorly and inferiorly (in order: retrosplenial cortex, PPA, middle occipital gyrus) showing gradually greater increases in *repeat* activity relative to *refresh* activity (see Figure 10.4B). This is consistent with the concept represented by the cones in the MEM framework (Figure 10.1A) – that executive and supervisor processes are capable of recruiting and influencing processes at the perceptual level of processing, though with decreasing efficacy at 'lower' (i.e. P-1) levels of perception. Of course, the fact that refreshing influences neural activity in areas involved in perception does not alone show that refreshing influences perception itself. However, the results of a study by Yi, Turk-Browne, Chun, and Johnson (2008) support the hypothesis that an act of refreshing can, in fact, exert an influence on perceptual processing.

Yi and colleagues (2008) scanned participants using fMRI during a refresh task involving scene stimuli. In each condition (see Figure 10.4C), trials began with the presentation of a novel scene stimulus with a fixation dot followed by a brief blank stimulus with a fixation point. Next, in the *repeat* condition, the same scene was presented a second time; in the *refresh* condition, participants saw a white dot on the fixation point, signaling them to think back to the scene that had just been presented; and in the *skip* condition, another novel scene stimulus was presented. In all three conditions, this sequence constituted the 'first presentation' trial. Thus, in the first presentation trial, scenes in the *repeat* condition had been seen twice, those in the *refresh* condition had been seen once and refreshed once, and those in the *skip* condition had been seen once. There were also 'second presentation' trials intermixed with these first presentation trials. In second presentation trials, a single scene stimulus was shown, which was the same as a scene that had appeared initially in a first presentation trial. There were also second presentation trials consisting of completely novel items that were seen only once.

The primary intent of this study was to compare repetition attenuation in the PPA for stimuli that had been refreshed to that of stimuli that had been repeated or presented only once. Repetition attenuation is a phenomenon where reduced neural activity is observed in stimulus-specific areas of cortex for stimuli that have been perceived before, compared to the activity for novel stimuli. It is thought to be a signature of neural tuning or sharpening of familiar representations or a reduction in the processing necessary for stimulus identification (Desimone, 1996; Grill-Spector, Henson, & Martin, 2006; Wiggs & Martin, 1998), and indeed greater repetition attenuation for a stimulus is associated with a greater likelihood of subsequent recognition (Turk-Browne, Yi, & Chun, 2006). Thus, as refreshing has been shown to modulate activity in perceptual regions (M. R. Johnson *et al.*, 2007) and is thought, like other reflective processes, to be able to influence perceptual processing (Johnson & Reeder, 1997), Yi and colleagues (2008) hypothesized that refreshing a stimulus would induce repetition attenuation during a subsequent presentation of the stimulus.

Analysing fMRI signal in the PPA during the 'second presentation' trials confirmed this hypothesis (see Figure 10.4C). In PPA, previously refreshed and repeated stimuli both showed a greater effect of repetition attenuation (i.e. lower overall signal) than stimuli in the *skip* condition that had previously been seen only once. The degree of repetition attenuation was similar for the *repeat* and *refresh* conditions, suggesting that reflection can sometimes have as much of an effect on later perceptual processing as perception itself. Since repetition attenuation in the ventral visual cortex can be considered a form of perceptual memory, this result supports a key prediction of the MEM framework, namely that subsystems interact. Of course, exactly how they interact remains to be clarified. For example, perception and reflection may both affect the same representations. Or, a cue may activate similar perceptually derived and reflectively generated representations, and this activation may be summed across both types of representations to yield a phenomenal experience or a response in a task.

Selection: The need for a new component?

A consequence of refreshing is, presumably, that the refreshed target is foregrounded (stands out) compared to other active representations, which can be considered a form of selection. To investigate the neural correlates of this selective aspect of refreshing, we conducted an fMRI study (Johnson *et al.*, 2005, Experiment 5; Raye, Mitchell, Reeder, Greene, & Johnson, 2008) in which participants on each trial saw either 1 or 3 words, followed by either a new word (*read* conditions) or a dot cuing them to refresh the single word (*refresh-1*) or one of the three words (*refresh-3*). Analyses identified four areas of frontal cortex where activity was greater when selectively refreshing 1 of 3 items than 1 of 1, but where the number of items presented did not affect activity in the *read* conditions. These were left DLPFC, left VLPFC, ACC, and a small area in right middle frontal gyrus.

Given that, other than DLPFC, these regions are not always associated with single-item refreshing, one might conclude that the *refresh-3* condition invokes a separate selection process that is a function of VLPFC and/or ACC (e.g. Jonides, Smith, Marshuetz, Koeppe, & Reuter-Lorenz, 1998; Thompson-Schill, D'Esposito, Aguirre, & Farah, 1997). However, while not always above threshold in an individual study, our meta-analysis suggests that these additional areas are frequently active to some extent during refreshing (Johnson *et al.*, 2005). Thus, the activity seen in the *refresh-3* condition may not reflect a separate selection process; instead, refreshing may involve a network of regions that are active to varying degrees depending on the information refreshed and the amount of competition among active representations. Furthermore, this network may always be engaged, to varying degrees, in the service of steering the stream of ongoing thought. Consistent with this idea, the pattern of activity found during selective refreshing is strikingly similar to the DLPFC-VLPFC-ACC network identified by Duncan and Owen (2000) as being activated by a wide range of cognitive tasks. The common patterns of activity that Duncan and Owen identified across studies may reflect a common reliance on one or more key component processes like refreshing.

In its current form, MEM contains no explicit representation of a selection process. An aspect of selection is already embodied in MEM's component processes (e.g. *refreshing* and *shifting* both imply targeting a single representation or process from among alternatives). That is, all of the MEM component processes may inherently involve some degree of selection. Hence, it is not clear what the definition of 'selection' would be outside of engaging one of the processes postulated in MEM. Alternatively, it may be that selection should be thought of as a complex action that can be broken down into a combination of extant MEM component processes (e.g. selective *refreshing* = *shifting* among available representations, *noting* the item that corresponds to the cue, and *refreshing* that representation). Or, perhaps we could more succinctly characterize the neural correlates of complex cognition if we add a separate *selecting* process to the MEM model that can be recruited in combination with certain other processes. Theory alone does not tell us whether selecting should be thought of as a mental activity that is inherently a feature of more basic processes, whether it consists of a combination of more basic processes, or whether it is itself a basic process. Neuroimaging data can help us decide among the alternatives by virtue of which explanation provides the most consistent and parsimonious account of the activation patterns observed. Neuroimaging data may also provide a common language for linking corresponding concepts in the literature. For example, Badre and Wagner (2002) have proposed that there is a difference between selecting from active representations and retrieving information from long-term semantic memory. In MEM, this would correspond to the difference between *refreshing* and *reactivating* (or *retrieving*), both of which inherently involve selection. If we operationalize these accounts and observe convergent neural correlates, that would constitute evidence for their conceptual equivalence.

We have found refresh-related areas of DLPFC and ACC that activate more in both *refresh-1* and *refresh-3* compared to their corresponding *read* conditions, but also 'selective refresh' areas of DLPFC, VLPFC and ACC exhibiting refresh-related activity only in the *refresh-3* condition (i.e. *refresh-1* activity did not exceed *read-1* activity; Johnson *et al.*, 2005, Experiment 5). One explanation is that selective refreshing causes an increase in activation extent relative to non-selective refreshing activations, producing above-threshold 'selective refresh' areas in nearby anatomical regions. On the other hand, if findings consistently show increased activation of a particular area or areas (e.g. Brodmann area 45) when the selection requirements for different cognitive processes are increased, that would support (but not alone require) the idea of selection as a separate component process. An analogy might be made if we imagine a MEM-like component process model of human movement containing processes like *walking*, *swimming*, and *climbing*. While *running* is clearly a more effortful analogue of *walking*, is *running* qualitatively different enough to merit being its own, separate component process? Ultimately, decisions about which constructs to include in a model rely on making judgements about which ideas capture observed phenomena most succinctly and intuitively. For now, we view selection as engaging a process (such as refreshing or retrieving) under conditions of competition. As further data emerge, perhaps it may become apparent that we should add selection as a separate component in the MEM framework.

Conclusions and future directions

The concept of 'executive function' has been central in theoretical accounts of behavioural studies of cognition and in describing the impact of certain types of brain damage. The MEM model provides a specific characterization of the concept of executive function in terms of component processes of reflection. Our findings suggest that functional neuroimaging has a level of resolution generally compatible with MEM's mid-level vocabulary of theoretical constructs. Consistent with MEM, neuroimaging has provided evidence that component processes such as *refreshing* (DLPFC), *initiating* (anterior PFC), and *rehearsing* (VLPFC) are differentially subserved by different regions of PFC, and that these regions' activity correlates differentially with other brain regions depending on the representations or other processes they interact with.

Refreshing is proposed to serve a broadly useful executive function in that it is a mechanism by which some information is foregrounded relative to other information so that the refreshed information has a competitive advantage. Thus, refreshing is a mechanism for selective attention to activated representations in the absence of ongoing sensory input (i.e. refreshing = reflective, as opposed to perceptual, attention). Consistent with this idea, we have shown that refreshing modulates activity in some of the same representational regions that are active during perception such as the parahippocampal place area and the fusiform face area. In addition, refreshing has functional consequences, e.g. benefiting subsequent long-term recognition memory (an explicit memory measure) and producing repetition attenuation during subsequent perception of the same stimulus again (an implicit memory measure). This latter finding is consistent with the idea that refreshing may serve as an important mechanism for the interaction between perception and reflection (e.g. bridging gaps between glances as a complex representation of a scene is built up, affecting what percepts are likely to persist in long-term memory, etc.). Interactions in MEM between processes or subsystems are proposed to be as important as the capacity of components to operate in a more modular fashion (Johnson, 1983). Further specifying how such interactions take place is a major challenge.

Although in our lab we have focused primarily on reflective component processes, the gradient we found showing a decrease in the difference in activity during perception and refreshing in visual processing areas, from middle occipital gyrus to parahippocampus to retrosplenial cortex to precuneus, raises interesting questions for further study and clarifying the MEM model. For example, do the representations/functions of these posterior areas map onto different functions of P-level processes in MEM, such as *resolving* and/or *locating* (middle occipital gyrus) vs. *identifying* (e.g. fusiform face area, parahippocampal place area) vs. *placing* objects in relation to each other (e.g. retrosplenial cortex)?

The neuroimaging data obtained to date suggest additional new questions regarding the relation of MEM component processes to other concepts. For example, as noted above, does the model need a separate process of *selecting* or is selectivity inherent in every cognitive operation? Does the maintenance activity conceptualized by Baddeley (1996) as the *visual-spatial sketchpad* have more in common with *refreshing* or *rehearsing*? With respect to the general question of the functional organization of PFC (e.g. Goldman-Rakic, 1995; Smith & Jonides, 1997), when are similar vs. different regions of PFC engaged in refreshing different types of information (e.g. Johnson *et al.*, 2003, 2005)? To what extent does the PFC region engaged to refresh a particular type of information depend on what other information is being processed and, more generally, what does this imply about the relation between brain activity and cognitive concepts?

A limited repertoire of component processes engaged in different combinations in different tasks could help account for the similarity in neural activity found across neuroimaging studies. For example, in 2006 alone, DLPFC activity was reported to be involved in tasks as widely varying as lexical retrieval (de Diego Balaguer *et al.*, 2006), task-set maintenance (Fassbender, Foxe, & Garavan, 2006), divided attention (J. A. Johnson & Zatorre, 2006), tactile decision making (Pleger *et al.*, 2006), episodic memory formation (Summerfield *et al.*, 2006), and temporal discrimination (Tregellas, Davalos, & Rojas, 2006). DLPFC activity could be due to these complex tasks all relying on one or more common component processes, or could be due to the recruitment of distinct component processes that each involve DLPFC (either different areas of DLPFC, or the same areas of DLFPC in concert with different other regions). Duncan and Owen (2000), in a meta-analysis, reported that a common network of mid-VLPFC, mid-DLPFC, and ACC was recruited in a wide range of tasks such as auditory discrimination (Holcomb *et al.*, 1998), visual divided attention (Vandenberghe *et al.*, 1997), self-paced response production (Jahanshahi *et al.*, 1995), task switching (Dove, Pollmann, Schubert, Wiggins, & von Cramon, 2000), spatial problem solving (Baker *et al.*, 1996), and semantic processing (Thompson-Schill *et al.*, 1997). Again, this could reflect commonality in component process(es) engaged in all of these tasks, or unique processes all involving this general network of regions. By clarifying specific proposed individual component processes, we should be able to address whether they represent a viable level of analysis for understanding cognitive and brain function in more complex tasks. Does each complex task generate a pattern of neural activity so unique as to challenge the concept of component processes? What types of evidence will justify inferring the operation of a specific cognitive process from a pattern of brain activity ('reverse inference', Poldrack, 2006; Poldrack & Wagner, 2004)?

As concepts of component processes are refined, including identifying their neural correlates, a component-process approach should be increasingly useful in providing more specific assessments, or 'biomarkers', in studies of cognitive impairment, e.g. from neurological damage (e.g. lesion-related losses of function) and psychiatric dysfunction (e.g. working memory impairments in schizophrenia [Goldman-Rakic, 1994, 1999]), as well as deficits that emerge in the course of normal, healthy aging (Craik & Jennings, 1992; Hasher & Zacks, 1988; Light, 1991). For example, older adults show a behavioural deficit in refreshing (i.e. relative to young adults, disproportionately slow response times to refresh than to read a word, as well as less long-term memory benefit, Johnson *et al.*, 2002) and they also show reduced activity, relative to young adults, in left DLPFC during refreshing (Johnson *et al.*, 2004). A recent study showing that TMS to left DLPFC slows refreshing in young adults provides converging evidence for the importance of this region for refreshing (Miller, Verstynen, Johnson, & D'Esposito, 2008). It is easy to see how dysfunction in one or two MEM component processes (e.g. *refreshing* and/or *initiating*), could lead to wide-ranging dysfunctions in all complex cognitive acts involving those components (e.g. Johnson *et al.*, 2004; Johnson *et al.*, 2002).

Of course, cognitive deficits of different etiologies have organic correlates that may lie at different levels of abstraction within the nervous system (e.g. systemic genetic/molecular abnormalities in schizophrenia [Owen, Williams, & O'Donovan, 2004] versus a lesion to a specific region of cortex in a stroke patient). Attempting to characterize cognitive dysfunction in terms of a common set of component processes should help connect these different levels of analysis.

In summary, a mid-level cognitive model such as MEM has both analytic and synthetic functions (Johnson, 2007), helping both to generate specific hypotheses and to organize major findings from multiple approaches (cognitive/behavioural, neuropsychological, neuroimaging). With respect to neuroimaging in particular, MEM provides hypotheses about the component processes we should look for in brain activity in particular experiments, and an integrative context for interpreting the brain activity we see across many experiments. Reciprocally, neuroimaging evidence affords us both opportunities to test our conceptual models and direction for revising them, and thus it should help adjudicate among alternative conceptualizations of component cognitive processes. We do not need neuroimaging to ask what we mean by general terms such as executive function, working memory, cognitive control, or reflection, and many elegant cognitive-behavioural experiments have helped clarify such concepts. However, the further agenda of linking cognitive processes to brain function provides one way of deconstructing those concepts for a more specific level of analysis, and may therefore result in a more complete science of cognition.

Acknowledgements

Preparation of this chapter was supported by NIH grants AG15793 and AG09253. We thank Marvin Chun, Carol Raye, Nicholas Turk-Browne, and Do-Joon Yi, as well as the editors and reviewers, for their comments on this manuscript.

References

Atkinson, R. C. & Juola, J. F. (1974). Search and decision processes in recognition memory. In D. H. Krantz, R. C. Atkinson, R. D. Luce, & P. Suppes (Eds), *Contemporary Developments in Mathematical Psychology: I. Learning, Memory, and Thinking* (pp. 243–293). Oxford, England: W. H. Freeman.

Awh, E., Jonides, J., Smith, E. E., Schumacher, E. H., Koeppe, R. A., & Katz, S. (1996). Dissociation of storage and rehearsal in verbal working memory: Evidence from positron emission tomography. *Psychological Science, 7,* 25–31.

Baddeley, A. D. (1982). Amnesia: A minimal model and an interpretation. In L. S. Cermak (Ed.), *Human Memory and Amnesia* (pp. 305–336). Hillsdale, NJ: Erlbaum.

Baddeley, A. D. (1984). The fractionation of human memory. *Psychological Medicine, 14*(2), 259–264.

Baddeley, A. D. (1992). Working memory. *Science, 255,* 556–559.

Baddeley, A. D. (1996). Exploring the central executive. *The Quarterly Journal of Experimental Psychology A: Human Experimental Psychology, 49A*(1), 5–28.

Baddeley, A. D. & Hitch, G. (1974). Working memory. In G. H. Bower (Ed.), *The Psychology of Learning and Motivation* (Vol. 8, pp. 47–90). San Diego, CA: Academic Press.

Baddeley, A. D., Lewis, V., & Vallar, G. (1984). Exploring the articulatory loop. *The Quarterly Journal of Experimental Psychology A: Human Experimental Psychology, 36A*(2), 233–252.

Baddeley, A. D. & Lieberman, K. (1980). Spatial working memory. In R. Nickerson (Ed.), *Attention and Performance VIII.* Hillsdale, NJ: Erlbaum.

Badre, D. & Wagner, A. D. (2002). Semantic retrieval, mnemonic control, and prefrontal cortex. *Behavioral and Cognitive Neuroscience Reviews, 1,* 206–218.

Baker, S. C., Rogers, R. D., Owen, A. M., Frith, C. D., Dolan, R. J., Frackowiak, R. S., *et al.* (1996). Neural systems engaged by planning: A PET study of the Tower of London task. *Neuropsychologia, 34*(6), 515–526.

Botvinick, M., Nystrom, L. E., Fissell, K., Carter, C. S., & Cohen, J. D. (1999). Conflict monitoring versus selection-for-action in anterior cingulate cortex. *Nature, 402*(6758), 179–181.

Braver, T. S. & Bongiolatti, S. R. (2002). The role of frontopolar cortex in subgoal processing during working memory. *NeuroImage, 15*(3), 523–536.

Carter, C. S., Braver, T. S., Barch, D. M., Botvinick, M. M., Noll, D., & Cohen, J. D. (1998). Anterior cingulate cortex, error detection, and the online monitoring of performance. *Science, 280*(5364), 747–749.

Chein, J. M. & Fiez, J. A. (2001). Dissociation of verbal working memory system components using a delayed serial recall task. *Cerebral Cortex, 11*(11), 1003–1014.

Christoff, K. & Gabrieli, J. D. E. (2000). The frontopolar cortex and human cognition: Evidence for a rostrocaudal hierarchical organization within the human prefrontal cortex. *Psychobiology, 28*(2), 168–186.

Cohen, J. D., Perlstein, W. M., Braver, T. S., Nystrom, L. E., Noll, D. C., Jonides, J., *et al.* (1997). Temporal dynamics of brain activation during a working memory task. *Nature, 386,* 604–608.

Cohen, N. J. & Squire, L. R. (1980). Preserved learning and retention of pattern-analyzing skill in amnesia: Dissociation of knowing how and knowing that. *Science, 210*(4466), 207–210.

Courtney, S. M. (2004). Attention and cognitive control as emergent properties of information representation in working memory. *Cognitive, Affective, & Behavioral Neuroscience*, *4*(4), 501–516.

Craik, F. I. M. & Jennings, J. M. (1992). Human memory. In F. I. M. Craik & T. A. Salthouse (Eds), *The Handbook of Aging and Cognition* (pp. 51–110). Hillsdale, NJ: Lawrence Erlbaum Associates.

Craik, F. I. M. & Lockhart, R. S. (1972). Levels of processing: A framework for memory research. *Journal of Verbal Learning and Verbal Behavior*, *11*, 671–684.

Curtis, C. E. & D'Esposito, M. (2003). Persistent activity in the prefrontal cortex during working memory. *Trends in Cognitive Sciences*, *7*(9), 415–423.

de Diego Balaguer, R., Rodriguez-Fornells, A., Rotte, M., Bahlmann, J., Heinze, H. J., & Munte, T. F. (2006). Neural circuits subserving the retrieval of stems and grammatical features in regular and irregular verbs. *Human Brain Mapping*, *27*(11), 874–888.

Desimone, R. (1996). Neural mechanisms for visual memory and their role in attention. *Proceedings of the National Academy of Sciences of the United States of America*, *93*(24), 13494–13499.

D'Esposito, M., Postle, B. R., Ballard, D., & Lease, J. (1999). Maintenance versus manipulation of information held in working memory: An event-related fMRI study. *Brain & Cognition*, *41*, 66–86.

Dove, A., Pollmann, S., Schubert, T., Wiggins, C. J., & von Cramon, D. Y. (2000). Prefrontal cortex activation in task switching: An event-related fMRI study. *Cognitive Brain Research*, *9*(1), 103–109.

Duncan, J. & Owen, A. M. (2000). Common regions of the human frontal lobe recruited by diverse cognitive demands. *Trends in Neurosciences*, *23*(10), 475–483.

Epstein, R. & Kanwisher, N. (1998). A cortical representation of the local visual environment. *Nature*, *392*(6676), 598–601.

Fassbender, C., Foxe, J. J., & Garavan, H. (2006). Mapping the functional anatomy of task preparation: Priming task-appropriate brain networks. *Human Brain Mapping*, *27*(10), 819–827.

Fodor, J. A. (1983). *The Modularity of Mind: An Essay on Faculty Psychology*. Cambridge, MA: MIT Press.

Friston, K. J. (1994). Functional and effective connectivity in neuroimaging: A synthesis. *Human Brain Mapping*, *2*(1–2), 56–78.

Goldman-Rakic, P. S. (1994). Working memory dysfunction in schizophrenia. *Journal of Neuropsychiatry & Clinical Neurosciences*, *6*(4), 348–357.

Goldman-Rakic, P. S. (1995). Architecture of the prefrontal cortex and the central executive. *Annals of the New York Academy of Sciences*, *769*, 71–83.

Goldman-Rakic, P. S. (1999). The physiological approach: Functional architecture of working memory and disordered cognition in schizophrenia. *Biological Psychiatry*, *46*(5), 650–661.

Grill-Spector, K., Henson, R., & Martin, A. (2006). Repetition and the brain: Neural models of stimulus-specific effects. *Trends in Cognitive Sciences*, *10*(1), 14–23.

Hasher, L. & Zacks, R. T. (1988). Working memory, comprehension, and aging: A review and a new view. In G. H. Bower (Ed.), *The Psychology of Learning and Motivation*, Vol. 22 (pp. 193–225). New York, NY: Academic Press.

Henson, R. (2005). What can functional neuroimaging tell the experimental psychologist? *The Quarterly Journal of Experimental Psychology: Section A*, *58*(2), 193–233.

Holcomb, H. H., Medoff, D. R., Caudill, P. J., Zhao, Z., Lahti, A. C., Dannals, R. F., *et al.* (1998). Cerebral blood flow relationships associated with a difficult tone recognition task in trained normal volunteers. *Cerebral Cortex*, *8*(6), 534–542.

Horwitz, B. (1994). Data analysis paradigms for metabolic-flow data: Combining neural modeling and functional neuroimaging. *Human Brain Mapping*, *2*(1–2), 112–122.

Jacoby, L. L. & Dallas, M. (1981). On the relationship between autobiographical memory and perceptual learning. *Journal of Experimental Psychology: General*, *110*(3), 306–340.

Jahanshahi, M., Jenkins, I. H., Brown, R. G., Marsden, C. D., Passingham, R. E., & Brooks, D. J. (1995). Self-initiated versus externally triggered movements. I. An investigation using measurement of regional cerebral blood flow with PET and movement-related potentials in normal and Parkinson's disease subjects. *Brain, 118*(Pt 4), 913–933.

Johnson, J. A. & Zatorre, R. J. (2006). Neural substrates for dividing and focusing attention between simultaneous auditory and visual events. *NeuroImage, 31*(4), 1673–1681.

Johnson, M. K. (1983). A multiple-entry, modular memory system. *The Psychology of Learning and Motivation: Advances in Research and Theory, 17,* 81–123.

Johnson, M. K. (1992). MEM: Mechanisms of recollection. *Journal of Cognitive Neuroscience, 4,* 268–280.

Johnson, M. K. (1997). Identifying the origin of mental experience. In M. S. Myslobodsky (Ed.), *The Mythomanias: The Nature of Deception and Self-deception* (pp. 133–180). Mahwah, NJ: Erlbaum.

Johnson, M. K. (2007). Memory systems: A cognitive construct for analysis and synthesis. In H. L. Roediger, III, Y. Dudai, & S. M. Fitzpatrick (Eds), *Science of Memory: Concepts* (pp. 353–357). New York: Oxford University Press.

Johnson, M. K. & Hirst, W. (1991). Processing subsystems of memory. In R. G. Lister & H. J. Weingartner (Eds), *Perspectives on Cognitive Neuroscience* (pp. 197–217). New York: Oxford University Press.

Johnson, M. K. & Hirst, W. (1993). MEM: Memory subsystems as processes. In A. F. Collins, S. E. Gathercole, M. A. Conway, & P. E. Morris (Eds), *Theories of Memory* (pp. 241–286). East Sussex, England: Lawrence Erlbaum Associates.

Johnson, M. K., Kim, J. K., & Risse, G. (1985). Do alcoholic Korsakoff's syndrome patients acquire affective reactions? *Journal of Experimental Psychology: Learning, Memory, & Cognition, 11,* 22–36.

Johnson, M. K., Mitchell, K. J., Raye, C. L., & Greene, E. J. (2004). An age-related deficit in prefrontal cortical function associated with refreshing information. *Psychological Science, 15*(2), 127–132.

Johnson, M. K., Raye, C. L., Mitchell, K. J., Greene, E. J., & Anderson, A. W. (2003). fMRI evidence for an organization of prefrontal cortex by both type of process and type of information. *Cerebral Cortex, 13,* 265–273.

Johnson, M. K., Raye, C. L., Mitchell, K. J., Greene, E. J., Cunningham, W. A., & Sanislow, C. A. (2005). Using fMRI to investigate a component process of reflection: Prefrontal correlates of refreshing a just-activated representation. *Cognitive, Affective, & Behavioral Neuroscience, 5*(3), 339–361.

Johnson, M. K. & Reeder, J. A. (1997). Consciousness as meta-processing. In J. D. Cohen & J. W. Schooler (Eds), *Scientific Approaches to Consciousness* (pp. 261–293). Mahwah, NJ: Erlbaum.

Johnson, M. K., Reeder, J. A., Raye, C. L., & Mitchell, K. J. (2002). Second thoughts versus second looks: An age-related deficit in reflectively refreshing just-activated information. *Psychological Science, 13*(1), 64–67.

Johnson, M. R., Mitchell, K. J., Raye, C. L., D'Esposito, M., & Johnson, M. K. (2007). A brief thought can modulate activity in extrastriate visual areas: Top-down effects of refreshing just-seen visual stimuli. *NeuroImage, 37,* 290–299.

Jonides, J., Smith, E. E., Marshuetz, C., Koeppe, R. A., & Reuter-Lorenz, P. A. (1998). Inhibition in verbal working memory revealed by brain activation. *Proceedings of the National Academy of Sciences of the United States of America, 95,* 8410–8413.

Kanwisher, N., McDermott, J., & Chun, M. M. (1997). The fusiform face area: A module in human extrastriate cortex specialized for face perception. *Journal of Neuroscience, 17,* 4302–4311.

Kerns, J. G., Cohen, J. D., MacDonald, A. W., III, Cho, R. Y., Stenger, V. A., & Carter, C. S. (2004). Anterior cingulate conflict monitoring and adjustments in control. *Science, 303*(5660), 1023–1026.

Kolers, P. A. & Roediger, H. L., III. (1984). Procedures of mind. *Journal of Verbal Learning and Verbal Behavior, 23,* 425–449.

Light, L. L. (1991). Memory and aging: Four hypotheses in search of data. *Annual Review of Psychology, 42*(1), 333–376.

MacDonald, A. W., III, Cohen, J. D., Stenger, V. A., & Carter, C. S. (2000). Dissociating the role of the dorsolateral prefrontal and anterior cingulate cortex in cognitive control. *Science*, *288*(5472), 1835–1838.

Mandler, G. (1980). Recognizing: The judgment of previous occurrence. *Psychological Review*, *87*, 252–271.

McClelland, J. L., McNaughton, B. L., & O'Reilly, R. C. (1995). Why there are complementary learning systems in the hippocampus and neocortex: Insights from the successes and failures of connectionist models of learning and memory. *Psychological Review*, *102*(3), 419–457.

McIntosh, A. R. & Gonzalez-Lima, F. (1994). Structural equation modeling and its application to network analysis in functional brain imaging. *Human Brain Mapping*, *2*(1–2), 2–22.

Miller, B. T., Verstynen, T., Johnson, M. K., & D'Esposito, M. (2008). Prefrontal and parietal contributions to refreshing: An rTMS study. *NeuroImage*, *39*, 436–440.

Miller, E. K. & Cohen, J. D. (2001). An integrative theory of prefrontal cortex function. *Annual Review of Neuroscience*, *24*, 167–202.

Miller, G. A., Galanter, E., & Pribram, K. H. (1960). *Plans and the Structure of Behavior*. New York: Holt, Rinehart, and Winston.

Mishkin, M. (1982). A memory system in the monkey. *Philosophical Transactions of the Royal Society of London – Series B: Biological Sciences*, *298*(1089), 83–95.

Miyashita, Y. (1993). Inferior temporal cortex: Where visual perception meets memory. *Annual Review of Neuroscience*, *16*, 245–263.

Norman, D. A. & Shallice, T. (1986). Attention to action: Willed and automatic control of behavior. In R. J. Davidson, G. E. Schwartz, & D. Shapiro (Eds), *Consciousness and Self-regulation*, *Vol. 4* (pp. 1–18). New York: Plenum Press.

Owen, M. J., Williams, N. M., & O'Donovan, M. C. (2004). The molecular genetics of schizophrenia: New findings promise new insights. *Molecular Psychiatry*, *9*(1), 14–27.

Passingham, D. & Sakai, K. (2004). The prefrontal cortex and working memory: Physiology and brain imaging. *Current Opinion in Neurobiology*, *14*(2), 163–168.

Petrides, M. (1994). Frontal lobes and working memory: Evidence from investigations of the effects of cortical excisions in nonhuman primates. In F. Boller & J. Grafman (Eds), *Handbook of Neuropsychology*, *Vol. 9* (pp. 59–82). Amsterdam: Elsevier Science.

Petrides, M. (2000). Dissociable roles of mid-dorsolateral prefrontal and anterior inferotemporal cortex in visual working memory. *Journal of Neuroscience*, *20*(19), 7496–7503.

Petrides, M., Alivisatos, B., Meyer, E., & Evans, A. C. (1993). Functional activation of the human frontal cortex during the performance of verbal working memory tasks. *Proceedings of the National Academy of Sciences of the United States of America*, *90*, 878–882.

Pleger, B., Ruff, C. C., Blankenburg, F., Bestmann, S., Wiech, K., Stephan, K. E., *et al.* (2006). Neural coding of tactile decisions in the human prefrontal cortex. *Journal of Neuroscience*, *26*(48), 12596–12601.

Poldrack, R. A. (2006). Can cognitive processes be inferred from neuroimaging data? *Trends in Cognitive Sciences*, *10*(2), 59–63.

Poldrack, R. A. & Packard, M. G. (2003). Competition among multiple memory systems: Converging evidence from animal and human brain studies. *Neuropsychologia*, *41*(3), 245–251.

Poldrack, R. A. & Rodriguez, P. (2004). How do memory systems interact? Evidence from human classification learning. *Neurobiology of Learning and Memory*, *82*(3), 324–332.

Poldrack, R. A. & Wagner, A. D. (2004). What can neuroimaging tell us about the mind? Insights from prefrontal cortex. *Current Directions in Psychological Science*, *13*(5), 177–181.

Ranganath, C. & D'Esposito, M. (2005). Directing the mind's eye: Prefrontal, inferior and medial temporal mechanisms for visual working memory. *Current Opinion in Neurobiology*, *15*(2), 175–182.

Raye, C. L., Johnson, M. K., Mitchell, K. J., Greene, E. J., & Johnson, M. R. (2007). Refreshing: A minimal executive function. *Cortex, 43*, 135–145.

Raye, C. L., Johnson, M. K., Mitchell, K. J., Reeder, J. A., & Greene, E. J. (2002). Neuroimaging a single thought: Dorsolateral PFC activity associated with refreshing just-activated information. *NeuroImage, 15*(2), 447–453.

Raye, C. L., Mitchell, K. J., Reeder, J. A., Greene, E. J., & Johnson, M. K. (2008). Refreshing one of several active representations: Behavioral and functional magnetic resonance imaging differences between young and older adults. *Journal of Cognitive Neuroscience, 20*(5), 852–862.

Reiser, B. J. (1986). The encoding and retrieval of memories of real-world experiences. In J. A. Galambo, R. P. Abelson, & J. B. Black (Eds), *Knowledge Structures* (pp. 71–99). Hillsdale, NJ: Lawrence Erlbaum Associates.

Ruchkin, D. S., Grafman, J., Cameron, K., & Berndt, R. S. (2003). Working memory retention systems: A state of activated long-term memory. *Behavioral & Brain Sciences, 26*(6), 709–728.

Salame, P. & Baddeley, A. D. (1982). Disruption of short-term memory by unattended speech: Implications for the structure of working memory. *Journal of Verbal Learning & Verbal Behavior, 21*, 150–164.

Smith, E. E. & Jonides, J. (1997). Working memory: A view from neuroimaging. *Cognitive Psychology, 33*(1), 5–42.

Smith, E. E. & Jonides, J. (1999). Storage and executive processes in the frontal lobes. *Science, 283*, 1657–1661.

Squire, L. R. & Alvarez, P. (1995). Retrograde amnesia and memory consolidation: A neurobiological perspective. *Current Opinion in Neurobiology, 5*(2), 169–177.

Stuss, D. T. & Benson, D. F. (1986). *The Frontal Lobes.* New York: Raven Press.

Summerfield, C., Greene, M., Wager, T., Egner, T., Hirsch, J., & Mangels, J. (2006). Neocortical connectivity during episodic memory formation. *PLoS Biology, 4*(5), e128.

Thompson-Schill, S. L., D'Esposito, M., Aguirre, G. K., & Farah, M. J. (1997). Role of left inferior prefrontal cortex in retrieval of semantic knowledge: A reevaluation. *Proceedings of the National Academy of Sciences of the United States of America, 94*(26), 14792–14797.

Tregellas, J. R., Davalos, D. B., & Rojas, D. C. (2006). Effect of task difficulty on the functional anatomy of temporal processing. *NeuroImage, 32*(1), 307–315.

Tulving, E. (1983). *Elements of Episodic Memory.* Oxford, England: Clarendon Press.

Tulving, E. (1985). Memory and consciousness. *Canadian Psychology, 26*, 1–12.

Tulving, E. & Schacter, D. L. (1990). Priming and human memory systems. *Science, 247*(4940), 301–306.

Turk-Browne, N. B., Yi, D.-J., & Chun, M. M. (2006). Linking implicit and explicit memory: Common encoding factors and shared representations. *Neuron, 49*(6), 917–927.

Uttal, W. R. (2001). *The New Phrenology: The Limits of Localizing Cognitive Processes in the Brain.* Cambridge, MA: The MIT Press.

Vandenberghe, R., Duncan, J., Dupont, P., Ward, R., Poline, J. B., Bormans, G., *et al.* (1997). Attention to one or two features in left or right visual field: A positron emission tomography study. *Journal of Neuroscience, 17*(10), 3739–3750.

Wiggs, C. L. & Martin, A. (1998). Properties and mechanisms of perceptual priming. *Current Opinion in Neurobiology, 8*(2), 227–233.

Yi, D.-J., Turk-Browne, N. B., Chun, M. M., & Johnson, M. K. (2008). When a thought equals a look: Refreshing enhances perceptual memory. *Journal of Cognitive Neuroscience, 20*(8), 1371–1380.

Yonelinas, A. P. (2002). The nature of recollection and familiarity: A review of 30 years of research. *Journal of Memory and Language, 46*(3), 441–517.

Chapter 11

The mid-ventrolateral frontal cortex and attentional control

Adrian M. Owen and Adam Hampshire

Introduction

For many years it has been known that medial temporal-lobe damage in humans produces profound memory impairments, while patients with frontal-lobe lesions often perform normally on many standard tests of memory (Lee *et al.*, 2000a; Petrides, 1994). The pattern that has emerged from functional neuroimaging studies in healthy volunteers is quite different, with increases in activity reported in medial temporal *and* frontal-lobe areas during many different memory tasks (Buckner *et al.*, 1995, 1999; Fletcher & Henson, 2001; Lee *et al.*, 2000a). One region that has been consistently activated is the mid-ventrolateral frontal cortex which, in humans, lies below the inferior frontal sulcus and includes Brodmann areas 45 and 47 (Brodmann, 1909) (see Figure 11.1). Activity in this region has been reported frequently during spatial, verbal and pattern *working* memory tasks (Owen *et al.*, 1996a, 2000; Stern *et al.*, 2000), but also during *episodic* memory tests of encoding and retrieval (Fletcher *et al.*, 1998; Lee *et al.*, 2000b; Owen *et al.*, 1996b).

Broadly speaking, these data support psychological models of memory in the sense that they confirm that certain common 'executive' or 'control' processes are vital to many different aspects of normal mnemonic processing. However, they go further than that in two important ways; first, by identifying that, within the frontal lobe, it is the mid-ventrolateral region that is central to this process or set of processes (e.g. Petrides, 1994; Owen 1997). Second, by demonstrating that activity in this region may just as easily map onto existing psychological models of other cognitive systems that are related to, but quite distinct from, theories of memory, e.g. *attention*. Thus, the fact that activation in the mid-ventrolateral frontal cortex has also been widely reported in tasks that do not place any significant demands on memory at all (e.g. Dove *et al.*, 2000, Cools *et al.*, 2002, Rushworth *et al.*, 1997) suggests that the function, or functions, of this region are not restricted to the memory domain, but rather, form part of a more general role in cognitive control processes. A corollary of this position, of course, is that these psychological systems may be less distinct (both functionally and neurally) than current cognitive models would have us believe.

In this chapter, we will review recent neuroimaging evidence that suggests that the mid-ventrolateral region of the frontal cortex plays a specific role in *intended action*; that is, any behaviour (e.g. an action or a thought), that is consciously *willed* by the agent responsible

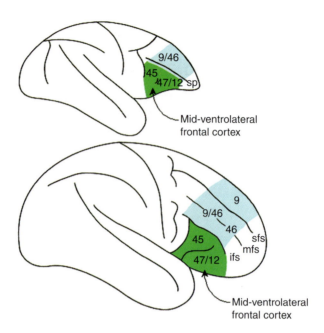

Figure 11.1 Schematic drawing of the lateral surface of the macaque brain (top) and the human brain (bottom), to indicate the location of the ventrolateral frontal cortex (areas 45, 47, 12). Adapted from Petrides and Pandya (1994). sp = sulcus principalis. ifs = inferior frontal sulcus. mfs = middle frontal sulcus. sfs = superior frontal sulcus.

for carrying out that behaviour. In this sense, it makes contributions to both memory and attention in a manner that cannot be predicted by current psychological models of either cognitive system. We will also argue that the basis for this role lies in the capacity that this region has for tuning rapidly to those aspects of any given task that are currently relevant, whilst becoming unresponsive to that same information when the task demands change. Although consistent with psychological models of memory and attention, these conclusions could not have been reached based solely on the predictions of those models. On this basis we argue that data from functional neuroimaging studies in healthy volunteers, neuropsychological investigations in patients and evidence from lesion and electrophysiological studies in the macaque have informed, and will continue to inform, psychological theories of memory.

The mid-ventrolateral frontal cortex and memory

Although many functional neuroimaging studies have activated the mid-ventrolateral frontal cortex in a variety of behavioural contexts, few have explicitly set out to investigate the role of this region directly. However, a significant number of early imaging studies did report activity in this region during tasks that emphasised the explicit retrieval of one, or a few, pieces of information and the sequencing of responses based directly on that stored information. For example, in one early positron emission tomography (PET) study (Jonides *et al.*, 1993; also see Smith *et al.*, 1995), healthy volunteers were required to remember the location of three simultaneously presented stimuli and then to decide whether or not a probe circle occupied one of those same three locations following a three second delay. Activation was observed in the mid-ventrolateral frontal cortex, but not in more dorsal regions of the frontal lobe. In a subsequent PET study of spatial span, the participants were required to remember a sequence of five previously presented locations, and then to respond directly by touching those same locations following a delay (Owen *et al.*, 1996a). The emphasis of the task was on the explicit encoding of spatial information and the uncued recall of this information following a short delay. A significant regional cerebral blood flow (rCBF) increase was observed in ventrolateral area 47 of the right hemisphere (Figure 11.2A), similar in location to that reported previously by Jonides at colleagues (1993). In a second task that required the volunteers to execute a fixed sequence of responses to eight previously learned locations, ventrolateral frontal area 47 was again significantly activated, bilaterally (Owen *et al.*, 1996a). During both of these tasks, rCBF changes within other frontal regions, including the dorsolateral frontal cortex did not approach significance. In a subsequent PET study, the 5-item spatial span task was used again, but compared with a variation on the more commonly used spatial '2-back' procedure (Owen *et al.*, 1999). Again, during the spatial span task, which (unlike the 2-back task) only required the retrieval and reproduction of stored information, a significant

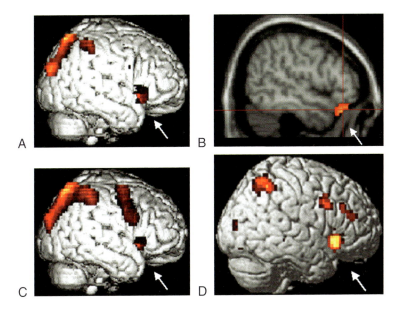

Figure 11.2 Four independent neuroimaging studies of memory activating an almost identical location within the mid-ventrolateral frontal cortex. (A) spatial span (adapted from Owen *et al.*, 1996a) (B) digit span (adapted from Owen *et al.*, 2000) (C) spatial span (adapted from Owen *et al.*, 1999). (D) Intentional retrieval of previously remembered abstract patterns (adapted from Dove *et al.*, 2006). Right hemisphere only is shown. Activity in the mid-ventrolateral frontal cortex is indicated with an arrow in each study.

rCBF increase was observed in the mid-ventrolateral prefrontal cortex at co-ordinates very similar to those reported previously (Jonides *et al.*, 1993; Owen *et al.*, 1996a) (Figure 11.2C).

To assess whether these effects were domain specific, a direct analogue of the spatial span task was developed (Owen *et al.*, 2000), based on the classic digit span paradigm. During one experimental task, subjects were required to hold a sequence of five auditorily presented numbers in memory (e.g. 7, 3, 8, 2, 9), and then to respond by (verbally) producing those numbers, in order, following a short delay. As predicted, when this digit span task was compared to a control task, significant activation was observed in right mid-ventrolateral area 47 at co-ordinates similar to those reported previously in studies of spatial span (Owen *et al.*, 1996a, 1999; see also, Jonides *et al.*, 1993; Smith *et al.*, 1995) (Figure 11.2B). In contrast, a backwards digit span task, identical in every respect (except the sequence had to be recalled in reverse order), activated both the mid-ventrolateral and the mid-dorsolateral frontal cortices.

In summary, these early imaging findings suggest that the mid-ventrolateral frontal cortex, but not more dorsal regions of the frontal lobe, is required for simple memory tasks that involve only the active encoding and/or retrieval of information. Moreover, this role appears to be independent of the modality of the stimuli to be remembered/recalled.

Given these results, it is somewhat surprising that patients with frontal-lobe lesions are typically unimpaired on such tasks (D'Esposito & Postle, 1999). One likely explanation for this apparent discrepancy is that the methods used to test patients on these types of task have not been sensitive enough to elicit existent (yet subtle) deficits. In support of this possibility, although most previous studies of spatial span have reported no significant deficit in frontal-lobe patients (Canavan *et al.*, 1989; Greenlee *et al.*, 1997; Miotto *et al.*, 1996; Owen *et al.*, 1990), in almost all cases these studies have reported a numerical decrease in the performance of the patients relative to the healthy controls. We have recently developed a more sensitive paradigm for measuring spatial span (Bor *et al.*, 2005), which employs a technique that allows for a continuum of span scores, unlike the method of testing that is more commonly used which produces discrete (integer) results. Using this task, the mean span score for a group of patients with large frontal-lobe lesions was shown to be significantly reduced compared to patients with smaller frontal-lobe lesions and a matched group of healthy controls (Bor *et al.*, 2005). Unfortunately, no direct relationship between the performance deficit and damage to the mid-ventrolateral part of the frontal cortex could be established; in fact, if anything, it was patients with more extensive damage to the mid-dorsolateral frontal cortex who were most impaired. However, in patient studies it is very difficult to establish which areas of the frontal cortex are involved in a given cognitive process with any degree of anatomical precision as the excisions are rarely confined to one, or even a few, cytoarchitectonic areas. In fact, we are not aware of any neuropsychological study in patients that has convincingly demonstrated a direct association between damage to the mid-ventrolateral region of the frontal cortex and a specific pattern of cognitive impairment. More generally, however, in the last 50 years, numerous neuropsychological studies have reported, or implied, a general dissociation between the performance of patients with frontal-lobe damage on tests of recognition and recall (for review, see Wheeler *et al.*, 1995). Such patients are more often impaired on memory tasks that require the active encoding and/or recall (especially free recall) of information, yet remain largely unimpaired on recognition memory tasks that can be solved on the basis of stimulus familiarity alone. Again, it has not been possible to relate this pattern of impairment to damage within any particular frontal-lobe region, although across the various studies, some of these patients will undoubtedly have sustained damage to the mid-ventrolateral frontal cortex.

Although the early imaging studies described above suggest that the mid-ventrolateral frontal cortex plays an important role in various types of span task, the long acquisition period of PET (typically 60–90 seconds per scan) precludes any more precise conclusions being drawn about the specific processes involved. Advances in event-related functional magnetic resonance imaging (fMRI) have made the measurement of transient cognitive events feasible by allowing short events with brief inter-stimulus-intervals to be estimated independently within a noisy background of other task-related events. In one recent fMRI study, (Dove *et al.*, 2006), colourful stimuli, based on examples of abstract art, were presented and volunteers were instructed on random trials either to just examine each piece ('incidental' encoding) or to try and remember it for later test ('intentional' encoding). Retrieval was examined by asking volunteers, on random trials, whether or not they remembered seeing specific pieces ('intentional' retrieval). In a fourth condition, designed to provide a control for these retrieval trials, volunteers were instructed to re-view stimuli that had been shown previously to elicit recognition ('incidental' re-viewing). Importantly, at the critical interval of each trial, i.e. when the stimulus was presented, all sensory and motor factors were held constant across all conditions. The only difference between conditions was how the volunteer chose to implement an *intention* based on a prior instruction. Intentional encoding led to significantly improved recall over incidental encoding, although, importantly, performance for incidentally encoded stimuli was significantly above chance. When incidental encoding was compared to the non-events, no significant activity was observed in the mid-ventrolateral frontal cortex, although significant increases in signal intensity were observed in the parahippocampal gyrus/hippocampus bilaterally. In contrast, when intentional encoding was compared to incidental encoding, significant signal intensity changes were observed in the mid-ventrolateral frontal cortex, but not in the parahippocampal gyrus/hippocampus. Thus, activity in the mid-ventrolateral frontal cortex was specifically associated with the act of *intentionally encoding* stimuli while non-intentional encoding (as indexed by later recognition performance), yielded no activity in this region. When incidental re-viewing and non-events were compared, again, no significant activity was observed in the mid-ventrolateral frontal cortex, although significant signal intensity changes were observed in the parahippocampal gyrus/hippocampus bilaterally. In contrast, when intentional retrieval was compared to incidental re-viewing, the mid-ventrolateral frontal cortex was activated bilaterally, but no significant differences in activity were observed in the medial temporal lobe (Figure 11.2D). Thus, activity in the mid-ventrolateral frontal cortex was specifically associated with the act of *intentionally recalling* whether stimuli had been seen previously, while re-viewing stimuli with no particular intention in mind, yielded no activity in this region.

In a follow-up study, these results were extended to examine the response of the mid-ventrolateral frontal cortex to a more diverse range of stimulus types, including abstract art, faces, and scenes (Dove et al., 2008). Again, this region was only significantly active in the conditions where the volunteer was explicitly instructed to try and remember, or recall, a stimulus regardless of its type (face, scenes, or abstract art). In contrast, stimulus-specific activity was observed in the fusiform face area (to faces) and the parahippocampal place area (to scenes), irrespective of whether an instruction to encode or recall had been given or not. In fact, the task instruction was the only factor that modulated activity in mid-ventrolateral cortex, whereas other factors such as stimulus type, task type, or stimulus repetition did not have any effect at all (Dove et al., in press).

The results of these two studies demonstrate that simply changing the task instructions at encoding and retrieval to encourage intentional processing results in an increase in signal intensity in the mid-ventrolateral frontal cortex, but not in other regions of the brain that are known to be involved in memory for those stimuli. These findings suggest that the implementation of an intended act, or plan to remember or recall, may be the common factor that underlies activation of the mid-ventrolateral frontal cortex during many previous neuroimaging studies of memory (e.g. Jonides et al., 1993; Owen et al., 1996a, 1999, 2000; Smith et al., 1995; Henson et al., 1999; Wagner et al., 1998; Courtney et al., 1997). In the case of short-term or working memory tasks, this might correspond to the relatively straightforward mapping of stimuli to responses such as that which occurs in spatial and digit span tasks (e.g. Owen et al., 1996a, 1999), or even simple delayed matching to sample paradigms (e.g. Elliott & Dolan, 1999). In the case of long-term episodic memory (e.g. verbal paired associate learning), these intentional encoding and retrieval processes might correspond to the active mapping and implementation of a somewhat arbitrary learned response (e.g. a category exemplar) to a specific stimulus (e.g. a category name) (e.g. Fletcher et al., 1998a, 1998b).

In summary, we suggest that an important factor for understanding the role that the mid-ventrolateral frontal cortex plays in memory and its relationship with more posterior regions (e.g. the medial temporal-lobe system) is the extent to which a volunteer explicitly *intends* to remember or retrieve a given stimulus and the changes in attentional control that may be consequent upon such an intention.

The mid-ventrolateral frontal cortex and tasks that do not require memory

Although all of the studies described above have reported activation in the mid-ventrolateral frontal cortex during tasks that place various demands on memory processes (see Figure 11.2), activity in this region has also been reported frequently during tasks that appear to make no direct demands on memory at all. For example, the mid-ventrolateral frontal cortex has been activated during stimulus selection (Rushworth et al., 1997), when judgements of word meaning are required (Kapur et al., 1994) during reversal learning (Cools et al., 2002), inhibition (Konishi et al., 1999), extra dimensional set-shifting (Nakahara et al., 2002; Hampshire & Owen, 2006) and task switching (Dove et al., 2000). Similarly, patients with frontal-lobe damage are impaired on many tasks, some of which have no obvious mnemonic component at all (e.g. Milner, 1964; Luria, 1966; Corkin, 1965; Semmes *et al.*, 1963). Whilst each of these tasks, arguably, require memory of some sort (if only to remember the task instructions), it seems unlikely that memory *per se*, or any specific mnemonic process, is the common feature that results in activation of the mid-ventrolateral frontal cortex, or an impairment in the patients with frontal-lobe damage. On the other hand, they do all require the self-initiated, conscious (i.e. intentional) selection of appropriate responses, often in the absence of external cues.

In one recent study, event-related fMRI was used to examine frontal-lobe activation in healthy human volunteers during performance of a probabilistic reversal learning task (Cools *et al.*, 2002). Reversal learning involves the adaptation of behaviour according to changes in stimulus-reward contingencies and places a relatively low load on memory. It is exemplified by visual discrimination tasks where subjects must learn to respond according to the opposite, previously irrelevant, stimulus-reward pairing. Reversal learning is disrupted following lesions of ventral prefrontal cortex in non-human primates (Iversen & Mishkin, 1970; Dias *et al.*, 1996). However, evidence of the same system being involved in reversal performance in humans is limited to two studies in patients with non-selective ventral prefrontal cortex damage (Rolls *et al.*, 1994; Rahman *et al.*, 1999). In the study by Cools *et al.* (2002), volunteers were required to respond to one of two stimuli according to probabilistic feedback; thus switches in the correct response were uncued in the sense that they could not be determined based on the feedback received on any given trial (e.g. the trial immediately prior to a switch). A significant signal change was observed in the right ventrolateral prefrontal cortex on trials when subjects decided to stop responding to the previously relevant stimulus and shifted responding to the newly relevant stimulus. Moreover, the response on the final reversal error, prior to shifting, was not modulated by the number of preceding reversal errors, indicating that error-related activity does not simply accumulate in this network, but rather, corresponds precisely to the exact moment when volunteers *decided to make the shift*. These data indicate that intentional shifting of lower-level stimulus-reward associations is sufficient to activate the ventrolateral prefrontal cortex. The study also concurs well with other, human brain imaging studies that have emphasized a role for the right ventrolateral prefrontal cortex in behavioural inhibition (or intentional stopping) using go-no go tasks (Garavan *et al.*, 1999; Konishi *et al.*, 1999).

Unfortunately in many studies that have used shifting tasks to examine attentional control, multiple discrete cognitive operations have been confounded within the design, making it impossible to define the exact contribution made by the mid-ventrolateral frontal cortex. For example, in the study by Cools *et al.* (2002) described above, volunteers were required to shift attention between two stimuli based on changes in partial reinforcement contingency. The same stimulus set was used repeatedly and consisted of complex stimuli; hence reversals, stimulus change, stimulus–response mapping change, and possibly even dimension change, were all confounded. In another relevant study (Dove *et al.*, 2000), isolation of the multiple components of switching was only achieved

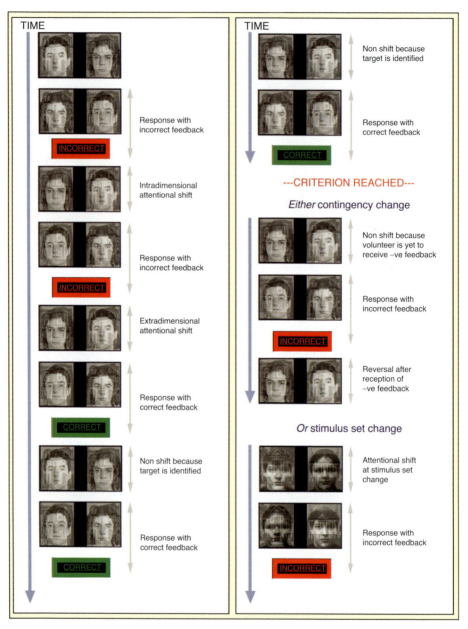

Figure 11.3 A typical series of trials from the study by Hampshire and Owen, (2006). In this example, the participant initially chooses the face in the left superimposed face/building pair and so indicates left with the button box by pressing the button with right index finger. When the response is made, the stimuli are removed from the screen and reappear after a short interval rearranged with the chosen face on the right of the screen superimposed on the other building; the participant therefore indicates right by pressing button with right middle finger. Because the face-building combinations swap from one trial to the next, the program can compute which item was selected and because (in this example) it is not the target, negative feedback

by confounding stimulus colour change, reversal of rule, and the reversal of response. Similarly, several previous fMRI studies that have used variants of the Wisconsin Card Sorting Test have confounded attentional switches between dimensions with reception of negative feedback, response inhibition, and updating working memory (e.g. Konishi *et al.*, 1998). Most importantly, all of these studies have focused on experimental manipulations (e.g. experimenter imposed shifts) rather than volunteer behaviour during the scanning session.

In one recent fMRI study, a novel approach was used in which the responses of the volunteer dictated the pace and order of experimental events (Hampshire and Owen, 2006 – see Figure 11.3 and legend for description). Hence, the focus of attention could be monitored and used to define the events (e.g. attentional shifts), rather than those events being dictated by the experimental design. This approach allowed the volunteers chosen decision-making strategies and attentional shifts to be functionally and behaviourally examined independent of the will of the experimenter. Many stimulus sets were used, each containing stimuli of two distinct types (faces and buildings). Switches of attention between stimuli of the same type (intra-dimensional shifts) and between stimuli of different types (extra-dimensional shifts) could therefore be modelled. Owing to the difficulty of intermixing extra- and intra-dimensional shifts without using unnatural cueing or fixed order event sequences, previous studies have often used blocked designs that allow only limited interpretation of the activation results (e.g. Rogers *et al.*, 2000). In the study by Hampshire and Owen (2006), these transient attentional control functions were intermixed and could therefore be contrasted at the event level in the current trial and error situation (see Figure 11.3). Thus, extra- and intra-dimensional shifts could be compared directly, effectively isolating the extra-dimensional component of shifting from other switch-related processes, such as inhibition of the previously relevant response

---

('INCORRECT') is given. Subsequently the stimuli reappear on the screen and the participant selects the other face (intra-dimensional, ID shift). Following the second response, negative feedback is given and the participant switches to select the building on the right of the screen (extra-dimensional, ED shift). Following the second response to the building, positive feedback ('CORRECT') is given because the participant has correctly identified the target item. When the stimuli reappear on the screen, the participant responds to the same building, as they now know that it is the target (early correct response). They receive positive feedback on the second response, and so continue to select the same building (late correct response). After responding correctly again they receive positive feedback and have now reached the criterion of six correct responses in a row. One of two things then happens; either a new stimulus set is presented, in which case the participant starts searching for the new target (set change). Alternatively, the reward contingency changes, in which case the participant responds twice more to the same building (because they have no way of knowing that anything has changed) before receiving negative feedback. They must then inhibit their responses to the recently rewarded target object, and start trying to identify which of the other three possible items has become the target (reversal). It is important to note that the extra- and intra-dimensional shift events, along with the feedback, do not always occur in the sequence shown because the order in which the stimuli are tested is determined entirely by the choices made by participants.

(Nakahara *et al.*, 2002). The novel partial feedback paradigm also enabled switch events and feedback events to be modelled separately, allowing regions involved in abstract reward processing and/or the implementation of attentional control to be measured independently.

The behavioural data demonstrated that moving attention between stimulus dimensions caused more errors than moving attention between stimuli of the same type. Since all target changes could logically be solved within the same number of trials, these differences must reflect the various strategies employed by the volunteers to solve the task. The main question for the imaging data, therefore, was whether this component of attentional control (extra-dimensional shifting) would be associated with any specific neural substrate. Accordingly, when shifts in the focus of attention between stimulus types (extra-dimensional shifts) were directly compared with shifts within stimulus type (intra-dimensional shifts), significant activation was observed only in the mid-ventrolateral frontal cortex (Figure 11.4).

This result clarifies and extends several previous imaging studies of set-shifting behaviour. For example, Nakahara *et al.* (2002) reported previously that the ventrolateral frontal cortex is involved in extra-dimensional shifting in both humans and macaques using a modified version of the Wisconsin Card Sorting Test. However, in that study, multiple processes were confounded in the set shift itself leading the authors to interpret the observed ventrolateral frontal cortex activity as 'related to inhibition of the previous

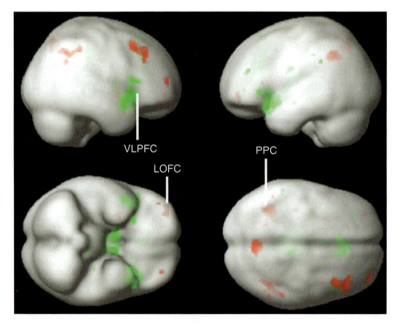

Figure 11.4 Adapted from Hampshire and Owen (2006). Results for the extra-dimensional shift component (green), and the reversal component (red) FDR corrected for the whole brain mass at p = 0.05. Extra-dimensional shifting was specifically associated with activity in the mid-ventrolateral frontal cortex. VLPFC = ventrolateral frontal cortex. LOFC = lateral orbitofrontal cortex. PPC = posterior parietal cortex.

relevant response'. The results of the study by Hampshire and Owen (2006) demonstrate that this is unlikely to have been the case. Thus, during reversals, where inhibition is maximal, there was no activation in the mid-ventrolateral frontal cortex compared to several other components of the task (see Figure 11.4). In addition, this region was not significantly activated when intra-dimensional shifting was compared to non-shifting trials.

On the basis of these findings, it was suggested that the commonly observed increase in reaction time for extra-dimensional shifting reflects the time taken for the ventrolateral frontal cortex to bias attentional processing between competing stimulus dimensions (Hampshire & Owen, 2006). Such attentional biasing, or 'tuning', while relevant to many components of set shifting, is likely to be maximal when a complete reconfiguration of the attentional set is required, as is the case during a shift from one dimension to another (competing) dimension (Figure 11.4).

The mid-ventrolateral frontal cortex and attentional control

In the two previous sections, we have reviewed evidence suggesting that the mid-ventrolateral frontal cortex plays an important role in intended thoughts and actions, whether that be in the active encoding and retrieval requirements of many memory tasks, or in the need to actively (or wilfully) shift attention between competing components of set-shifting tasks.

Broadly speaking, the findings from lesion and electrophysiological studies in the monkey also suggest that the mid-ventrolateral frontal cortex makes a polymodal contribution to a variety of different tasks that require the initiation and execution of intended actions. In the macaque, the mid-ventrolateral frontal cortex lies below the sulcus principalis on the inferior convexity and comprises areas 12 or 47/12 and 45 (Carmicheal & Price, 1994; Petrides & Pandya, 1994). Lesions of the ventrolateral frontal cortex, but not the more dorsal cortex surrounding the *sulcus principalis*, cause impairments in non-spatial delayed-matching-to-sample for single items (Mishkin & Manning, 1978; Passingham, 1975), spatial and non-spatial delayed alternation (Mishkin *et al.*, 1969), the learning of arbitrary stimulus-response associations (Gaffan, 1994; Petrides, 1994; Murray & Wise, 1997) switching attention to behaviourally relevant aspects of the world (e.g. Dias *et al.*, 1996), and even impair object matching when the sample and the match are simultaneously present and there is no delay component (Rushworth *et al.*, 1997). Thus, once a simultaneous version of the task has been relearned, the imposition of a delay between sample and match poses no more of a problem for a monkey with a ventrolateral frontal lesion than it does prior to surgery (Rushworth *et al.*, 1997). Electrophysiological data from the monkey also support a role for this region in the initiation of a variety of explicit cognitive processes. For example, Sakagami and Niki (1994) trained monkeys to either make or withhold a response depending on which stimulus they were shown. On some blocks of trials the relevant dimension of the stimulus was its colour, on other trials it was its position or shape. Ventrolateral neurons appeared to encode the stimulus dimension of current interest to the monkey. Similarly, Rao *et al.* (1997) identified neurons ventral to the principal sulcus, that encoded either, or both, the location and the identity of stimuli presented in a novel delayed response procedure.

Remarkably, some neurons adapted (or 'tune') flexibly as the emphasis of the task changed during its various stages. Thus, once a target object's identity was no longer relevant many of the 'what-and-where' cells no longer coded for object identity but switched to code for object location. This finding suggests that the response of ventrolateral prefrontal 'memory cells' is flexible, i.e. they can code different stimulus attributes at different times according to task demands. In other words, they will respond to a stimulus, irrespective of the modality and whenever there is an explicit requirement and an associated intention to do so. In categorisation tasks, similar properties have been described for lateral frontal neurons; e.g. Freedman *et al.* (2001) identified neurons within the monkey lateral frontal cortex that tune to respond selectively to just those categories that are currently relevant, whilst becoming unresponsive to those same categories when the task demands change.

We have recently investigated whether regions of the human frontal lobe can also be shown to selectively adapt to represent currently relevant information during a simple attentional task – monitoring for a target item in a series of non-targets (Hampshire, Duncan, & Owen, 2007). Volunteers were instructed to simply look for a previously defined target item (e.g. a particular face) within sequences of non-target items. Non-targets are drawn from either the same category (e.g. another face) or a different category (e.g. a building) as the current target item, allowing categorical similarity to be used as a

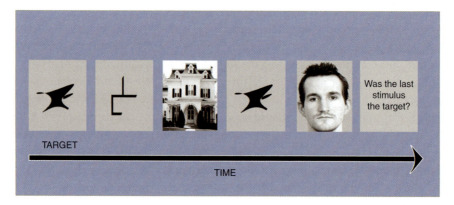

Figure 11.5 Adapted from Hampshire *et al.* (2007). Volunteers looked for the presentation of a target item within sequences of visually displayed non-target items. At the beginning of a sequence, the current target item appeared with the word 'target'. Sequence lengths were varied from 1 to 8 stimuli in a row, and the target could be presented at one, many, or none of those positions. At the end of each sequence the question 'Was the last stimulus the target?' appeared on the screen and the volunteer was required to respond yes or no, using a button box. Target and non-target items were taken from a pool of stimuli, consisting of pictures from each of four distinct categories: faces, buildings, abstract line figures, and abstract shapes. The stimuli monitored could therefore be categorised according to whether they were the target item, non-targets from the same category as the target item, or non-targets from one of the other three categories.

metric for comparing how selective the neural response in different frontal and non-frontal sub-regions actually is (Figure 11.5).

Using fMRI, we searched the brain for regions that followed either a tightly tuned profile, responding selectively to just the current target item, or a more widely tuned profile, responding to all stimuli from the same category as that target. The results demonstrated that the mid-ventrolateral frontal cortex, bilaterally, followed a tightly tuned response function; thus, activation was tightly tuned to the presentation of just the target stimulus, with no significant differences between responses to non-targets from the same or different categories as the target (Figure 11.6). In contrast, both the mid-dorsolateral frontal cortex and the posterior parietal cortex followed a more widely tuned response function, responding to all stimuli from the current target category, regardless of whether it was the actual target that was presented or not (Figure 11.6). These results confirm that, even in a simple target detection task, the role of the mid-ventrolateral frontal cortex can be dissociated from other frontal and parietal regions, according to their differential responses to targets and target category non-targets. More importantly, they suggest that the mid-ventrolateral frontal cortex acts specifically by biasing or 'tuning' attentional processing to the representations that are most relevant to the task at hand. Thus, activation within this region will be maximal whenever an intended thought or action requires a discrete (or 'tight') focus of attention, either on a specific stimulus, or on a particular

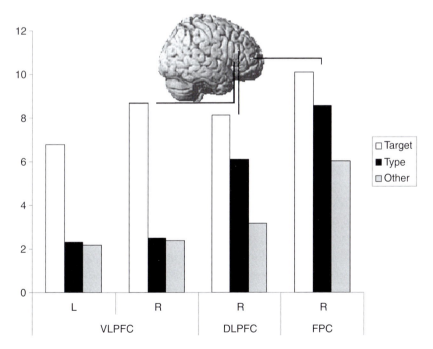

Figure 11.6 Adapted from Hampshire et al. (2007). Activation levels in the frontal cortex for targets, target category non-targets (labelled 'type') and non-target category non-targets (labelled 'other'). Unlike other areas, the mid-ventrolateral frontal cortex is tightly tuned to the target with little activity in response to same type or other distractors.

aspect of the task in hand. Such a requirement is, of course, central to many memory tasks in which the memoranda need to be attended to, either for intentional encoding or for active retrieval, but is also an important component of many non-memory tasks that require that some stimuli are the targets of attention, while others are ignored (e.g. many attentional set-shifting tasks). In this context, it is perhaps not surprising that the ventro-lateral frontal cortex is particularly active during extra dimensional shifting (Hampshire & Owen, 2006) given that the focus of attention needs to be shifted entirely, i.e. from one stimulus of a particular dimension to an entirely different stimulus from an unrelated dimension (see Figure 11.4).

Conclusions

In summary, the studies reviewed here demonstrate how finely tuned experiments in both humans and in non-human primates, which are guided by psychological observations and theories, can sharpen our view of both the functional architecture and the neural bases of specific cognitive processes. For example, a wealth of data exists from neuroimaging to suggest that the mid-ventrolateral frontal cortex plays a crucial role in intended thoughts and actions across multiple cognitive domains. Crucially, the tests that were used to probe those cognitive domains were derived largely from predictions based on psychological theories and models. On the other hand, the neuroimaging data feed back into the psychological models by revealing hidden processes (e.g. fMRI events that correspond to the BOLD response in a particular task) or intervening variables within the observed behaviour. For example, in one of the neuroimaging studies described above (Hampshire & Owen, 2006 – see Figure 11.3), it was shown that the brain regions that contribute to shifting behaviour continue to be involved beyond the point at which the stimulus ceases to be novel – suggesting that there may be parallel systems, within the frontal-lobe system that remain involved, but become redundant, with familiarity. In that case, the fMRI data analysis was driven by internal events that can not be observed directly and therefore, would be impossible to predict based on psychological theories alone. Indeed, the findings are not obviously predicted by the results of lesion studies in humans or monkeys either.

The neuroimaging data have also revealed a mechanism of action for the mid-ventrolateral frontal cortex in mnemonic and attentional processes; this region appears to operate by biasing or 'tuning' attentional processing between competing representations in modality-specific posterior regions in order to maintain their relevance to current behavioural goals. Such a view is anatomically plausible given the strong bi-directional connections between many posterior cortical association areas and the mid-ventrolateral frontal region, which, in turn, is closely interconnected with the entire lateral prefrontal cortex (Petrides, 1994). Moreover, a frontal module with such properties has been proposed recently (O'Reilly et al., 2002; Frank et al., 2004; see also, Dehaene et al., 1998), although in those computational models the critical region was defined rather more generally as the 'lateral prefrontal cortex'. Flexible tuning of task relevant variables within the mid-ventrolateral frontal cortex would be consistent with accounts of prefrontal function that emphasise its importance in switching (Cools *et al.*, 2002; Konishi *et al.*, 1999; Nakahara *et al.*, 2002; Dove *et al.*, 2000; Hampshire & Owen, 2006) and the 'top-down' modulation of attention (e.g. Owen *et al.*, 1991, 1993; Knight, 1994; Desimone & Duncan, 1995; Dias *et al.*, 1996). Moreover, compromising such a function would be expected to affect a wide variety of tasks, but particularly any behaviour (e.g. an action or a thought), that derives from the subject's plans and intentions (Petrides, 1994).

References

Bor, D., Duncan, J., Lee, A. C. H., Parr, A., & Owen, A. M. (2005). Frontal Lobe Involvement In Spatial Span: Converging Studies Of Normal And Impaired Function. *Neuropsychologia*, *44*(2), 229–237.

Brodmann, K. (1909). *Vergleichende Lokalisationslehre der Grosshirnrinde in ihren Prinzipien dargestellt auf Grund des Zellaufbaus*. Leipzig: J. A. Barth.

Buckner, R. L., Petersen, S. E., Ojemann, J. G, Miezin, F. M., Squire, L. R., & Raichle, M. E. (1995). Functional anatomical studies of explicit and implicit memory retrieval tasks. *Journal of Neuroscience*, *15*, 12–29.

Buckner, R. L., Kelley, W. M., & Petersen, S. E. (1999). Frontal cortex contributes to human memory formation. *Nature Neuroscience*, *2*(4), 311–314.

Canavan, A. G., Passingham, R. E., Marsden, C. D., Quinn, N., Wyke, M., and Polkey, C. E. (1989). Sequence ability in parkinsonians, patients with frontal lobe lesions and patients who have undergone unilateral temporal lobectomies. *Neuropsychologia*, *27*(6), 787–798.

Carmicheal, S. T. & Price, J. L. (1994). Architectonic subdivision of the orbital and medial prefrontal cortex in the macaque monkey. *The Journal of Comparative Neurology*, *346*, 366–402.

Cools, R., Clark, L., Owen, A. M., & Robbins, T. W. (2002). Defining the neural mechanisms of probabilistic reversal learning using event-related functional magnetic resonance imaging. *Journal of Neuroscience*, *22*, 4563–4567.

Corkin, S. (1965). Tactually-guided maze learning in man: effects of unilateral cortical excisions and bilateral hippocampal lesions. *Neuropsychologia*, *3*, 339–351.

Courtney, S. M., Ungerleider, L. G., Keil, K. K., & Haxby, J. V. (1997). Transient and sustained activity in a distributed system for human working memory. *Nature*, *386*, 608–611.

Dehaene, S., Kerszberg, M., & Changeux, J. (1998). A neuronal model of a global workspace in effortful cognitive tasks. *Neurobiology*, *95*(24), 14529–14534.

D'Esposito, M. & Postle, B. R. (1999). The dependence of span and delayed-response performance on prefrontal cortex. *Neuropsychologia*, *37*(11), 1303–1315.

Desimone, R. & Duncan, J. (1995). Neural Mechanisms of selective visual attention. *Annual Review of Neuroscience*, *18*, 193–222.

Dias, R., Robbins, T. W., & Roberts, A. C. (1996). Dissociation in prefrontal cortex of affective and attentional shifts. *Nature*, *380*, 69.

Dove, A., Pollmann, S., Schubert, T., Wiggins, C. J., & von Cramon, D. Y. (2000). Prefrontal cortex activation in task switching: an event-related fMRI study. *Brain Research. Cognitive Brain Research*, *9*, 103–109.

Dove, A., Brett, M. Cusack, R., & Owen, A. M. (2006). Dissociable contributions of the mid-ventrolateral frontal cortex and the medial temporal-lobe system to human memory. *Neuroimage*, *31*(4), 1790–1801.

Dove, A., Manly, T., Epstein, R. A., & Owen, A. M. (2008). The engagement of mid-ventrolateral prefrontal cortex and posterior brain regions in intentional cognitive activity. *Human Brain Mapping*, *29*(1), 107–119.

Elliot, R. and Dolan, R. J. (1999). Differential neural responses during performance of matching and nonmatching to sample tasks at two delay intervals. *Journal of Neuroscience, 19*(12), 5066–5073.

Fletcher, P. C. and Henson, R. N. A. (2001). Frontal lobes and human memory. *Insights from functional neuroimaging. Brain, 124*, 849–881.

Fletcher, P., Shallice, T., & Dolan, R. J. (1998a). The functional roles of prefrontal cortex in episodic memory. *I. Encoding. Brain, 121*, 1239–1248.

Fletcher, P., Shallice, T., Frith, C. D., Frackowiak, R. S. J., & Dolan, R. J. (1998b). The functional roles of prefrontal cortex in episodic memory. II Retrieval. *Brain, 121*, 1249–1256.

Frank, M. J., Seeberger, L., & O'Reilly, R. C. (2004). By carrot or by stick: Cognitive reinforcement learning in Parkinsonism. *Science, 306*, 1940–1943.

Freedman, D. J., Riesenhuber, M., Poggio, T., & Miller, E. K. (2001). Categorical representation of visual stimuli in the primate prefrontal cortex. *Science, 291*, 312–316.

Gaffan, D. (1994). Interaction of the temporal lobe and frontal lobe in memory. In: A.-M. Thierry, J. Glowinski, P. S. Goldman-Rakic, & Y. Christen (Eds), *Research and Perspectives in the Neurosciences, 3: Motor and Cognitive Functions of the Prefrontal Cortex* (pp. 129–139). New York: Springer-Verlag.

Garavan, H., Ross, T., & Stein, E. (1999). Right hemispheric dominance of inhibitoty control: An event-related functional MRI study. *Proceedings of the National Academy of Sciences of the United States of America, 96*, 8301–8306.

Greenlee, M. W., Koessler, M., Cornelissen, F. W., & Mergner, T. (1997). Visual discrimination and short-term memory for random patterns in patients with a focal cortical lesion. *Cerebral Cortex, 7*(3), 253–267.

Hampshire, A. & Owen, A. M. (2006). Fractionating attentional control using event related fMRI. *Cerebral Cortex, 16*(12), 1679–1689.

Hampshire, A., Duncan, J., & Owen, A. M. (2007). Frontoparietal information coding at different levels of abstraction. *Journal of Neuroscience, 7*(23), 6219–6223.

Henson, R. N., Shallice, T., & Dolan, R. J. (1999). Right prefrontal cortex and episodic memory retrieval: a functional MRI test of the monitoring hypothesis. *Brain, 122*(Pt 7), 1367–1381.

Iversen, S. & Mishkin, M. (1970). Perseverative interference in monkeys following selective lesions of the inferior prefrontal convexity. *Experimental Brain Research, 11*, 376–386.

Jonides, J., Smith, E. E., Koeppe, R. A., Awh, E., Minoshima, S., & Mintun, M. A. (1993). Spatial working memory in humans as revealed by PET. *Nature, 363*, 623–625.

Kapur, S., Craik, F. I. M., Tulving, E., Wilson, A. A., Houle, S., & Brown, G. M. (1994). Neuroanatomical correlates of encoding in episodic memory: levels of processing effect. *Proceedings of the National Academy of Sciences of the United States of America, 91*, 2008–2011.

Knight, R. T. (1994). Attention regulation and human prefrontal cortex. In: A.-M. Thierry, J. Glowinski, P. S. Goldman-Rakic, & Y. Christen (Eds), *Motor and Cognitive Functions of the Prefrontal Cortex* (pp. 161–173). Berlin Heidelberg: Springer Verlag,

Konishi, S., Nakajima, K., Uchida, I., *et al.* (1998). Transient activation of inferior prefrontal cortex during cognitive set shifting. *Nature Neuroscience, 1*, 80–84.

Konishi, S., Nakajima, K., Uchida, I., Kikyo, H., Kameyama, M., & Miyashita, Y. (1999). Common inhibitory mechanisms in human inferior prefrontal cortex revealed by event-related functional MRI. *Brain, 122*, 981–991.

Lee, A. C. H., Robbins, T. W., & Owen, A. M. (2000a). Episodic memory meets working memory in the frontal lobes: functional neuroimaging studies of encoding and retrieval. *Critical Reviews in Neurobiology, 14*, 165–197.

Lee, A. C. H., Robbins, T. W., Pickard, J. D., & Owen, A. M. (2000b). Asymmetric frontal activation during episodic memory: the effects of stimulus type on encoding and retrieval. *Neuropsychologia, 38*, 677–692.

Luria, A. R. (1966). *Higher Cortical Functions in Man.* New York: Basic.

Milner, B. (1964). Some effects of frontal lobectomy in man. In: J. M. Warren & K. Akert (Eds), *The Frontal Granular Cortex and Behaviour* (pp. 313–331). New York: McGraw-Hill.

Miotto, E. C., Bullock, P., Polkey, C. E., & Morris, R. G. (1996). Spatial working memory and strategy formation in patients with frontal lobe excisions. *Cortex, 32*(4), 613–630.

Mishkin, M. & Manning, F. J. (1978). Non-spatial memory after selective prefrontal lesions in monkeys. *Brain Research, 143*, 313–323.

Mishkin, M., Vest, B., Waxler, M., & Rosvold, H. E. (1969). A re-examination of the effects of frontal lesions on object alternation. *Neuropsychologia, 7*, 357–363.

Murray, E. A. & Wise, S. P. (1997). Role of orbitoventral prefrontal cortex in conditional motor learning. *Society for Neuroscience Abstracts, 27*, 12.1.

Nakahara, K., Hayashi, T., Konishi, S., & Miyashita, Y. (2002). Functional MRI of macaque monkeys performing a cognitive set-shifting task. *Science, 295*, 1532–1536.

O'Reilly, R. C., Noelle, D. C., Braver, T. S., & Cohen, J. D. (2002). Prefrontal cortex in dynamic categorization tasks: Representational organization and neuromodulatory control. *Cerebral Cortex, 12*, 246–257.

Owen, A. M. (1997). The functional organization of working memory processes within human lateral frontal cortex: the contribution of functional neuroimaging. *The European Journal of Neuroscience, 9*, 1329–1339.

Owen, A. M., Downes, J. J., Sahakian, B. J., Polkey, C. E., & Robbins, T. W. (1990). Planning and spatial working memory following frontal lobe lesions in man. *Neuropsychologia, 28*, 1021–1034.

Owen, A. M., Roberts, A. C., Polkey, C. E., Sahakian, B. J., & Robbins, T. W. (1991). Extra-dimensional versus intra-dimensional set shifting performance following frontal lobe excisions, temporal lobe excisions, or amygdalohippocampelectomy in man. *Neuropsychologia, 29*, 993–1006.

Owen, A. M., Roberts, A. C., Hodges, J. R., Summers, B. A., Polkey, C. E., & Robbins, T. W. (1993). Contrasting mechanisms of impaired attention: set-shifting in patients with frontal lobe damage or Parkinson's disease. *Brain, 116*, 1159–1175.

Owen, A. M., Evans, A. C., & Petrides, M. (1996a). Evidence for a two-stage model of spatial working memory processing within the lateral frontal cortex: a positron emission tomography study. *Cerebral Cortex, 6*, 31–38.

Owen, A. M. Milner, B., Petrides, M., & Evans, A. (1996b). A specific role for the right parahippocampal region in the retrieval of object-location: A positron emission tomography study. *Journal of Cognitive Neuroscience, 8*, 588–602.

Owen, A. M., Herrod, N. J., Menon, D. K., Clark, J. C., Downey, S. P. M. J., Carpenter, T. A., Minhas, P. S., Turkheimer, F. E., Williams, E. J., Robbins, T. W., Sahakian, B. J., Petrides, M., & Pickard, J. D. (1999). Redefining the functional organisation of working memory processes within human lateral prefrontal cortex. *European Journal of Neuroscience, 11*, 567–574.

Owen, A. M., Lee, A. C. H., & Williams. (2000). Dissociating aspects of verbal working memory within the human frontal lobe: Further evidence for a 'process-specific' model of lateral frontal organization. *Psychobiology, 28*(2), 146–155.

Passingham, R. E. (1975). Delayed matching after selective prefrontal lesions in monkeys. *Brain Research, 92*, 89–102.

Petrides, M. (1994). Frontal lobes and working memory: evidence from investigations of the effects of cortical excisions in nonhuman primates. In: F. Boller & J. Grafman (Eds), *Handbook of Neuropsychology, Vol. 9* (pp. 59–81). Amsterdam: Elsevier Science.

Petrides, M. & Pandya, D. N. (1994). Comparative architectonic analysis of the human and the macaque frontal cortex. In: F. Boller & J. Grafman (Eds), *Handbook of Neuropsychology Vol. 9* (pp. 17–58). Amsterdam: Elsevier Science B.V.

Rahman, S., Sahakian, B., Hodges, J., Rogers, R., & Robbins, T. (1999). Specific cognitive deficits in mild frontal variant frontotemporal dementia. *Brain, 122*, 670–673.

Rao, S. R., Rainer, G., & Miller, E. K. (1997). Integration of what and where in the primate prefrontal cortex. *Science, 276*, 821–823.

Rogers, R. D., Andrews, T. C., Grasby, P. M., Brooks, D. J., & Robbins, T. W. (2000). Contrasting cortical and subcortical activations produced by attentional-set shifting and reversal learning in humans. *Journal of Cognitive Neuroscience, 12*, 142–162.

Rolls, E. T., Hornak, J., Wade, D., & McGrath, J. (1994). Emotion-related learing in patients with social and emotional changes associated with frontal lobe damage. *Journal of Neurology*, Neurosurgery, and Psychiatry, 57, 1518–1524.

Rushworth, M. F. S., Nixon, P. D., Eacott, M. J., & Passingham, R. E. (1997). Ventral prefrontal cortex is not essential for working memory. *Journal of Neuroscience, 17*, 4829–4838.

Sakagami, M. & Niki, H. (1994). Encoding of behavioral significance of visual stimuli by primate prefrontal neurons: relation to relevant task conditions. *Experimental Brain Research, 97*, 423–436.

Semmes, J., Weinstein, S., Ghent, L., & Tueber, H.-L. (1963). Correlates of impaired orientation in personal and extrapersonal space. *Brain, 86*, 747–772.

Smith, E. E., Jonides, J. J., Koeppe, R. A., Awh, E., Schumacher, E. H., & Minoshima, S. (1995). Spatial versus object working memory: PET investigations. *Journal of Cognitive Neuroscience, 7*(3), 337–356.

Stern, C. E., Owen, A. M., Petrides, M., Look, R. B., Tracey, I., & Rosen, B. R. (2000). Activity in ventrolateral and mid-dorsolateral prefrontal cortex during non-spatial visual working memory processing: Evidence from functional magnetic resonance imaging. *Neuroimage, 11*, 392–399.

Wagner, A. D., Schacter, D. L., Rotte, M., Koutstaal, W., Maril, A., Dale, A. M., Rosen, B., & Buckner, R. L. (1998). Building memories: Remembering and forgetting of verbal experiences as predicted by brain activity. *Science, 281*, 1188–1191.

Wheeler, M. A., Stuss, D. T., & Tulving, E. (1995). Frontal lobe damage produces episodic memory impairment. *Journal of the International Neuropsychological Society, 1*, 525–536.

Chapter 12

Mechanisms underlying the short-term retention of information

Bradley R. Postle

Introduction

Can neuroimaging data inform psychological theories of short-term and working memory? The blood oxygen level-dependent (BOLD) signal measured with functional magnetic resonance imaging (fMRI), when measured while a subject performs a task, is a dependent measure whose interpretability - whose 'value' - is determined by the theory, the design, and the methodological rigor of the experiment that produced it. In this way fMRI data are not inherently different from such behavioural measures as reaction time (RT) or accuracy, or such other physiological measures as galvanic skin response or electroencephalogram (EEG)/event-related potentials (ERP). Nor do they differ in this regard from data produced by non-human animals or by humans selected because of a neurological or psychiatric diagnosis. This chapter will illustrate this point by reviewing a series of experiments investigating the short-term retention of visual information, also known as the storage component of short-term or working memory. Although all contributing to the same research enterprise, some of the hypotheses featured here will be more 'cognitive' in nature and some more 'neural'. This will highlight a second theme of this chapter, which is that the distinction between strictly cognitive vs. strictly neural science is often no longer appropriate.

The psychological construct that is the focus of this chapter, working memory, refers to the ability to retain information in an active state when it is not present in the environment, to transform it when necessary, and to use it to guide behaviour. This ability has been of interest to behavioural scientists at least since the 1930s, when Jacobsen (1935, 1936) highlighted its dysfunction as a core deficit produced by damage to the frontal lobes. In the 1970s, the linkage between working memory and the frontal cortex, particularly the prefrontal cortex (PFC), was reinforced by the observation that individual neurons in PFC of the monkey demonstrate sustained activity throughout the delay period of a delayed-response task (Fuster, 1973; Fuster & Alexander, 1971; Niki, 1974). At around the same time, independent of the neuroscience work that preceded it, Baddeley and Hitch (1974) articulated the multiple-component model of working memory. This cognitive model described a working memory system comprising two independent buffers for the storage of verbal and of visuospatial information, and a Central Executive to control attention and to manage information in the buffers. For the next several years, neuroscience and cognitive investigations of working memory proceeded largely independently of each other. The next important conceptual advance in working memory research illustrates the analytic power that can be gained by synthesizing across neural and cognitive data: Goldman-Rakic (1987, 1990) proposed that the sustained delay-period activity in PFC that was studied by neuroscientists and the storage buffers of the (cognitive) multiple-component model were cross-species manifestations of the same fundamental mental phenomenon. One proposal to arise from this insight was that the organization of the visual system into discrete pathways relatively specialized for the analysis of information about 'what' vs. 'where' in the visual environment, a tenet of visual neuroscience (Ungerleider & Haxby, 1994; Ungerleider & Mishkin, 1982), might also characterize the organization of visual working memory.

This chapter will focus on studies of the short-term retention (STR) of information during the delay between the presentation of to-be-remembered information and the end of the trial, at which point the subject's memory for this information is tested. Another fact about working memory that has been highlighted by human and non-human neuro-scientific studies is that different patterns of neurophysiological and/or neuroanatomical recruitment can be associated with each of these three trial epochs. Where appropriate, I will use "STR" rather than more commonly used formulations such as 'storage', 'maintenance', or 'rehearsal', because the former is non-committal with regard to what processes may be active during the delay period. (Indeed, it is non-committal as to whether the STR of information even requires an active delay-period process.)

Neuropsychological investigations of visual working memory

The first studies to be reviewed in this chapter investigated evidence for a *what/where* organization of visual working memory by comparing the performance of patients with Parkinson's disease (PD) with that of healthy control subjects (HCS). This work followed similarly motivated studies of single-unit electrophysiological activity in the PFC of monkeys (Wilson, O'Scalaidhe, & Goldman-Rakic, 1993), and experimental psychological (Hecker & Mapperson, 1997; Smith *et al.*, 1995; Tresch, Sinnamon, & Seamon, 1993), positron emission tomography (PET, Smith *et al.*, 1995), and ERP (Mecklinger & Muller, 1996) studies in humans. We reasoned that PD offered a good model with which to study this question because previous studies of spatial working memory (but that had not included a comparable test of working memory for objects) had found impairment in PD compared to HCS (e.g. Freedman & Oscar-Berman, 1986; Owen *et al.*, 1992; Taylor, Saint-Cyr, & Lang, 1986). And because early PD is characterized by a systematic pattern of neurodegeneration - targeting some brain systems while leaving others relatively intact - evidence for a selective deficit in working memory for locations, but not objects, could provide valuable information about the neural bases of the STR of these two kinds of information. One study was a test of delayed recognition of visually presented stimuli (Postle, Jonides, Smith, Corkin, & Growdon, 1997). Each trial began with the presentation of two difficult-to-name polygons ('targets') followed by a 3 s delay period, followed by a memory probe that matched the identity of one of the two targets with $p = .5$. Target exposure duration was calibrated individually to equate for perceptual difficulty across subjects. Type of memory required - stimulus location or stimulus shape - was blocked, but only the instructions differentiated the two trial types. A second study used a conditional-associative learning task that required the learning of arbitrary associations between two locations or between two difficult-to-name objects (Postle, Locascio, Corkin, & Growdon, 1997).

For both studies we found that PD patients were selectively impaired on the spatial task. We interpreted this as evidence that the STR of location information and of object information differ in that only the former depends on brain systems that are compromised early in the course of PD. This was corroborated by a study from a different group that compared spatial vs. object working memory performance in patients with early- vs. advanced-stage PD, and found the selective spatial deficit only in the early-stage group. (The advanced-stage PD group was impaired on both measures relative to HCS [Owen, Iddon, Hodges, Summers, & Robbins, 1997].) Thus, these studies implicated the dorsolateral head and body of the caudate nucleus, a neostriatal region that participates, via monosynaptic inputs from posterior parietal cortex (PPC) and dorsolateral PFC and its role in a PFC-basal ganglia-thalamic network, in the processing of the cortical dorsal stream. Their results were complementary with the electrophysiological, behavioural, and neuroimaging results that have already been summarized, and they implicated a brain region that the others had not.

One result of all these studies, plus others not reviewed here, was that the multiple component model of working memory was adjusted such that its visuospatial component was divided into 'visual cache' and 'inner scribe' components for representing object and spatiotemporal information, respectively (Baddeley & Logie, 1999; Logie, 1995). That is, knowledge gained from neuroscience experiments prompted a refinement in a cognitive model.

fMRI investigations of visual working memory

The PD studies performed by the author of this chapter were followed by a series of fMRI studies designed to evaluate the (fundamentally neuroscientific) hypothesis that STR of visuospatial vs. visuoobject information is supported by discrete dorsolateral vs. ventrolateral portions of the PFC, respectively (Postle & D'Esposito, 1999b; Postle, Stern, Rosen, & Corkin, 2000). Although these studies failed to find evidence for this functional organization in PFC, they did find evidence for a dorsal/ventral segregation of working memory for locations vs. objects, respectively, in posterior cortical regions. Additionally, because the PD studies had suggested an important role for dorsolateral caudate nucleus in the STR of locations, we also focused on this structure with an ROI-based analysis of the data from the task that permitted the isolation of delay-period activity. This task, inspired by a monkey electrophysiology study (Rao, Rainer, & Miller, 1997), required the STR of 'what'-then-'where' (and of 'where'-then-'what') visual characteristics with a two-delay procedure that permitted the assessment of the STR of location information when it would, and would not, be the basis for the behavioural response (Postle & D'Esposito, 1999b). Our analyses revealed greater spatial delay-period activity in the caudate nucleus when the response depended on this memory than when it did not (Figure 12.1). Perhaps, then, the

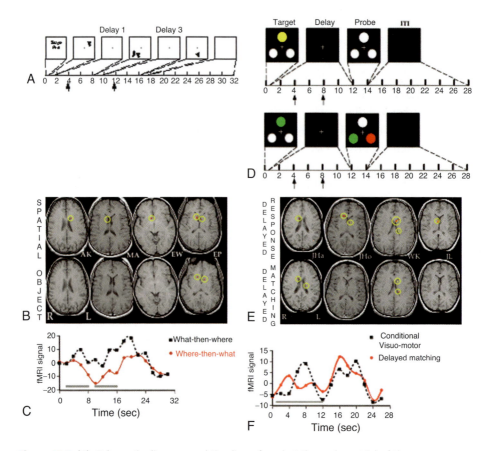

Figure 12.1 (A). Schematic diagram and timeline of a what-then-where trial of the delayed-recognition task featured in Postle & D'Esposito (1999a). Each box represents a stimulus display event, and the dotted lines connecting each box to the timeline represent the sequence and duration of each of these events. The numbers along the timeline represent seconds, and the two arrows indicate the positioning of the two delay-sensitive independent variables in our statistical model. A where-then-what trial would be formally identical, but with the instructions reading 'location first', one of the two intermediate stimuli occupying the same location on the screen as the initial target, and neither of the two intermediate stimuli matching the feature identity of the initial target. (B). Results of single subject analyses in the four subjects from Postle & D'Esposito (1999a) exhibiting significantly greater caudate nucleus activity during spatial delay 2 than during spatial delay 1. (C). Superimposed trial averaged BOLD fMRI data from what-then-where and where-then-what trials for the suprathreshold voxels identified in the *[spatial delay 2 - spatial delay 1]* contrast for subject EP from Panel B. The gray bars represent the two delay periods of each trial; the time on the horizontal axis corresponds to the diagram of trial events presented in Panel A. Note that spatial delay-period activity is higher in what-then-where than in where-then-what trials, whereas object delay activity is at a comparable level during the two conditions. (D). Schematic diagram and timeline for the delayed conditional visuo-motor and delayed-matching tasks featured in Postle & D'Esposito (1999a). (E). Results of single subject analyses in the four subjects exhibiting significantly greater caudate nucleus activity during the early delay than the late delay in the delayed conditional visuo-motor task. Analogous activity was not observed in the delayed-matching task for subjects

deficit that we had observed in PD patients reflected a role for the caudate nucleus in spatially dependent motor preparation. We assessed this possibility with an ROI-based analysis of a second task that contrasted delayed recognition of colour (requiring the STR of colour information) vs. a colour-based visuomotor association task that permitted the subject to prepare his/her response during the delay period. Consistent with our hypothesis, delay-period activity of the caudate nucleus in this second task showed greater time dependence in the visuomotor association task than in the colour memory task that featured the same response contingencies (Postle & D'Esposito, 1999a). Together, these results suggested that a working-memory function of the caudate nucleus may be in the integration of spatially coded mnemonic information with motor preparation to guide behaviour. More broadly, it pointed to the possibility that spatial working memory features greater interaction with the motor system than does non-spatial working memory.

Based on these results, which were reanalyses of data that had been generated to test other hypotheses, we designed a prospective test of the hypothesis that the caudate nucleus would be preferentially recruited by a spatial delayed-recognition task employing egocentrically defined stimuli, which were amenable to transformation into a motor code, as contrasted with allocentrically defined stimuli, which were not (Figure 12.2; (Postle & D'Esposito, 2003). The results revealed greater delay-period activity during egocentric than during allocentric trials in the caudate nucleus and trends in the same direction in the putamen and the lateral premotor cortex (PMC). Response-related activity was greater for egocentric trials in the lateral PMC. We interpreted these results as evidence that the neostriatum, possibly interacting with the PMC, contributed to the sensorimotor transformation necessary to establish a prospective motor code. This motor representation could contribute to spatial working memory by representing the to-be-remembered location with the metrics of the saccade (or, in other settings, the grasp or some other action) that could acquire the target. In this way, a succession of neuropsychological and neuroimaging studies gave rise to a cognitive hypothesis that will be detailed in the subsequent section: One way that we represent location information in working memory is via a *prospective motor code*. First, however, an aside about another mechanism hypothesized to support the STR of location information.

Attention-based rehearsal

Attention-based rehearsal refers to the covert allocation of attention to the location at which a stimulus appeared, as a means of remembering that location (Awh & Jonides, 2001).

JHo and JL. Subjects JHa and WK also exhibited greater early-than-late delay-period activity in the delayed-matching task; note that suprathreshold conditional visuo-motor and delayed-matching voxels are overlapping for these two subjects. (F). Superimposed trial averaged BOLD fMRI data from conditional visuo-motor and delayed-matching trials from the suprathreshold voxels identified in the *[conditional visuo-motor early delay - conditional visuo-motor late delay]* contrast for subject JHo. The gray bar represents the delay period of each trial; the time on the horizontal axis corresponds to the diagram of trial events presented in Panel D. Note that conditional visuo-motor delay-period activity is higher in the first portion of the delay period, whereas delayed-matching delay-period activity is relatively stable throughout the delay period.

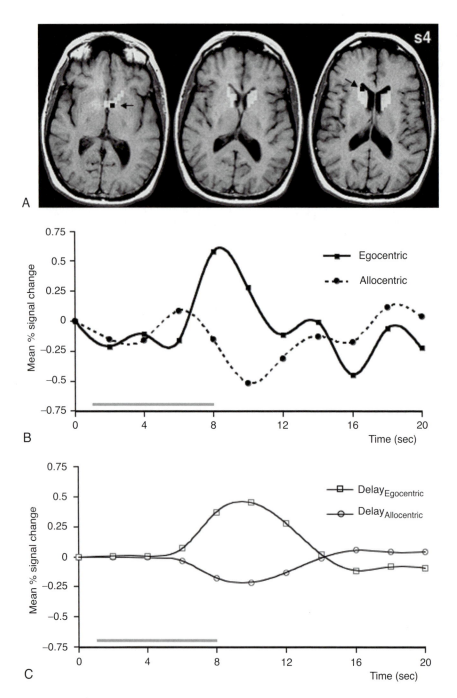

Figure 12.2 Significantly greater ego- than allocentric delay-epoch activity in the caudate nucleus of a participant in (Postle & D'Esposito, 2003). (A). Locus of activation of the two suprathreshold voxels (black squares identified with arrows; $\underline{t}(1204) = 5.0$, $\underline{p} < .0001$). The caudate nucleus ROI is depicted in translucent white overlaid on the structural T-1 images; 'gaps' in ROI in the right hemisphere reflect areas in which fMRI signal was too low to measure due

Although considerable behavioural (Awh, Jonides, & Reuter-Lorenz, 1998) and neuro-physiological (Awh, Anllo-Vento, & Hillyard, 2000; Awh *et al.*, 1999) data had been marshaled as evidence for this mechanism, we performed an event-related fMRI study to better characterize its neural bases. In this study, subjects fixated centrally throughout the trial and observed the following sequence of events: presentation of a target stimulus in one of two visual fields; followed by a delay period that was filled with a rapidly flickering checkerboard; followed by a memory probe. The logic was that the covert allocation of attention to a location in space has the well-established effect of boosting the visually evoked response in brain regions that represent that location in space. The attention-based rehearsal hypothesis, therefore, predicted that the delay-period STR of a location would selectively increase the checkerboard-evoked visual response in the hemisphere contralateral to the visual field of target presentation. The results were consistent with this prediction, revealing a gradient of decreasing contralateral bias in delay-period activity as one proceeded rostrally from extrastriate visual areas 18 and 19, through intraparietal sulcus and superior parietal lobule, and finally premotor cortex. There was no evidence of this delay-period bias in dorsolateral or ventrolateral prefrontal cortex, although these regions did demonstrate delay-period activity (Postle, Awh, Jonides, Smith, & D'Esposito, 2004).

Multiple encoding in visual working memory

Our neuropsychological and neuroimaging work with visual working memory not only gave rise to the prospective motor coding hypothesis, but also gave rise to a hypothesis about a *non-visual* representational code for the identity of visually presented objects (i.e. for 'what'): The STR of visual object information may necessarily entail its recoding into a verbal code. That is, in addition to the well-established role of inherently *visual* representational codes supported by the ventral visual stream (e.g. Della Sala, Gray, Baddeley, Allamano, & Wilson, 1999; Ranganath, 2006; Smith *et al.*, 1995; Tresch, Sinnamon, & Seamon, 1993), the STR of 'what' information about objects also recruits verbal (and, perhaps, semantic) representations. This theoretical proposition arose from our experience with the spatial/object studies reviewed up to this point - we observed that participants often adopted a strategy of verbally encoding stimuli in the object condition, even though the tasks used relatively 'non-verbalizable' shapes (Attneave & Arnoult, 1956; Vanderplas & Garvin, 1959). Perhaps, we reasoned, because object recognition

---

to susceptibility artifact. (B). fMRI time series data from these two voxels, trial averaged for each of the two trial types; gray bar represents the duration of the delay epoch. (C). Illustration of the least-squares solution of the GLM for the delay-epoch effects from these two voxels. Each plot represents a delay-epoch covariate scaled by its parameter estimate. These covariates model delay-epoch activity taking place at time 4; note how they take into account the sluggishness of this participant's haemodynamic response, which peaks approximately 6 sec after onset. The slight negative weighting on the Delay$_{Allocentric}$ covariate indicates that there was no detectable delay-epoch activity in these voxels on allocentric trials. Gray bar represents the duration of the delay epoch.

entails the association of visually perceived information with preexisting knowledge, STR of information about a visually presented object entails the activation (Potter, 1993) and retention of this semantic information. In our initial direct test of this hypothesis we employed a dual-task procedure that paired *n*-back working memory tasks with domain-specific distractor trials inserted into each interstimulus interval of the *n*-back tasks (Postle, D'Esposito, & Corkin, 2005). In two experiments, object *n*-back performance demonstrated greater sensitivity to verbal distraction, whereas spatial *n*-back performance demonstrated greater sensitivity to motion distraction.

Together, these two hypothesized *non-visual* mechanisms hypothesized to contribute to the STR of visually presented information - prospective motor coding and verbal recoding - illustrate the principle of *multiple encoding*: Humans will recode information and represent it in parallel in as many mental codes as are afforded by the stimulus (Postle, 2006; Wickens, 1973). The behavioural and fMRI studies with which we evaluated evidence for multiple encoding in working memory are the final studies that will be reviewed in this chapter.

Non-visual codes and non-visual brain areas support visual working memory

These studies, like the Postle *et al.* (2005) study, drew on the logic of dual-task interference. They were administered as a delayed-recognition tasks that required memory for the location or the shape of a target stimulus, crossed with three levels of delay-period distraction: endogenously guided saccades; rapid serial presentation of concrete nouns; and no distraction. Testing was conducted in a dark room in which all sources of light (with the exception of the screen of the computer monitor that displayed stimuli) were occluded. Additionally, the 'brightness' setting on the monitor was set to 0 in order to prevent the gray-black glow that typically emanates from a computer monitor that is displaying a uniformly blank screen. The effect for the participant was to be sitting in a room in which nothing was visible except for the periodic appearance of instructions and stimuli. The intent of this procedure was to minimize the likelihood that non-motoric factors could explain the selective disruption that saccadic distraction was expected to produce. Because participants were seated in absolute darkness during the distraction portion of the delay period, and because the source of the auditory 'start' and 'stop' signals was 0 degree with respect to trunk and head position, there were no possible sources of perceptual distraction. Saccades were endogenously generated, and participants had never been trained to guide them with, for example, a visual array of targets. Therefore, the likelihood that participants guided their saccades with internally generated mental images was minimized to the greatest extent possible.

Behavioural evidence for multiple encoding

The initial behavioural study produced a crossover interaction revealing the selective disruption of spatial-task performance by saccadic distraction and of shape-task performance by the rapid serial visual presentation of words (Postle, Idzikowski, Della Salla, Logie, & Baddeley, 2006). Although consistent with both the prospective motor coding and the verbal recoding hypotheses, this procedure left open the possibility that the source of the word interference on the STR of shape information was visual, not verbal. In a follow-up behavioural study, therefore, we replicated this procedure with the modification that the verbal distraction was presented auditorily rather than visually (Postle & Hamidi, 2007). The patterns of selective interference were replicated (Figure 12.3). But although this second result ruled out the most obvious alternative to the verbal recoding interpretation, another remained. It was possible that, upon hearing the verbal distraction, subjects generated mental images of these concrete nouns, and the interference with object working memory, by this alternative account, occurred between *visual* representations of the object memoranda and *visual* mental images generated as a result of the verbal distraction items. The adjudication between these two alternatives, as we shall see, was convincingly effected in the fMRI study of this task.

fMRI evidence for multiple encoding

The critical 2 (memory domain: location; object) x 2 (distraction: saccades; passive listening) arrangement in these experiments was embedded in an overall design that had three levels per factor, because the factor of memory domain also had a 'no memory' level, and the factor of distraction also had a 'no distraction' level. This was important for the fMRI study in particular, because our underlying hypothesis for spatial working memory, for example was that oculomotor codes contribute even to the simple, undistracted STR of location information. Thus, the analysis strategy was to first identify voxels showing delay-period activity on undistracted trials, then to evaluate the effect on the delay-period activity of these voxels of concurrent distraction (Postle & Hamidi, 2007).

The results from the fMRI study produced a neural double dissociation: a neural interference effect in frontal oculomotor regions (the FEF and supplementary eye fields [SEF]) for saccadic distraction of location memory, but no analogous effect for passive-listening distraction of object memory; and in left hemisphere superior temporal and Sylvian cortex for passive-listening distraction of object memory, but no analogous effect for saccadic distraction of location memory (Figure 12.3). In both cases the neural interference effect was characterized by a relative increase of delay-period activity (vs. no-distraction trials) for the behaviourally interfering distractor relative to the behaviourally non-interfering distractor. These results were further bolstered by individual differences analyses: The magnitude of the neural interference effect in FEF and SEF predicted the magnitude of the behavioural inference effect of concurrent saccades on spatial delayed recognition; and the neural interference effect in left Sylvian cortex increased as a function of the magnitude of the behavioural inference effect of concurrent passive listening on object delayed recognition (although this effect did not achieve statistical reliability). Further, this brain-behaviour trend in left Sylvian cortex differed significantly from the analogous regression of the behavioural interference effect against the neural interference effect in right inferior occipitotemporal cortex (IOTC). That is, although the IOTC showed strong object delay-period activity in this experiment, the neural interference effect in this region was unrelated to the behavioural interference effect of passive listening on object delayed recognition. These analyses of the fMRI results resolved the *verbal* vs. *visual* ambiguity of

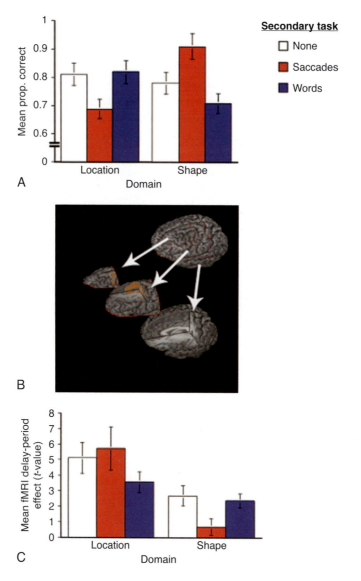

Figure 12.3 Multiple encoding in visual delayed recognition (Postle & Hamidi, 2007).
(A). Behavioural results illustrating the selective interference of concurrent saccades on the STR of locations and of concurrent passive listening to nouns on the STR of shapes. (B). Loci of memory-delay responses in the *no distraction* conditions for location (orange) and object (green) memoranda, in a single subject (#9). The top-left cutout features activity in the FEF and the SEF; the bottom-right cutout in the left Sylvian fissure. (C). Group data from frontal oculomotor location memory-delay ROI and left Sylvian shape memory-delay ROI, illustrating a region by secondary-task interaction. This neural double dissociation mirrors the behavioural double dissociation illustrated in (A), and illustrates that interference-specific neural effects are anatomically specific.

the behavioural passive-listening effect by demonstrating that the neural correlates of the effect localized to a region associated with the STR of phonological representations (e.g. Buchsbaum, Olsen, Koch, & Berman, 2005), and not to regions associated with the STR of visual representations. (It is also noteworthy that the Sylvian locus of the neural interference effect corresponded closely to a neural locus [from a previous set of studies] of the irrelevant speech effect [Gisselgard, Petersson, Baddeley, & Ingvar, 2003; Gisselgard, Petersson, & Ingvar, 2004], an unambiguously 'verbal' effect that is characteristic of verbal working memory [Repovs & Baddeley, 2006].)

Conclusions

The research summarized in this chapter highlights processes of recoding and parallel representation (i.e., of multiple encoding) in the STR of visually perceived information. For the STR of locations, it provides evidence for two mechanisms - attention-based rehearsal and prospective motor coding. (As has been noted elsewhere [Postle, 2006], it remains to be seen whether or not these two constructs may reduce to one underlying principle of recurrent interaction between 'perceptual' and 'motor' centers of the brain.) For the STR of object features, it also provides evidence for two mechanisms - one perceptual, one verbal. Together, these results demand changes to extant psychological theory of working memory. A cautious approach would be to consider whether the multiple-component model can be refined to accommodate these results. It can, by adding mechanistic specificity to the constructs of the *inner scribe* and the *visual cache*. To the former, it specifies a mechanism - prospective oculomotor coding - and a neural substrate - the dorsolateral caudate nucleus and the FEF. To the latter, it suggests that the function of the *visual cache* can be supplemented by the *phonological loop*, provided that the memoranda afford verbal recoding. This verbal recoding is hypothesized to be mediated via the association of visual stimuli with long-term knowledge, which, in turn, activates a lexical representation. This author's preference, however, has been to use the results described in this chapter (along with 'neuroscientific' and 'psychological' results from several other groups) as evidence for an alternative theoretical perspective.

A cognitive neuroscience research program yields a new theory of human working memory

An alternative to memory-systems accounts of working memory is an emergent property framework. The neuropsychological, neuroimaging, and behavioural studies summarized in this chapter support the view that the STR information arises from the allocation of sustained attention to any and all mental representations engendered and/or engaged by the task in question. Thus, if a task engages, for example, oculomotor control and/or visual perception and/or semantic knowledge and/or the phonological lexicon and/or speech production, the nominally 'non-memory' systems that support these functions are sufficient, with the aid of selective attention, to also support the STR of oculomotor and/or visual and/or semantic and/or phonological information in the service of behavioural goals (Postle, 2006). From this perspective there is no need to invoke specialized working memory buffers (such as a *visual cache* or a *phonological loop*) to accomplish the STR of information. Rather, working memory is simply a functionality of the cognitive system/nervous system. (To put it another way, there is no more need to appeal to a specialized working memory system(s) than there is to appeal to a specialized 'thinking system' that is independent of the representations and processes that make up thoughts.)

This review of 10 years of working memory research has illustrated instances in which neuropsychological, neuroimaging, and behavioural studies have each informed both cognitive and neural hypotheses, which, in turn, have prompted new studies that have sometimes been best addressed with the same type of method, and sometimes with a different type of method. In some instances, such as with the question of the basis of the interfering effect of passive listening to nouns on the STR of object information, we have seen that the distinction between a 'cognitive' answer and a 'neural' piece of evidence is blurred.

Acknowledgements

The author is supported by NIH grant MH064498.

References

Attneave, F. & Arnoult, M. D. (1956). Methodological considerations in the quantitative study of shape and pattern perception. *Psychological Bulletin, 53*, 221–227.

Awh, E., Anllo-Vento, L., & Hillyard, S. A. (2000). The role of spatial selective attention in working memory for locations: evidence from event-related potentials. *Journal of Cognitive Neuroscience, 12*, 840–847.

Awh, E. & Jonides, J. (2001). Overlapping mechanisms of attention and spatial working memory. *Trends in Cognitive Sciences, 5*, 119–126.

Awh, E., Jonides, J., & Reuter-Lorenz, P. A. (1998). Rehearsal in spatial working memory. *Journal of Experimental Psychology: Human Perception & Performance, 24*, 780–790.

Awh, E., Jonides, J., Smith, E. E., Buxton, R. B., Frank, L. R., Love, T., *et al.* (1999). Rehearsal in spatial working memory: evidence from neuroimaging. *Psychological Science, 10*, 433–437.

Baddeley, A. D. & Hitch, G. J. (1974). Working Memory. In G. H. Bower (Ed.), *The Psychology of Learning and Motivation* (Vol. 8, pp. 47-89). New York: Academic Press.

Baddeley, A. D. & Logie, R. H. (1999). Working memory: the multiple-component model. In A. Miyake & P. Shah (Eds), *Models of Working Memory* (pp. 28-61). Cambridge, U.K.: Cambridge University Press.

Buchsbaum, B. R., Olsen, R. K., Koch, P., & Berman, K. F. (2005). Human dorsal and ventral auditory streams subserve rehearsal-based and echoic processes during verbal working memory. *Neuron, 48*, 687–697.

Della Sala, S., Gray, C., Baddeley, A., Allamano, N., & Wilson, L. (1999). Pattern span: a tool for unwelding visuo-spatial memory. *Neuropsychologia, 37*, 1189–1199.

Freedman, M. & Oscar-Berman, M. (1986). Selective delayed response deficits in Parkinson's and Alzheimer's disease. *Archives of Neurology, 43*, 886–890.

Fuster, J. M. (1973). Unit activity in prefrontal cortex during delayed-response performance: neuronal correlates of transient memory. *Journal of Neurophysiology, 36*, 61–78.

Fuster, J. M. & Alexander, G. E. (1971). Neuron activity related to short-term memory. *Science, 173*, 652–654.

Gisselgard, J., Petersson, K. M., Baddeley, A. D., & Ingvar, M. (2003). The irrelevant speech effect: a PET study. *Neuropsychologia, 41*, 1899–1911.

Gisselgard, J., Petersson, K. M., & Ingvar, M. (2004). The irrelevant speech effect and working memory load. *NeuroImage, 22*, 1107–1116.

Goldman-Rakic, P. S. (1987). Circuitry of the prefrontal cortex and the regulation of behavior by representational memory. In V. B. Mountcastle, F. Plum, & S. R. Geiger (Eds), *Handbook of Neurobiology* (pp. 373-417). Bethesda: American Physiological Society.

Goldman-Rakic, P. S. (1990). Cellular and circuit basis of working memory in prefrontal cortex of nonhuman primates. In H. B. M. Uylings, C. G. V. Eden, J. P. C. DeBruin, M. A. Corner, & M. G. P. Feenstra (Eds), *Progress in Brain Research* (Vol. 85, pp. 325-336). Amsterdam: Elsevier Science Publishers.

Hecker, R. & Mapperson, B. (1997). Dissociation of visual and spatial processing in working memory. *Neuropsychologia, 35*, 599–603.

Jacobsen, C. F. (1935). Functions of frontal association areas in primates. *Archives of Neurology and Psychiatry, 33*, 558–560.

Jacobsen, C. F. (1936). The functions of the frontal association areas in monkeys. *Comparative Psychology Monographs, 13*, 1–60.

Logie, R. H. (1995). *Visuo-Spatial Working Memory*. Hove, UK: Erlbaum.

Mecklinger, A. & Muller, N. (1996). Dissociations in the processing of "what" and "where" information in working memory: an event-related potential analysis. *Journal of Cognitive Neuroscience, 8*, 453–473.

Niki, H. (1974). Differential activity of prefrontal units during right and left delayed response trials. *Brain Research, 70*, 346–349.

Owen, A. M., Iddon, J. L., Hodges, J. R., Summers, B. A., & Robbins, T. W. (1997). Spatial and non-spatial working memory at different stages of Parkinson's disease. *Neuropsychologia, 35*, 519–532.

Owen, A. M., James, M., Leigh, P. N., Summers, B. A., Marsden, C. D., Quinn, N. P., *et al.* (1992). Fronto-striatal cognitive deficits at different stages of Parkinson's disease. *Brain, 115*, 1727–1751.

Postle, B. R. (2006). Working memory as an emergent property of the mind and brain. *Neuroscience, 139*, 23–38.

Postle, B. R., Awh, E., Jonides, J., Smith, E. E., & D'Esposito, M. (2004). The where and how of attention-based rehearsal in spatial working memory. *Cognitive Brain Research, 20*, 194–205.

Postle, B. R. & D'Esposito, M. (1999a). Dissociation of caudate nucleus activity in spatial and nonspatial working memory: an event-related fMRI study. *Cognitive Brain Research, 8*, 107–115.

Postle, B. R. & D'Esposito, M. (1999b). "What" - then - "where" in visual working memory: an event-related fMRI study. *Journal of Cognitive Neuroscience, 11*, 585–597.

Postle, B. R. & D'Esposito, M. (2003). Spatial working memory activity of the caudate nucleus is sensitive to frame of reference. *Cognitive, Affective, and Behavioral Neuroscience, 3*, 133–144.

Postle, B. R., D'Esposito, M., & Corkin, S. (2005). Effects of verbal and nonverbal interference on spatial and object visual working memory. *Memory & Cognition, 33*(2), 203–212.

Postle, B. R. & Hamidi, M. (2007). Nonvisual codes and nonvisual brain areas support visual working memory. *Cerebral Cortex, 17*, 2134–2142.

Postle, B. R., Idzikowski, C., Della Salla, S., Logie, R. H., & Baddeley, A. D. (2006). The selective disruption of spatial working memory by eye movements. *Quarterly Journal of Experimental Psychology, 59*, 100–120.

Postle, B. R., Jonides, J., Smith, E., Corkin, S., & Growdon, J. H. (1997). Spatial, but not object, delayed response is impaired in early Parkinson's disease. *Neuropsychology, 11*, 1–9.

Postle, B. R., Locascio, J. J., Corkin, S., & Growdon, J. H. (1997). The time course of spatial and object visual learning in early Parkinson's disease. *Neuropsychologia, 35,* 1413–1422.

Postle, B. R., Stern, C. E., Rosen, B. R., & Corkin, S. (2000). An fMRI investigation of cortical contributions to spatial and nonspatial visual working memory. *NeuroImage, 11,* 409–423.

Potter, M. C. (1993). Very short-term conceptual memory. *Memory & Cognition, 21,* 156–161.

Ranganath, C. (2006). Working memory for visual objects: Complementary roles of inferior temporal, medial temporal, and prefrontal cortex. *Neuroscience, 139,* 277–289.

Rao, S. C., Rainer, G., & Miller, E. K. (1997). Integration of what and where in the primate prefrontal cortex. *Science, 276,* 821–824.

Repovs, G. & Baddeley, A. D. (2006). The multi-component model of working memory: explorations in experimental cognitive psychology. *Neuroscience, 139,* 5–21.

Smith, E. E., Jonides, J., Koeppe, R. A., Awh, E., Schumacher, E. H., & Minoshima, S. (1995). Spatial vs. object working memory: PET investigations. *Journal of Cognitive Neuroscience, 7,* 337–356.

Taylor, A. E., Saint-Cyr, J. A., & Lang, A. E. (1986). Frontal lobe dysfunction in Parkinson's disease. The cortical focus of neostriatal outflow. *Brain, 109,* 845–883.

Tresch, M. C., Sinnamon, H. M., & Seamon, J. G. (1993). Double dissociation of spatial and object visual memory: Evidence from selective interference in intact human subjects. *Neuropsychologia, 31,* 211–219.

Ungerleider, L. & Haxby, J. (1994). 'What' and 'where' in the human brain. *Current Opinion in Neurobiology, 4,* 157–165.

Ungerleider, L. G. & Mishkin, M. (1982). Two cortical visual systems. In D. J. Ingle, M. A. Goodale, & R. J. W. Mansfield (Eds), *Analysis of Visual Behavior* (pp. 549-586). Cambridge, MA: MIT Press.

Vanderplas, J. M. & Garvin, E. A. (1959). The association value of random shapes. *Journal of Experimental Psychology, 57,* 147–163.

Wickens, D. D. (1973). Some characteristics of word encoding. *Memory & Cognition, 1,* 485–490.

Wilson, F. A. W., O'Scalaidhe, S. P., & Goldman-Rakic, P. S. (1993). Dissociation of object and spatial processing domains in primate prefrontal cortex. *Science, 260,* 1955–1958.

Chapter 13

Interrelationships between working memory and long-term memory

Charan Ranganath

Introduction

The advent of functional neuroimaging has brought about an explosion of research in cognitive neuroscience, which in turn has had a significant impact on both cognitive psychology and neuroscience. At the same time, many have expressed concern about whether neuroimaging has ultimately revealed anything about the brain or about cognition (e.g. Coltheart, 2006; Uttal, 2001). This concern is not trivial, and points to a conundrum faced by all cognitive neuroscientists. In order to make inferences about brain function, researchers often rely on manipulations whose effects on cognitive processing seem to be well-understood based on behavioural studies. However, one can argue that cognitive psychology has yet to conclusively specify the component processes that support any aspect of complex behaviour (Uttal, 2001). To the extent that a behavioural manipulation affects multiple processes that are not yet known or understood, it could be easy to misinterpret the functional significance of a corresponding change in brain activity. An alternative application of neuroimaging is to use patterns of brain activity elicited during task performance as the basis for making inferences about the underlying cognitive processes that must be engaged. This approach is called 'reverse inference', and it relies on the tenuous assumption that the engagement of a particular brain region can be used to determine whether or not a given process is occurring. Unfortunately, it is not clear that we understand the functions of any brain region well enough to assume that activation of that region means that a particular process is being implemented and no other (Poldrack, 2006). Furthermore, if a particular brain area is involved in more than one process or if it consists of multiple, functionally dissociable subregions, then the inference may be invalid. To sum up, both cognitive processes and brain organization are currently underspecified, and this ultimately limits the degree to which one can be used to conclusively inform the other.

Based on the concerns outlined above, a pessimist might conclude that neuroimaging results have no relevance to cognitive psychology, or that principles and paradigms from cognitive psychology have no relevance to neuroimaging. From here it is only a small leap to argue that psychologists should return to treating the brain as a black box, and neuroscientists should stick to understanding the behaviour of molecules, rather than minds. I suspect, however, that most psychologists or neuroscientists would see this conclusion as a bit extreme.

I believe that the question of whether an imaging finding *necessitates* a theoretical shift in cognitive psychology (or vice versa) is somewhat ill-posed. To me, the more relevant question is whether the exchange of ideas between imagers and cognitive psychologists can be fruitful, despite the fact that both fields are still evolving. My research has been guided by the principle that findings and theories from cognitive psychology can yield insights into brain organization, even if our understanding of cognitive processes is imperfect, and that neuroimaging evidence can contribute to the development of psychological theories and inspire novel research, even if our understanding of brain function is imperfect. To illustrate this point, I will consider how imaging research on the relationship between working- and long-term memory has contributed to, and benefited from, cognitive psychology.

Terminology

Before proceeding, it is important to clarify the terminology that will be used in this chapter. In particular, it is essential to avoid confusing *measures* of memory performance with the hypothetical *processes* that might support performance. The terms 'working memory' (WM) or 'short-term memory' are often used to describe memory tasks with short retention intervals and also to describe hypothetical processes or systems that might support performance in such tasks. Interestingly, in psychology, these terms have been used to refer to processes as attention and executive control (R. Atkinson & Shiffrin, 1968; Kane, Bleckley, Conway, & Engle, 2001), short-term maintenance (Vogel, Woodman, & Luck, 2001), as well as to encoding and retrieval that support temporary, goal-directed information processing (Ericsson & Kintsch, 1995; Jolicoeur & Dell'Acqua, 1998; Jonides et al., 2008; Miller, 1956). In contrast, in most neuroscience research, WM refers primarily to active maintenance processes which are thought to be supported by persistent activity (Curtis & D'Esposito, 2003; Goldman-Rakic, 1992).

In this chapter, I will use the term 'working memory' to refer to goal-directed processes that allow information to be retained in a hyper-accessible state and/or transformed (i.e. manipulated) in order to guide behaviour. According to this definition, a WM process could facilitate accessibility of information without necessarily requiring rehearsal or active maintenance. Furthermore, the term can encompass encoding processes that support the processing of information 'in' WM (Jolicoeur & Dell'Acqua, 1998; Miller, 1956) and retrieval processes that support the use of WM to guide behaviour (Jonides et al., 2008; Sternberg, 1966). The present chapter will review imaging results pertinent to WM encoding, maintenance, manipulation, and retrieval, thereby highlighting the complexity of WM.

In the text, I will also use the term 'long-term memory'. By this term, I mean simply *measures* of memory tested over retention intervals of minutes or longer, during which on-line processing of memoranda would likely have ceased. Of course, there are numerous models of the processes or representations that contribute to performance on long-term memory measures, but I have chosen this operational definition because it is relatively neutral with respect to the question of how WM and LTM might be related.

I realize that this approach differs from more common definitions that either implicitly or explicitly assume that WM and LTM are inherently separate. For instance, one popular definition is that WM should refer to rehearsal-based memory, whereas LTM should refer to all forms of memory that are not supported by rehearsal. This is related to the idea that WM should only refer to 'activity-based' memory, whereas all LTM is 'weight-based', in that it is encoded through changes in synaptic efficiency. This definition is misleading, however, because some events can elicit changes in synaptic efficiency that last at most for a few minutes (Zucker & Regehr, 2002), so this kind of synaptic plasticity could be a mechanism that supports WM. Another implicit definition adopted by many is that LTM should refer more to memory that is supported by the medial temporal lobe region. This definition, however, leads to circular reasoning, such that if the medial temporal lobes are found to contribute to any putative WM task, then the finding is re-interpreted as evidence that the task really tests LTM at a very short retention interval.

Representational basis of WM

In the 1960's and early 1970's, this was an active topic of research (e.g. R. Atkinson & Shiffrin, 1968), but evidence of neuropsychological double dissociations led to a growing consensus that WM and LTM are supported by functionally and neurally distinct processes/systems. For example, one recent book notes that, 'While many early notions held that short-term memory is the gateway to the long-term store (for any kind of long-term memory), there is evidence that working memory can be fully dissociated from long-term memory...amnesic patients with damage to the hippocampal system have no difficulty holding information in consciousness... Conversely, patients with other types of brain damage have selective deficits in working memory... these findings have led many to consider working memory a distinct memory system...' (Eichenbaum & Cohen, 2001, pp.471,472). Citing similar neuropsychological dissociations, a recent textbook remarked, 'these data do demonstrate a clear dissociation between long-term memory ability and short-term retention of information' (Gazzaniga, Ivry, & Mangun, 2002, p. 311). A book aimed at a more popular audience also concluded that, '...working memory depends on a different network of brain structures than long-term memory systems do' (Schacter, 1996, p. 43).

In short, popular accounts of memory read by specialists, students, and laypeople generally convey a common message - that WM and LTM are fully independent. Indeed, psychological theories and research have generally considered WM and LTM in isolation. For instance, the WM model of Baddeley and Hitch (1974) focused primarily on explaining the control and maintenance processes that support STM, whereas theories such as 'levels of processing' (F. Craik & Lockhart, 1972) focused on explaining the relationship between control processes engaged during encoding, and their effects on subsequent LTM formation. Building on those frameworks, neuroscientists have generally examined WM and LTM in isolation, with WM research focused on the role of the prefrontal cortex (P. S. Goldman-Rakic, 1987), and LTM research focused on regions of the medial temporal lobes (Squire & Knowlton, 2000).

To sum up, the finding that medial temporal lobe amnesia seemingly spares WM led both psychologists and neuroscientists to treat WM and LTM as completely separate systems. It should be noted, however, that the initial neuropsychological studies of WM in amnesia examined short-term retention of simple stimuli or recall of sequences of simple digits or spatial locations (i.e. 'immediate serial recall'). These studies suggest that patients with medial temporal lobe damage can show severe impairments in LTM but still retain simple information across short delays (e.g. Cave & Squire, 1992). One important caveat to this conclusion is that amnesic patients with medial temporal lobe damage typically suffer from a relatively specific deficit in the ability to form new memories for events or facts. They do not lose other forms of LTM, such as the ability to understand the sound or meaning of words or numbers, to use strategies or skills, or to recognize or use objects (although there is increasing evidence that the medial temporal region may contribute to some aspects of visual perception, e.g. Lee *et al.*, 2005). Thus, if one construes 'memory' in a broad sense, many forms of LTM may be represented in cortical areas outside of the medial temporal region (see Postle's chapter in this volume for further discussion). If one assumes that the medial temporal lobe region plays a critical role in rapid formation of *new* declarative memory representations, then this region might contribute to maintenance and/or manipulation of novel materials that lack a stable representation in other brain regions (Hasselmo & Stern, 2006; Ranganath & Blumenfeld, 2005). Accordingly, it might be more appropriate to investigate WM by using novel materials that are more likely to be uniquely processed by the medial temporal region.

Two neuroimaging studies published in 2001 investigated this question. The first, by Stern and colleagues (2001), investigated the neural correlates of WM for novel scenes. Activity was examined while participants performed a '2-back' task that required them to decide whether each scene was the same as the one presented two trials previously. The hippocampus, a region in the medial temporal lobes, showed increased activity during blocks with novel scenes, as compared to blocks with scenes that were highly familiar. Stern *et al.* also examined activation in the hippocampus during performance of a target detection task that placed minimal demands on WM maintenance. Hippocampal activation did not differentiate between blocks of target detection with novel stimuli and blocks with highly familiar stimuli. This finding suggests that hippocampal activation during the WM task was not driven by passive processing of novel stimuli, but rather by the demand to actively maintain these stimuli.

In a separate study, we (Ranganath & D'Esposito, 2001) used event-related FMRI to investigate the neural correlates of WM for novel faces (Figure 13.1A). In the first experiment, participants performed a delayed recognition task, in which a novel sample face was presented for 1 s. This face was to be maintained across a 7 s delay. Next, a probe face was presented, and participants were required to decide whether this face matched the one that was held in memory. The faces presented on each trial were novel and not repeated on subsequent trials. We hypothesized that if the hippocampus is recruited during active maintenance of novel stimuli, then we should see increased hippocampal activation during the memory delay. As shown in Figure 13.1B, this is exactly what we observed.

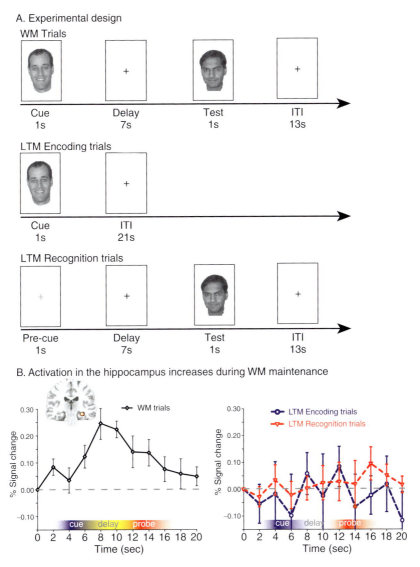

A. Experimental design

WM Trials

Cue
1s

Delay
7s

Test
1s

ITI
13s

LTM Encoding trials

Cue
1s

ITI
21s

LTM Recognition trials

Pre-cue
1s

Delay
7s

Test
1s

ITI
13s

B. Activation in the hippocampus increases during WM maintenance

Figure 13.1 Hippocampal activity during active maintenance of novel information (Ranganath & D'Esposito, 2001). (A). Participants were scanned while performing WM and LTM tasks that required encoding and retrieval of novel face stimuli. The figure schematically illustrates example stimuli and the relative timing of events for each trial type. (B). Activation in a region of the right anterior hippocampus is plotted for WM (left) and LTM (right) trials. Percent signal change is plotted as a function of time (in seconds) following trial onset. A colour bar at the bottom of each plot shows when MRI signal related to neural processing during cue (blue), delay (yellow), or probe (red) period would be expected to peak, based on the sluggishness of the haemodynamic response. Hippocampal activation was increased during the delay period, when participants were likely maintaining a mental image of the cue face in anticipation of the upcoming test probe.

We also included a comparison condition, in which participants were asked to encode a series of faces or perform recognition decisions on these faces we did not see reliable changes in hippocampal activation in this condition (Figure 13.1B). Of course, this finding should not be interpreted to suggest that hippocampal activity is uncorrelated with successful LTM encoding and retrieval. Numerous studies have shown that, hippocampal activity during encoding is predictive of whether the item will be successfully recollected on a long-term memory task (Diana, Yonelinas, & Ranganath, 2007; Eichenbaum, Yonelinas, & Ranganath, 2007). In the Ranganath *et al.* (2001) study, however, we could not separately average the data between subsequently recollected and subsequently forgotten items. The point of including the face encoding and retrieval trials in this experiment was simply to determine whether activation during the delay period of WM trials might have reflected passive perceptual processing of the sample face or anticipation of the test face, and the results ruled out that possibility. In a second experiment, we replicated our previous finding of hippocampal activation during maintenance of novel faces in a new sample of participants, and extended it by demonstrating that delay period activation in the same region was increased during maintenance of novel faces, as compared with familiar faces.

As described earlier, most arguments for neurally distinct short- and long-term memory stores were based in large part on reported neuropsychological studies showing that the medial temporal lobe lesions affected LTM, but not WM (Alvarez, Zola-Morgan, & Squire, 1994; A. Baddeley, 1986; Cave & Squire, 1992; Ryan & Cohen, 2004). However, our findings, along with those of Stern *et al.* (2001) seemed to suggest that the hippocampus is recruited during the maintenance of novel, complex stimuli. Accordingly, these results challenged the prevailing assumption that the medial temporal lobes are involved in LTM, but not WM, thereby undermining the claim that the two forms of memory are independent.

The findings from the studies by Ranganath & D'Esposito (2001) and Stern *et al.* (2001) prompted several groups to re-examine the question of whether WM is intact following medial temporal lobe damage. For example, one group ran a study aimed at replicating our FMRI findings (Ranganath & D'Esposito, 2001) and then tested performance of amnesic patients using essentially the same paradigm (Nichols, Kao, Verfaellie, & Gabrieli, 2006). Consistent with our study, they also found that activity in the hippocampus was increased during maintenance of novel faces. Additionally, amnesic participants with medial temporal lobe damage due to anoxia or encephalitis were impaired at performing the task at a 7 s delay. A similar study conducted by Olson and colleagues also found that amnesic patients with medial temporal damage were impaired at retaining novel faces across a 4s delay (Olson, Moore, Stark, & Chatterjee, 2006).

As noted earlier, the Baddeley & Hitch model of WM suggests that maintenance processes are independent from LTM (A. Baddeley, 1986, 2003). Other models, however, differ, in that they suggest that working memory processes reflect activation of representations that can also support LTM (e.g. Cowan, 1997; Jonides *et al.*, 2008; Ruchkin, Grafman, Cameron, & Berndt, 2003). According to the latter view, hippocampal activation during maintenance of novel stimuli makes sense, because the hippocampus may be needed to rapidly encode representations of novel stimuli that are not well represented in other parts of the brain (O'Reilly, Braver, & Cohen, 1999). These representations could then be transiently reactivated after a long delay, thereby supporting LTM, or persistently activated following encoding, thereby supporting WM maintenance. If so, we would expect that activation of the hippocampus during WM maintenance should be correlated with LTM for novel stimuli. Consistent with this prediction, hippocampal activation has been associated with both WM maintenance and LTM formation in studies using faces (Nichols *et al.*, 2006), scenes (Schon, Hasselmo, Lopresti, Tricarico, & Stern, 2004), and complex, novel 3D objects (Ranganath, Cohen, & Brozinsky, 2005).

Are there other conditions under which the medial temporal lobes might contribute to WM? Some research suggests that, in addition to processing novel information, the hippocampus and other medial temporal lobe regions may be needed to process and bind relations between items in WM. The basis for this idea comes from models suggesting that the hippocampus is critical for encoding representations of arbitrary relationships between specific aspects of an event (e.g. remembering where you put your keys, the name associated with a familiar face, etc.) in a manner that can support episodic LTM (Cohen & Eichenbaum, 1993; Diana *et al.*, 2007; Eichenbaum *et al.*, 2007). If the hippocampus rapidly encodes representations of arbitrary relationships, these representations could support short-term retention of these relationships (Hannula, Tranel, & Cohen, 2006; Olson, Page, Moore, Chatterjee, & Verfaellie, 2006; Ranganath & D'Esposito, 2001).

An alternative idea proposed by Baddeley (2002) is that there is a system for temporary retention of relational information that is independent of LTM, which he has termed the 'episodic buffer' (A. D. Baddeley, 2000). According to this account, the episodic buffer is a workspace for temporary storage of information in an integrated, multimodal format, which is separate from LTM. This model would not predict involvement of the medial temporal lobes in relational WM processing.

Evidence from recent imaging and patient studies, however, suggests that the hippocampus may be critical for temporary retention of relational information. For example, three imaging studies have reported hippocampal activation during WM tasks that required temporary retention of object-location associations (Hannula & Ranganath, 2008; Mitchell, Johnson, Raye, & D'Esposito, 2000; Piekema, Kessels, Mars, Petersson, & Fernandez, 2006). In one such study, we demonstrated that hippocampal activation was not only correlated with relational WM processing, but that the activation was predictive of whether or not relational information could be accurately retained across a short delay (Hannula & Ranganath, 2008). In this task, participants viewed a rendering of four objects, each presented in one of nine possible spatial locations of a three-dimensional grid (Figure 13.2). Participants were to mentally rotate the grid and maintain the rotated representation in anticipation of a test stimulus - a rendering of the grid, rotated 90 degrees from the original viewpoint. The test stimulus was either a 'match' display, in which object-location relations were intact, or a mismatch display, in which one object occupied a new,

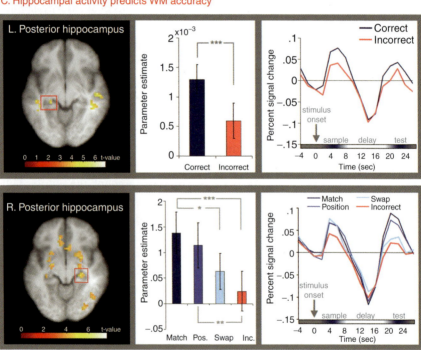

A. Example of a single short-term memory trial

| Sample (3 sec) | Delay (11 sec) | Test (3 sec) | ITI (9,11, or 13 sec) |

1 = Match   2=Mismatch Position   3 = Mismatch-Swap

B. Examples of the 3 test displays

Match   Mismatch-position   Mismatch-swap

C. Hippocampal activity predicts WM accuracy

L. Posterior hippocampus

0 1 2 3 4 5 6 t-value

R. Posterior hippocampus

0   2   4   6 t-value

Figure 13.2 Hippocampal activation predicts accurate WM for spatial relations (Hannula & Ranganath, 2008). (A). Example stimuli and relative timing of events on each trial. In this task, participants maintained the locations of four objects in a grid, and were tested with a rendering of the grid that was rotated 90 degrees clockwise. A 'match' probe is shown in this example. (B). Three examples of probe displays are shown. (C) Activation in the posterior hippocampus during the cue (top) and probe (bottom) phases differentiated correct from incorrect trials.

previously unfilled, location ('mismatch-position'), or two objects had swapped locations ('mismatch-swap'). During presentation of the test stimulus, participants indicated with a button press whether the stimulus was a match, a mismatch-position, or a mismatch-swap display. Thus, in order to perform accurately on the task, participants needed to retain a flexible representation of object-location bindings in each array.

Analyses of the FMRI data revealed that hippocampal activation during encoding of the sample display and processing of the test display predicted accuracy on the WM decision (Figure 13.2C). Notably, activation in these posterior hippocampal regions was also sensitive to the degree to which object-location bindings were preserved in the test stimulus: activation was greatest for correctly identified match displays (in which all bindings were intact), followed by correctly identified mismatch-position displays (in which one binding was changed), and finally correctly identified mismatch-swap displays (in which 2 bindings were changed). This finding is remarkable, because neither match nor mismatch test displays were perceptually identical to the cue (because of the 90 degree viewpoint rotation; see Figure 13.2A-B). Therefore, hippocampal activity parametrically signaled the *relational* match between the sample and test displays, despite the fact that they were visually dissimilar.

Another aspect of this data that was interesting is that although frontal and parietal brain areas showed persistent activity increases during the delay period, there were *no* brain areas for which activation during the delay period was correlated with successful working memory binding. Thus, our data suggest that short-term retention of the kinds of relationships tested here might reflect transient 'weight-based' processes possibly due to short-acting changes in synaptic efficiency (Zucker & Regehr, 2002), rather than relying an active maintenance/rehearsal process driven by persistent activity. Although this interpretation is speculative, our results do clearly suggest that hippocampal activity may reflect the formation and activation of relational memory representations that support WM.

Studies of amnesic patients with medial temporal damage converge with the imaging results described above, and suggest that the medial temporal lobes may play an essential role in WM for relational information. For example, Hannula *et al.* found that amnesics with damage limited to the hippocampus showed impaired *immediate* memory for the locations of objects within a complex scene (Hannula *et al.*, 2006). In a follow-up study, these researchers demonstrated that the effect was not limited to spatial relations by showing that patients were also impaired when tested on immediate memory for arbitrary associations between faces and scenes. A different research group also found that amnesic patients were impaired at memory for object-location associations (Olson, Page *et al.*, 2006). This study used a paradigm adapted from an imaging study (Mitchell *et al.*, 2000), in which subjects remembered the locations of line drawings of objects in a 2-dimensional 3x3 grid. Comparisons of patients with controls revealed that amnesic patients with medial temporal damage were significantly impaired at retaining the object-location associations across an eight second delay. Collectively, the studies of Olson *et al.* and Hannula *et al.* are not consistent with the idea that short-term retention of relational information must be separated from long-term retention, as suggested by Baddeley (2000).

In summary, before neuroimaging, neuropsychological evidence led to the development of psychological and neuroscientific theories proposing that WM and LTM are supported by separate systems. The neuroimaging results described above, combined with the neuropsychological studies that they inspired, suggest that the medial temporal lobe region contributes to, and is necessary for, accurate WM under many conditions. Such results do not necessarily suggest that it is wrong to propose fundamental differences between mechanisms for WM and LTM. The imaging results do suggest, however, that prior evidence for independence between WM and LTM needs to be re-evaluated. Indeed, the imaging results described above have led to a substantial shift in the way both psychologists and neuroscientists view WM, such that models proposing commonality between mechanisms that support WM and LTM task performance (Cowan, 1997; Hasselmo & Stern, 2006; Jonides *et al.*, 2008; Ruchkin *et al.*, 2003) are receiving renewed attention.

Working memory control processes and LTM formation

In the 1960's, a major theme of psychological research was to examine the relationship between short-term retention of information and the ability to subsequently remember that information after a long delay. Initially, this issue was the focus of a number of models which proposed that the amount of time spent during online (WM) processing should be correlated with subsequent LTM performance (e.g. R. Atkinson & Shiffrin, 1968; R. C. Atkinson & Shiffrin, 1971). Subsequent research was guided by the Levels of Processing Framework (F. Craik & Lockhart, 1972), which emphasized that successful LTM formation depends on the way in which items are processed. More specifically, it was asserted that if an item is processed in its basic sensory form, then maintaining that information for increasing periods of time ('maintenance rehearsal') should have a minimal effect on LTM formation. In contrast, increasing time spent on more extensive processing of an item ('elaborative rehearsal') should significantly improve memory performance. As an example, if one is trying to remember an auditorily presented word, rehearsing the sound of the word will have little impact on memory, whereas elaborating on the meaning of the word, engaging in visual imagery, etc. should have a strong effect on subsequent memory. A strength of the levels of processing framework is that it prompted researchers to think carefully about how information is encoded (F. I. Craik, 2002). Furthermore, it is clear that elaborative processing generally elicits much higher levels of LTM performance, as compared to maintenance rehearsal.

A more controversial prediction emerging from the levels of processing framework is that increasing the amount of time spent on maintenance rehearsal should not improve LTM, a prediction which contrasts with other models (e.g. R. Atkinson & Shiffrin, 1968). Consistent with this prediction, some studies have failed to find a relationship between maintenance rehearsal and LTM, particularly when LTM is tested by free recall (F. I. Craik & Watkins, 1973; Nairne, 1983), but other studies have observed that maintenance rehearsal improves LTM, even when elaboration was minimized (Greene, 1987).

As noted above, neuroimaging studies have correlated activation during maintenance rehearsal with subsequent LTM performance (Blumenfeld & Ranganath, 2006; Davachi,

Maril, & Wagner, 2001; Nichols *et al.*, 2006; Schon *et al.*, 2004). In one of these studies, activation in several cortical areas that are typically engaged during phonological rehearsal (Smith, Jonides, Marshuetz, & Koeppe, 1998) was correlated with subsequent LTM, leading the authors to conclude that WM maintenance does, in fact, contribute to successful LTM formation (Davachi *et al.*, 2001). This conclusion, however, relies on the reverse inference that if the 'rehearsal network' is engaged more for items that are subsequently remembered, then rehearsal must support successful LTM. Although this is a reasonable hypothesis, it would be helpful to reveal a more direct link between rehearsal and LTM formation.

Most imaging and behavioural studies of maintenance rehearsal and LTM formation are designed under the assumption that WM maintenance is a static and constant process, such that the processing that occurs during the first 1-2 seconds of maintenance is equivalent to the processing that occurs later in rehearsal. Results from one of our imaging studies, however, led us to question this assumption. In this study, participants were scanned while performing a WM task with novel 3D objects (Figure 13.3A). After the scan session, they were given a surprise LTM recognition test on the objects that they had previously seen in the scanner, allowing us to examine whether activity during WM maintenance was correlated with successful LTM formation (Paller & Wagner, 2002).

Consistent with our initial predictions, we did find that activity in the prefrontal cortex and hippocampus during the memory delay was increased during maintenance of objects that were subsequently remembered, as compared with activity during maintenance of objects that were later forgotten. We were surprised, however, when we looked at the time course of activation during each trial. Our experiment incorporated a variable-length memory delay in order to assess whether activity in many regions persisted throughout the delay. With this design, one would expect that, as the delay length increased, so should the duration of BOLD signal increases during the memory delay. This was true in some areas, but interestingly, in most areas that showed subsequent memory effects (e.g. prefrontal cortex and hippocampus), activity was increased only during the early part of the memory delay and gradually subsided over the course of the trial (Figure 13.3B). This finding suggested to us that there might have been cognitive processing that occurred specifically during the initial few seconds of the memory delay, and that this processing might have contributed to successful LTM formation.[1]

Although this idea was a speculation, it was bolstered by findings from behavioural studies of WM. For example, Jolicoeur and Dell'Acqua (1998) demonstrated that performance of a simple tone discrimination task was slowed for the first 500–1000 ms of processing of an item in WM. Their explanation is that when new information must be processed in WM, it must undergo a controlled process called 'short-term consolidation',

---

[1] In a recent study, we measured slow brain potentials elicited during the same task, in order to more precisely determine whether the critical activity occurred during the delay or during initial stimulus processing (Khader, Ranganath, Seemuller, & Rosler, 2007). Consistent with the FMRI study, our results showed that brain potentials during the first 1–2 seconds of the delay period differentiated between objects that were subsequently remembered and those that were subsequently forgotten.

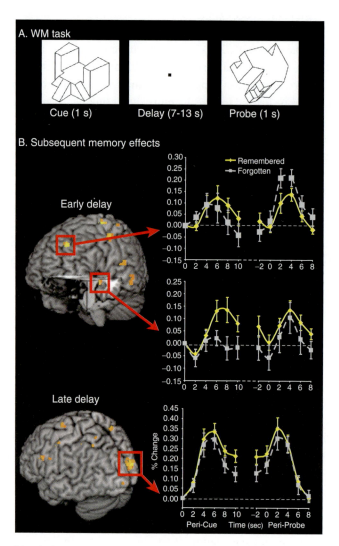

Figure 13.3 Activity during WM maintenance predicts successful LTM formation (Ranganath et al., 2005). (A) Example stimuli and relative timing of events on each WM trial. (B) FMRI subsequent memory effects. At left, regions are shown where activation during the early (top) or late (bottom) parts of the WM delay was predictive of subsequent LTM performance. At right, the time course of activation during WM trials is plotted separately for objects that were subsequently remembered (yellow) or subsequently forgotten (gray). The time course plots depict percent signal change as a function of time relative to onset of the cue (left) or probe (right) stimulus. In most cortical areas, activation differences between remembered and forgotten objects were apparent during the early part of the delay, whereas during the late delay, subsequent memory effects were primarily restricted to visual cortical areas.

by which sensory information may be transformed into a code that can be maintained in a manner that is robust in the face of interference. This idea may be similar to the proposal that initial WM processing may involve 'recoding' of external stimuli (Miller, 1956), or that previously active representations must be 'refreshed' (M.K. Johnson, 1992; M. K. Johnson, Mitchell, Raye, & Greene, 2004; M. K. Johnson, Raye, Mitchell, Greene, & Anderson, 2003; M. K. Johnson, Reeder, Raye, & Mitchell, 2002; Raye, Johnson, Mitchell, Reeder, & Greene, 2002; see also Johnson, this volume). All of these proposals have in common the idea that there is some kind of initial, controlled processing that occurs initially during WM maintenance, and that subsequent maintenance may proceed relatively automatically.

Based on our imaging results, we considered the possibility that processing during the initial stage of WM maintenance might disproportionately increase LTM performance, as compared with processing that occurred later in the memory delay. Results from two previous behavioural studies (Naveh-Benjamin & Jonides, 1984a, 1984b) suggested that this might be the case. In these studies, it was shown that increasing the number of times a word was rehearsed from 1 to 4 or 5 times significantly increased the likelihood that it would be subsequently remembered. Interestingly, when the number of rehearsals was further increased to 10, it did not result in additional improvements in subsequent LTM performance. These findings are consistent with the idea that processing during the initial stage of WM maintenance may be fundamentally different than processing that occurs during later stages.

To sum up, our analysis of the imaging data led us to discover a convergence between different strands of behavioural research on WM and behavioural research on LTM. Consideration of these behavioural results, in turn, suggested a straightforward explanation of the data from our FMRI experiment: That is, participants actively constructed a mental image of the object that they had previously seen during the initial part of the memory delay, and this processing led to the development of a stable, detailed mnemonic representation of the object. Subsequent maintenance of the mental image across the remainder of the delay period, however, had little further impact on memory formation. Based on this reasoning, we generated a novel prediction: interfering with processing early in the memory delay should disproportionately impair LTM formation, as compared to interference with processing later in the memory delay.

We tested this prediction in a subsequent behavioural experiment (Figure 13.4A) which was similar to the imaging experiment, except that, while performing the WM task, subjects were additionally instructed to perform a secondary task. Specifically, they were informed that, on most trials, an array of lines would be shown during the memory delay. When this happened, they were instructed to verbally indicate the number of lines shown in the array. The onset of the interference array was varied such that it was presented either early (1 s), in the middle (4 s), or late (7 s) in the memory delay. On the remaining trials, no distracter was presented during the delay. After the WM task was completed, subjects were given a surprise LTM test on the previously rehearsed objects. With this design, we were able to analyze subsequent LTM performance as a function of the presence

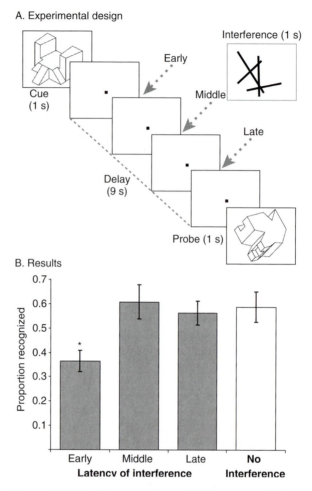

Figure 13.4 Interfering with WM maintenance impairs LTM formation. (A). Design of behavioural experiment performed by Ranganath et al. (2005). Participants performed a WM task, but on some trials, an array of lines was shown either early, in the middle of, or late in the delay period. When this occurred, participants were required to say aloud the number of lines on the screen. (B). Results of the subsequent LTM test. Subsequent memory was significantly impaired if interference occurred early in the delay, but no significant impairment was observed if interference occurred in the middle of, or late in the memory delay.

and temporal onset of interference with WM processing. The early delay interference probe was presented precisely at the time when we would expect subjects to be actively constructing internal representations of each object in WM (Jiang, 2004). We therefore hypothesized that interference during the early stage of WM maintenance (i.e. early in the memory delay) should impair subsequent LTM performance. The results, shown in Figure 13.4b, were fully consistent with this hypothesis: interfering with processing early in the delay period significantly and disproportionately impaired subsequent LTM performance, whereas interfering with processing later in the delay had no observable effect on subsequent LTM.

The results described above exemplify the synergistic effect of considering psychological research and results from imaging studies. From inspection of the unexpected activation timecourses in our study, we discovered a link between psychological theories of WM and LTM. This link was made explicit in the two-component model of maintenance rehearsal previously proposed by Naveh-Benjamin & Jonides (1984b), but the model was not previously well known. Results from our behavioural experiment confirmed the prediction of the two-component model, thereby demonstrating that processing during the initial stage of WM maintenance directly and disproportionately contributes to successful LTM formation. The findings suggest that some previous behavioural studies did not find a relationship between rehearsal and LTM because they did not specifically examine processing during the initial stage of WM maintenance.

In other studies, we have used psychological theories to construct unified models to explain how specific brain regions contribute to WM and LTM (Blumenfeld & Ranganath, 2007; Ranganath & Blumenfeld, 2009). As mentioned earlier, a great deal of research in cognitive neuroscience has been geared towards understanding the role of the prefrontal cortex in WM. Much of this research suggests that the prefrontal cortex may be critical for implementing control processes that are linked with the 'central executive' component of the Baddeley and Hitch WM model (D'Esposito, Postle, & Rypma, 2000; Ranganath & Blumenfeld, 2009) (see chapter by Owen, this volume). Furthermore, much of this research suggests that the prefrontal cortex may consist of multiple, functionally dissociable subregions. The most common distinction that has been drawn is between dorsolateral prefrontal regions (DLPFC) lying on the middle and superior frontal gyri (Brodmann's areas 9 and 46) and ventrolateral prefrontal regions (VLPFC) lying on the inferior frontal gyri (D'Esposito et al., 2000; Ranganath & Blumenfeld, 2009) (see also chapter by Owen, this volume).

Neuroimaging studies have shown that VLPFC activation is increased when a task requires inhibition of irrelevant or potentially distracting items (Aron, Robbins, & Poldrack, 2004; Konishi et al., 1999; Zhang, Feng, Fox, Gao, & Tan, 2004), resolution of proactive interference (Jonides & Nee, 2006), resolution of competition amongst competing linguistic representations (Thompson-Schill, D'Esposito, Aguirre, & Farah, 1997; Wagner, Pare-Blagoev, Clark, & Poldrack, 2001), or maintenance of an item representation (i.e. WM maintenance, Curtis & D'Esposito, 2003). These findings suggest that the VLPFC may be a source of top-down signals that select (i.e. enhance or reduce the activation of) item representations in posterior cortical areas based on current task demands.

Unlike VLPFC, DLPFC is not robustly recruited during tasks that solely require selection of task-relevant information. Instead, evidence from neuroimaging studies suggests that DLPFC is involved in using rules to activate, inhibit, or transform relationships amongst items that are active in WM. For example, DLPFC activation is reported in 'manipulation' tasks that involve sequencing of information that is being maintained in WM (Barde & Thompson-Schill, 2002; Blumenfeld & Ranganath, 2006; Crone, Wendelken, Donohue, van Leijenhorst, & Bunge, 2006; D'Esposito, Postle, Ballard,

& Lease, 1999; Mohr, Goebel, & Linden, 2006; Postle, Berger, & D'Esposito, 1999; Wagner, Maril, Bjork, & Schacter, 2001) or monitoring of previous responses when selecting a future response (A.M. Owen, 1997; A. M. Owen et al., 1999). DLPFC activation has also been reported in 'chunking' studies which involve processing of relationships to build higher-level groupings amongst items that are active in memory (Bor, Cumming, Scott, & Owen, 2004; Bor, Duncan, Wiseman, & Owen, 2003; Bor & Owen, 2007). One parsimonious explanation for this diverse array of findings is that DLPFC may implement selection processes that accentuate or inhibit representations of relationships amongst items that are active in memory.

Based on the findings from WM studies, one would expect that the recruitment of DLPFC and VLPFC should be correlated with successful LTM formation. Imaging studies have generally shown that similar prefrontal regions are recruited during WM and LTM tasks (Braver et al., 2001; Cabeza, Dolcos, Graham, & Nyberg, 2002; Nyberg, Forkstam, Petersson, Cabeza, & Ingvar, 2002; Nyberg et al., 2003; Ranganath et al., 2003), but that does not necessarily mean that prefrontal recruitment during WM processing actually improves LTM formation. To address this question, in 2006, we (Blumenfeld & Ranganath, 2006, 2007; Ranganath & Blumenfeld, 2009) reviewed results from event-related fMRI studies that investigated LTM encoding by identifying 'subsequent memory' or 'difference due to memory' effects. In these studies, activation during encoding of a particular item or set of items is analysed as a function of later memory success or failure (for review, see Paller & Wagner, 2002). Regions where activation is increased during encoding of items that are subsequently remembered (relative to activation during encoding of items that are subsequently forgotten) are thought to play a role in promoting successful LTM formation.

As shown in Figure 13.5, studies using the subsequent memory paradigm have demonstrated significant prefrontal involvement in LTM encoding. Inspection of the spatial distribution of activation peaks (or 'local maxima') from these studies indicates a clear link between VLPFC activity and successful LTM formation. Out of 150 local maxima associated with subsequent memory within PFC, 132 fall within VLPFC. Furthermore, all but two studies that reported subsequent memory effects reported local maxima within VLPFC. Given that the ability to select relevant item information is essential for many forms of goal-directed cognitive processing, including memory encoding, it makes sense that VLPFC activity should be strongly linked to memory encoding in a wide variety of behavioural contexts.

The imaging literature suggested a different story about DLPFC. Out of 150 local maxima throughout the PFC, only 18 were within DLPFC. Furthermore, some studies reported that DLPFC activation was increased during encoding of items that were subsequently forgotten, as compared with those that were subsequently remembered (i.e. a 'subsequent forgetting' effect). This pattern of findings is consistent with at least two possibilities: (1) DLPFC implements processes that do not typically promote successful LTM formation, or (2) most previous studies were insensitive to detect the way in which DLPFC contributes to LTM formation.

Based on the findings from studies of WM control processes, it seemed unlikely that DLPFC does not contribute to successful LTM formation. I therefore began to question

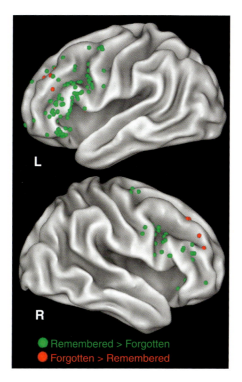

Figure 13.5 Prefrontal activations reported in 37 fMRI studies of LTM formation (Blumenfeld & Ranganath, 2007). Each green dot represents an activation peak in an analysis that reported increased activation during encoding of items that were subsequently remembered, as compared with items that were subsequently forgotten (i.e. a 'subsequent memory effect'). Each red dot represents an activation peak in an analysis that reported increased activation during encoding of items that were subsequently forgotten, as compared with items that were subsequently remembered (i.e. 'a subsequent forgetting effect'). Of the 150 local maxima associated with subsequent memory, only 18 fall within DLPFC (BA 46 and 9) compared with 132 in VLPFC (BA 6, 44, 45, and 47). Furthermore, 10 of the 11 local maxima associated with subsequent forgetting fall within DLPFC. L, Left; R, right.

the central assumptions that guided most imaging investigations of LTM encoding. As I noted earlier, most of these studies (e.g. Baker, Sanders, Maccotta, & Buckner, 2001; Otten, Henson, & Rugg, 2001; Otten & Rugg, 2001; Wagner *et al.*, 1998) drew inspiration from the levels of processing framework, in which memory encoding can be essentially characterized on a unidimensional continuum from 'shallow' to 'deep'. Other behavioural findings, however, suggest that the engagement of different kinds of control processes can affect memory traces in different ways that are not easily accounted for by the levels of processing framework. For example, Hunt & Einstein (1981) noted that some 'deep' encoding tasks promote memory by orienting subjects towards distinctive features of relevant items ('item-specific' encoding), whereas others promote memory by highlighting similarities amongst items to be learned ('relational encoding'). They manipulated these two factors and found that they had an additive effect on memory - suggesting that relational and item-specific encoding promote LTM in different ways. Further insight into this issue comes from studies by Bower (1970a), who demonstrated that relational and item-specific encoding of word pairs yielded equivalent memory for the words in each pair, but relational processing additionally elicited increased memory for the associations between the words. Again, this finding suggests that relational processing may promote LTM by strengthening associations between items, whereas item-specific processing may promote LTM by producing a more distinctive item representation, and thereby reducing interference during item recognition.

The findings from psychological studies of encoding led us to consider whether the kind of encoding and retrieval tests used to investigate memory encoding in imaging studies were appropriate for investigating the way in which the DLPFC might contribute to successful LTM formation. As noted above, neuroimaging investigations of WM control processes suggest that the dorsolateral prefrontal cortex may be involved in using rules to activate, inhibit, or transform relationships amongst items that are active in WM (D'Esposito et al., 1999; Postle et al., 1999; Wagner, Maril et al., 2001). This process is similar to the relational encoding tasks that were used in the LTM encoding studies described above (Bower, 1970a; Hunt & Einstein, 1981). Accordingly, it seemed that the WM control processes implemented by the DLPFC might facilitate LTM by strengthening representations of relationships between items that are encoded. Most imaging studies of LTM encoding, however, examined encoding of single items studied in isolation, using encoding tasks that orient attention towards specific attributes of a study item, and away from relationships between items. In these studies, it is unlikely that participants would spontaneously process relationships amongst items in the study list, and engagement of relational processing might have even been deleterious to later memory performance (i.e. because allocating resources towards processing the relationships amongst items might take attentional resources away from processing the distinctive features of the items themselves). The retrieval tests used in subsequent memory paradigms might also be a relevant factor. Most imaging studies of encoding assess successful LTM formation with tests of item recognition memory. However, processing of relationships between items facilitates memory by enhancing inter-item associations, and item recognition memory tests may not be sensitive to detecting these effects (Bower, 1970b). Thus, sorting encoding activation by subsequent item recognition performance might mask the role of DLPFC in successful LTM encoding.

If DLPFC contributes to LTM encoding through its role in relational processing, the ability to detect this contribution may depend on the kinds of encoding and retrieval tasks that are used. Indeed, in imaging studies that used encoding tasks that encouraged relational processing or retrieval tests that are sensitive to memory for associations amongst items, DLPFC activity during encoding predicts subsequent memory (Addis & McAndrews, 2006; Blumenfeld & Ranganath, 2006; Murray & Ranganath, 2007; Staresina & Davachi, 2006; Summerfield et al., 2006). In the first study to directly address this issue (Blumenfeld & Ranganath, 2006), we scanned participants while they performed two WM tasks (Figure 13.6A) and then examined prefrontal activation during these tasks as a function of subsequent LTM performance. During the 'rehearse' task, participants were presented with a set of three words and required to maintain the set

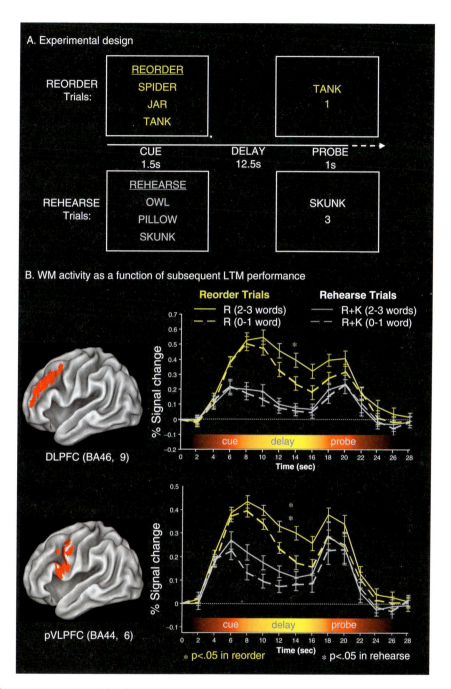

Figure 13.6 DLPFC activity during relational WM processing predicts successful LTM formation (Blumenfeld & Ranganath, 2006). (A). Schematic depiction of the tasks performed during FMRI scanning. (B). FMRI data showing that DLPFC (top) activation was increased during the delay period of reorder trials for which 2-3 items were subsequently remembered (solid yellow), relative to trials in which 0-1 items were remembered (dashed yellow). No such effect is seen on rehearse trials (gray lines). At bottom, activation in a region of posterior VLPFC ('pVLPFC') is plotted, showing that delay period activation in this region during both rehearse and reorder trials was predictive of subsequent memory performance.

across a 12 s delay period, in anticipation of a question probing memory for the identity and serial position of the items. During the 'reorder' task, participants were required to rearrange a set of three words based on the weight of the object that each word referred to. They maintained this information across a 12 s delay period in anticipation of a question probing memory for serial order of the items in the rearranged set. Although both rehearse and reorder trials required maintenance of the three item set, reorder trials additionally required participants to compare the items in the set and transform the serial order of the items. Thus, reorder trials forced participants to actively process relationships between the items in the memory set, whereas rehearse trials simply required maintenance of the memory set across a delay. Analyses of subsequent recognition memory performance showed that there were significantly more reorder trials in which all three items were recollected than would be expected based on the overall item hit-rates alone. The same was not true for memory for rehearse trials, for which the proportion of trials on which all three items were subsequently recollected was no different than would be expected by the item hit-rates alone. These findings suggest that, on reorder trials, processing of the relationships amongst the items in each memory set resulted in successful encoding of the associations amongst these items.

Consistent with the idea that the DLPFC is involved in processing of relationships between items in WM, FMRI data revealed that DLPFC activation was increased during reorder trials, as compared with rehearse trials (Figure 13.6b). Furthermore, DLPFC activation during reorder, but not rehearse trials, was positively correlated with subsequent memory performance. Specifically, DLPFC activation was increased on reorder trials for which 2-3 items were later recollected, as compared with trials for which 1 or 0 items were later recollected. Critically, no such relationship was evident during rehearse trials. In contrast, activation in a posterior region of left VLPFC (BA 44/6) was correlated with subsequent memory performance on both rehearse and reorder trials.

The results from Blumenfeld & Ranganath (2006) were consistent with the idea that DLPFC activation may specifically promote successful LTM formation through its role in processing of relationships amongst items, whereas VLPFC activation may promote LTM formation under a broader range of conditions. Nonetheless, this conclusion could be criticized because the reorder task involved more semantic processing, was more difficult, and yielded more item memory than did the rehearse task. We therefore ran a subsequent study (Murray & Ranganath, 2007) that addressed these concerns and more specifically linked the DLPFC to processing of and memory for inter-item relations (Figure 13.7). In this study, participants were scanned while during sequential encoding of unrelated word pairs. During presentation of the second ('target') word in each pair, subjects either made a semantic judgement specific to the target word ('item-specific' trials), or a semantic judgement that involved a comparison between the target word and the first word in the pair ('relational' trials). After scanning, participants were tested on memory for the individual words presented during the study phase, and for the associations between the word pairs. Behaviourally, item recognition memory for target words was equivalent between the two trial types, but associative recognition of studied word pairs was significantly greater for relational trials (Figure 13.7B). These results demonstrate that although

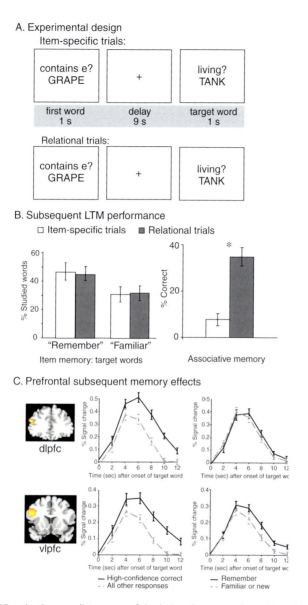

Figure 13.7 DLPFC activation predicts successful relational memory formation (Murray & Ranganath, 2007). (A). Example stimuli and timing of events for item-specific (top) and relational (bottom) encoding trials. (B). The graph at left shows that the proportion of target words that were either remembered or recognized on the basis of familiarity did not differ between the item-specific (open bars) and relational (shaded bars) conditions.

item-specific and relational processing had an equivalent effect on memory for the target word, memory for the association between the first word and the target word was significantly increased on relational trials.

Based on our previous results (Blumenfeld & Ranganath, 2006), we predicted that DLPFC activation should be (1) greater during relational trials than during item-specific trials, and (2) predictive of subsequent associative memory. Consistent with these predictions, our analyses (Figure 13.7C) showed that DLPFC activity during processing of the target word was greater during relational, as compared with item-specific encoding, and that DLPFC activity predicted successful memory for associations but not successful item memory. In contrast, activity in VLPFC was also greater for relational compared to item-specific encoding, but VLPFC activation predicted successful memory for both associations and items. Considered collectively, these findings support the hypothesis that the DLPFC is critical for active processing of relationships between items in WM, which in turn may promote LTM for associations (Murray & Ranganath, 2007).

This research demonstrates how theoretical concepts in cognitive psychology can be used to generate new hypotheses about brain organization that can be directly tested in imaging studies. Previous studies comparing the effects of relational and item-specific encoding processes led us to new insights into the results of imaging studies of LTM formation. In addition to allowing us to develop a unified model to explain prefrontal contributions to WM and LTM, this line of research has led us to consider the extent to which imaging studies might be missing critical aspects of memory functioning. Previous imaging studies probably failed to link DLPFC activity to successful LTM formation because these studies minimized relational processing at encoding and de-emphasized the role of inter-item associations at retrieval. Given that memory for complex real-life episodes relies on the ability to remember for inter-item associations, this is a topic that clearly demands further attention in cognitive neuroscience.

Concluding comments

The research reviewed here exemplifies how functional neuroimaging can contribute to and benefit from cognitive psychology. The idea that WM and LTM are functionally independent has, until recently, been accepted as dogma by many psychologists and neuroscientists. Evidence from functional imaging studies has led many to question that idea. We are now only beginning to understand the relationship between working- and long-term memory, but it is likely that evolving concepts in both psychology and neuroscience will contribute to future developments in this area.

References

Addis, D. R. & McAndrews, M. P. (2006). Prefrontal and hippocampal contributions to the generation and binding of semantic associations during successful encoding. *Neuroimage, 33*(4), 1194–1206.

Alvarez, P., Zola-Morgan, S., & Squire, L. R. (1994). The animal model of human amnesia: long-term memory impaired and short-term memory intact. *Proceedings of the National Academy of Sciences of the United States of America, 91*(12), 5637–5641.

Aron, A. R., Robbins, T. W., & Poldrack, R. A. (2004). Inhibition and the right inferior frontal cortex. *Trends in Cognitive Science, 8*(4), 170–177.

Atkinson, R. & Shiffrin, R. (1968). Human memory: a proposed system and its control processes. In (K. Spence & J. Spence (Eds)), *The Psychology of Learning and Motivation* (Vol. 2, pp. 89–105). New York: Academic Press.

Atkinson, R. C. & Shiffrin, R. M. (1971). The control of short-term memory. *Scientific American, 225*(2), 82–90.

Baddeley, A. (1986). *Working Memory*. New York: Oxford University Press.

Baddeley, A. (2003). Working memory: looking back and looking forward. *Nature Reviews. Neuroscience, 4*(10), 829–839.

Baddeley, A. & Hitch, G. J. (1974). Working memory. In G. Bower (Ed.), *Recent Advances in Learning and Motivation* (Vol. VIII, pp. 47–90). New York: Academic Press.

Baddeley, A. & Wilson, B. A. (2002). Prose recall and amnesia: implications for the structure of working memory. *Neuropsychologia, 40*(10), 1737–1743.

Baddeley, A. D. (2000). The episodic buffer: a new component of working memory? *Trends in Cognitive Sciences, 20*(11), 417–423.

Baker, J. T., Sanders, A. L., Maccotta, L., & Buckner, R. L. (2001). Neural correlates of verbal memory encoding during semantic and structural processing tasks. *Neuroreport, 12*(6), 1251–1256.

Barde, L. H. & Thompson-Schill, S. L. (2002). Models of functional organization of the lateral prefrontal cortex in verbal working memory: evidence in favor of the process model. *Journal of Cognitive Neuroscience, 14*(7), 1054–1063.

Blumenfeld, R. S. & Ranganath, C. (2006). Dorsolateral prefrontal cortex promotes long-term memory formation through its role in working memory organization. *Journal of Neuroscience, 26*(3), 916–925.

Blumenfeld, R. S. & Ranganath, C. (2007). Prefrontal cortex and long-term memory encoding: An integrative review of findings from neuropsychology and neuroimaging. *The Neuroscientist, 13*(3), 280–291.

Bor, D., Cumming, N., Scott, C. E., & Owen, A. M. (2004). Prefrontal cortical involvement in verbal encoding strategies. *The European Journal of Neuroscience, 19*(12), 3365–3370.

Bor, D., Duncan, J., Wiseman, R. J., & Owen, A. M. (2003). Encoding strategies dissociate prefrontal activity from working memory demand. *Neuron, 37*(2), 361–367.

Bor, D. & Owen, A. M. (2007). A Common Prefrontal-Parietal Network for Mnemonic and Mathematical Recoding Strategies within Working Memory. *Cerebral Cortex, 17*(4), 778–786.

Bower, G. H. (1970a). Imagery as a relational organizer in associative learning. *Journal of Verbal Learning and Behavior, 9*, 529–533.

Bower, G. H. (1970b). Organizational factors in memory. *Cognitive Psychology, 1*, 18–46.

Braver, T. S., Barch, D. M., Kelley, W. M., Buckner, R. L., Cohen, N. J., Miezin, F. M., *etal.* (2001). Direct comparison of prefrontal cortex regions engaged by working and long-term memory tasks. *Neuroimage, 14*(1), 48–59.

Cabeza, R., Dolcos, F., Graham, R., & Nyberg, L. (2002). Similarities and Differences in the Neural Correlates of Episodic Memory Retrieval and Working Memory. *Neuroimage, 16*, 317–330.

Cave, C. B. & Squire, L. R. (1992). Intact verbal and nonverbal short-term memory following damage to the human hippocampus. *Hippocampus, 2*(2), 151–163.

Cohen, N. J. & Eichenbaum, H. (1993). *Memory, Amnesia, and the Hippocampal System*. Cambridge, MA: MIT Press.

Coltheart, M. (2006). What has functional neuroimaging told us about the mind (so far)? *Cortex, 42*(3), 323–331.

Cowan, N. (1997). *Attention and Memory* (Vol. 26). New York: Oxford University Press.

Craik, F. & Lockhart, R. (1972). Levels of processing: a framework for memory research. *Journal of Verbal Leaning and Behavior, 11*, 671–684.

Craik, F. I. (2002). Levels of processing: past, present. and future? *Memory, 10*(5–6), 305–318.

Craik, F. I. & Watkins, M. J. (1973). The role of rehearsal in short-term memory. *Journal of verbal learning and behavior, 12*, 599–607.

Crone, E. A., Wendelken, C., Donohue, S., van Leijenhorst, L., & Bunge, S. A. (2006). Neurocognitive development of the ability to manipulate information in working memory. *Proceedings of the National Academy of Sciences of the United States of America, 103*(24), 9315–9320.

Curtis, C. E. & D'Esposito, M. (2003). Persistent activity in the prefrontal cortex during working memory. *Trends in Cognitive Science*, 7(9), 415–423.

D'Esposito, M., Postle, B. R., Ballard, D., & Lease, J. (1999). Maintenance versus manipulation of information held in working memory: an event-related fMRI study. *Brain and Cognition*, 41(1), 66–86.

D'Esposito, M., Postle, B. R., & Rypma, B. (2000). Prefrontal cortical contributions to working memory: evidence from event-related fMRI studies. *Experimental Brain Research*, 133(1), 3–11.

Davachi, L., Maril, A., & Wagner, A. D. (2001). When keeping in mind supports later bringing to mind: neural markers of phonological rehearsal predict subsequent remembering. *Journal of Cognitive Neuroscience*, 13(8), 1059–1070.

Diana, R. A., Yonelinas, A. P., & Ranganath, C. (2007). Imaging recollection and familiarity in the medial temporal lobe: a three-component model. *Trends in Cognitive Science*, 11(9), 379–386.

Eichenbaum, H. & Cohen, N. J. (2001). *From Conditioning to Conscious Recollection: Memory Systems of the Brain*. New York: Oxford University Press.

Eichenbaum, H., Yonelinas, A. R., & Ranganath, C. (2007). The Medial Temporal Lobe and Recognition Memory. *Annual Review of Neuroscience*, 30, 123–152.

Ericsson, K. A. & Kintsch, W. (1995). Long-term working memory. *Psychological Review*, 102(2), 211–245.

Gazzaniga, M. S., Ivry, R., & Mangun, G. R. (2002). *Cognitive Neuroscience* (2nd Edn). New York: W.W. Norton.

Goldman-Rakic. (1992). Working Memory and the Mind. *Scientific American Magazine*, 267, 111–117.

Goldman-Rakic, P. S. (1987). Circuitry of the prefrontal cortex and the regulation of behavior by representational memory. In F. Plum & V. Mountcastle (Eds), *Handbook of Physiology. Sec 1. The Nervous System. Vol 5.* (Section I, Vol. V, Part 1, pp. 373–417). Bethesda: Americal Physiological Society.

Greene, R. L. (1987). Effects of maintenance rehearsal on human memory. *Psychological Bulletin*, 102(3), 403–413.

Hannula, D. E. & Ranganath, C. (2008). Medial temporal lobe activity predicts successful relational memory binding. *Journal of Neuroscience*, 28(1), 116–124.

Hannula, D. E., Tranel, D., & Cohen, N. J. (2006). The long and the short of it: relational memory impairments in amnesia, even at short lags. *Journal of Neuroscience*, 26(32), 8352–8359.

Hasselmo, M. E. & Stern, C. E. (2006). Mechanisms underlying working memory for novel information. *Trends in Cognitive Science*, 10(11), 487–493.

Hunt, R. R. & Einstein, G. O. (1981). Relational and item-specific information in memory. *Journal of Verbal Learning and Behavior*, 20, 497–514.

Jiang, Y. (2004). Time window from visual images to visual short-term memory: consolidation or integration? *Experimental Psychology*, 51(1), 45–51.

Johnson, M. K. (1992). MEM: Mechanisms of recollection. *Journal of Cognitive Neuroscience*, 4(3), 268–280.

Johnson, M. K., Mitchell, K. J., Raye, C. L., & Greene, E. J. (2004). An age-related deficit in prefrontal cortical function associated with refreshing information. *Psychological Science*, 15(2), 127–132.

Johnson, M. K., Raye, C. L., Mitchell, K. J., Greene, E. J., & Anderson, A. W. (2003). FMRI evidence for an organization of prefrontal cortex by both type of process and type of information. *Cerebral Cortex*, 13(3), 265–273.

Johnson, M. K., Reeder, J. A., Raye, C. L., & Mitchell, K. J. (2002). Second thoughts versus second looks: an age-related deficit in reflectively refreshing just-activated information. *Psychological Science*, 13(1), 64–67.

Jolicoeur, P. & Dell'Acqua, R. (1998). The demonstration of short-term consolidation. *Cognitive Psychology*, *36*(2), 138–202.

Jonides, J., Lewis, R. L., Nee, D. E., Lustig, C. A., Berman, M. G., & Moore, K. S. (2008). The mind and brain of short-term memory. *Annual Review of Psychology*, *59*, 193–224.

Jonides, J. & Nee, D. E. (2006). Brain mechanisms of proactive interference in working memory. *Neuroscience*, *139*(1), 181–193.

Kane, M. J., Bleckley, M. K., Conway, A. R., & Engle, R. W. (2001). A controlled-attention view of working-memory capacity. *Journal of Experimental Psychology. General*, *130*(2), 169–183.

Khader, P., Ranganath, C., Seemuller, A., & Rosler, F. (2007). Working memory maintenance contributes to long-term memory formation: evidence from slow event-related brain potentials. *Cognitive, Affective & Behavioral Neuroscience*, *7*(3), 212–224.

Konishi, S., Nakajima, K., Uchida, I., Kikyo, H., Kameyama, M., & Miyashita, Y. (1999). Common inhibitory mechanism in human inferior prefrontal cortex revealed by event-related functional MRI. *Brain*, *122*(Pt 5), 981–991.

Lee, A. C., Bussey, T. J., Murray, E. A., Saksida, L. M., Epstein, R. A., Kapur, N., *etal.* (2005). Perceptual deficits in amnesia: challenging the medial temporal lobe 'mnemonic' view. *Neuropsychologia*, *43*(1), 1–11.

Miller, G. A. (1956). The Magical Number Seven, Plus or Minus Two: Some Limits on Our Capacity for Processing Information. *Psychological Review*, *63*, 81–97.

Mitchell, K. J., Johnson, M. K., Raye, C. L., & D'Esposito, M. (2000). fMRI evidence of age-related hippocampal dysfunction in feature binding in working memory. *Brain Research. Cognitive Brain Research*, *10*(1–2), 197–206.

Mohr, H. M., Goebel, R., & Linden, D. E. (2006). Content- and task-specific dissociations of frontal activity during maintenance and manipulation in visual working memory. *Journal of Neuroscience*, *26*(17), 4465–4471.

Murray, L. J. & Ranganath, C. (2007). The dorsolateral prefrontal cortex contributes to successful relational memory encoding. *Journal of Neuroscience*, *27*(20), 5515–5522.

Nairne, J. S. (1983). Associative processing during rote rehearsal. *Journal of Experimental Psychology. Learning, Memory, and Cognition*, *9*(1), 3–20.

Naveh-Benjamin, M. & Jonides, J. (1984a). Cognitive load and maintenance rehearsal. *Journal of Verbal Learning and Behavior*, *23*, 494–507.

Naveh-Benjamin, M. & Jonides, J. (1984b). Maintenance rehearsal: A two-component analysis. *Journal of Experimental Psychology. Learning, Memory, and Cognition*, *10*(3), 369–385.

Nichols, E. A., Kao, Y. C., Verfaellie, M., & Gabrieli, J. D. (2006). Working memory and long-term memory for faces: Evidence from fMRI and global amnesia for involvement of the medial temporal lobes. *Hippocampus*, *16*(7), 604–616.

Nyberg, L., Forkstam, C., Petersson, K. M., Cabeza, R., & Ingvar, M. (2002). Brain imaging of human memory systems: between-systems similarities and within-system differences. *Brain Research. Cognitive Brain Research*, *13*(2), 281–292.

Nyberg, L., Marklund, P., Persson, J., Cabeza, R., Forkstam, C., Petersson, K. M., *etal.* (2003). Common prefrontal activations during working memory, episodic memory, and semantic memory. *Neuropsychologia*, *41*(3), 371–377.

O'Reilly, R. C., Braver, T. S., & Cohen, J. D. (1999). A biologically based computational model of working memory. In (A. Miyake & P. Shah (Eds)), *Models of Working Memory: Mechanisms of Active Maintenance of Executive Control* (pp. 375–411). Cambridge: Cambridge University Press.

Olson, I. R., Moore, K. S., Stark, M., & Chatterjee, A. (2006). Visual working memory is impaired when the medial temporal lobe is damaged. *Journal of Cognitive Neuroscience*, *18*(7), 1087–1097.

Olson, I. R., Page, K., Moore, K. S., Chatterjee, A., & Verfaellie, M. (2006). Working memory for conjunctions relies on the medial temporal lobe. *Journal of Neuroscience, 26*(17), 4596–4601.

Otten, L. J., Henson, R. N., & Rugg, M. D. (2001). Depth of processing effects on neural correlates of memory encoding: relationship between findings from across- and within-task comparisons. *Brain, 124*(Pt 2), 399–412.

Otten, L. J. & Rugg, M. D. (2001). Task-dependency of the neural correlates of episodic encoding as measured by fMRI. *Cerebral Cortex, 11*(12), 1150–1160.

Owen, A. M. (1997). The functional organization of working memory processes within human lateral frontal cortex: the contribution of functional neuroimaging. *The European Journal of Neuroscience, 9*(7), 1329–1339.

Owen, A. M., Herrod, N. J., Menon, D. K., Clark, J. C., Downey, S. P., Carpenter, T. A., *et al.* (1999). Redefining the functional organization of working memory processes within human lateral prefrontal cortex. *The European Journal of Neuroscience, 11*(2), 567–574.

Paller, K. A. & Wagner, A. D. (2002). Observing the transformation of experience into memory. *Trends in Cognitive Sciences, 6*(2), 93–102.

Piekema, C., Kessels, R. P., Mars, R. B., Petersson, K. M., & Fernandez, G. (2006). The right hippocampus participates in short-term memory maintenance of object-location associations. *Neuroimage, 33*(1), 374–382.

Poldrack, R. A. (2006). Can cognitive processes be inferred from neuroimaging data? *Trends in Cognitive Sciences, 10*(2), 59–63.

Postle, B. R., Berger, J. S., & D'Esposito, M. (1999). Functional neuroanatomical double dissociation of mnemonic and executive control processes contributing to working memory performance. *Proceedings of the National Academy of Sciences of the United States of America, 96*(22), 12959–12964.

Ranganath, C. & Blumenfeld, R. S. (2005). Doubts about double dissociations between short- and long-term memory. *Trends in Cognitive Sciences, 9*(8), 374–380.

Ranganath, C. & Blumenfeld, R. S. (2009). Prefrontal cortex and memory. In H. Eichenbaum and J. H. Byrne (Ed.), *Concise learning and memory: The editor's selection.* (pp. 169–188). Oxford, UK: Elsevier.

Ranganath, C., Cohen, M. X., & Brozinsky, C. J. (2005). Working memory maintenance contributes to long-term memory formation: Neural and behavioral evidence. *Journal of Cognitive Neurosciences, 17*(7), 994–1010.

Ranganath, C. & D'Esposito, M. (2001). Medial temporal lobe activity associated with active maintenance of novel information. *Neuron, 31*, 865–873.

Ranganath, C., Yonelinas, A. P., Cohen, M. X., Dy, C. J., Tom, S. M., & D'Esposito, M. (2003). Dissociable correlates of recollection and familiarity within the medial temporal lobes. *Neuropsychologia, 42*(1), 2–13.

Raye, C. L., Johnson, M. K., Mitchell, K. J., Reeder, J. A., & Greene, E. J. (2002). Neuroimaging a single thought: dorsolateral PFC activity associated with refreshing just-activated information. *Neuroimage, 15*(2), 447–453.

Ruchkin, D. S., Grafman, J., Cameron, K., & Berndt, R. S. (2003). Working memory retention systems: a state of activated long-term memory. *The Behavioral and Brain Sciences, 26*(6), 709–728; discussion 728–777.

Ryan, J. D. & Cohen, N. J. (2004). Processing and short-term retention of relational information in amnesia. *Neuropsychologia, 42*(4), 497–511.

Schacter, D. L. (1996). *Searching for Memory.* New York: BasicBooks.

Schon, K., Hasselmo, M. E., Lopresti, M. L., Tricarico, M. D., & Stern, C. E. (2004). Persistence of parahippocampal representation in the absence of stimulus input enhances long-term encoding:

a functional magnetic resonance imaging study of subsequent memory after a delayed match-to-sample task. *Journal of Neuroscience, 24*(49), 11088–11097.

Smith, E. E., Jonides, J., Marshuetz, C., & Koeppe, R. A. (1998). Components of verbal working memory: Evidence from neuroimaging. *Proceedings of the National Academy of Sciences in the United States of America, 95*, 876–882.

Squire, L. R. & Knowlton, B. J. (2000). The medial temporal lobe, the hippocampus, and the memory systems of the brain. In M. S. Gazzaniga (Ed.), *The New Cognitive Neurosciences* (2nd Edn, pp. 765–779). Cambridge: MIT Press.

Staresina, B. P. & Davachi, L. (2006). Differential encoding mechanisms for subsequent associative recognition and free recall. *Journal of Neuroscience, 26*(36), 9162–9172.

Stern, C. E., Sherman, S. J., Kirchhoff, B. A., & Hasselmo, M. E. (2001). Medial temporal and prefrontal contributions to working memory tasks with novel and familiar stimuli. *Hippocampus, 11*, 337–346.

Sternberg, S. (1966). High-speed scanning in human memory. *Science, 153*, 652–654.

Summerfield, C., Greene, M., Wager, T., Egner, T., Hirsch, J., & Mangels, J. (2006). Neocortical connectivity during episodic memory formation. *PLoS Biology, 4*(5), e128.

Thompson-Schill, S. L., D'Esposito, M., Aguirre, G. K., & Farah, M. J. (1997). Role of left inferior prefrontal cortex in retrieval of semantic knowledge: a reevaluation. *Proceedings of the National Academy of Sciences of the United States of America, 94*(26), 14792–14797.

Uttal, W. R. (2001). *The New Phrenology: The Limits of Localizing Cognitive Processes in the Brain.* Cambridge MA: MITPress.

Vogel, E. K., Woodman, G. F., & Luck, S. J. (2001). Storage of features, conjunctions and objects in visual working memory. *Journal of Experimental Psychology. Human Perception and Performance, 27*(1), 92–114.

Wagner, A. D., Maril, A., Bjork, R. A., & Schacter, D. L. (2001). Prefrontal contributions to executive control: fMRI evidence for functional distinctions within lateral Prefrontal cortex. *Neuroimage, 14*(6), 1337–1347.

Wagner, A. D., Pare-Blagoev, E. J., Clark, J., & Poldrack, R. A. (2001). Recovering meaning: left prefrontal cortex guides controlled semantic retrieval. *Neuron, 31*(2), 329–338.

Wagner, A. D., Schacter, D. L., Rotte, M., Koutstaal, W., Maril, A., Dale, A. M., *etal.* (1998). Building memories: remembering and forgetting of verbal experiences as predicted by brain activity. *Science, 281*(5380), 1188–1191.

Zhang, J. X., Feng, C., Fox, P. T., Gao, J., & Tan, L. (2004). Is left inferior frontal gyrus a general mechanism for selection? *Neuroimage, 23*(2), 596–603.

Zucker, R. S., & Regehr, W. G. (2002). Short-term synaptic plasticity. *Annual Review of Physiology, 64*, 355–405.

Chapter 14

Is there anything special about working memory?

Bradley R. Buchsbaum and Mark D'Esposito

Introduction

In a recent article entitled 'What has functional neuroimaging told us about the mind (so far)?' Coltheart (2006) concludes that the answer to this question is: 'nothing'. The essential reason for this gloomy assessment about the value of functional neuroimaging for cognitive psychology boils down to this basic argument, namely, that since psychological theories do not make predictions about the brain, it follows that such theories are necessarily consistent with all possible brain imaging results. Of course, while this statement is true, it is also tautological – i.e. it is true by definition. Coltheart's conclusion rests on the premise that psychological theories do not and cannot make predictions about the brain. A hypothetical philosopher of metaphysics might ask the question: 'What has physics told us about metaphysics?' to which he might answer that because metaphysics is the science of the non-physical, physics by definition has nothing to say about metaphysics. Unlike metaphysics and physics, however, most would agree that the study of the mind and the study of the brain are fundamentally related if not, indeed, one and the same endeavour. There is therefore absolutely no reason why psychological theories should not refer to and make explicit predictions about brain function, nor is there any reason to think such theories would, upon making contact with neuroscience, somehow cease to be 'psychological'. Indeed, the four chapters in this section all stand out as examples, contra to Coltheart claims, that psychological theories can and do make predictions about the brain, and that, in the words of Postle (Chapter 8, p. 2), 'the distinction between strictly cognitive vs. strictly neural science is often no longer appropriate'.

New insights on short- and long-term memory

One of the classic divisions used by memory researchers, as well as clinicians caring for patients with memory disorders, is that between short- and long-term memory. Short-term memory is defined as the ability to store information temporarily (for seconds) before it is consolidated into long-term memory. Clinicians often examine short-term memory with a test such as digit span (e.g. repeat these digits immediately back to me: 4, 3, 7, 1, 5, 0, 6). The concept of short-term memory has evolved into 'working memory' which refers to the temporary maintenance of information that was just experienced or just retrieved from long-term memory but no longer exists in the external environment. These internal representations are short-lived, but can be maintained for longer periods of time through active rehearsal strategies, and can be subjected to various operations that manipulate the information in such a way that makes it useful for goal-directed behaviour. In contrast, long-term memory is defined as the ability to learn new information and recall (or recognize) this information after some time has passed. Clinicians often examine long-term memory by asking the patient to learn items that must be retrieved after an interval with some distraction (e.g. recall of three items – cat, apple, table – after one minute of performing some other task). The term amnesic syndrome, as used by clinicians, refers to the loss of long-term memory only.

The report of patient H.M. by Scoville and Milner (Scoville & Milner, 1957) provided support for this sensible distinction of memory function. Patient H.M. had intractable epilepsy and underwent bilateral surgical excision of the hippocampus and amygdala. Following surgery, H.M. suffered a dense and isolated impairment in episodic memory that that still persists today. However, H.M. did not exhibit a short-term memory deficit since he was reported as having a normal digit span. In contrast, a number of years later, several patients were reported (Vallar & Baddeley, 1984; Warrington & Shallice, 1969) with the opposite deficit – impaired short-term memory and intact long-term memory. The combination of these two patterns of memory deficits – which together constituted a *double dissociation* – amounted to a powerful argument for the independence of short- and long-term memory stores in the brain. These conclusions drawn from human lesion data were further bolstered by contemporaneous information processing models in cognitive psychology that also postulated separate and independent short- and long-term memory systems (Atkinson & Shiffrin, 1968). This convergence of evidence supporting a two-system view of memory made it the dominant paradigm in memory research over the past 50 years.

The data presented in all of the chapters in this section in one way or another buck this trend in that they emphasize *commonalities* in the processes underlying short- and long-term memory rather than differences. Moreover, much of the impetus for this more unified treatment of human memory comes directly from functional neuroimaging data. Thus, Ranganath (Chapter 9) reviews the recent history of neuroimaging studies that seemed to demonstrate what had previously been nearly unthinkable – that the hippocampus is important for active maintenance of information in working memory. Ranganath further describes how these neuroimaging findings led to a renewed interest in testing patients with hippocampal lesions on tests of short-term memory, and consequently, to a reappraisal of earlier conclusions. Also, in an elegant set of functional MRI (fMRI) studies Ranganath challenged the long-held view that rehearsal in working memory plays no role in long-term memory formation. Specifically, these studies demonstrated that processing during the initial stage of working memory maintenance directly and disproportionately contributes to successful long-term memory formation. In our opinion, this neuroimaging study has told us something about the 'mind' by testing predictions derived from purely behavioural studies and providing data that helps to shape and modify cognitive theory.

In the chapter by Johnson and Johnson, a similar effort is made to escape the strait-jacket of the two-system view of memory. In their presentation of the Multiple-Entry, Modular (MEM) model, the authors develop a framework that consists of a set of core cognitive processes that are marshaled in various contexts and combinations in the service of cognitive control. This means that less emphasis is placed on the traditional short- and long-term memory systems, but rather on the constituent operations that are required for 'reflective' cognitive operations. For instance, 'noting', 'refreshing', 'reactivation', 'rehearsal', and 'retrieval' comprise the cognitive vocabulary of the MEM model, and each of these operations may play a role in working memory and long-term memory, depending on the context. In this chapter they have primarily focused on one of these operations – that of 'refreshing' just-presented perceptual information – and have linked this operation to the dorsolateral prefrontal cortex (DLPFC). An important aspect of their work is that while the MEM model has a distinctive cognitive psychological 'flavour' to it, the authors have made clear predictions about its relation to functional neuroanatomy.

Indeed, the explicit neuroanatomical link drawn between 'refreshing' and the DLPFC in the MEM model brings it in to direct competition with the ideas of Owen and Hampshire (Chapter 7), who ascribe a similar, but more general, function to the mid ventrolateral prefrontal cortex (VLPFC). Thus, Owen and Hampshire review recent evidence that suggests that the mid VLPFC plays a specific role in *intended action* – that is, 'any behaviour that is consciously willed by the agent responsible for carrying out that behaviour' (p. 3). Owen and Hampshire, like the other chapters in this section, pursue a hypothesis about frontal lobe function that goes beyond the memory systems approach. For instance, they note that both short-term memory (e.g. 'digit span') and long-term memory tasks, as well as 'cognitive control' type tasks with no clear memory component at all, appear to recruit the mid VLPFC in equal measure. They also show that the mid VLPFC is active during both memory *encoding* and memory *retrieval* – two aspects of long-term memory that are often considered apart – provided that the subjects had been instructed to attend to the mnemonic stimuli with the *intention* of storing it for later use or remembering its prior occurrence. Finally, Owen and Hampshire show that in a task requiring shifts of attention both within ('intradimensional shift') and across ('extradimensional shift') stimulus categories, the mid VLPFC was most active in the latter case, wherein a complete reconfiguration of attentional set is required. This kind of cross-category set shifting, they argue, is mediated by a top-down biasing or 'tuning' process that modulates activity in modality-specific posterior regions, according to the currently relevant behavioural goal. It remains to be seen how other models of VLPFC function (Badre & Wagner, 2007; Thompson-Schill, D'Esposito, Aguirre, & Farah, 1997), which emphasize selection and controlled retrieval processes, can be reconciled with this view. In addition, one wonders whether the 'refresh' operation of the MEM model might also depend on this kind of attentional biasing; and, if so, to what extent this mechanism is a general capability of the prefrontal cortex or whether there are true dissociations between DLPFC and VLPFC as is implied by both Owen and Hampshire, and Johnson and Johnson.

In the chapter by Postle, we are shown how the study of short-term memory has benefited from an intra-disciplinary approach – from cognitive psychology, to monkey electrophysiology, to clinical neurology, to human functional neuroimaging. The Working Memory model of Baddeley and Hitch (1974) initially distinguished between short-term retention of visual and verbal information. Neurobiological investigations of the functional anatomy of the visual system, however, supported a dissociation between object and spatial processing ('what/where') streams in both perception (Ungerleider & Mishkin, 1982) and delayed response tasks (Goldman-Rakic, 1987). Postle and colleagues hypothesized that Parkinson's disease (PD) offered a good model to study this object/spatial dichotomy in the context of working memory because of its systematic pattern of neurodegeneration and because previous studies had found impairment in PD patients in tasks of spatial working memory. They found that PD patients were selectively impaired in memory for spatial location information (relative to information about object identity), arguing for a dissociation between object and spatial working memory that was dependent on the prefrontal-basal ganglia circuit that is compromised in PD. These results stimulated fMRI studies on object and spatial working memory that showed a greater role for the caudate nucleus (a region compromised in PD) for spatial working memory, as well as dissociations in the posterior neocortex. These and other studies ultimately led Baddeley and Logie to fractionate the visual subsystem of the Working Memory model into a 'visual cache' and 'inner scribe' for the representation of object and spatial information, respectively. Ultimately, then, the chapter by Postle shows how the willingness to pursue an idea using different research styles and methodologies – even those that cut across traditional disciplines – may generate new evidence and insights that can then 'ripple back' and change the very theoretical framework from which the original research question was formed.

Neuroimaging begets neuroimaging

An important thread running through each of the chapters in this section is that the models of brain function that they advance have emerged not just from ideas borrowed from cognitive psychology and basic neuroscience, but rather have (at least partly) derived from an empirical study of prior neuroimaging research. Thus, while the first generation of functional neuroimaging studies was overwhelmingly focused on 'brain mapping' and relied heavily on other disciplines for theoretical guidance, such research nevertheless supplied a mountain of empirical data from which a second generation of functional neuroimaging research could mine for patterns and commonalities that would lead to the formulation new hypotheses about the function of the brain; and thus, in the last few years, the functional neuroimaging community has truly begun to 'eat its own dog food'. Indeed, three of the four articles (Ranganath, Johnson & Johnson and Owen & Hampshire) cite functional neuroimaging meta-analyses that they or others carried out as leading to new insights or contributing to the generation of new hypotheses about the role of certain brain regions in the domain of memory and cognitive control.

For instance, in trying to address the role of the DLPFC in long-term memory encoding, Ranganath and Blumenfield examined a large number of neuroimaging studies that had examined so-called 'subsequent memory' effects. What they found was that the overwhelming majority of such studies found these effects in the VLPFC while very few were found in the DLPFC. Far from concluding that the DLPFC is unimportant for long-term memory formation, the result of the meta-analysis, coupled with previous work implicating the DLPFC in relational memory processing, led Ranganath to hypothesize that the reason previous studies had not observed subsequent memory effects in DLPFC was because they had not used a task that had required relational processing at encoding. This speculation turned out to be correct, as Ranganath demonstrated that when relational or associative processing was required at encoding, activation in DLPFC predicted subsequent memory performance.

Despite the apparent success of using neuroimaging data to provide valuable insight regarding the brain basis of memory function, this method cannot provide all the answers. Other neuroscientific methods can offer different temporal and spatial resolution as well as provide data that can support different types of inferences that can be drawn from it. Undoubtedly, data obtained addressing a single question but derived from multiple methods will provide more comprehensive and inferentially sound conclusions. Functional neuroimaging studies support inferences about the association of a particular brain system with a cognitive process. However, it is difficult to prove in such a study that the observed activity is necessary for an isolated cognitive process because perfect control over a subject's cognitive processes during a functional neuroimaging experiment is never possible. Even if the task a subject performs is well designed, it is difficult to demonstrate conclusively that he or she is differentially engaging a single, identified cognitive process. The subject may engage in unwanted cognitive processes that either have no overt, measurable effects or are perfectly confounded with the process of interest. Consequently, the neural activity measured by functional neuroimaging may result from some confounding neural computation that is itself not necessary for executing the cognitive process seemingly under study. It is important to note that the limitations in the inferences that can be drawn from functional neuroimaging studies such as fMRI apply to all methods of physiological measurement (e.g. EEG or MEG).

The inference that a particular brain region is necessary for a cognitive process cannot be made without showing that inactivating that brain region disrupts the cognitive process in question. When the results from lesion and functional neuroimaging studies are combined, a stronger level of inference emerges. If a lesion of a specific brain region causes impairment of a given cognitive process and when engaged by an intact individual, that cognitive process evokes neural activity in the same brain region, the inference that this brain region is computationally necessary for the cognitive process is stronger than data derived from each study performed in isolation. Thus, lesion and functional neuroimaging studies are complementary, each providing inferential support that the other lacks.

Although none of the chapters in this section presented data obtained from the same paradigm in both healthy individuals and those with focal lesions, several authors consider their fMRI data in the context of lesion data collected in other contexts. For example, Ranganath notes that his fMRI findings showing hippocampal activity during the temporary retention of relational information is consistent with studies of amnesics that have found that damage limited to the hippocampus exhibit impairments in immediate memory for stimuli that require relations processing such as the locations of objects within a complex scenes (Hannula, Tranel, & Cohen, 2006). Other functional neuroimaging data presented in these chapters have not been linked to lesion data but would benefit from such a comparison. For example, two authors attribute seemingly different cognitive processes to DLPFC function. Ranganath proposes that DLPFC is involved in 'processing of relationships between items in working memory' whereas Johnson and colleagues proposes that the DLPFC is involved in refreshing: the act of thinking of, or foregrounding, a representation of a thought or percept which was activated just a moment earlier and has not yet become inactive. Perhaps studies of patients with focal lesions to subregions of the PFC can reconcile these different viewpoints derived from imaging data.

Conclusions

Each of the four chapters in this section illustrate how psychological theory and functional neuroimaging (and other methods as well) are no longer 'strange bedfellows'. From the standpoint of memory research, the data presented herein is a part of a broader trend in the cognitive neuroscience community that is moving beyond the strict two-system view of memory. From the multiple encoding framework of Postle, to Ranganath's investigations of the role of the hippocampus in working memory, to Owen and Hampshire's examination of the VLPFC in digit span and long-term encoding and retrieval, and Johnson and Johnson's investigations of the refresh operation, 'memory' is increasingly being seen as a by-product of some more basic neural mechanisms. Indeed, this view was advocated by Joaquin Fuster in his monograph entitled, *Memory in the Cerebral Cortex* (Fuster, 1995) which he begins with the following sentence: 'This book is about the *memory of systems*, not about *systems of memory*'. He went on to elaborate with a paragraph that captures the spirit of the four chapters in this section and with which we will close: 'Memory is a functional property, among others, of each and all of the areas of the cerebral cortex, and thus all cortical systems. This cardinal cognitive function is inherent in the fabric of the entire cortex and cannot be ascribed exclusively to any of its parts. Furthermore, as the cortex engages in representing and acting on the world, memory in one form or another is an integral part of all operations. In this respect, what distinguishes one cortical area from another is it *kind* (i.e. the content and history) of memory; in the temporal domain, it is the *state* of memory, active or inactive or somewhere in between. Thus, as one of the cognitive functions of the cerebral cortex, memory is global and nonlocalizable. Its most concrete contents, however, those that are inextricable from specific sensory or motor functions, are well localized.'

References

Atkinson, R. C. & Shiffrin, R. M. (1968). Human Memory: A proposed system and its control processes. In K. W. Spence (Ed.), *The Psychology of Learning and Motivation: Advances in Research and Theory* (Vol. 2, pp. 89–195). New York: Academic Press.

Baddeley, A. D. & Hitch, G. J. (1974). Working Memory. In G. Bower (Ed.), *The Psychology of Learning and Motivation* (Vol. 7, pp. 47–90). New York: Academic Press.

Badre, D. & Wagner, A. D. (2007). Left ventrolateral prefrontal cortex and the cognitive control of memory. *Neuropsychologia, 45*(13), 2883–2901.

Coltheart, M. (2006). What has functional neuroimaging told us about the mind (so far)? *Cortex, 42*(3), 323–331.

Fuster, J. M. (1995). Memory in the Cerebral Cortex. Cambridge: The MIT Press.

Goldman-Rakic, P. S. (1987). Circuitry of primate prefrontal cortex and regulation of behavior by representational memory. In F. Plum (Ed.), Handbook of Physiology – the Nervous System (Vol. 5, pp. 373–417). Bethesda, MD: American Physiological Society.

Hannula, D. E., Tranel, D., & Cohen, N. J. (2006). The long and the short of it: relational memory impairments in amnesia, even at short lags. *Journal of Neuroscience, 26*(32), 8352–8359.

Scoville, W. B. & Milner, B. (1957). Loss of recent memory after bilateral hippocampal lesions. *Journal of Neurology, Neurosurgery and Psychiatry, 20*(1), 11–21.

Thompson-Schill, S. L., D'Esposito, M., Aguirre, G. K., & Farah, M. J. (1997). Role of left inferior prefrontal cortex in retrieval of semantic knowledge: a reevaluation. *Proceedings of the National Academy of Sciences of the United States of America, 94*(26), 14792–14797.

Ungerleider, L. & Mishkin, M. (1982). Two cortical visual systems. In D. Ingle, M. A. Goodale, & R. J. W. Mansfield (Eds), *Analysis of Visual Behavior* (pp. 549–586). Cambridge, MA: MIT Press.

Vallar, G. & Baddeley, A. (1984). Fractionation of Working Memory: Neuropsychological Evidence for a Phonological Short-Term Store. *Journal of Verbal Learning and Verbal Behavior, 23*, 151–161.

Warrington, E. & Shallice, T. (1969). Selective Impairment of Auditory Verbal Short-Term Memory. *Brain, 92*, 885-&.

Part 4

Long-term memory representations

Chapter 15

Retrieving pictures from long-term memory

Alumit Ishai

Introduction

'At the present time, one of the major deficiencies in cognitive psychology is the lack of explicit theories that encompass more than a single experimental paradigm. The lack of such theories and some of the unfortunate consequences have been discussed by Allport (1975) and Newell (1973). Two important points are made by Newell: First, research in cognitive psychology is motivated and guided by phenomena (e.g. those of the Sternberg paradigm and the Brown-Peterson paradigm). Second, attempts to theorize result in the construction of binary oppositions (e.g. serial vs. parallel, storage vs. retrieval, and semantic vs. episodic). Thus, an appreciable portion of research in cognitive psychology can be described as testing binary oppositions within the framework of a particular experimental paradigm. This style of research does not emphasize or encourage theory constructions; but without theory, it is almost impossible to relate experimental paradigms or to substantiate claims that the same processes underlie different experimental paradigms. Furthermore, the concern with binary oppositions tends to obscure the more interesting aspects of data, such as the form of functional relations' (Ratcliff, 1978, p. 59).

Three decades have passed since these words have been written. Despite the functional brain imaging revolution, which transformed cognitive psychology to cognitive neuroscience, we still do not have a theory of human memory, we are still guided by phenomena, and we still test binary oppositions. The contemporary neuroimaging literature on human memory is saturated with studies that contrast encoding with retrieval, recollection with familiarity, remembered with forgotten items, and correct with incorrect responses. These contrasts result in statistical maps that identify the location of activation in some brain areas during some experimental conditions. At best, these functional brain imaging studies are designed to test a specific hypothesis, but hypotheses do not comprise a unified theory of human memory. Perhaps the best example of how psychological theories have provided insights into functional brain imaging studies is Baddeley's influential model of working memory and its subsequent revision due to novel neuroimaging data, from which new predictions derived (see chapters by Postle and Ranganath). It has been argued that the collection of large-scale fMRI data do not represent an intellectual integration (Savoy, 2001). It has also been suggested that we have to accept the assumption that there is a systematic mapping from cognitive function to brain structure and that neuroimaging data comprise an independent variable that can be used to construct and test competing theories (Henson, 2005). In this chapter, several fMRI studies, designed to elucidate the neural correlates of retrieving pictorial information from long-term memory (LTM), are described. Although these studies were originally designed to test binary oppositions (e.g. perception vs. imagery; short- vs. long-term memory; old vs. new), I argue that the complex activation patterns observed when subjects generate mental images of faces and objects or perform recognition memory tasks provide us with valuable information that is essential for the formulation of any theories or models of human memory. As visual imagery and recognition memory are mediated by activation in distributed cortical networks that include visual, parietal, limbic, and prefrontal structures, I further argue that an integrative theory of human memory has to account for wide spread patterns of activation and for the dynamics and effective connectivity within these cortical networks.

Visual perception, imagery, and effective connectivity

Visual imagery is the ability to generate percept-like images in the absence of retinal input and therefore is a vivid demonstration of retrieving pictorial information from memory. The subjective similarity of seeing and imagining suggests that perception and imagery share common internal representations. Psychophysical and brain-imaging studies have demonstrated functional similarities between visual perception and visual imagery, to the extent that common mechanisms appear to be activated by both (Roland et al., 1987; Farah et al., 1988; Goldenberg et al., 1989; Ishai & Sagi 1995). Numerous neuroimaging studies have shown that visual imagery, like visual perception, evokes activation in occipito-parietal and occipito-temporal visual association areas (Mellet et al., 1996; D'Esposito et al., 1997). In some studies, the primary visual cortex (Le Bihan et al., 1993; Kosslyn et al., 1993, 1999) and the lateral geniculate nucleus (Chen et al., 1998) were activated during imagery, suggesting that the generation of mental images may involve sensory representations at the earlier processing stages in the visual pathway. Studies of patients with brain damage have demonstrated a dissociation of visual-object and visual-spatial imagery (Levine et al., 1985), indicating that different parts of the visual system mediate 'where' and 'what' imagery, a dissociation that parallels the two anatomically distinct visual systems proposed for visual perception (Ungerleider & Mishkin, 1982).

Functional MRI studies have reported that within the ventral object vision pathway faces and other objects, such as outdoor scenes, houses, chairs, animals, and tools, have distinct representations (Kanwisher et al., 1997; Epstein & Kanwisher, 1998; Aguirre et al., 1998; Chao et al., 1999). In particular, it has been shown that faces, houses, and chairs evoke maximal responses in distinct occipital and ventral temporal regions with a highly consistent topological arrangement across subjects (Ishai et al., 1999, 2000a). As each category was associated with its own differential pattern of responses across a broad expanse of cortex, it has been proposed that the representation of objects in the ventral stream is not restricted to discrete, highly selective patches of cortex, but, rather, is comprised of distributed representation of information about object form (Ishai et al., 1999, 2000a; Haxby et al., 2001). Inspired by the consistent topology of the response to faces, houses, and chairs, we investigated whether visual imagery of these objects would evoke content-related activation within the same extrastriate ventral regions that are activated during perception. Furthermore, we asked which brain regions, activated during imagery, provide the top-down signal to visual extrastriate cortex. To that end, we designed an fMRI study with the following experimental conditions: Perception, in which subjects viewed pictures of faces, houses, and chairs; Perception-control, in which subjects viewed scrambled pictures; Imagery, in which subjects were instructed to generate vivid mental images of familiar houses, faces, and chairs from LTM while viewing a gray square, and to press a button when ready with a vivid image; and Imagery-control, in which subjects were asked to press the button from time to time while viewing the gray square. Conventional Statistical Parametric Mapping (SPM) analysis revealed differential activation in medial fusiform, lateral fusiform, and inferior temporal gyri during the perception of houses, faces, and chairs, respectively. During visual imagery, content-related patterns of activation were found, but this activity was restricted to small sectors of the regions that responded differentially during perception. Thus, the generation of mental images of familiar faces from LTM evoked activation within small subsets of the lateral fusiform gyrus, a face-responsive region, whereas generating mental images of houses and chairs evoked activation within subsets of the medial fusiform and inferior temporal gyri, respectively. Visual perception and visual imagery evoked activity with opposite patterns of hemispheric asymmetry in ventral temporal cortex, with stronger responses in the right hemisphere during perception, and stronger responses in the left hemisphere during imagery. Contrasting responses evoked by visual imagery and responses evoked during the imagery control condition revealed activation within a network of parietal and frontal regions. This 'imagery network' included the precuneus, intraparietal sulcus (IPS) and inferior frontal gyrus (IFG), regions that were implicated in various attention and retrieval from episodic memory tasks (e.g. Fletcher *et al.*, 1995; Buckner *et al.*, 1996; Mellet *et al.*, 1998). We interpreted these findings to suggest that retrieval of content-specific memory traces, stored in the ventral pathway, is top-down controlled by a parieto-frontal network that mediates the generation and maintenance of mental images (Ishai *et al.*, 2000b).

To investigate the neuronal interactions and effective connectivity that mediate the category-specific responses in the visual cortex, we used Dynamic Causal Modeling (DCM), a relatively new analytic approach that allows the assessment of effective connectivity within cortical networks (Friston *et al.*, 2003). The aim of DCM is to estimate and make inferences about the coupling among brain areas, and how that coupling is influenced by changes in experimental context (e.g. stimuli or tasks). Consistent with a previous DCM study, which showed that category effects in occipito-temporal cortex were mediated by forward connections from early visual areas (Mechelli *et al.*, 2003), we hypothesized that the category-specific patterns of activation observed in occipito-temporal cortex during visual perception of faces and objects could be explained by a selective enabling of forward connectivity from early visual areas. We also predicted that content-related activation observed during visual imagery would be associated with category-dependent changes in backward connectivity from parietal and frontal areas. Finally, we examined whether the DCM analysis would reveal different patterns of effective connectivity during imagery of faces, houses, and chairs in parietal and frontal cortices, as our original SPM analysis did not show category-specific imagery activation within these regions (Ishai *et al.*, 2000b). We found that during visual perception, when subjects viewed gray-scale pictures of faces, houses, and chairs, the category-selective effects in occipito-temporal cortex were mediated by forward connections from early visual areas. In contrast, during visual imagery, when subjects generated mental images of faces, houses, and chairs from LTM, the category-selective effects in the visual cortex were mediated by backward connections from prefrontal cortex. Interestingly, the backward connections from prefrontal, but not from parietal cortex, to occipito-temporal cortex were category-selective (Figure 15.1). Thus, the DCM analysis revealed that dynamic neuronal interactions between occipito-temporal, parietal, and frontal regions are task- and stimulus-dependent. Sensory representations of faces and objects in ventral extrastriate cortex are mediated by bottom-up mechanisms arising in early visual areas during

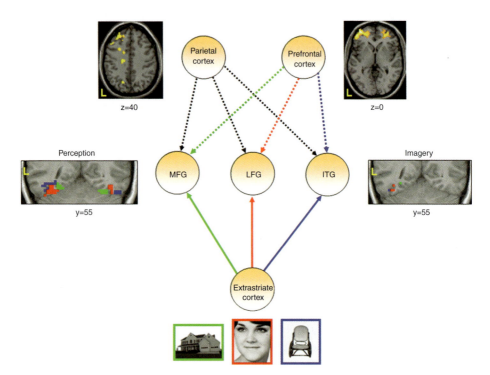

Figure 15.1 Category-selective effects during visual perception and visual imagery. Dynamic Causal Modeling (DCM) analysis revealed that category-selective effects observed in occipito-temporal cortex during perception of houses, faces, and chairs are mediated by forward connections from early visual areas (green, red, and blue arrows, respectively). During visual imagery, the backward connections from prefrontal cortex were category-selective (dashed green, red, and blue arrows), whereas the backward connections from parietal cortex (dashed black arrows) were not content-specific. MFG = medial fusiform gyrus; LFG = lateral fusiform gyrus; ITG = inferior temporal gyrus. (This figure summarizes data published in Ishai *et al.*, 1999, 2000a, 2000b; Mechelli *et al.*, 2003, 2004).

perception, and top-down mechanisms originating in prefrontal cortex during imagery. Additionally, non-selective, top-down processes, originating in superior parietal areas, contribute to the generation of mental images and their maintenance in the 'mind's eye' (Mechelli *et al.*, 2004).

Behavioural studies have reported differential effects of visual imagery on the performance of a perceptual task: visual recall from short-term memory (STM) facilitated task performance, whereas visual recall from LTM interfered with performance, suggesting that imagery-induced facilitation and interference are memory-dependent (Ishai & Sagi 1995, 1997a, 1997b). Moreover, the type of memory (short- or long-term) required for the generation of mental images seems to be a crucial factor in the 'V1 debate', namely the controversy about the extent to which the primary visual cortex is activated during visual imagery. In the vast majority of studies reporting activation during visual imagery in the primary visual cortex, the imagery tasks were based on recall from STM (e.g. Le Bihan *et al.*, 1993; Kosslyn *et al.*, 1993, 1999; Chen *et al.*, 1998; O'Craven & Kanwisher, 2000). To investigate whether similar or different cortical regions are activated during visual imagery generated from STM and from LTM, we had to use a special class of stimuli: famous faces (Ishai *et al.*, 2002). We chose faces of contemporary Hollywood celebrities, assuming that as a result of exposure to these faces in everyday life, subjects would have pictorial representations in memory that could be retrieved by way of visual imagery. Moreover, giving the same visual cue, i.e. a famous name, an image could be generated from either LTM or STM. For example, one could imagine Marilyn Monroe without seeing her picture before the imagery task (LTM), or one could memorize a specific picture of Marilyn Monroe and shortly after generate a mental image of that picture (STM). We also tested the effect of focal attention during visual imagery. Numerous fMRI studies have shown that selective attention to particular attributes of visual stimuli, such as colour or motion, enhanced the activity in regions of extrastriate cortex that process these attributes (e.g. Corbetta *et al.*, 1990). We therefore hypothesized that focusing attention on features of a mental image, rather than on the global configuration of that image, might also result in increased activation. We also speculated that focal attention to mental images would evoke activation in primary visual cortex, based on a model suggested by Sakai and Miyashita (1994), according to which visual imagery is implemented by the interactions between memory retrieval of representations stored in higher visual association areas, and the effect of focal attention on early visual areas. To test all these predictions, our experimental design included the following imagery conditions: Imagery from STM, in which subjects were presented with names of famous faces they had seen and memorized shortly before, and were instructed to generate vivid images of the exact same faces; Imagery from LTM, in which subjects were presented with names of famous faces they had not seen during the experiment, and were instructed to generate any vivid images of these faces; Imagery from STM + Attention, in which subjects were presented with names of famous faces they had seen and memorized shortly before, and were instructed to generate vivid images of these faces and then to answer questions about some facial feature (e.g. 'thick lips?'); and Imagery from LTM + Attention, in which subjects were presented with names of famous faces they had not seen during the experiment, and were instructed to generate vivid images of these faces and then answer questions about some facial feature (e.g. 'big nose?'). We found that visual perception of famous faces activated the inferior occipital gyrus, lateral fusiform gyrus, the superior temporal sulcus (STS), and the amygdala, regions of the distributed network that mediates face perception (Haxby et al., 2000; Ishai et al., 2005; Fairhall & Ishai, 2007), whereas visual imagery of famous faces activated small subsets of these face-responsive regions. Visual imagery of famous faces activated a network of regions that included the calcarine, precuneus, hippocampus, IPS, and IFG. In all these regions, imagery generated from STM evoked more activation than imagery generated from LTM (Ishai et al., 2002). Furthermore, during imagery generated from both STM and LTM, focusing attention on features of the imagined faces resulted in increased activation in the right IPS and right IFG, consistent with reports on activation in these regions during sustained attention (e.g. Pardo et al., 1990).

Our findings propose a new perspective on the neural basis of visual imagery. We found evidence for content-related activation in ventral temporal cortex: small sectors of extrastriate regions that participate in visual perception of faces and objects are also involved in representing perceptual information retrieved from LTM during visual imagery of faces and objects (Ishai et al., 2000b, 2002; Mechelli et al., 2004). As imagery evoked activity in small portions of the regions that participate in perception, it is possible that stored information evoked by imagery is simply weaker than equivalent representations evoked by actual visual input. Alternatively, only a specific subset of cortical regions may be dedicated to mental imagery, allowing perception and imagery to operate simultaneously. These results suggest that sensory representations of faces and objects stored in ventral temporal cortex are reactivated during the generation of visual images, consistent with electrophysiological and other fMRI studies, which have reported content-specific activation in sensory areas during imagery and memory retrieval (Buckner & Wheeler, 2001; Kreiman et al, 2000; Wheeler et al., 2000). Interestingly, electric stimulation of regions in the temporal lobe of humans results in imagery recall, suggesting that memory traces are localized in these regions (Penfield & Perot, 1963). Similarly, studies in non-human primates indicate that the temporal lobe is the memory storehouse for visual representations of complex stimuli (Miyashita & Chang, 1988; Miyashita, 1988).

Visual imagery of faces and objects also activated several parietal and frontal regions that were previously implicated in 'top-down' control functions. These parietal and frontal regions may mediate the retrieval of object representations from LTM, their maintenance in a working memory 'buffer', and the attention required to generate those mental images. Interestingly, a similar network of prefrontal areas was activated during motion imagery (Goebel et al., 1998). On the basis of our effective connectivity analysis, we suggest that this 'imagery network' is composed of a general attentional mechanism arising in parietal cortex, and a content-sensitive mechanism originated in prefrontal cortex. Numerous studies of spatial and non-spatial attention tasks have shown activation in parietal cortex (e.g. Corbetta et al., 1998; Kastner et al., 1999; Wojciulik & Kanwisher, 1999). Moreover, parietal activation has been reported in a variety of mental imagery tasks (Mellet et al., 2000; Ishai et al., 2002). It is therefore reasonable to assume that regions in parietal cortex mediate the attentional processes required to perform the imagery task, irrespective of stimulus-content. Electrophysiological and lesion studies have shown that the prefrontal cortex is not only crucial for object recognition (Bechevalier & Mishkin, 1986), but importantly, that category-selective responses exist in the monkey prefrontal cortex (Freedman *et al.*, 2001). Current models of visual working memory (Miller *et al.* 1996; Fuster & Bauer, 1974) posit that visual working memory is mediated by neuronal interactions between prefrontal and occipito-temporal cortices. Evidence for the existence of similar mechanism in the human brain comes from working memory studies showing that the retrieval of visual information is mediated by a top-down flow of information from prefrontal cortex to category-selective regions in the ventral stream (e.g, Druzgal & D'Esposito, 2003). Our visual imagery studies further show that content-specific imagery effects in the ventral stream are mediated by top-down mechanisms arising in prefrontal cortex (Ishai *et al.*, 2000b, 2002; Mechelli *et al.*, 2004).

Recognition memory and visual similarity

The neural mechanism that mediates the retrieval of newly learned pictures from memory is currently unknown. We conducted a series of event-related fMRI studies to investigate how novel pictorial representations are formed in the cortex and retrieved from LTM. As recognition memory requires matching new items with stored ones, we tested whether matching between new and old pictures depends on their visual similarity. In the first study, the experimental approach combined explicit category learning with a recognition memory task, and original sets of stimuli, namely portraits, landscapes, and abstract compositions by six painters with a unique style (Modigliani, Renoir, Pissarro, Van Gogh, Kandinsky, and Miro). In the training session, subjects were told that paintings from each artist belonged to a category of paintings with a characteristic style and were instructed to memorize these pictures. Four days later, a memory retrieval session was conducted in the MR scanner. Subjects were presented with old and new pictures and indicated whether they had seen these pictures before. The new paintings were either visually similar to the old ones, somewhat similar (ambiguous), or visually different (Figure 15.2). We predicted fast and accurate responses to the new, visually different items, and slower, less accurate responses to the new, similar and ambiguous pictures, due to their visual resemblance to the old items. Moreover, we predicted that activation in the visual cortex and in parietal and prefrontal regions would be modulated by the degree of visual similarity and expected reduced activity with decreased visual similarity between the new and the old pictures. The behavioural data showed that about 70% of the old paintings were correctly recognized and that responses to the new pictures depended on their visual similarity to the old ones. Subjects responded faster and more accurately to new, visually different items, and longer latencies were associated with the new, similar pictures. We found activation in a distributed cortical network that included regions in visual, parietal, and prefrontal cortices, where responses evoked by the new items were modulated by their visual similarity to the old pictures (Figure 15.2). In the visual cortex, the paintings evoked activation in face- and object-responsive regions, where old pictures elicited stronger

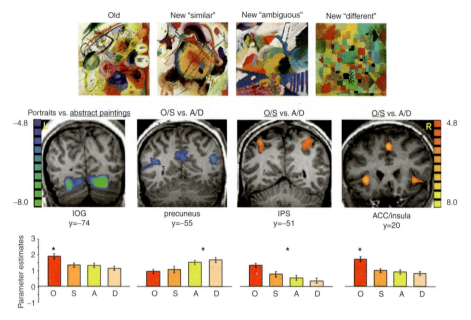

Figure 15.2 Recognition memory is modulated by visual similarity. Subjects memorized art paintings and four days later, a memory retrieval session was conducted in the MR scanner. The old paintings (O) were mixed with new ones that were visually similar (S), ambiguous (A), or different (D), and subjects indicated whether they had seen each picture before. The fMRI data analysis revealed activation within a distributed cortical network. In the inferior occipital gyrus (IOG), an extrastirate visual region, the old pictures evoked stronger activation than all new items, regardless of their visual similarity. When the old and new, visually similar pictures were contrasted with the new, visually ambiguous and different pictures (O+S vs. A+D), modulation by visual similarity was found in the precuneus, where the new, visually different items evoked the strongest activation, and in the intraparietal sulcus (IPS), where activation was reduced with decreased visual similarity to the old paintings. In the insula and the anterior cingulate cortex (ACC), the old paintings evoked stronger activation than all the new ones. The paintings: 'Black Lines' (old); 'Panel' (new, visually similar); 'Church' (new, ambiguous) by Kandinsky; 'Tunisian Garden' by Klee (new, different).

activation than all new pictures, regardless of their visual similarity. Consistent with our hypothesis, in the IPS and superior parietal lobule (SPL), responses evoked by new pictures were reduced with decreased similarity to the old ones. In memory-related areas, two patterns of activation were observed: in the caudate, insula, and anterior cingulate cortex (ACC), the old pictures elicited stronger activation than the new items, whereas in the precuneus, superior temporal, and superior frontal gyri (STG and SFG) the new, visually different pictures evoked stronger activation than both the old and the new, visually similar pictures. Finally, in the hippocampus, the new, similar pictures evoked weaker activation than the new, ambiguous, and different items. These findings suggest that recognition memory is mediated by activation in a cortical network that includes regions in visual cortex where stimulus-specific representations are stored, attention-related areas where visual similarity to old pictures is detected, and memory-related areas where new items are classified as a match or a mismatch based on their similarity to the old pictures (Yago & Ishai, 2006).

Our old-new recognition memory tasks did not address the issue of memory processes and the extent to which the observed behavioural and neural responses were due to recollection- or familiarity-based memory decisions. To test whether recollection and familiarity judgments were influenced by the degree of visual similarity between old and new pictures, we conducted a behavioural study. A new group of subjects memorized the paintings and four days later returned for a memory test in which they had to indicate whether they remembered the picture, the picture looked familiar, or the picture was new. Consistent with our hypothesis, subjects correctly recognized more new, visually different items and the response latency was significantly shorter than responses to the new, similar, or ambiguous paintings. We found that the proportion of false alarms, namely Remember and Know responses to new pictures, was reduced with reduced visual similarity between the new pictures and the old ones. The number of Know responses to the new, similar items was significantly higher than the number of Know responses to the ambiguous and different paintings. It therefore seems that mistaking new pictures for old ones is associated with feelings of familiarity, not recollection (Ishai & Wiesmann, 2007).

Our study with art paintings has shown that recognition memory of newly learned, visually similar items is associated with many false alarms, namely erroneous responses subjects make, mistaking new items for old ones. To further investigate the neural correlates of false memory, we conducted a second study with unfamiliar South Korean faces. Caucasian subjects, who had limited exposure to Asian faces in their environment, memorized unfamiliar neutral and happy South Korean faces, and four days later performed a recognition memory task in the MR scanner. Previously seen faces were recognized faster and more accurately than new faces. Response latencies for misses were significantly longer than the response latencies for hits, and response latencies for hits were significantly longer than the latencies for false alarms. These behavioural data suggest that it took subjects longer to decide whether a face was new, probably due to the high visual similarity between the South Korean faces. The recognition memory task elicited activation within a distributed cortical network that included visual, parietal, and prefrontal regions. Within all regions, previously seen faces evoked stronger activation than new faces and the response to happy faces was very similar to the response to neutral faces. In parietal and prefrontal cortices, activation during correct trials was stronger than activation during incorrect trials. Finally, in the hippocampus, false alarms to happy faces evoked stronger activation than false alarms to neutral faces (Ishai & Yago, 2006).

Recognition memory of portraits, landscapes, abstract paintings, and South Korean faces evoked activation in face- and object-responsive regions in the visual cortex. In the lateral fusiform gyrus, a face-responsive region (Kanwisher et al., 1997), portraits elicited stronger activation than landscapes and abstract paintings. In the medial fusiform and parahippocampal gyri, regions that respond to houses and places, respectively (Aguirre et al., 1998; Epstein & Kanwisher, 1998; Ishai et al., 1999), landscapes evoked stronger activation than portraits and abstract paintings. In the posterior fusiform gyrus, abstract paintings evoked stronger activation than portraits and landscapes. Finally, landscapes and abstract paintings evoked stronger responses than portraits in dorsal occipital cortex. Within these face- and object-selective regions, previously seen pictures evoked stronger responses than the new items. The patterns of activation observed in the visual cortex indicate that explicit encoding of pictures results in stimulus-specific representations, consistent with numerous category learning (Reber *et al.*, 1998), visual imagery (Ishai *et al.*, 2000b; Mechelli *et al.*, 2004), working memory (Druzgal & D'Esposito, 2003) and associative memory retrieval (Ranganath *et al.*, 2004) studies, which showed stimulus-specific memory traces in the human visual ventral stream.

Activation in parietal cortex during recognition memory of paintings revealed stronger responses to the old pictures than to the new items. Furthermore, confirming our hypothesis, activation within these regions was reduced with decreased similarity between the new paintings and the old ones. The IPS and the SPL, regions of the dorsal frontoparietal attention network, were implicated in many cognitive studies of attention. In particular, both regions were activated in target detection tasks (Corbetta *et al.*, 2000; Shulman *et al.*, 2001; Kincade *et al.*, 2005). The old items, for which the correct response was 'Yes, I had seen these pictures before', were randomly mixed with new, never seen before pictures. It is highly likely that subjects were searching for and detecting these old paintings as 'targets'. We observed shorter reaction times and decreased amplitudes of the fMRI signal with decreased similarity to the old items. The enhanced activation evoked by the old pictures and the reduced activity elicited by the new, visually different pictures suggest that the IPS and SPL process the segmentation of old from new items (Pollmann *et al.*, 2003). Thus, recognition of familiar pictures and target detection seem to be mediated by similar neural correlates within the attentional network. Numerous recognition memory studies have further shown that posterior parietal cortex does not merely 'detect old items' but, rather, mediates higher order cognitive processes associated with memory retrieval (Konishi *et al.*, 2000; Wheeler & Buckner, 2003; Shannon & Buckner, 2004). Our data also support the 'mnemonic accumulator' hypothesis, according to which recognition memory decisions are based on the integration of sensory signals (Wagner *et al.*, 2005).

Explicit encoding and recognition of the paintings, revealed activation in multiple memory-related areas, with two distinct patterns of response: stronger activation for the old pictures in the caudate, ACC and the insula, and stronger activation for new, visually different items in the precuneus, STG, and the SFG. Some of these regions were implicated in previous studies of category learning (e.g. Reber *et al.*, 2002; Vogels *et al.*, 2002). Our study revealed differential activation within these regions as a function of visual similarity between old and new pictures. In the caudate, ACC, and insula, the old paintings evoked stronger activation than all new items, regardless of their visual similarity. These regions therefore likely mediate the correct classification of the old items, consistent with previous reports about their role in memory retrieval, target detection, and category learning (Poldrack *et al.*, 1999; Seger & Cincotta, 2002). It is of interest that the pattern of activation in the caudate, ACC, and insula resembles that of the face- and object-responsive regions in the visual cortex, where old pictures evoked stronger responses than new ones. The enhanced activation elicited by the old items is consistent with visual categorization studies in monkeys that showed stronger responses to familiar prototypes in IT and PFC (Freedman *et al.*, 2003). Moreover, it has been shown that during associative learning in monkeys, rapid learning-related responses in the caudate precedes slower responses in the PFC, further suggesting that output from the basal ganglia also modulates PFC activation during learning (Pasupathy & Miller, 2005). An fMRI study in humans has shown that the caudate has two functional roles in category learning: the body and tail mediate classification, whereas the head processes feedback during learning (Seger & Cincotta, 2005). It therefore seems that in addition to stimulus-specific representations stored in visual and prefrontal regions, recognition of familiar pictures requires output signals from the striatum. In the precuneus, STG, and SFG, regions implicated in many studies of memory retrieval (e.g. Fletcher *et al.*, 1995; Shannon & Buckner, 2004; Yonelinas *et al.*, 2005), the new, visually different exemplars evoked stronger activation than both the old and the new, visually similar pictures. Behaviourally, responses to the new, visually different pictures were faster and more accurate than responses to the visually similar ones. It is likely that the visually different, or mismatch items were classified as new within these regions.

Recognition memory of South Korean faces revealed activation in the IFG, insula, and ACC. Within these regions, responses during correct trials, regardless of stimulus type (old or new faces) were stronger than responses during incorrect trials. Previous functional brain imaging studies have implicated the prefrontal cortex in memory formation (Buckner *et al.*, 1999) and monitoring during retrieval (Buckner & Wheeler, 2001). Enhanced activation in parietal and prefrontal regions in response to old items has been reported in numerous fMRI studies (e.g., Kahn *et al.*, 2004). This 'old-new' parieto-frontal effect is also consistent with the ERP correlates of recollection, namely a positive shift in waveforms elicited by correctly classified old items relative to the waveforms evoked by new items in the left parietal cortex, and a sustained positive shift elicited by old items in the right prefrontal cortex (Rugg *et al.*, 2002). Most functional brain imaging studies of episodic memory retrieval have used written words, and not pictures, as stimuli (Cabeza *et al.*, 2003; Rugg & Wilding, 2000). Moreover, our task required a simple 'Yes-No' recognition, whereas other studies of episodic retrieval employed the 'Remember-Know' procedure (Rugg & Yonelinas, 2003). Finally, the ERP and fMRI techniques detect different signals, namely scalp electrical activity and the haemodynamic response, which reflect direct and indirect measures of neuronal activity, respectively. Hemispheric asymmetries should therefore be carefully interpreted.

In both recognition memory studies we found differential patterns of activation in the hippocampus. The new, visually similar paintings evoked less activation than both the old and the new, visually different items. Moreover, activation evoked by false alarms to happy South Korean faces was stronger than activation elicited by false alarms to neutral faces, suggesting that emotional faces are more susceptible to be mistaken as familiar faces and are therefore likely to induce illusory memories. Activation in the hippocampus has been observed in various memory-related processes, including recognition memory (Stark & Squire, 2001), maintenance in working memory (Ranganath & D'Esposito, 2001), source memory (Davachi *et al.*, 2003), generation of visual images from STM (Ishai *et al.*, 2002), and explicit categorization (Reber *et al.*, 2003). Although it is currently unclear to what extent the hippocampus mediates the recovery of true and false memory traces (Cabeza *et al.*, 2001; Slotnick & Schacter, 2004), our findings suggest that true and false memories result in differential patterns of activation within this region. It has been reported that false memory can be induced by way of visual imagery. When subjects generate mental images of objects based on a corresponding word-cue and on some trials pictures of these objects are presented after the imagery task, some words are later falsely remembered as pictures. Interestingly, these false memories are associated with more positive posterior brain potentials (Gonsalves & Paller, 2000).

Taken collectively, our recognition memory studies have shown that retrieving pictures from LTM is mediated by a distributed cortical network, where activation is modulated by the visual similarity between old and new pictures: Face- and object-responsive regions in the visual cortex store stimulus-specific representations; parietal, and prefrontal regions mediate the retrieval and classification of old and new items; and the hippocampus mediates the recovery of true memory traces.

Conclusions

Retrieving pictures from LTM is mediated by a distributed neural system that includes visual, limbic, parietal, and prefrontal regions. Cognitive factors such as memory type (short- or long-term), attention, and visual similarity modulate the neural responses within these regions. The identification of distributed patterns of activation and their effective connectivity provides useful clues for theory building, however, bridging the gap between correlational data and a theory of human memory is not trivial and remains a challenge. Although my own research was tailored to test binary oppositions, the empirical findings described here clearly demonstrate the importance of understanding and integrating large-scale fMRI data. Thus, regardless of whether mental images are 'pictorial' or 'propositional', or whether 'recollection' and 'familiarity' are independent memory processes, the wide spread patterns of activation in the human brain during memory retrieval suggest that we should pursue cortical connectivity instead of dichotomies. Cognitive theories should therefore take into account the dynamics and modulation of neural coupling among nodes in distributed networks.

In order to develop functional, testable theories that go beyond mere localization of cognitive functions, we need new cognitive models. A few years ago, Mel has written: 'The need for modeling in neuroscience is particularly intense because what most neuroscientists ultimately want to know about the brain *is* the model – that is, the laws governing the brain's information processing functions. The brain as an electrical system, or a chemical system, is simply not the point. In general, the model as a research tool is more important when the system under study is more complex. In the extreme case of the brain, the most complicated machine known, the importance of gathering more facts *about* the brain through empirical studies must give way to efforts to relate brain facts to each other, which requires models matched to the complexity of the brain itself.' (Mel, 2000). With the advent of brain-imaging technology and novel analytic tools, mapping higher cognitive functions is a feasible task, and better understanding of brain-imaging data would hopefully lead to the formulation of refined network models of the human brain.

Acknowledgments

The author is supported by the Swiss National Science Foundation grant 3200B0-105278 and by the Swiss National Center for Competence in Research: Neural Plasticity and Repair.

References

Aguirre, G. K., Zarahn, E., & D'Esposito, M. (1998). An area within human ventral cortex sensitive to "building" stimuli: Evidence and implications. *Neuron, 21*, 1–20.

Bachevalier, J. & Mishkin, M. (1986). Visual recognition impairment follows ventromedial but not dorsolateral prefrontal lesions in monkeys. *Behavioural Brain Research, 20*, 249–261.

Buckner, R. L., Kelly, W. M., & Petersen, S. E. (1999). Frontal cortex contributes to human memory formation. *Nature Neuroscience, 2*, 311–314.

Buckner, R. L., Raichle, M. E., Miezin, F. M., & Petersen, S. E. (1996). Functional anatomic studies of memory retrieval for auditory words and visual pictures. *Journal of Neuroscience, 16*, 6219–6235.

Buckner, R. L. & Wheeler, M. E. (2001). The cognitive neuroscience of remembering. *Nature Reviews Neuroscience, 2*, 624–634.

Cabeza, R., Rao, S. M., Wagner, A. D., Mayer, A. R., & Schacter, D. L. (2001). Can medial temporal lobe regions distinguish true from false? An event-related functional MRI study of veridical and illusory recognition memory. *Proceedings of the National Academy of Sciences, USA, 98*, 4805–4810.

Cabeza, R., Locantore, J. K., & Anderson, N. D. (2003). Lateralization of prefrontal activity during episodic memory retrieval: evidence for the production-monitoring hypothesis. *Journal of Cognitive Neuroscience, 15*, 249–259.

Chao, L. L., Haxby, J. V., & Martin, A. (1999). Attribute-based neural substrates in posterior temporal cortex for perceiving and knowing about objects. *Nature Neuroscience, 2*, 913–919.

Chen, W., Kato, T., Zhu, X. H., Ogawa, S., Tank, D. W., & Ugurbil, K. (1998). Human primary visual cortex and lateral geniculate nucleus activation during visual imagery. *Neuroreport, 9*, 3669–3674.

Corbetta, M., Miezin F. M., Dobmeyer, S., Shulman, G. L., & Petersen, S. E. (1990). Attentional modulation of neural processing of shape, color, and velocity in humans. *Science, 248*, 1556–1559.

Corbetta, M., Akbudak, E., Conturo, T. E., Snyder, A. Z., Ollinger, J. M., *et al.* (1998). A common network of functional areas for attention and eye movements. *Neuron, 21*, 761–773.

Corbetta, M., Kincade, J. M., Ollinger, J. M., McAvoy, M. P., & Shulman, G. L. (2000). Voluntary orienting is dissociated from target detection in human posterior parietal cortex. *Nature Neuroscience, 3*, 292–297.

Davachi, L., Mitchell, J. P., & Wagner, A. D. (2003). Multiple routes to memory: distinct medial temporal lobe processes build item and source memories. *Proceedings of the National Academy of Sciences, USA, 100*, 2157–2162.

Druzgal, T. J. & D'Esposito, M. (2003). Dissecting contributions of prefrontal cortex and fusiform face area to face working memory. *Journal of Cognitive Neuroscience, 15*, 771–784.

D'Esposito, M., Deter, J. A., Aguirre, G. K., Stallcup, M., Alsop, D. C., Tippet, L. J., & Farah, M. J. (1997). A functional MRI study of mental image generation. *Neuropsychologia, 35*, 725–730.

Epstein, R. & Kanwisher, N. (1998). A cortical representation of the local visual environment. *Nature, 392*, 598–601.

Fairhall, S. L. & Ishai, A. (2007). Effective connectivity within the distributed cortical network for face perception. *Cerebral Cortex, 17*, 2400–2406.

Farah, M., Peronnet, F., Gonon, M. A., & Giard, M. H. (1988). Electrophysiological evidence for a shared representational medium for visual images and visual percepts. *Journal of Experimental Psychology: General, 117*, 248–257.

Fletcher, P. C., Frith, C. D., Baker, S. C., Shallice, T., Frackowiak, R. S. J., & Dolan, R. J. (1995). The mind's eye – precuneus activation in memory-related imagery. *Neuroimage, 2,* 195–200.

Freedman, D. J., Riesenhuber, M., Poggio, T., & Miller, E. K. (2001). Categorical representation of visual stimuli in the primate prefrontal cortex. *Science, 291,* 312–316.

Freedman, D. J., Riesenhuber, M., Poggio, T., & Miller, E. K. (2003). A comparison of primate prefrontal and inferior temporal cortices during visual categorization. *Journal of Neuroscience, 23,* 5235–5246.

Friston, K. J., Harrison, L., & Penny, W. (2003). Dynamic causal modeling. *NeuroImage, 19*(4), 1273–1302.

Fuster, J. M. & Bauer, R. (1974). Visual short-term memory deficit from hypothermia of frontal cortex. *Brain Research, 81,* 393–400.

Goebel, R., Khorram-Sefat, D., Muckli, L., Hacker, H., & Singer, W. (1998). The constructive nature of vision: Direct evidence from functional magnetic resonance imaging studies of apparent motion and motion imagery. *European Journal of Neuroscience, 10,* 1563–1573.

Goldenberg, G., Poderka, I., Steiner, M., Willmes, K., Suess, E., & Deecke, L. (1989). Regional cerebral blood flow patterns in visual imagery. *Neuropsychologia, 27,* 641–664.

Gonsalves, B. & Paller, K. A. (2000). Neural events that underlie remembering something that never happened. *Nature Neuroscience, 3,* 1316–1321.

Haxby, J. V., Hoffman, E. A., & Gobbini, I. M. (2000). The distributed human neural system for face perception. *Trends in Cognitive Sciences, 4,* 223–233.

Haxby, J. V., Gobbini, M. I., Furey, M. L., Ishai, A., Schouten, J. L., & Pietrini, P. (2001). Distributed and overlapping representations of faces and objects in ventral temporal cortex. *Science, 293,* 2425–2430.

Henson, R. (2005). What can functional neuroimaging tell the experimental psychologuist? *The Quarterly Journal of Experimental Psychology, 58*A, 193–233.

Ishai, A. & Sagi, D. (1995). Common mechanisms of visual imagery and perception. *Science, 268,* 1772–1774.

Ishai, A. & Sagi, D. (1997a). Visual imagery facilitates visual perception: Psychophysical evidence. *Journal of Cognitive Neuroscience, 9,* 476–489.

Ishai, A. & Sagi, D. (1997b). Visual imagery: Effects of short- and long-term memory. *Journal of Cognitive Neuroscience, 9,* 734–742.

Ishai, A., Ungerleider, L. G., Martin, A., Schouten, J. L., & Haxby, J. V. (1999). Distributed representation of objects in the human ventral visual pathway. *Proceedings National Academy of Sciences USA, 96,* 9379–9384.

Ishai, A., Ungerleider, L. G., Martin, A., & Haxby, J. V. (2000a). The representation of objects in the human occipital and temporal cortex. *Journal of Cognitive Neuroscience, 12,* 35–51.

Ishai, A., Ungerleider, L. G., & Haxby, J. V. (2000b). Distributed neural systems for the generation of visual images. *Neuron, 28,* 979–990.

Ishai, A., Haxby, J. V., & Ungerleider, L. G. (2002). Visual imagery of famous faces: effects of memory and attention revealed by fMRI. *NeuroImage, 17,* 1729–1741.

Ishai, A., Schmidt, C. F., & Boesiger, P. (2005). Face perception is mediated by a distributed cortical network. *Brain Research Bulletin, 67,* 87–93.

Ishai, A. & Yago, E. (2006). Recognition memory of newly learned faces. *Brain Research Bulletin, 71,* 167–173.

Ishai, A. & Wiesmann, M. (2007). Recollection, familiarity, and visual similarity. *Perception, 36*(Supplement), 1001–1001,

Kahn, I. Davachi, L., & Wagner, A. D. (2004). Functional-neuroanatomic correlates of recollection: implications for models of recognition memory. *Journal of Neuroscience, 24,* 4172–4180.

Kanwisher, N., McDermott, J., & Chun, M. M. (1997). The fusiform face area: A module in human extrastriate cortex specialized for face perception. *Journal of Neuroscience*, *17*, 4302–4311.

Kastner, S., Pinsk, M. A., De Weerd, P., Desimone, R., & Ungerleider, L. G. (1999). Increased activity in human visual cortex in the absence of visual stimulation. *Neuron*, *22*, 751–761.

Kincade, J. M., Abrams, R. A., Astafiev, S. V., Shulman, G. L., & Corbetta, M. (2005). An event-related functional magnetic resonance imaging study of voluntary and stimulus-driven orienting of attention. *Journal of Neuroscience*, *25*, 4593–4604.

Konishi, S., Wheeler, M. E., Donaldson, D. I., & Buckner, R. L., (2000). Neural correlates of episodic retrieval success. *NeuroImage*, *12*, 276–286.

Kosslyn, S. M., Alpert, N. M., Thompson, W. L., Maljkovic, V., Weise, S. B., Chabris, C. F., Hamilton, S. E., Rauch, S. L., & Buonanno, F. S. (1993). Visual mental imagery activates topographically organized visual cortex: PET investigations. *Journal of Cognitive Neuroscience*, *5*, 263–287.

Kosslyn, S. M., Pascual-Leone, A., Felician, O., Camposano, S., Keenan, J. P., Thompson, W. L., Ganis, G., Sukel, K. E., & Alpert, N. M. (1999). The role of area 17 in visual imagery: Convergent evidence from PET and rTMS. *Science*, *284*, 167–170.

Kreiman, G., Koch, C., & Fried, I. (2000). Category-specific visual responses of single neurons in the human medial temporal lobe. *Nature Neuroscience*, *3*, 946–953.

Le Bihan, D., Turner, R., Zeffiro, T., Cuendo, C., Jezzard, P., & Bonnerot, V. (1993). Activation of human primary visual cortex during visual recall: A magnetic resonance imaging study. *Proceedings National Academy of Sciences USA*, *90*, 11802–11805.

Levine, D. N., Warach, J., & Farah, M. (1985). Two visual systems in mental imagery: Dissociation of "what" and "where" in imagery disorders due to bilateral posterior cerebral lesions. *Neurology*, *35*, 1010–1018.

Mechelli, A., Price, C. J., Noppeney, U., & Friston, K. J. (2003). A dynamic causal modeling study on category effects: bottom-up or top-down mediation? *Journal of Cognitive Neuroscience*, *15*, 925–934.

Mechelli, A., Price, C. J., Friston, K. J., & Ishai, A. (2004). Where bottom-up meets top-down: neuronal interactions during perception and imagery. *Cerebral Cortex*, *14*, 1256–1265.

Mel, B. W. (2000). In the brain, the model is the goal. *Nature Neuroscience*, *3*, 1183.

Mellet, E., Tzourio, N., Crivello, F., Joliot, M., Denis, M., & Mazoyer, B. (1996). Functional anatomy of spatial mental imagery generated from verbal instructions. *Journal of Neuroscience*, *16*, 6504–6512.

Mellet, E., Petit, L., Mazoyer, B., Denis, M., & Tzourio, N. (1998). Reopening the mental imagery debate: Lessons from functional anatomy. *Neuroimage*, *8*, 129–139.

Mellet, E., Tzourio-Mazoyer, N., Bricogne, S., Mazoyer, B., Kosslyn, S. M., & Denis, M. (2000). Functional anatomy of high-resolution visual mental imagery. *Journal of Cognitive Neuroscience*, *12*, 98–109.

Miller, E. K., Erickson, C. A., & Desimone, R. (1996). Neural mechanisms of visual working memory in prefrontal cortex of the macaque. *Journal of Neuroscience*, *16*, 5154–5167.

Miyashita, Y. (1988). Neural correlate of visual associative long-term memory in the primate temporal cortex. *Nature*, *335*, 817–820.

Miyashita, Y. & Chang, H. S. (1988). Neural correlate of pictorial short-term memory in the primate temporal cortex. *Nature*, *331*, 68–70.

O'Craven, K. & Kanwisher, N. (2000). Mental imagery of faces and places activates corresponding stimulus-specific brain regions. *Journal of Cognitive Neuroscience*, *12*, 1013–1023.

Pardo, J. V., Fox, P. T., & Raichle, M. E. (1990). Localization of a human system for sustained attention by positron emission tomography. *Nature*, *349*, 61–64.

Pasupathy, A. & Miller, E. K. (2005). Different time courses of learning-related activity in the prefrontal cortex and striatum. *Nature, 433*, 873–876.

Penfield, W. & Perot, P. (1963). The brain's record of auditory and visual experience. *Brain 86*, 595–697.

Poldrack, R. A., Prabhakaran, V., Seger, C. A., & Gabrieli, J. D. (1999). Striatal activation during acquisition of a cognitive skill. *Neuropsychology, 13*, 564–574.

Pollmann, S., Weidner, R., Humphreys, G. W., Olivers, C. N., Muller, K., Lohmann, G., Wiggins, C. J., & Watson, D. G. (2003). Separating distractor rejection and target detection in posterior parietal cortex – an event-related fMRI study of visual marking. *NeuroImage, 18*, 310–323.

Ranganath, C. & D'Esposito, M. (2001). Medial temporal lobe activity associated with active maintenance of novel information. *Neuron, 31*, 865–873.

Ranganath, C., Cohen, M. X., Dam, C., & D'Esposito, M. (2004). Inferior temporal, prefrontal, and hippocampal contributions to visual working memory maintenance and associative memory retrieval. *Journal of Neuroscience, 24*, 3917–3925.

Ratcliff, R. (1978). A theory of memory retrieval. *Psychological Review, 85*, 59–108.

Reber, P. J., Stark, C. E., & Squire, L. R. (1998). Contrasting cortical activity associated with category memory and recognition memory. *Learning and Memory, 5*, 420–428.

Reber, P. J., Wong, E. C., & Buxton, R. B. (2002). Comparing the brain areas supporting nondeclarative categorization and recognition memory. *Brain Research, Cognitive Brain Research, 14*, 245–257.

Reber, P. J., Gitelman, D. R., Parrish, T. B., & Mesulam, M. M. (2003). Dissociating explicit and implicit category knowledge with fMRI. *Journal of Cognitive Neuroscience, 15*, 574–583.

Roland, P. E., Eriksson, L., Stone-Elander, S., & Widen, L. (1987). Does mental activity change the oxidative metabolism of the brain? *Journal of Neuroscience, 7*, 2373–2389.

Rugg, M. D. & Wilding, E. L. (2000). Retrieval processing and episodic memory. *Trends in Cognitive Sciences, 4*, 108–115.

Rugg, M. D., Otten, L. J., & Henson, R. N. (2002). The neural basis of episodic memory: evidence from functional neuroimaging. *Philosophical Transactions of the Royal Society of London: Series B. Biological Sciences, 357*, 1097–1110.

Rugg, M. D. & Yonelinas, A. P. (2003). Human recognition memory: a cognitive neuroscience perspective. *Trends in Cognitive Sciences, 7*, 313–319.

Sakai, K. & Miyashita, Y. (1994). Visual imagery: An interaction between memory retrieval and focal attention. *Trends in Neuroscience, 17*, 287–289.

Savoy, R. (2001). History and future directions of human brain mapping and functional neuroimaging. *Acta Psychologica, 107*, 9–42.

Seger, C. A. & Cincotta, C. M. (2002). Striatal activity in concept learning. *Cognitive, Affective and Behavioral Neuroscience, 2*, 149–161.

Seger, C. A. & Cincotta, C. M. (2005). The roles of the caudate nucleus in human classification learning. *Journal of Neuroscience, 25*, 2941–2951.

Shannon, B. J. & Buckner, R. L. (2004). Functional-anatomic correlates of memory retrieval that suggest nontraditional processing roles for multiple distinct regions within posterior parietal cortex. *Journal of Neuroscience, 24*, 10084–10092.

Shulman, G. L., Ollinger, J. M., Linenweber, M., Petersen, S. E., & Corbetta, M. (2001). Multiple neural correlates of detection in the human brain. *Proceedings National Academy of Sciences USA, 98*, 313–318.

Slotnick, S. D. & Schacter, D. L. (2004). A sensory signature that distinguishes true from false memories. *Nature Neuroscience, 7*, 664–672.

Stark, C. E. & Squire, L. R. (2001). Simple and associative recognition memory in the hippocampal region. *Learning and Memory, 8*, 190–197.

Ungerleider, L. G. & Mishkin, M. (1982). Two cortical visual systems. In: D.J. Ingle, M.A. Goodale, & R.J.W. Mansfield (Eds), *Analysis of Visual Behavior*. Cambridge, MA: MIT Press.

Vogels, R., Sary, G., Dupont, P., & Orban, G. A. (2002). Human brain regions involved in visual categorization. *NeuroImage*, *16*, 401–414.

Wagner, A. D., Shannon, B. J., Kahn, I., & Buckner, R. L. (2005). Parietal lobe contributions to episodic memory retrieval. *Trends in Cognitive Sciences*, *9*, 445–453.

Wheeler, M. E., Petersen, S. E., & Buckner, R. L. (2000). Memory's echo: Vivid remembering reactivates sensory-specific cortex. *Proceedings National Academy of Sciences USA*, *97*, 11125–11129.

Wheeler, M. E., & Buckner, R. L. (2003). Functional dissociation among components of remembering: control, perceived oldness, and content. *Journal of Neuroscience*, *23*, 3869–3880.

Wojciulik, E. & Kanwisher, N. (1999). The generality of parietal involvement in visual attention. *Neuron*, *23*, 747–764.

Yago, E. & Ishai, A. (2006). Recognition memory is modulated by visual similarity. *NeuroImage*, *31*, 807–817.

Yonelinas, A. P., Otten, L. J., Shaw, K. N., & Rugg, M. D. (2005). Separating the brain regions involved in recollection and familiarity in recognition memory. *Journal of Neuroscience*, *25*, 3002–3008.

Chapter 16

Content specificity of long-term memory representations

Patrick Khader and Frank Rösler

Introduction

Since the late 19th century psychologists try to understand how memories are stored and retrieved (Ebbinghaus, 1966). One of the key issues in this enterprise has been and still is the question whether all memory contents are stored in one uniform or rather in distinct, material-specific 'codes'. Several experimental findings suggest a fundamental distinction between visual-spatial and linguistic memory contents. Results from mental rotation and mental imagery experiments support the notion that visual input is preferentially stored in an analog manner which preserves most physical attributes of an encoded scene (Shepard & Metzler, 1971; Kosslyn, 1994), while studies on sentence and text comprehension suggest a more abstract, propositional form of encoding for verbal material (Kintsch, 1974; Kintsch & van Dijk, 1978). This claim of two distinct coding principles (Paivio, 1986) is also supported by dual-task studies of working memory (WM), which revealed that memory for visual-spatial material is impeded more by a competing visual-spatial task than by a competing verbal task and vice versa (Logie, 1986). Consistent with such findings, it has been assumed that there are at least two distinct WM 'compartments', a 'phonological loop', in which verbal information is maintained in an auditory-phonological form, and a 'visual-spatial sketchpad', in which visual-spatial information is maintained in an analogue, visual form (Baddeley & Hitch, 1974). An equivalent distinction seems also to be valid for long-term memory (LTM) contents, as shown by Heil, Rösler, Rauch, and Hennighausen (1998). They observed that retrieval of verbal LTM contents was hampered more by a secondary verbal task (grammatical gender decision) than a secondary visual-spatial task (mental rotation), while the opposite held for retrieval of spatial material from LTM. Thus, distinct representations for verbal and visual-spatial information seem to exist for both WM and LTM.

Content-specific representations

With the advent of electrophysiological and neuroimaging methods, the question of whether distinct memory systems exist for different types of information has also been studied on a functional neuroanatomical level. Several studies provided evidence that anatomically distinct cortical areas are involved when verbal and visual-spatial information are encoded, stored, and retrieved (for reviews, see Jonides *et al.*, 2003;

Rösler & Heil, 2003). Distinct neural networks have also been proposed for more specific categories like faces (de Renzi, 2000; Maguire, Frith, & Cipolotti, 2001; McNeil & Warrington, 1993), buildings (Epstein & Kanwisher, 1998; Maguire *et al.*, 2001), tools and animals (Damasio, Grabowski, Tranel, Hichwa, & Damasio, 1996; Damasio *et al.*, 1996), fruits and vegetables (Hart, Berndt, & Caramazza, 1985), and living vs. non-living entities (Warrington & Shallice, 1984). However, it is so far unsettled whether these areas are specialized for representing entities of specific stimulus categories, or whether they represent specific perceptual features that are relevant for various distinct categories. In support of the first view, two highly specialized areas have been reliably identified in the inferior temporal lobe, the fusiform face area (FFA) and the parahippocampal place area (PPA) (Epstein & Kanwisher, 1998; Maguire *et al.*, 2001; McCarthy, Puce, Gore, & Allison, 1997). Gauthier, Behrmann, and Tarr (1999), however, failed to find a dissociation of face recognition and recognition of other kinds of object stimuli in two prosopagnostic patients with lesions in the inferior temporal lobe. Therefore, they proposed that the FFA is not specialized for faces *per se*, but rather for expert within-category discrimination of highly similar exemplars. However, two recent fMRI studies found that the FFA cannot be a processing module for generic within-category identification or expert individuation, but that it is specialized for perceiving and discriminating face stimuli as such (Grill-Spector, Knouf, & Kanwisher, 2004; Rhodes, Byatt, Michie, & Puce, 2004). In these studies, within-category identification for non-face objects was correlated with activation in regions of the ventral occipito-temporal cortex anatomically distinct from the FFA. A completely different model of object representation has been proposed by Haxby *et al.* (2001) on the basis of brain-imaging data. They found strongly overlapping, but clearly separable activation *patterns* for different visual categories (faces, scissors, chairs, etc.) in a 1-back visual WM task, and they integrated these findings in their 'object form topography hypothesis'. In its essence, the hypothesis says that cell assemblies in the inferior temporal cortex represent attributes of object form that are differently combined to multivariate feature vectors representing exemplars of the one or the other object category.

Reactivation theory of long-term memory contents

The 'object form topography hypothesis' is consistent with a more general theory on where and how long-term memories are represented in the brain (Damasio, 1989b; McClelland, McNaughton, & O'Reilly, 1995). Its basic assumption is that engrams are permanently formed in those cortical cell assemblies that also mediate the online processing of the very same information during perception, imagery, reasoning, motor planning, and other mental activities, i.e., memory contents that are experienced as wholistic entities (e.g. a face), are not stored as a wholistic entity in a certain brain region, but rather as a set of representational fragments in multiple and separate regions. Accordingly, retrieving a stimulus or an episode from LTM should invoke brain areas that were activated during the initial sensory processing and encoding of that very item. Therefore, stimuli processed in different cortical networks during perception should also be dissociable during memory retrieval. For example, faces and other visual objects should activate the primary and secondary visual areas of the occipital and temporal cortex during memory retrieval, whereas the retrieval of spatial information should activate regions of the parietal cortex in which information about spatial positions and coordinates is processed (Mishkin, Ungerleider, & Macko, 1983; Ungerleider & Mishkin, 1982). Furthermore, engrams comprise different perceptual and functional properties like colour, shape, orientation, and position, and these are represented by distinct cell assemblies. These specialized regions are supposed to become activated simultaneously, forming 'coherence ensembles' via mutual neural activation (Damasio, 1989a; Paller, 2003). According to Damasio (1989a), there also exist specialized 'convergence zones', which are spread throughout the neocortex and serve to synchronize the distributed neural activity from different brain regions that encode different stimulus fragments. A possible neurophysiological basis for such a synchronization process can be seen in coherent firing patterns of spatially separated neuron ensembles (Eckhorn et al., 1988; Gray, König, Engel, & Singer, 1989).

Brain activation patterns during memory retrieval

From what has been outlined so far follows that the same neocortical areas should be activated during encoding and retrieval of the same type of information, whereas distinct types of information should activate distinct brain areas. Consistent with this notion, neuroimaging research has demonstrated that domain-specific sensory cortices engaged during encoding become reactivated if the same stimulus is retrieved from memory. For example, Nyberg, Habib, McIntosh, and Tulving (2000) found that remembering visually presented words that had been paired with sounds at the time of encoding activated some of the auditory brain regions that were found to be active during encoding. Furthermore, Nyberg et al. (2001) found that retrieval of verbal action phrases was associated with an activation of motor brain regions if the actions had been performed overtly or covertly during encoding (see also Heil et al., 1999). In an fMRI study, Wheeler and Buckner (2003) presented word-sound (e.g. train + sound of a train) or word-picture pairs (e.g. apple + picture of an apple) during encoding, but the words only at the time of retrieval, and found stronger brain activations for those words that had been associated with pictures in object-sensitive regions of the inferior temporal cortex. Accordingly, Wheeler, Petersen, and Buckner (2000) found with a similar paradigm that remembering pictures and sounds activated subsets of those regions of the auditory and visual cortex that were found to be active during their perception.

Many studies that tried to separate functionally and anatomically distinct memory partitions focused on the distinction between a dorsal and a ventral stream ('where' and 'what' pathway) that are assumed to be specialized for either processing spatial or object information within the visual system (Ungerleider & Mishkin, 1982). According to findings derived from visual discrimination and delayed-matching to sample tasks with animals (Funahashi, Bruce, & Goldman-Rakic, 1989; Pesaran, Pezaris, Sahani, Mitra, & Andersen, 2002; Desimone, Albright, Gross, & Bruce, 1984; Miller, Li, & Desimone, 1993), it was assumed that an equivalent distinction should also be found by means of neuroimaging tools for human WM tasks. A number of studies indeed provided strong evidence in support of this hypothesis. For example, the prominent role of the parietal cortex for spatial WM has been demonstrated by Smith, Jonides, and Koeppe (1996), who found a bilateral activation the posterior parietal and premotor cortex in a spatial 3-back WM task, in which the positions of letters, appearing successively at random locations, had to be compared. In comparable object memory tasks, sustained neural activity was found in the inferior temporal cortex with fMRI (Ranganath, Cohen, Dam, & D'Esposito, 2004). Other studies directly compared the retrieval of spatial and object information. In a delayed recognition task, in which participants had to store either the location or the shape of visual objects, Postle and D'Esposito (1999) found fMRI activation in the superior parietal cortex for the spatial task and in the ventral posterior temporal cortex for the object task (see also Moscovitch, Kapur, Köhler, & Houle, 1995, for related results).

The modified fan paradigm

The studies alluded to in the previous section mostly used WM tasks to separate anatomically distinct storage networks. Therefore, the activation patterns obtained are functionally related to short-living processes as perceptual encoding, priming, and brief episodes of WM maintenance, but they are not necessarily related to retrieval of more permanent LTM representations. In order to test the neocortical reactivation theory with respect to LTM representations, a retrieval paradigm has to be employed that separates encoding and retrieval for at least several hours, and that also separates perceptual and retrieval processes proper. In delayed recognition tasks, such as n-back or matching-to-sample tasks, participants see in the retrieval situation stimuli that are either identical to or different from previously encountered stimuli. Therefore, the same or similar sensory and perceptual processes must necessarily take place, and it will be impossible to decide whether obtained activation patterns in EEG or fMRI are caused by the perceptual analysis of the stimuli or by the reactivation of stored representations. In order to separate these processes, it is necessary to separate cue processing and memory retrieval proper in time. Moreover, qualitatively different memory representations (e.g. positions and objects) should always be cued by the very same type of perceptual stimulus in order to keep these more transient effects constant across conditions.

To meet these requirements, Heil and colleagues (Heil *et al.*, 1996; Heil, Rösler, & Hennighausen, 1997; Rösler *et al.*, 1995) used a modified version of the so-called fan paradigm (Anderson, 1974). They first trained their subjects with a set of paired associates. The pairs comprised always a picture as a cue and either one or two spatial positions (visual-spatial information) or one or two words as targets (verbal information). During recall, that took place one day later, two pictures were presented and participants had to decide whether the pictures were linked to each other via one and the same associated target, i.e., a spatial position or face. Depending on the number of learned associations, participants had to compare two, three, or four spatial positions or words, resulting in three levels of 'associative fan'. Therefore, it was possible to manipulate both the quality and the quantity of LTM retrieval without changing any other aspect of the experiment. Moreover, as the retrieval cue was always the same (i.e., two pictures), while the associated and to be retrieved targets were different, as intended, perceptual processes were kept constant while access to distinct memory domains was varied systematically.

Using this paradigm, Heil and colleagues were able to demonstrate that a functional dissociation between verbal and visual-spatial information does also exist for LTM representations. They measured slow event-related brain potentials as an indicator of cortical activation and they found that slow-potential topography during LTM retrieval was clearly distinct for spatial and verbal information, with a parietal maximum for positions and a left frontal maximum for words. Furthermore, consistent with the reactivation theory the most negative amplitudes for the different stimulus categories were found over those cortical areas that are assumed to play a prominent role during encoding of these stimuli, i.e., parietal regions for spatial positions and left frontal areas for verbal information. Most importantly, the peak amplitudes of these code-specific topographic maxima were found to increase significantly with the number of reactivated stimulus representations. Thus, the study revealed that topographically clearly distinct cortical activation patterns are evoked if distinct materials must be retrieved from LTM. Moreover, the amplitude of these activations was found to be systematically related to retrieval effort.

Reactivation of spatial and object information with the modified fan paradigm

In two more recent EEG experiments (Khader, Heil, & Rösler, 2005; Khader *et al.*, 2007), we pursued this idea further and tested whether the fundamental dissociation between the dorsal and ventral visual processing pathways, which was found during perception and WM maintenance, can also be observed if representations of objects and locations have to be retrieved from LTM. Basically, we used the same paradigm as Heil *et al.* (1996, 1997), but rather than using pictures we used words as cues and either faces and spatial positions (Khader, Heil, *et al.*, 2005), or objects (i.e. pictures of cups) and spatial positions (Khader *et al.*, 2007) as targets (see Figure 16.1). These contrasts imply also a more thorough test of the claim that distinct activation patterns during memory retrieval become manifest in brain-imaging data, because areas processing and storing objects and locations might be less clearly separated topographically than areas that are specialized for processing words and spatial locations.

As expected, slow potentials dissociated topographically during the retrieval of object and spatial information in both experiments, with a maximum over parietal scalp sites for positions and over left frontal sites for faces and objects. Consistently, slow wave amplitude increased monotonically with the number of to-be-reactivated associations, with the most pronounced effect for positions over parietal and for faces and objects over left frontal scalp sites. These findings of clearly different scalp topographies for different stimulus types are further empirical support for the reactivation account of LTM retrieval, and they substantiate the claim that stored representations of objects and positions are reactivated in material-specific cortical cell assemblies that overlap with the areas of the dorsal and the ventral stream used for online processing of such materials.

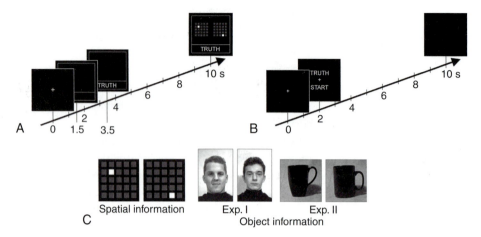

C   Spatial information   Exp. I   Exp. II

Object information

Figure 16.1 Trial structure and stimulus material used in the modified fan paradigm to test reactivation from LTM. Stimulus sequence of acquisition (A) and recall (B) trials. (C) Examples of spatial positions, faces, and objects that had to be encoded during acquisition and retrieved during the recall phase (modified from Khader, Heil, *et al.*, 2005; Khader, Burke, *et al.*, 2005; Khader *et al.*, 2007).

Furthermore, despite the considerable difference between the stimuli that were used to trigger memory retrieval, i.e. pictures in the Heil *et al.* vs. written nouns in the Khader *et al.* studies, topographically distinct LTM representations were systematically activated with both types of cues, and the parietal topography for spatial information that had been found in the earlier studies was fully replicated. This generalization across cues shows that the location and dynamics of cortical cell assemblies where code-specific information becomes reactivated are independent from the stimulus that is used to access this information.

Although different slow wave topographies are evidence for spatially distinct neural generators (McCarthy & Wood, 1985; Khader, Schicke, Röder, & Rösler, 2008), the method does not allow for determining exactly which brain regions cause the observed topographic differences. In order to identify the involved brain regions more precisely, we repeated the same retrieval procedure with the same set of participants also in the fMRI scanner. By so doing, corresponding fMRI data were obtained from most of our participants of the face/position study (Khader, Burke, Bien, Ranganath, & Rösler, 2005) and the object/position study (Khader *et al.*, 2007).

The fMRI analysis revealed a broadly distributed network of cortical areas that were found to be differently activated during recall of positions, faces, and objects, and that comprised the parietal and precentral cortex for positions, the left prefrontal, occipito-temporal, and posterior cingulate cortex for faces, and the left temporal and prefrontal cortex for cups (see Figure 16.2). These activations were material-specific along the dorsal and ventral visual pathways (i.e. the parietal cortex was active during retrieval of positions, the occipital and fusiform gyrus during retrieval of faces, and the middle temporal gyrus during retrieval of cups). Furthermore, in a subset of these areas the BOLD response

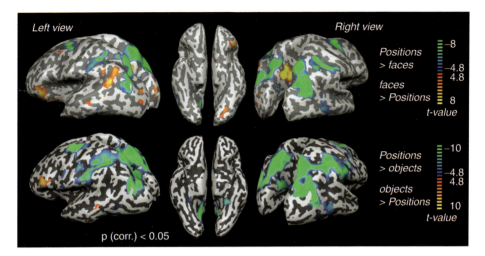

Figure 16.2 fMRI contrast of recalling positions vs. faces (upper line of activation maps) and positions vs. objects (lower row of activation maps), independent of the number of to-be-retrieved associations. Activations are projected on the partially inflated cortex reconstruction of one participant shown in three different orientations (left, inferior, and right view) (modified from Khader, Burke, *et al.*, 2005; Khader *et al.*, 2007).

was found to increase monotonically for each stimulus type with the number of the to-be-reactivated associations, indicating that the activity level of stimulus-specific cell assemblies increased the more representations had to be accessed. These areas also dissociated topographically for positions, faces, and objects (Figure 16.3). The left superior parietal lobe and bilateral precentral cortex were found to be more strongly activated by the fan manipulation for positions compared to faces and objects, whereas the left inferior prefrontal cortex was more active for faces and objects compared to positions. Furthermore, the posterior cingulate cortex was found to be activated by this contrast only in case of faces. Thus, there were two material-specific effects, one that became apparent in an overall contrast or main effect of the distinct materials, and one revealed by a parametric comparison of the difficulty levels within one material. Both findings clearly show that material-specific cortical networks are systematically activated during LTM retrieval that overlap with areas that also become activated by positions and objects during perceptual and WM tasks. Moreover, EEG and fMRI data revealed highly corresponding activation patterns that could also be formally related by means of fMRI-derived source localizations, in which equivalent dipoles in EEG source models were seeded based on the fMRI activations (Khader *et al.*, 2007).

To conclude, the studies reviewed in this section strongly support the neocortical model of material-specific memory storage and retrieval. They also demonstrate that a functional-anatomical dissociation seems not only to be valid for verbal vs. visual-spatial information, i.e. for categories that are traditionally separated by psychological theories (e.g. Paivio, 1986), but similar dissociations seem also to be valid for more subtle category distinctions within the domain of visually processed items, such as objects, faces, and spatial locations.

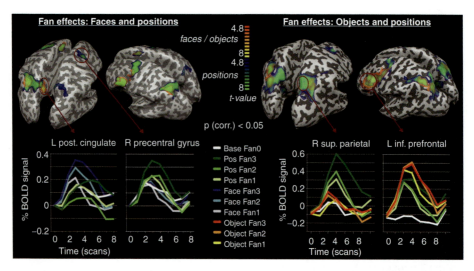

Figure 16.3 Brain areas showing a monotonic activation increase with increasing associative fan. Superimposed are the fMRI fan contrasts (3 > 2 > 1 > 0) for recalling faces and positions (left side) and for recalling objects and positions (right side). Below are illustrative sample plots of event-related BOLD signals (averaged to cue onset) from brain areas showing a material-specific gradual increase with increasing fan during retrieval of positions, faces, and objects (modified from Khader, Burke, *et al.*, 2005; Khader *et al.*, 2007).

Control processes during LTM retrieval

The cortical reactivation theory assumes that internal or external stimuli can reinstate the complete pattern of cortical activity that represents the memory episode of which the triggering stimulus is part of (Damasio, 1989b; McClelland *et al.*, 1995; Squire, 1992). After reactivation, memory traces are supposed to remain in an active state as long as they are not disturbed or overwritten by other external or internal stimulus patterns. The theory, however, says little about processes that guide and control retrieval, e.g. processes that direct attention to certain features of the engram, that suppress distracting, irrelevant activations, that maintain the activation pattern when the triggering input is no longer available, or that evaluate the relevance of retrieved engrams with respect to the task at hand (e.g. Buckner & Wheeler, 2001; Rugg & Wilding, 2000). According to Buckner and Wheeler (2001), such control processes are distinguishable from reactivation processes proper, and they are most likely embodied in areas which are distinct form the memory networks where engrams are reactivated. Results of brain imaging, neuropsychological, and neurophysiological studies suggest that the prefrontal cortex (PFC) exerts such control functions by interacting with more posterior parietal and temporal areas (Buckner, 2003; Ranganath *et al.*, 2004; Ranganath, Johnson, & D'Esposito, 2003; Wheeler, Stuss, & Tulving, 1995).

The important role of the PFC for maintaining information in the absence of sensory stimulation has been substantiated by transient lesion studies in monkeys

(Goldman-Rakic, 1995; Goldman-Rakic, Ó'Scalaidhe, & Chafee, 2000), which revealed that prefrontal neurons persistently fire during the delay period of a delayed matching-to-sample task, but not prior to or after the delay. This suggests that the maintenance of an active representation is controlled by the PFC. Furthermore, neuropsychological studies showed that retrograde amnesia occurs not only in patients with medial temporal lobe lesions, but also when frontal regions are damaged (e.g. Kopelman, Stanhope, & Kingsley, 1999), and that patients with lesions in the frontal lobe are impaired in memory tests that require the evaluation and manipulation of activated representations (Wheeler, Stuss, & Tulving, 1995). In the context of free recall tests, the frontal cortex seems to be especially important for retrieving source information about a recalled episode (Janowsky, Shimamura, & Squire, 1989; Ranganath, Johnson, & D'Esposito, 2000).

Using fMRI in humans, many studies found persisting neural activity in the PFC during WM tasks (e.g. Courtney, Petit, Maisog, Ungerleider, & Haxby, 1998; Zarahn, Aguirre, & D'Esposito, 1999). In a review of these studies, Curtis and D'Esposito (2003) concluded that the dorsolateral PFC supports the maintenance of information by directing attention to representations that are stored in more posterior brain regions. In the special case of WM for visual information, the PFC is supposed to facilitate maintenance by top-down modulation of inferior-temporal object representations. For example, selective cooling of the PFC in monkeys was found to reduce behavioural performance and delay-period activity in inferior temporal neurons during a delayed matching-to-sample task (Fuster, Bauer, & Jervey, 1985), suggesting that prefrontal regions are critical for 'directing the mind's eye' (Ranganath & D'Esposito, 2005), i.e. keeping representation in the inferior temporal cortex in an activated state.

In addition to prefrontal control processes, others (Farah, 2000; Kosslyn & Koenig, 1992; Kosslyn, 1994) have postulated the existence of specialized cell assemblies in the parietal and occipital cortex that are involved in the transformation and maintenance of visual information during mental imagery. Parietal activations were found, e.g., when spatial memory traces had to be modified during the delay in a delayed matching-to-sample-task (Rolke, Heil, Hennighausen, Häussler, & Rösler, 2000), when participants had to scan a certain distance on an imagined map (Mellet et al., 2002; Schicke et al., 2006), or when participants had to match two imagined clocks in a mental rotation task (Trojano et al., 2000). According to Kosslyn and Koenig (1992), the posterior imagery buffer in the occipital and parietal lobes is supposed to interact with the prefrontal control system, forming a functionally connected network for visual imagery. Whereas the posterior buffer is supposed to store visual-spatial information over brief periods of time – and is thus equivalent to what Baddeley termed the 'visual-spatial sketchpad' (Baddeley, 2003; Baddeley & Hitch, 1974) – the prefrontal executive modules are supposed to read and rewrite information from and to the buffer and to modify the stored information.

Content specificity of control processes

Although material specificity of memory representations in the brain is beyond doubt, much less agreement exists whether the mentioned control systems also exhibit material specificity. Based on lesion and electrophysiological data from delayed matching-to-sample tasks in monkeys, Goldman-Rakic and colleagues have proposed a specialization of the dorsolateral and more anterior PFC (Brodmann areas 9, 10, and 46) for spatial information, and of the ventrolateral and more posterior PFC (Brodmann areas 6/8, 44, 45, and 47) for object information (Goldman-Rakic et al., 2000; Levy & Goldman-Rakic, 2000). In humans, a study by Banich et al. (2000) found material-specific dissociations within the PFC while participants performed a shape and location version of the Stroop task, in which task-relevant information was kept constant (i.e. words), whereas the task-irrelevant information (i.e. either the word's colour or the word's position) was made either congruent or incongruent. The spatial version of this task elicited more dorsal and the colour task more ventral activations within the PFC. Quite similar, we found in our fMRI study on LTM retrieval of faces and positions (Khader, Burke, et al., 2005) that, in addition to the posterior differences along the dorsal and ventral visual pathways, differences appeared also in the left PFC, with stronger activity for positions in the dorsolateral and for faces in the ventrolateral left PFC. However, these prefrontal dissociations proved as less consistent than the more posterior dissociations. For example, in our study in which we contrasted spatial locations with pictures of drinking cups instead of pictures of faces we did not find a more ventral frontal activation for the objects (Khader et al., 2007). This result accords with a review on the material specificity of the PFC by D'Esposito (2001). He concluded that the only methodically sound and well controlled study that found a material-specific dissociation in the PFC (Courtney et al., 1998) had contrasted spatial information with *faces*, while all other studies that did not find material specificity of PFC areas had contrasted other objects than faces with spatial information (see also D'Esposito et al., 1998; Nystrom et al., 2000; Owen, 2000, for other reviews suggesting that there is no consistent evidence for a material-specific organization of the PFC in humans).

Recent evidence from neurophysiological and neuroimaging studies suggest that the diverging results on material specificity of the PFC are possibly due to confounding material and task (Johnson, Raye, Mitchell, Greene, & Anderson, 2003; Ranganath & D'Esposito, 2005) and that the results could be integrated by assuming that the ventral and/or posterior PFC is specialized for activating representations of task-relevant items (e.g. objects, words, etc.), whereas the dorsal and/or anterior PFC is specialized for activating spatial and non-spatial relations between items that are active in memory (see Ranganath & D'Esposito, 2005, for further discussion).

Conclusions

This chapter summarized evidence supporting the idea that different types of concepts are stored and reactivated in multiple, content-specific memory systems. Topographic dissociations were found for rather global stimulus categories, such as verbal vs. spatial or motor vs. visual representations, but also for less distinct stimulus categories, such as spatial vs. object information, or for even more fine-grained distinctions, such as faces, buildings, tools, chairs, houses, etc. These dissociations have been substantiated not only by behavioural experiments (e.g. dual task conditions), but also by different topographies of brain activation processes as measured by event-related EEG or BOLD signals. Such material-specific topographies were observed across a wide range of distinct tasks, including storage, rehearsal, and transformation of representations in WM as well as storage and retrieval of representations in intermediate or long-term memory.

With respect to the question of how brain-imaging studies can inform psychological theories of memory, three implications can be derived from this pattern of results: (1) Engrams are most likely not stored in an abstract material-independent code, such as, e.g., propositions. Rather, memory representations are encoded and retrieved in a material-specific manner, i.e. they preserve the sensory features and context associations that were relevant during encoding. Different categories seem to be stored and reactivated always in those areas in which they are also processed perceptually. This implies (2) that a memory representation is not stored and retrieved as a narrowly circumscribed entity. The highly distributed activation patterns observed in brain-imaging studies during memory tasks suggest that always very widely distributed cell assemblies are involved. Translated into psychological terms this means that memory contents are most likely represented by a set of features which is simultaneously reactivated if a triggering cue is presented. Even if this cue triggers directly only one specific aspect of the whole engram, it will nevertheless result in an activation of the full associative network that defines this memory episode. (3) Activation patterns in posterior and temporal areas seem to be more specific for certain material types (faces, objects, locations, etc.) rather than for particular memory tasks. These patterns show substantial overlap irrespective of whether they are triggered by WM tasks, as delayed matching-to-sample or by LTM task, such as paired associate retrieval. This supports the psychological claim that WM and LTM contents are not structurally separated in that they are housed within distinct compartments and transferred from one in the other depending on the task, but rather that WM and LTM contents differ only with respect to the activation state of the engrams (Cowan, 1999).

Code-specific activation patterns were not only observed in posterior projection areas or anterior motor areas, but also in other brain regions, e.g. the frontal lobes. However, these frontal areas, as well as some areas in the parietal cortex, showed not only material-specific, but in some studies also material-unspecific activation patterns in memory retrieval tasks. All of these activations have to be distinguished from memory reactivation processes proper, and they are functionally related to control processes as direction of attention, suppression of irrelevant information, maintaining activation patterns without external stimuli, or evaluation of reactivated information with respect to the task demands. For the time being, it is not clear whether these inconsistencies in material specificity vs. unspecificity are simply due to methodological differences, e.g. differences in spatial resolution of the imaging tools, whether both types of control processes, material-unspecific and material-specific, do actually exist, or whether the categorical distinctions valid for posterior areas do not apply for executive areas in PFC. These questions will have to be studied in more detail in future experiments. Whatever the eventual results will be, they will have consequences for the formulation of psychological theories. Given that truly material-unspecific control processes are embodied in some brain areas, e.g. PFC, it has to be explained in psychological terms how material-unspecificity and material specificity are mapped onto each other, i.e., it has to be explained how a more abstract address code is extracted and used to access material-specific representations. On the other hand, if also material-specific control processes are identified by corresponding activation patterns, it has to be explained how these processes interact with the more abstract material-independent processes and, likewise, if the categorical distinctions that dissociate activation patterns in frontal and more posterior areas are incongruent to each other, it has to be explained how these distinct mapping rules are related to each other.

Acknowledgments

The empirical studies of Khader *et al.* cited in this chapter were supported by grant FOR254/2 of the German Research Foundation (DFG).

References

Anderson, J. R. (1974). Retrieval of propositional information from long-term memory. *Cognitive Psychology*, 6, 451–474.

Baddeley, A. (2003). Working memory: looking back and looking forward. *Nature Reviews Neuroscience*, 4, 829–839.

Baddeley, A. D. & Hitch, G. (1974). Working Memory. In G. A. Bower (Ed.), *The Psychology of Learning and Motivation* (Vol. 8, pp. 47–89). New York: Academic Press.

Banich, M. T., Milham, M. P., Atchley, R., Cohen, N. J., Webb, A., Wszalek, T., Kramer, A. F., Liang, Z. P., Wright, A., Shenker, J., & Magin, R. (2000). fMRI studies of Stroop tasks reveal unique roles of anterior and posterior brain systems in attentional selection. *Journal of Cognitive Neuroscience*, 12, 988–1000.

Buckner, R. L. (2003). Functional-anatomic correlates of control processes in memory. *Journal of Neuroscience*, 23, 3999–4004.

Buckner, R. L. & Wheeler, M. E. (2001). The cognitive neuroscience of remembering. *Nature Reviews Neuroscience*, 2, 624–634.

Courtney, S. M., Petit, L., Maisog, J. M., Ungerleider, L. G., & Haxby, J. V. (1998). An area specialized for spatial working memory in human frontal cortex. *Science*, 279, 1347–1351.

Cowan, N. (1999). An embedded-processes model of working memory. In A. Miyake & P. Shah (Eds), *Models of Working Memory: Mechanisms of Active Maintenance and Executive Control* (pp. 62–101). New York: Cambridge University Press.

Curtis, C. E. & D'Esposito, M. (2003). Persistent activity in the prefrontal cortex during working memory. *Trends in Cognitive Sciences*, 7, 415–423.

D'Esposito, M. (2001). Functional Neuroimaging of Working Memory. In R. Cabeza & A. Kingstone (Eds), *Handbook of Functional Neuroimaging of Cognition* (pp. 293–327). Cambridge: MIT Press.

D'Esposito, M., Aguirre, G. K., Zarahn, E., Ballard, D., Shin, R. K., & Lease, J. (1998). Functional MRI studies of spatial and nonspatial working memory. *Cognitive Brain Research*, 7, 1–13.

Damasio, A. R. (1989a). The brain binds entities and events by multiregional activation from convergence zones. *Neural Computation*, 1, 123–132.

Damasio, A. R. (1989b). Time-locked multiregional retroactivation: a systems-level proposal for the neural substrates of recall and recognition. *Cognition*, 33, 25–62.

Damasio, H., Grabowski, T. J., Tranel, D., Hichwa, R. D., & Damasio, A. R. (1996). A neural basis for lexical retrieval. *Nature*, 380, 499–505.

de Renzi, E. (2000). Prosopagnosia. In M. J. Farah & T. E. Feinberg (Eds.), *Patient-Based Approaches to Cognitive Neuroscience* (pp. 85–95). Cambridge, MA: MIT Press.

Desimone, R., Albright, T. D., Gross, C. G., & Bruce, C. (1984). Stimulus-selective properties of inferior temporal neurons in the macaque. *Journal of Neuroscience*, 4, 2051–2062.

Ebbinghaus, H. (1966). *Über das Gedächtnis [On memory]* (Original work published 1885). Amsterdam, Netherlands: E. J. Bonset.

Eckhorn, R., Bauer, R., Jordan, W., Brosch, M., Kruse, W., Munk, M., & Reitboeck, H. J. (1988). Coherent oscillations: A mechansim of feature linking in the visual cortex? Multiple electrode and correlation analysis in the cat. *Biological Cybernetics*, 60, 121–130.

Epstein, R. & Kanwisher, N. (1998). A cortical representation of the local visual environment. *Nature*, 392, 598–601.

Farah, M. J. (2000). The neural bases of mental imagery. In M. S. Gazzaniga (Ed.), *The New Cognitive Neurosciences* (2nd Edn, pp. 965–975). Cambridge, MA: MIT Press.

Funahashi, S., Bruce, C. J., & Goldman-Rakic, P. S. (1989). Mnemonic coding of visual space in the monkey's dorsolateral prefrontal cortex. *Journal of Neurophysiology*, 61, 331–349.

Fuster, J. M., Bauer, R. H., & Jervey, J. P. (1985). Functional interactions between inferotemporal and prefrontal cortex in a cognitive task. *Brain Research*, 330, 299–307.

Gauthier, I., Behrmann, M., & Tarr, M. J. (1999). Can face recognition really be dissociated from object recognition? *Journal of Cognitive Neuroscience*, 11, 349–370.

Goldman-Rakic, P. S. (1995). Architecture of the prefrontal cortex and the central executive. J. Grafman, K. J. Holyoak, & F. Boller (Eds), *Structure and Functions of the Human Prefrontal Cortex* (Annals of the New York Academy of Sciences Edn, Vol. 769, pp. 71–83). New York: New York Academy of Science.

Goldman-Rakic, P. S., Ó'Scalaidhe, S. P., & Chafee, M. V. (2000). Domain specificity in cognitive systems. In M. Gazzaniga (Ed.), *The New Cognitive Neurosciences* (pp. 845–866). Cambridge, MA: MIT Press.

Gray, C. M., König, P., Engel, A. K., & Singer, W. (1989). Oscillatory responses in cat visual cortex exhibit inter-columnar synchronization which reflects global stimulus properties. *Nature*, 338, 334–337.

Grill-Spector, K., Knouf, N., & Kanwisher, N. (2004). The fusiform face area subserves face perception, not generic within-category identification. *Nature Neuroscience*, 7, 555–562.

Hart, J., Berndt, R. S., & Caramazza, A. (1985). Category-specific naming deficit following cerebral infarction. *Nature*, 316, 439–440.

Haxby, J. V., Gobbini, M. I., Furey, M. L., Ishai, A., Schouten, J. L., & Pietrini, P. (2001). Distributed and overlapping representations of faces and objects in ventral temporal cortex. *Science*, 293, 2425–2430.

Heil, M., Rösler, F., & Hennighausen, E. (1996). Topographically distinct cortical activation in episodic long-term memory: the retrieval of spatial versus verbal information. *Memory and Cognition*, 24, 777–795.

Heil, M., Rösler, F., Rauch, M., & Hennighausen, E. (1998). Selective interference during the retrieval of spatial and verbal information from episodic long-term memory. *International Journal of Psychology*, 33, 249–257.

Heil, M., Rösler, F., & Hennighausen, E. (1997). Topography of brain electrical activity dissociates the retrieval of spatial versus verbal information from episodic long-term memory in humans. *Neuroscience Letters*, 222, 45–48.

Heil, M., Rolke, B., Engelkamp, J., Rösler, F., Özcan, M., & Hennighausen, E. (1999). Event-related brain potentials during recognition of ordinary and bizarre action phrases following verbal and subject-performed encoding conditions. *European Journal of Cognitive Psychology*, 11, 261–280.

Janowsky, J. S., Shimamura, A. P., & Squire, L. R. (1989). Source memory impairment in patients with frontal lobe lesions. *Neuropsychologia, 27*, 1043–1056.

Johnson, M. K., Raye, C. L., Mitchell, K. J., Greene, E. J., & Anderson, A. W. (2003). FMRI evidence for an organization of prefrontal cortex by both type of process and type of information. *Cerebral Cortex, 13*, 265–273.

Jonides, J., Sylvester, C. Y. C., Lacey, S. C., Wager, T. D., Nichols, T. E., & Awh, E. (2003). Modules of working memory. In R. H. Kluwe, G. Lüer, & F. Rösler (Eds), *Principles of Learning and Memory* (pp. 113–134). Cambridge, MA: Birkhäuser.

Khader, P., Burke, M., Bien, S., Ranganath, C., & Rösler, F. (2005). Content-specific activation during associative long-term memory retrieval. *Neuroimage, 27*, 805–816.

Khader, P., Heil, M., & Rösler, F. (2005). Material-specific long-term memory representations of faces and spatial positions: Evidence from slow event-related brain potentials. *Neuropsychologia, 43*, 2109–2124.

Khader, P., Knoth, K., Burke, M., Bien, S., Ranganath, C., & Rösler, F. (2007). Topography and dynamics of associative long-term memory retrieval in humans. *Journal of Cognitive Neuroscience, 19*, 493–512.

Khader, P., Schicke, T., Röder, B., & Rösler, F. (2008). On the relationship between slow cortical potentials and BOLD signal changes in humans – A review. *International Journal of Psychophysiology, 67*, 252–261.

Kintsch, W. (1974). *The Representation of Meaning in Memory*. Hillsdale, NJ: Lawrence Erlbaum.

Kintsch, W. & van Dijk, T. A. (1978). Toward a model of text comprehension and production. *Psychological Review, 85*, 363–394.

Kopelman, M. D., Stanhope, N., & Kingsley, D. (1999). Retrograde amnesia in patients with diencephalic, temporal lobe or frontal lesions. *Neuropsychologia, 37*, 939–958.

Kosslyn, S. M. & Koenig, O. (1992). *Wet Mind*. New York: Free Press.

Kosslyn, S. M. (1994). *Image and Brain: The Resolution of the Imagery Debate*. Cambridge, MA: MIT Press.

Levy, R. & Goldman-Rakic, P. S. (2000). Segregation of working memory functions within the dorsolateral prefrontal cortex. *Experimental Brain Research, 133*, 23–32.

Logie, R. H. (1986). Visuo-spatial processes in working memory. *Quarterly Journal of Experimental Psychology, 38A*, 229–247.

Maguire, E. A., Frith, C. D., & Cipolotti, L. (2001). Distinct neural systems for the encoding and recognition of topography and faces. *Neuroimage, 13*, 743–750.

McCarthy, G. & Wood, C. C. (1985). Scalp distributions of event-related potentials: an ambiguity associated with analysis of variance models. *Electroencephalography and Clinical Neurophysiology, 62*, 203–208.

McCarthy, G., Puce, A., Gore, J. C., & Allison, T. (1997). Face-specific processing in the human fusiform gyrus. *Journal of Cognitive Neuroscience, 9*, 605–610.

McClelland, J. L., McNaughton, B. L., & O'Reilly, R. C. (1995). Why there are complementary learning systems in the hippocampus and neocortex: insights from the successes and failures of connectionist models of learning and memory. *Psychological Review, 102*, 419–457.

McNeil, J. E. & Warrington, E. K. (1993). Prosopagnosia: a face-specific disorder. *Quarterly Journal of Experimental Psychology A, 46*, 1–10.

Mellet, E., Bricogne, S., Crivello, F., Mazoyer, B., Denis, M., & Tzourio-Mazoyer, N. (2002). Neural basis of mental scanning of a topographic representation built from a text. *Cerebral Cortex, 12*, 1322–1330.

Miller, E. K., Li, L., & Desimone, R. (1993). Activity of neurons in anterior inferior temporal cortex during a short-term memory task. *Journal of Neuroscience, 13*, 1460–1478.

Mishkin, M., Ungerleider, L. G., & Macko, K. A. (1983). Object vision and spatial vision: Two cortical pathways. *Trends in Neurosciences*, 6, 414–417.

Moscovitch, C., Kapur, S., Köhler, S., & Houle, S. (1995). Distinct neural correlates of visual long-term memory for spatial location and object identity: a positron emission tomography study in humans. *Proceedings of the National Academy of Sciences, USA*, 92, 3721–3725.

Nyberg, L., Habib, R., McIntosh, A. R., & Tulving, E. (2000). Reactivation of encoding-related brain activity during memory retrieval. *Proceedings of the National Academy of Sciences of the United States of America*, 97, 11120–11124.

Nyberg, L., Petersson, K. M., Nilsson, L. G., Sandblom, J., Aberg, C., & Ingvar, M. (2001). Reactivation of motor brain areas during explicit memory for actions. *NeuroImage*, 14, 521–528.

Nystrom, L. E., Braver, T. S., Sabb, F. W., Delgado, M. R., Noll, D. C., & Cohen, J. D. (2000). Working memory for letters, shapes, and locations: fMRI evidence against stimulus-based regional organization in human prefrontal cortex. *Neuroimage*, 11, 424–446.

Owen, A. M. (2000). The role of the lateral frontal cortex in mnemonic processing: the contribution of functional neuroimaging. *Experimental Brain Research*, 133, 33–43.

Paivio, A. (1986). *Mental Representations*. New York: Oxford University Press.

Paller, K. A. (2003). The principle of cross-cortical consolidation of declarative memories. In R. H. Kluwe, G. Lüer, & F. Rösler (Eds), *Principles of Learning and Memory* (pp. 155–169). Cambridge, MA: Birkhäuser.

Pesaran, B., Pezaris, J. S., Sahani, M., Mitra, P. P., & Andersen, R. A. (2002). Temporal structure in neuronal activity during working memory in macaque parietal cortex. *Nature Neuroscience*, 5, 805–811.

Postle, B. R. & D'Esposito, M. (1999). "What-Then-Where" in visual working memory: an event-related fMRI study. *Journal of Cognitive Neuroscience*, 11, 585–597.

Ranganath, C., Cohen, M. X., Dam, C., & D'Esposito, M. (2004). Inferior temporal, prefrontal, and hippocampal contributions to visual working memory maintenance and associative memory retrieval. *Journal of Neuroscience*, 24, 3917–3925.

Ranganath, C. & D'Esposito, M. (2005). Directing the mind's eye: prefrontal, inferior and medial temporal mechanisms for visual working memory. *Current Opinion in Neurobiology*, 15, 175–182.

Ranganath, C., Johnson, M. K., & D'Esposito, M. (2000). Left anterior prefrontal activation increases with demands to recall specific perceptual information. *The Journal of Neuroscience*, 20, 108RC.

Ranganath, C., Johnson, M. K., & D'Esposito, M. (2003). Prefrontal activity associated with working memory and episodic long-term memory. *Neuropsychologia*, 41, 378–389.

Rhodes, G., Byatt, G., Michie, P. T., & Puce, A. (2004). Is the fusiform face area specialized for faces, individuation, or expert individuation?. *Journal of Cognitive Neuroscience*, 16, 189–203.

Rolke, B., Heil, M., Hennighausen, E., Häussler, C., & Rösler, F. (2000). Topography of brain electrical activity dissociates the sequential order transformation of verbal versus spatial information in humans. *Neuroscience Letters*, 282, 81–84.

Rugg, M. D. & Wilding, E. L. (2000). Retrieval processing and episodic memory. *Trends in Cognitive Sciences*, 4, 108–115.

Rösler, F., Heil, M., & Hennighausen, E. (1995). Distinct cortical activation patterns during long-term memory retrieval of verbal, spatial, and color information. *Journal of Cognitive Neuroscience*, 7, 51–65.

Schicke, T., Muckli, L., Beer, A. L., Wibral, M., Singer, W., Goebel, R., Rösler, F., & Röder, B. (2006). Tight covariation of BOLD signal changes and slow ERPs in the parietal cortex in a parametric spatial imagery task with haptic acquisition. *European Journal of Neuroscience*, 23, 1910–1918.

Shepard, R. N. & Metzler, J. (1971). Mental rotation of three dimensional objects. *Science*, 171, 701–703.

Smith, E. E., Jonides, J., & Koeppe, R. A. (1996). Dissociating verbal and spatial working memory using PET. *Cerebral Cortex*, 6, 11–20.

Squire, L. R. (1992). Memory and the hippocampus: a synthesis from findings with rats, monkeys, and humans. *Psychological Review, 99*, 195–231.

Trojano, L., Grossi, D., Linden, D. E., Formisano, E., Hacker, H., Zanella, F. E., Goebel, R., & Di Salle, F. (2000). Matching two imagined clocks: the functional anatomy of spatial analysis in the absence of visual stimulation. *Cerebral Cortex, 10*, 473–481.

Ungerleider, L. G. & Mishkin, M. (1982). Two cortical visual systems. In D. J. Ingle, M. A. Goodale, & R. J. Mansfield (Eds), *Analysis of Visual Behavior* (pp. 549–580). Cambridge, MA: MIT Press.

Warrington, E. & Shallice, T. (1984). Category specific semantic impairments. *Brain, 107*, 829–854.

Wheeler, M. A., Stuss, D. T., & Tulving, E. (1995). Frontal lobe damage produces episodic memory impairment. *Journal of the International Neuropsychological Society, 1*, 525–536.

Wheeler, M. E. & Buckner, R. L. (2003). Functional dissociation among components of remembering: control, perceived oldness, and content. *Journal of Neuroscience, 23*, 3869–3880.

Wheeler, M. E., Petersen, S. E., & Buckner, R. L. (2000). Memory's echo: vivid remembering reactivates sensory-specific cortex. *Proceedings of the National Academy of Sciences*, USA, 97, 11125–11129.

Zarahn, E., Aguirre, G. K., & D'Esposito, M. (1999). Temporal isolation of the neural correlates of spatial mnemonic processing with fMRI. *Cognitive Brain Research, 7*, 255–268.

Chapter 17

Multivariate methods for tracking cognitive states

Kenneth A. Norman, Joel R. Quamme,
and Ehren L. Newman

Introduction

Most fMRI studies of memory focus on relating the activity of specific, localized brain regions to task conditions or to behaviour. Based on this information, one can make inferences about how these regions contribute to memory, and about cognitive processes more generally.[1] In this paper, we describe a different, complementary approach: Multi-voxel pattern analysis (MVPA). Instead of trying to characterize the functional properties of individual brain voxels (volumetric pixels), MVPA involves applying pattern-classification algorithms to *multi-voxel* patterns of brain activity, and training these classifiers to detect the spatially distributed neural correlates of specific cognitive states. Once a pattern classifier has been trained to detect the neural manifestation of a particular cognitive state, the classifier can be used to track the comings and goings of that state over time. For recent reviews of MVPA research, see Norman, Polyn, Detre, and Haxby (2006b) and Haynes and Rees (2006). The idea of analysing multi-voxel patterns has a long history in fMRI data analysis (e.g. Friston & Buchel, 2003; Friston, Harrison, & Penny, 2003; McIntosh, Bookstein, Haxby, & Grady, 1996; McIntosh & Lobaugh, 2004; Calhoun, Adali, Pearlson, & Pekar, 2001). The difference between MVPA and other multivariate analysis methods is, in large part, one of emphasis: Other multivariate techniques have focused on characterizing functional relationships between brain regions, whereas MVPA is more focused on decoding the informational contents of particular brain states.

   Importantly, the same pattern classification approach can be applied to other types of neuroimaging data besides fMRI; we discuss applications to EEG in this paper. To accommodate the fact that pattern analysis can be applied to multiple imaging modalities, the term MVPA can be construed more broadly as *multivariate* pattern analysis (to refer to the fact that MVPA factors in multiple aspects of the signal, whatever that signal might be), not just multi-voxel pattern analysis.

---

[1] For discussion of the kinds of inferences that one can (and cannot) make about cognitive processes based on localized fMRI activations, see Henson (2005) and Poldrack (2006).

This paper is divided into three sections: In the first section, we provide a general overview of the MVPA approach, drawing on our recent review of MVPA methods (Norman *et al.*, 2006b). In the second section, we show how MVPA can be used to address theoretically meaningful questions about memory. The key idea here is that having a time-varying readout of the subject's cognitive state makes it possible to more directly test hypotheses about how specific cognitive states are related to behavioural outcomes. Finally, in the third section we will discuss these findings and we will point out some future directions of research.

Overview of the MVPA approach

Patterns in the brain

The central idea that underlies the MVPA approach is that (to a first approximation) each cognitive state is associated with a characteristic pattern of brain activity. A study by Haxby *et al.* (2001) provides a useful illustration of how multi-voxel patterns of activity can be used to distinguish between cognitive states. Subjects viewed faces, houses, and a variety of object categories (e.g. chairs, shoes, bottles, etc.). The data were split in half for each subject (based on odd vs. even scanner runs), and the multi-voxel pattern of response to each category in ventral temporal (VT) cortex was characterized separately for each half. By correlating the first-half patterns with the second-half patterns (within a particular subject), Haxby *et al.* (2001) were able to show that each category was associated with a reliable, distinct pattern of activity in VT cortex (e.g. the first-half 'shoe' pattern matched the second-half 'shoe' pattern more than it matched the patterns associated with other categories; for similar results, see Spiridon & Kanwisher, 2002; Tsao, Freiwald, Knutsen, Mandeville, & Tootell, 2003; Carlson, Schrater, & He, 2003; Cox & Savoy, 2003; Hanson, Matsuka, & Haxby, 2004; O'Toole, Jiang, Abdi, & Haxby, 2005).

Sensitively detecting brain patterns

Given the goal of detecting the presence of a particular mental representation in the brain, the primary advantage of MVPA methods over individual-voxel-based methods is increased sensitivity. Conventional fMRI analysis methods try to find voxels that show a statistically significant response to the experimental conditions. To increase sensitivity to a particular condition, these methods spatially average across voxels that respond significantly to that condition. While this approach reduces noise, it also reduces signal in two important ways: First, voxels with weaker (i.e. non-significant) responses to a particular condition might carry some information about the presence/absence of that condition. Second, spatial averaging blurs out fine-grained spatial patterns that might discriminate between experimental conditions (Kriegeskorte, Goebel, & Bandettini, 2006).

Like conventional methods, the MVPA approach also seeks to boost sensitivity by looking at the contributions of multiple voxels. However, to avoid the signal-loss issues mentioned above, MVPA does not routinely involve spatial averaging of voxel responses. Instead, MVPA uses pattern classification algorithms, derived from computer science and statistics, to aggregate the (possibly weak) information that is present in the responses of individual voxels. Because MVPA analyses focus on high-spatial-frequency (and often idiosyncratic) patterns of response, MVPA analyses are typically conducted within individual subjects.

MVPA methods

The basic MVPA method is a straightforward application of pattern classification techniques, where the patterns to be classified are typically vectors of voxel activity values. To illustrate these standard MVPA procedures, assume (for the purposes of this example) that we want to be able to decode whether the subject is viewing shoes or bottles based on fMRI activity.

The first step of an MVPA analysis is *feature selection*: Deciding which voxels to include in the pattern classification analysis (Figure 17.1A). As mentioned above, one of the defining features of MVPA is that it can make use of information provided by voxels that (on their own) do not meet conventional criteria for statistical significance. However, there is a cost to being too inclusive: If a voxel is especially noisy, the harmful effects of added noise (from this voxel) might outweigh the beneficial effects of added signal. As such, removing voxels with an especially poor signal-to-noise ratio prior to classification can greatly improve classification performance. There are several approaches to feature selection. Many studies use voxel-wise tests to weed out noisy voxels (e.g. Polyn, Natu, Cohen, & Norman, 2005). Another approach that is gaining popularity is to sweep a spherical 'searchlight' around the brain and choose voxels based on whether the pattern of activity within the searchlight discriminates between the conditions of interest (Kriegeskorte *et al.*, 2006). See Norman *et al.* (2006b) and Mitchell *et al.* (2004) for additional discussion of feature selection methods. The second step in an MVPA analysis, *pattern assembly*, involves sorting the data into discrete 'brain patterns' corresponding to the pattern of activity across the selected voxels at a particular time in the experiment (Figure 17.1B). Brain patterns are labeled according to which experimental condition generated the pattern. This labeling procedure needs to account for the fact that the haemodynamic response measured by the scanner is delayed and smeared out in time, relative to the instigating neural event.

The third step, *classifier training*, involves feeding a subset of these labeled patterns into a multivariate pattern classification algorithm. Based on these patterns, the classifier learns a function that maps between voxel activity patterns and the labels (Figure 17.1C). Most MVPA studies have used *linear classification algorithms* such as linear support vector machines (Kamitani & Tong, 2005; Cox & Savoy, 2003; Mitchell *et al.*, 2004) and neural network classifiers without a hidden layer (Polyn *et al.*, 2005). Linear classifiers compute a weighted sum of voxel activity values. In some classifiers, this weighted sum is then passed through a decision function, which effectively creates a threshold for saying whether or not a category is present. The linear classifiers listed above all adjust weights in order to optimize the network's ability to predict the labels of the training data; the details of how the weights are adjusted vary from classifier to classifier. For further discussion of how linear classifiers and other (non-linear) classifiers have been applied to neuroimaging data, see Norman *et al.* (2006b).

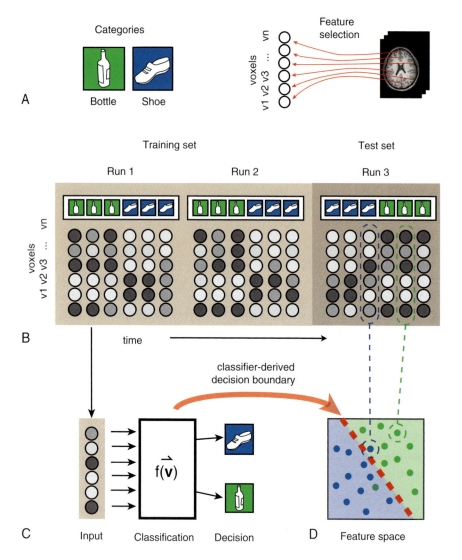

Figure 17.1 Illustration of a hypothetical experiment and how it could be analysed using MVPA. (A) Subjects view stimuli from two object categories (bottles and shoes). A feature selection procedure is used to determine which voxels will be included in the classification analysis. (B) The fMRI time series is decomposed into discrete brain patterns that correspond to the pattern of activity across the selected voxels at a particular point in time. Each brain pattern is labeled according to the corresponding experimental condition (bottle vs. shoe). The patterns are divided into a training set and a testing set. (C) Patterns from the training set are used to train a classifier function that maps between brain patterns and experimental conditions. (D) The trained classifier function $f(\vec{v})$ defines a decision boundary (red dashed line) in the high-dimensional space of voxel patterns (collapsed here to 2-D for illustrative purposes). Each dot corresponds to a pattern, and the colour of the dot indicates its category. The background colour of the figure corresponds to the guess the classifier makes for patterns in that region. The trained classifier is used to predict category membership for patterns from the test set. The figure shows one example of the classifier correctly identifying a bottle pattern (green dot) as a bottle, and one example of the classifier misidentifying a shoe pattern (blue dot) as a bottle. Figure reprinted from Norman *et al.* (2006b) with permission from Elsevier.

The fourth step is *generalization testing*. In this step, the classifier is given new patterns of brain activity that were not presented at training (and were not used for feature selection). For each pattern, the classifier is asked to generate an estimate of the subject's cognitive state (Figure 17.1D). If the new brain patterns have already been labeled (in this example, as shoes vs. bottles), we can evaluate the classifier's performance by seeing whether it predicts the correct label. However, for many MVPA applications the brain patterns in the generalization set have not been labeled (i.e. we do not know the 'ground truth' of which cognitive state the subject is in at that moment). In this case, we can evaluate the classifier based on whether its estimate of the subject's cognitive state predicts the subject's behaviour. This point is discussed in further detail below.

MVPA examples

Over the past several years, MVPA methods have been applied to a very wide range of problems, ranging from decoding the direction of movement of a viewed field of dots (Kamitani & Tong, in press) to decoding whether a subject intends to perform an addition or subtraction operation on two numbers (Haynes *et al.*, 2007). For a more complete listing of MVPA studies, see Norman *et al.* (2006b) and Haynes and Rees (2006).

Generating a temporal trace

Importantly, the increased sensitivity afforded by MVPA methods makes it possible to measure the presence/absence of cognitive states based on only a few seconds' worth of brain activity. If the cognitive states in question are sufficiently distinct from one another, discrimination can be well above chance based on single brain scans (acquired over a period of approximately 2–4 s) (Haynes & Rees, 2005a, 2005b; Polyn *et al.*, 2005; Mitchell *et al.*, 2004; O'Toole *et al.*, 2005; Carlson *et al.*, 2003; LaConte *et al.*, 2003; LaConte, Strother, Cherkassky, Anderson, & Hu, 2005; Strother *et al.*, 2004; Mourao-Miranda, Bokde, Born, Hampel, & Stetter, 2005). This increase in temporal resolution makes it possible to create a temporal trace of the waxing and waning of a particular cognitive state over the course of the experiment, which (in turn) can be related to subjects' ongoing behaviour. For example, MVPA has been used to predict ongoing recall behaviour in a free recall task (Polyn *et al.*, 2005) (see *Case Study 1*, below), and it has also been used to predict changes in perceived stimulus dominance during a binocular rivalry task (Haynes & Rees, 2005b). The results of the 2006 Pittsburgh brain activity interpretation competition provide another example of how MVPA can be used to predict time-varying aspects of subjects' cognitive state (see http://www.ebc.pitt.edu/2006/competition.html). For this competition, subjects were scanned while they watched three episodes of the television show 'Home Improvement' and then rated several aspects of their experience (e.g. subjects generated time-varying, real-valued ratings of how amused they were while watching the show, etc.). The winning entrants in this competition were able to decode several time-varying aspects of subjects' cognitive state, raging from subjective factors (amusement ratings) to more 'objective' factors (whether tools were being used on screen).

Testing psychological theories of memory with MVPA

The above discussion of MVPA illustrates how this method can be used to track subjects' cognitive state over time. The rest of the chapter is focused on how we can use this 'thought-tracking' ability to test psychological theories of memory.[2] At a high level, psychological theories can be construed as collections of 'if-then' statements: *If* the subject is in a particular cognitive state, *then* a particular outcome should take place. The standard, behavioural approach to testing theories is to set up experimental conditions that you expect will bring about the cognitive state of interest, and then look for the predicted outcome. The difficulty with this approach is that the mapping between experimental conditions and cognitive states is not perfect: Within a particular condition, subjects might slip in and out of the cognitive state of interest. As such, when the predicted outcome is not observed, there are always two possible explanations for this failure:

• The first explanation is that the theory is incorrect (i.e. the cognitive state in question does not elicit the predicted outcome).

• The second explanation is that the experiment did not succeed in eliciting the cognitive state of interest. In this case, the experiment's failure to elicit the predicted outcome does not speak to the validity (or lack thereof) of the theory in question.

One way of summarizing this point is that there is almost always variability in subjects' cognitive state, above and beyond the variability that is directly driven by the experimental manipulation. In analyses that focus on comparing experimental conditions, this extra variability is treated as a source of noise and makes it harder to see the predicted effect.

MVPA gives us a way of addressing this problem: Instead of simply assuming that experimental conditions are effective in eliciting the cognitive state of interest, we can use MVPA to track that cognitive state and relate it to outcomes of interest. In paradigms where there is extensive uncontrolled variance in subjects' cognitive state, this approach gives us a much more sensitive way of testing theories of how cognitive states drive behaviour. Another benefit of MVPA is that it allows for more unconstrained designs: Instead of trying to lock in subjects' cognitive state, MVPA gives us the option of letting subjects' cognitive state 'float' more naturally. So long as the classifier has been trained to detect fluctuations in the cognitive states of interest, we can use the classifier to soak up variance in the subject's cognitive state and explore the consequences of these fluctuations.

[2] There are other ways to apply MVPA to theory-testing, in addition to tracking thoughts over time. For example, MVPA can be used to test theories regarding the *similarity-structure* of cognitive states. To a first approximation, similar cognitive states should be associated with similar brain states. As such, it should be possible to make inferences about cognitive similarity (e.g. whether bottles are more similar to scissors than to faces) based on the similarity of the multi-voxel patterns associated with these states. For an example of this approach, see O'Toole *et al.* (2005), and for a review of relevant studies see Norman *et al.* (2006b).

Case studies

In the remaining part of section, we will present three case studies from our laboratory of how MVPA can be used to test psychological theories of memory.

All three experiments consist of two distinct parts:

- *Data for classifier training*: One part of the experiment is devoted to strongly and unambiguously eliciting the cognitive states of interest. Data from this part of the experiment are used to train the classifier to recognize these cognitive states.
- *Data for theory testing*: In the other part of the experiment, the trained classifier is then applied to new data (not presented at training) where the cognitive state(s) of interest are more variable. We then relate classifier's readout of the subject's cognitive state during this period to the subject's behaviour, in order to test whether the subject's cognitive state predicts behaviour in the manner predicted by the theory being tested.

The three case studies are as follows: In the first case study, we discuss how MVPA can be used to evaluate *contextual reinstatement* theories of recall (Polyn *et al.*, 2005). In the second, we use MVPA to test some basic predictions of dual-process models of recognition (Quamme & Norman, 2006). In the third, we discuss how pattern classification methods can be applied to EEG data to track the fine-grained temporal dynamics of competition between mental representations (Newman & Norman, 2006). We also discuss how this approach can be used to test theories of how competition drives learning. Note that the latter two case studies report preliminary data. Our focus here is primarily on explaining the logic of the studies and demonstrating the feasibility of the MVPA approach to theory-testing.

Case study 1: Testing contextual reinstatement

A recent study by Polyn *et al.* (2005) set out to test the *contextual reinstatement* hypothesis of memory search (Tulving & Thompson, 1973; Bartlett, 1932). This hypothesis states that subjects target memories from a particular episode (or type of episode) by trying to reactivate characteristic patterns of mental activity from the to-be-remembered event. To the extent that subjects succeed in aligning the pattern of mental activity at recall with the general pattern of mental activity that was present at study, this will trigger recall of specific details from the event. The contextual reinstatement hypothesis can be framed as an 'if-then' statement in the following manner: If the subject's cognitive state at test matches the general properties of their cognitive state at study, then specific details should come to mind.

To test this hypothesis, MVPA methods were used to calculate the degree to which patterns of brain activity recorded during recall matched those seen during the initial encoding phase, on a time-varying basis. During the initial part of the experiment, subjects studied celebrity faces, famous locations, and common objects. Each stimulus category was studied using a different encoding task (for faces, subjects were asked how much they liked the celebrity; for locations, subjects were asked how much they would like to visit that location; and for objects subjects were asked how often they encounter that object). A neural network classifier was trained (separately for each subject) to recognize the pattern of brain activity corresponding to studying faces, locations, and objects. Then, subjects were asked to recall (in any order they liked, over a three-minute period) the names of all of the faces, locations, and objects that they had studied earlier in the experiment, and the classifier was used to track the re-emergence (during this recall period) of brain patterns from the study phase.

This design conforms to the general design principles outlined earlier: The classifier is trained using data from a part of the experiment where cognitive states are relatively well-controlled (the study phase), and the trained classifier is used to track mental activity from a part of the experiment where cognitive states are more variable (the recall phase).

There were two key predictions: (1) During the recall period, subjects' brain state should come into alignment with brain states associated with studying faces, locations, and objects. (2) Reinstatement of study-phase activity associated with a particular category should predict recall of specific items from that category. Also, to the extent to that reinstatement is (at least in part) causing recall of specific items, reinstatement of category-specific study-phase activity should start to occur before recall of items from that category.

One thing to note about this design is that (because of MVPA) we can test the contextual reinstatement hypothesis without specifically asking subjects to reinstate context: Rather, we can let subjects' cognitive state fluctuate and explore the extent to which contextual reinstatement occurs naturally.

In keeping with the idea that subjects think about general event properties in order to remember specific details, Polyn *et al.* (2005) found that fluctuations in the strength of 'neural reinstatement' over time were highly correlated with subjects' recall behaviour. Figure 17.2A illustrates the close correspondence between classifier estimates of category-specific reinstatement and recall behaviour in a single representative subject. Also, in keeping with the idea that reinstatement precedes (and triggers) recall, Polyn *et al.* (2005) found that – on average – category-specific patterns of brain activity (associated with studying faces, locations, and objects) started to emerge approximately 5 s before recall of specific items from that category (Figure 17.2B). This study is not the first to show reinstatement of study-phase brain activity during recall (Wheeler, Petersen, & Buckner, 2000; Nyberg, Habib, & Tulving, 2000; Wheeler & Buckner, 2003; Kahn, Davachi, & Wagner, 2004; Smith, Henson, Dolan, & Rugg, 2004). The main difference between the Polyn *et al.* study and these other studies is that, because of the increased sensitivity of the MVPA approach, Polyn *et al.* were able to track the temporal dynamics of reinstatement over the course of the recall period and relate these dynamics to second-by-second changes in behaviour.

Methodologically, the Polyn *et al.* (2005) study is significant insofar as it provides 'proof of concept' that we can track cognitive states during an unconstrained memory retrieval task. Theoretically, the finding that reinstatement precedes recall provides some initial evidence in support of the contextual reinstatement hypothesis. However, more work is needed to evaluate this hypothesis. Insofar as the to-be-recalled items in the

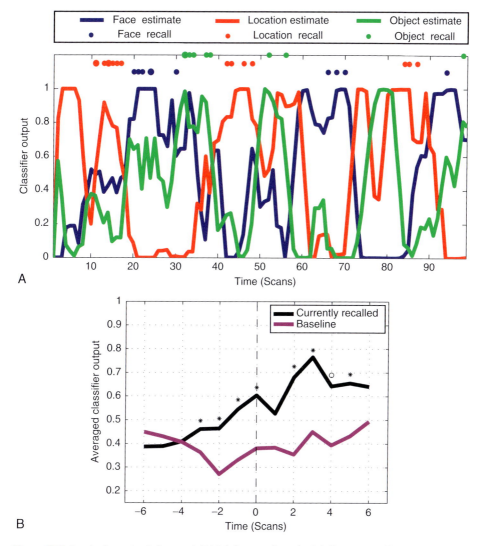

Figure 17.2 Results from the Polyn *et al.* (2005) free recall study. (A) Illustration of how brain activity during recall relates to recall behaviour, in a single subject. Each point on the x-axis corresponds to a single brain scan (acquired over a period of 1.8 seconds, during the 3 min recall period). The blue, red, and green lines correspond to the classifier's estimate as to how strongly the subject is reinstating brain patterns characteristic of face-study, location-study, and object-study at that point in time. The blue, red, and green dots indicate time points where subjects recalled faces, locations, and objects; the dots were shifted forward by three time-points, to account for the lag in the peak haemodynamic response. The graph illustrates the strong correspondence between the classifier's estimate of category-specific brain activity, and the subject's actual recall behaviour. (B) Event-related average (incorporating data from nine subjects) of the classifier's estimates of category-specific brain activity, for the time intervals surrounding recall events. This graph shows that the classifier starts to detect the to-be-recalled category several seconds before recall occurs. The dotted line at t = 0 represents the time point at which the verbal recall was made. The Currently Recalled plot (black line) shows average classifier activity for the category that was recalled at t = 0. The Baseline plot (purple line) shows average classifier activity for the two categories that were not recalled at t = 0. Points marked with stars and circles differ from baseline at p < 0.01 and p < 0.05, respectively. For additional details of how the plot was computed see Polyn *et al.* (2005). Parts a and b both adapted with permission from Polyn *et al.* (2005).

Polyn *et al.* (2005) study came from different semantic categories, it is possible that reinstatement effects in that study simply reflect subjects thinking about the semantic (categorical) properties of the items themselves, as opposed to subjects reinstating their 'mindset' from the study phase (which should include information about how items were processed at study and how they were presented, in addition to core semantic features of the items). A much stronger test of the contextual reinstatement hypothesis would be to design an experiment where the same types of items are presented in different 'contexts' (e.g. stimuli could be randomly selected words), and the only thing that differs across contexts is how the items are presented perceptually at study (e.g. words could be presented on top of different backgrounds) and/or how they are processed at study (e.g. different encoding tasks could be used for the different contexts). Experiments that fit this description are presently underway in our laboratory. We are also running studies that track contextual reinstatement in paradigms other than free recall (Frankel, Robison, & Norman, 2006).

Case study 2: Testing dual-process models of recognition

In the second case study, we explore how MVPA can be used to help test *dual-process* theories of recognition memory. The basic idea behind these theories is that recognition judgements can be driven by two distinct sources of information: Recollection of specific studied details and non-specific feelings of familiarity. For a review of dual-process theories, see Yonelinas (2002). In recent years, researchers have started to develop computational models of recollection and familiarity, such as the Complementary Learning Systems (*CLS*) model (Norman & O'Reilly, 2003) and the Source of Activation Confusion (*SAC*) model (Reder *et al.*, 2000). These models can be used to generate specific predictions about how a given manipulation will affect recollection and familiarity.

The major challenge that arises in testing the predictions of dual-process models of recognition is deciding how to combine the recollection and familiarity signals, in order to generate predictions about overall recognition performance (Wixted & Stretch, 2004). Put another way, how much should subjects 'weight' recollection vs. familiarity when making a recognition decision?

Most dual-process models use very simple decision-making rules, where subjects' use of recollection vs. familiarity does not vary as a function of situational factors. For example, Jacoby, Yonelinas, and Jennings (1997) and Norman and O'Reilly (2003) use a decision rule whereby subjects always consult recollection first; if the level of recollection is below a pre-specified threshold, then subjects consult familiarity. However, contrary to this view of dual-process decision-making (whereby recollection always takes precedence over familiarity), extant data suggest that numerous situational factors can influence the extent to which subjects rely on recollection. For example, Malmberg and Xu (2007) explored subjects' utilization of recollection in an associative recognition paradigm, where subjects have to discriminate studied word pairs from *re-paired lures* generated by re-combining words from studied pairs. In this paradigm, familiarity and recollection have opposing effects on false recognition of re-paired lures: The fact that the individual items in the pair are familiar pushes subjects to say 'old' but recollection of the actual pairs that were studied (i.e. 'I studied window-banana, not window-shoebox') pushes subjects to say 'new'. To measure how strongly subjects were relying on recollection vs. familiarity, Malmberg and Xu (2007) measured how repeating pairs at study affects false recognition of re-paired lures: To the extent that subjects rely on familiarity, repeating pairs at study should boost false alarms (by making the items in re-paired lures more familiar). However, to the extent that subjects utilize recollection, repeating pairs at study should reduce false alarms (by increasing the odds that subjects will recollect the pairs they actually studied when given a re-paired lure at test).

The key finding from Malmberg and Xu (2007) was that subjects' use of recollection was modulated by various aspects of the test procedure: Asking subjects to give confidence ratings at test and asking subjects to delay their responses both increased subjects' use of recollection. Also, adding novel-item lures to the test (in addition to re-paired lures) reduced the extent to which subjects relied on recollection for the re-paired lures. Intuitively, the presence of novel items at test makes familiarity more useful (overall) as a basis for discriminating studied items vs. lures, reducing subjects' incentive to use recollection.

Variability in subjects' use of recollection can be explained in terms of two ideas: First, several studies have demonstrated that (over the course of a retrieval attempt) information about stimulus familiarity becomes available more quickly than recollected details (e.g. Hintzman & Curran, 1994; Gronlund & Ratcliff, 1989; Rotello & Heit, 1999). As such, recollection should play less of a role when subjects are responding relatively quickly. Second, using recollection requires more cognitive effort than using familiarity. For example Gruppuso, Lindsay and Kelley (1997) found that dual-task demands hurt recollection-based responding more than familiarity-based responding. The idea that there is an 'effort cost' associated with recollection-based responding implies that subjects will only draw upon recollection to the extent that the benefits (in terms of increased performance) outweigh the costs (in terms of increased effort and time).

Implications for theory-testing

The fact that subjects can strategically vary their use of recollection makes it difficult to test behavioural predictions of dual-process models. For example, the Complementary Learning Systems (CLS) model predicts that increasing *list strength* (i.e. strengthening some items on the list but not others) should impair recollection of non-strengthened studied items, but it should not impair subjects' ability to discriminate non-strengthened studied items from lures based on familiarity. To the extent that both recollection and familiarity contribute to recognition and increasing list strength impairs recollection, this implies that list strength should also impair overall recognition sensitivity. However, several studies have failed to find a list strength effect for overall recognition sensitivity (e.g. Ratcliff, Clark, & Shiffrin, 1990). As discussed by Norman (2002), there are two possible interpretations of this finding:

• The first possibility is that the model is wrong, and that list strength does not affect recollection or familiarity.

- The second possibility is that the model is correct (i.e. list strength does affect recollection) but, for whatever reason, subjects were not making use of recollection in the studies that failed to find a list strength effect.

Put another way: 'Use of recollection' is an uncontrolled variable in these studies and this makes it difficult to evaluate predictions about the properties of recollection (when it is being used). To address this problem, it is necessary to take steps to eliminate this uncontrolled variance.

There are two ways to address this uncontrolled variance: The standard approach is to adjust the paradigm in order to boost subjects' use of recollection. For example, to specifically address how list strength affects recollection, Norman (2002) explored list strength effects using a *plurality recognition* paradigm. In this paradigm, subjects have to discriminate between studied items, unrelated lures, and also switched-plurality lures (e.g. study 'rats', test with 'rat'). Prior work with this paradigm has established that discrimination of studied items and switched-plurality lures relies heavily on recollection of plurality information (familiarity is not useful insofar as switched-plurality lures are also familiar; Hintzman, Curran, & Oppy, 1992; Hintzman & Curran, 1994; Curran, 2000). To the extent that plurality discrimination depends on recollection, and list strength impairs recollection, increasing list strength should impair plurality discrimination. This prediction was confirmed by Norman (2002).

A different approach to the problem of uncontrolled variance in 'use of recollection' is to use MVPA to extract a time-varying measure (based on brain activity) of whether subjects are using recollection. This approach potentially has several advantages over the first approach (i.e. adjusting the paradigm to boost subjects' reliance on recollection):

- The first advantage is that MVPA can be used to study the properties of recollection in a wider range of situations. So long as subjects are using recollection on some fraction of the test trials, we can use the classifier's readout of 'use of recollection' to restrict the analysis to those trials.

- A second, related advantage is that this approach lets us collect data on how subjects vary their use of recollection on their own (i.e. when their strategies are not being strongly constrained), which will help us refine our theories of dual-process decision-making.

- A final point is that there are limits on our ability to control recollection: Even in the plurality paradigm, it seems likely that the level of effort that subjects expend on trying to retrieve specific details will wax and wane over time, which has implications for their behaviour.

Paradigm details

Here, we present results from our initial attempt to use MVPA to track subjects' use of recollection (Quamme & Norman, 2006). Our long-term goal is to use this technology to test sophisticated predictions of dual-process models, such as the list strength prediction described above. However, for our initial foray into this area, we decided to focus on a basic and relatively uncontroversial prediction of dual-process models: the idea (discussed above) that recollection of studied details can be used to oppose the familiarity of lures that are similar to studied items, thereby helping subjects avoid false recognition of these items.

To explore this idea, we used the plurality recognition paradigm described above (Hintzman *et al.*, 1992). In this paradigm, familiarity pushes subjects to respond 'old' to switched plurality lures, but recollection of studied plurality information pushes subjects to say 'new' to these items. Thus, the straightforward prediction is that *if* subjects are using recollection, *then* they will be less likely to false alarm to switched-plurality lures.

As with our previous case study, this study used a two-phase design:

The goal of phase 1 was to train the classifier to recognize brain states associated with intentionally using recollection to make recognition judgements vs. making recognition judgements based on familiarity. Subjects studied singular and plural words. For each stimulus, subjects were asked to mentally picture multiple objects if the word was plural and single objects if the word was singular (e.g. picture multiple shoes for the word 'shoes' and a single shoe for the word 'shoe'). After the study phase, subjects were scanned while they were given recognition tests comprised of studied items (rats) and unrelated lures (bicycle); subjects were not given switched-plurality lures during this phase of the experiment. The key manipulation was to divide up the test into *recollection blocks* and *familiarity blocks*. For recollection blocks, subjects were told that they should try to recall specific details of the metal image they formed at study, and respond 'yes' only if they were successful. For familiarity blocks, subjects were instructed to say 'yes' if the word seemed familiar, and to ignore any details that they might recollect from the study phase. The classifier was trained to discriminate between brain patterns from recollection blocks and brain patterns from familiarity blocks.

Note that, although subjects were asked to focus on either recollection or familiarity (but not both) during phase 1, the classifier training procedure does not assume that recollection and familiarity are mutually exclusive. The only assumption that we make is that subjects rely relatively more on recollection during recollection blocks vs. familiarity blocks. The output of a classifier trained using this procedure indicates the *relative extent* to which subjects are relying on recollection vs. familiarity (i.e. does the pattern of brain activity more closely resemble the pattern associated with *relatively high* use of recollection, or does it more closely resemble the pattern associated with *relatively low* use of recollection).

The goal of phase 2 was to use the trained classifier to explore subjects' use of recollection and familiarity, and to relate the classifier activity to behaviour. Here, subjects were scanned while they were given a recognition test containing studied items, unrelated lures, and switched-plurality lures. Crucially, during this phase, subjects were not given any specific advice about whether to use recollection vs. familiarity to make their judgements. The trained classifier was used to estimate (on a scan-by-scan basis) how closely the subject's brain state resembled their brain state during recollection blocks vs. familiarity blocks from phase 1.

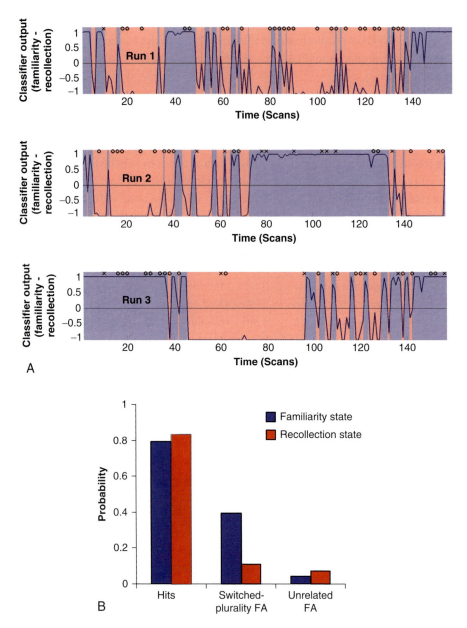

Figure 17.3 Classification results for phase two (plurals test) data from a single subject. (A) Classifier output as a function of time for three runs of the plurality recognition task (each time point corresponds to a single brain scan, acquired over a 2 s period) The output measure plotted on the y-axis is the classifier's estimate of how well the brain activity matches the 'familiarity state' from phase 1, minus the classifier's estimate of how well brain activity matches the 'recollection state' from phase 1. Blue regions indicate time points where, according to the classifier, the subject is in a familiarity state (familiarity > recollection); red regions indicate time points where, according to the classifier, the subject is in a recollection state (recollection > familiarity). Symbols ('o' and 'x') at the top of each panel indicate time points when switched-plurality lures were presented. An 'o' indicates a correct rejection by the subject

Predictions

As discussed above, we predicted that subjects would be more likely to falsely recognize switched-plurality lures when their brain is in a familiarity state vs. when their brain is in a recollection state. Importantly, while we expected an effect of familiarity vs. recollection state on responding to switched-plurality lures, we did not expect to see an effect of familiarity vs. recollection state on responding to studied items. For studied items, familiarity and recollection push responding in the same direction (i.e. they both push subjects to make an 'old' response), so responding to studied items should be similar regardless of how much subjects are utilizing familiarity vs. recollection. The same logic applies to unrelated lures: These items are associated with low familiarity values and low levels of recollection. Both of these factors should push subjects to say 'new', so responding to unrelated lures should be generally similar when subjects are utilizing familiarity vs. recollection.

Results

The first step in the classification analysis was to assess whether the classifier was able to reliably discriminate between brain states associated with recollection blocks vs. familiarity blocks in phase 1. If the classifier is unable to discriminate between recollection and familiarity blocks in phase 1, there is no reason to expect that the classifier will be able to accurately track subjects' use of recollection vs. familiarity in phase 2. To assess phase 1 accuracy, we trained the classifier on 3/4 of the phase 1 data and tested its ability to classify individual brain scans from the remaining 1/4 of the data. Across all 10 subjects, average classification accuracy was 0.59, which was significantly above 0.50 (chance), $p < 0.01$. Inspection of individual accuracy scores revealed that classification was well above chance for 6/10 subjects (accuracy > 0.60), and classification was basically at chance (accuracy between 0.48 and 0.53) for the remaining 4/10 subjects.[3] All subsequent analyses (exploring how a classifier trained on phase 1 generalizes to phase 2) were only run on the six subjects who showed above-chance classification performance on the phase 1 data. Representative results from phase 2 (the plurals test) from one of these six subjects are shown in Figure 17.3. Part A plots (over time) the classifier's readout of whether the

---

[3] We hypothesize that chance performance in these subjects was due to high rates of involuntary recollection during 'familiarity blocks'. In more recent versions of the experiment, we have tried to reduce involuntary recollection by speeding up the stimulus presentation rate at test during phase 1. This change has led to a substantial improvement in classification accuracy (in the updated version of the experiment, mean accuracy = 0.71 across 12 subjects, $SEM = 0.03$).

---

and an 'x' indicates a false alarm. These labels have been shifted forward by three time-points, to account for the lag in the peak haemodynamic response. (B) Bar graph showing the proportion of hits (correct 'old' responses to studied items) and false alarms (FA; incorrect 'old' responses to switched plurality lures and unrelated lures), as a function of whether (according to the classifier) the subject was in a familiarity state or a recollection state for that item. The figure shows that false alarms for switched-plurality lures were greater when the subject was in a familiarity state vs. a recollection state, but that no such difference was present for hits or for unrelated lure false alarms.

subject's current brain state more closely resembles the 'familiarity' brain state from phase 1 or the 'recollection' brain state from phase 1. Part B plots (for this subject) the rate of saying 'old' to studied items, switched-plurality lures, and unrelated lures, as a function of whether (according to the classifier) the subject was relying on recollection vs. familiarity. As predicted, false recognition of switched-plurality lures was higher when the subject was in a familiarity brain state vs. a recollection brain state, but responding to studied items and unrelated lures was relatively unaffected by whether the subject was in a familiarity brain state vs. a recollection brain state. We used non-parametric Monte Carlo statistical procedures to test the significance of individual-subject results. These procedures involve randomly scrambling the data and assessing the likelihood of obtaining the observed differences between 'recollection state' vs. 'familiarity state' behaviour, assuming no actual difference between conditions (for additional details regarding our non-parametric statistical procedures, see Polyn et al., 2005). For the subject shown in Figure 17.3, the difference in switched-plurality false alarms was significant ($p = 0.014$), as was the interaction between trial type (studied item, switched-plurality lure, and unrelated lure) and recollection/familiarity state ($p = 0.025$), indicating that recollection/familiarity state differentially affects responding to switched-plurality lures. We also ran a group analysis (across the 6 subjects who showed above-chance phase 1 classification) using standard parametric statistics (an ANOVA on the per-subject means) and obtained the same pattern of results: There was a significant effect of recollection/familiarity state on switched-plurality false alarms and a significant trial type X recollection/familiarity interaction; the effect of recollection/familiarity state on responding to studied items and unrelated lures was not significant.

Discussion

The pilot results presented above provide preliminary evidence that we can track subjects' use of recollection. Here, we discuss two current & future directions for this work. One major direction is *functional localization*: using MVPA to map out which brain regions contribute to subjects' use of recollection vs. familiarity, and how these regions contribute. We also briefly describe how we can extend our analysis procedure to address more complex types of strategic variability.

With regard to functional localization: Numerous studies have used conventional, individual-voxel-based fMRI analysis methods to identify brain regions that are differentially activated when subjects are orienting to recollected details (e.g. judging the source of an item) vs. responding to item familiarity (see Wagner et al., 2005 for a review). These studies have identified a network of parietal regions (including the precuneus, retrosplenial cortex, posterior cingulate, and lateral parietal areas in and around the intraparietal sulcus) and frontal regions that are differentially recruited by tasks that place demands on recollection vs. familiarity. At this point in time, however, it is unclear *how* these regions are contributing. As discussed by Wagner et al. (2005), there are at least two reasons why a brain region might activate more strongly when subjects are trying to recollect details: One possibility is that the region helps to establish an *internally directed attentional state* ('listening for recollection') that amplifies hippocampal output. Another possibility is that the region implements processes that *operate on retrieved information*. For example, several researchers have argued that parietal regions may serve to accumulate evidence during decision-making (e.g. Huk & Shadlen, 2005; Ploran *et al.*, 2007; Shadlen & Newsome, 2001).

To specify which regions contribute and how they contribute, we are currently running a variant of the pilot study described above, where – instead of applying the classifier to whole-brain patterns of activity – we are applying the classifier to patterns of activity from localized brain regions. Specifically, we are using the 'searchlight' procedure mentioned in the *MVPA methods* section above (Kriegeskorte *et al.*, 2006). This procedure involves sweeping a spherical searchlight (radius = 3 voxels) around the brain. For each location of the searchlight, we apply our two-phase classifier analysis (train on phase 1, generalize to phase 2) to the pattern of activity within the searchlight. The goal of this analysis is to find searchlight locations where the pattern of activity within the searchlight reliably discriminates between recollection vs. familiarity blocks during phase 1, and where the output of the classifier during phase 2 predicts behaviour in the manner specified previously (i.e. classifier output indicating 'recollection state' is associated with a decrease in false alarms to switched-plurality lures, but hits and unrelated-lure false alarms are relatively unaffected).

This searchlight procedure tells us, in an unbiased fashion, which regions carry information about subjects' use of recollection. Importantly, we should also be able to gain insight into how these regions contribute by examining *when* (relative to stimulus onset) classifier activity predicts behaviour. If a brain region contributes to internally-directed attention, it should be possible to use the pattern of activity *prior to stimulus onset* to determine whether the subject is 'listening to recollection' at that point in time. This information should (in turn) give us some ability to predict how the subject will respond to a test item, *before the test item actually appears*. In contrast, if a brain region is involved in processing recollected information, then the pattern of activity in that region should predict behaviour *after* stimulus onset but not *before* stimulus onset. Importantly, it may be that some of the brain regions identified in the Wagner *et al.* (2005) review show timing profiles consistent with internally directed attention, and other regions show timing profiles that are more consistent with some kind of post-retrieval processing. We are examining these possibilities in our current work (Quamme, Weiss, & Norman, 2007).

In addition to exploring functional localization, we also plan to explore more complex models of strategic variability. As described earlier, our current paradigm allows us to measure the relative extent to which subjects are relying on recollection vs. familiarity. This measurement procedure assumes that subjects' recognition strategies vary along a single dimension (indicating the relative mix of recollection vs. familiarity). We consider this simple model to be a good starting point for our investigations of strategic processes in recognition memory, but we also acknowledge the possibility that subjects' strategies may vary along multiple dimensions. In particular, subjects may be able to independently vary their use of recollection and their use of familiarity (see, e.g. Wixted & Stretch, 2004). To accommodate this more complex model, we could add a third, 'baseline' condition to phase 1. During baseline blocks, subjects would be asked to make simple perceptual judgements about studied and non-studied words instead of recognition memory judgements. The presence of this third condition would force the classifier to discriminate recollection and familiarity states (individually) from the brain pattern that is present when subjects are not trying to use recollection *or* familiarity. During phase 2, a classifier trained in this fashion should be able to separately compute the strength of the recollection pattern vs. baseline and the strength of the familiarity pattern vs. baseline.

One final point regarding this case study is that, while we have focused on recollection and familiarity, the approach described here is quite general: In principle, it can be applied to any situation where there are multiple sources of information that could be used in making a decision, and subjects can choose to rely on some sources of information more than others.

Case study 3: Classifying EEG and tracking competitive dynamics

The fMRI classification methods described above are appropriate for tracking cognitive processes that vary on the order of seconds. This level of temporal resolution makes it possible to test theories about how cognitive processes vary across trials (or how cognitive processes vary across an extended recall attempt, as in the Polyn *et al.*, 2005 study). However, temporal resolution of fMRI pattern classification is insufficient to address hypotheses about within-trial dynamics. For example, building on work by Anderson (2003) and others, Norman, Newman, and Detre (2007) developed a computational model of how competition between stored memory representations during a retrieval attempt can drive strengthening or weakening of the competing memories. To directly test this theory, we need a way of tracking the activation of memory representations as they compete, over the course of a single trial. Insofar as the retrieval competition plays out on the order of tens of milliseconds (as opposed to seconds), there is no easy way to accomplish this goal using fMRI.

To address this problem, we have started to explore ways of extending our pattern classification methods to other imaging modalities with better temporal resolution than fMRI (in particular, EEG). Pattern classification of EEG has a long history; most applications of EEG pattern-classification have focused on decoding movement-related activity (e.g. Peters, Pfurtscheller, & Flyvbjerg, 1998; Parra *et al.*, 2002; Muller-Putz, Scherer, Pfurtscheller, & Rupp, 2005; Vallabhaineni & He, 2004; Wang, Deng, & He, 2004), although a few recent studies have used pattern classifiers to decode perceptually-related cognitive states (Philiastides & Sajda, 2006; Philiastides, Ratcliff, & Sajda, 2006).

This case study is divided up into two parts: First, we describe our preliminary attempts to classify subjects' cognitive state based on EEG data. Second, we describe how we plan to use these methods to test theoretical accounts of how competitive dynamics drive learning. All of the results presented below were initially reported by Newman and Norman (2006).

Classifying EEG

In our initial explorations of EEG classification, we used a delayed match to sample task, where subjects saw a *sample* stimulus (a photo of a face, a house, a chair, or a shoe), followed by a 500 ms mask, followed by a *probe* stimulus (see Figure 17.4 parts A and B). When the probe stimulus appeared, subjects had to judge whether the probe stimulus matched the sample stimulus. The probe was either the same photo (in which case subjects were instructed to respond 'yes') or a photo of a different item from the same category (in which case subjects were instructed to respond 'no').

The goal of our preliminary analyses was to see whether we could train a classifier (based on EEG data collected during the sample stimulus presentation) to discriminate between trials where subjects were viewing a face, a house, a chair, or a shoe (for related work, see Philiastides & Sajda, 2006 and Philiastides *et al.*, 2006, who showed that it is possible to decode whether a subject is viewing a face or a car based on single-trial EEG). EEG data were collected using a 79 electrode cap, using a 1000 Hz sampling rate. After removing trials with excessive noise or blinks, we ran a wavelet decomposition on the data for each electrode to extract (for each EEG sample) oscillatory power at 49 frequency bands between 2 and 128 Hz. Then, for each trial, we computed the average oscillatory power value (for each frequency/electrode combination) for each of the 20 ms 'time bins' relative to the onset of the stimulus.

In the fMRI classification analyses described in *Case Studies 1 and 2*, the 'brain patterns' that we fed into the classifier were vectors of voxel activity values (see Figure 17.1). For our EEG classification analyses, we applied a classifier to vectors of oscillatory power values, where each 'feature' in the vector corresponds oscillatory power at a particular frequency, electrode, and time bin (relative to stimulus onset). As in our fMRI analyses, we did not run our classification analyses on the entire feature set: Only features that individually showed significant discrimination between categories (as indexed by a non-parametric statistical procedure) were used for classification. Finally, in keeping with the idea that different features could discriminate at different time points in the trial, we trained a separate classifier for each time bin (so, one classifier was trained to discriminate between stimulus categories based on data collected 0–20 ms post-stimulus-onset; another classifier was trained to discriminate based on data collected 20–40 ms post-stimulus-onset; and so on).

To test the classifier's generalization performance, we used a cross-validation procedure where the classifier was trained on 9/10 of the data and then tested on the remaining 1/10 of the data. Figure 17.4C plots generalization accuracy (averaged across 9 subjects) as a function of time bin. Average classification accuracy peaked at approximately 0.50 (chance = 0.25) at around 200 ms post-stimulus-onset. In light of data showing that face stimuli elicit distinctive EEG patterns (Jeffreys, 1989; Itier & Taylor, 2004; Philiastides & Sajda, 2006), one might speculate that classification performance was being driven entirely by the face/non-face distinction (e.g. perfect face/non-face discrimination, but no ability to discriminate between non-face categories, would yield perfect accuracy for faces and 0.33 accuracy for the three non-face categories, leading to 0.50 overall accuracy). To address this hypothesis, we ran a follow-up analysis where we computed accuracy by category; average accuracy for the non-face categories was 0.42. This result shows that the classifier was picking up some information about the non-face categories (albeit less than it was picking up for faces).

Testing the competitor weakening hypothesis: Applications to negative priming

The above results show that we can decode category information with well-above-chance accuracy based on 20 ms time bins of EEG data. Here, we discuss how this ability to track activation dynamics at a fine time scale can be used to test theories of how competitive dynamics affect learning.

Over the past decade, several researchers (see Anderson, 2003) have argued that retrieving a memory can have lasting consequences on memory strength, whereby the retrieved memory (the 'winner' of the competition) is strengthened and other, 'losing' memories are weakened. Crucially, Anderson has argued that this weakening effect is *competition-dependent*, such that the degree of weakening for a particular 'losing' memory is proportional to how strongly it competes at retrieval. Recently, Norman *et al.* (2007) presented a neural network model that provides a concrete neural mechanistic account of competition-dependent forgetting, and relates this phenomenon to neural oscillations (see also Norman, Newman, Detre, & Polyn, 2006a for a discussion of how competition-dependent forgetting can boost the capacity of neural networks).

A large number of semantic memory and episodic memory findings can be explained in terms of competition-dependent weakening (for reviews, see Anderson, 2003; Norman *et al.*, 2007). For example, Anderson, Bjork, and Bjork (1994) had subjects study word pairs like Fruit-Apple, Fruit-Kiwi, and Fruit-Pear; they found that practicing retrieval of Pear (using the cue Fruit-Pe) impaired subsequent retrieval of Apple (a taxonomically strong Fruit) but not Kiwi (a taxonomically weak Fruit). Anderson *et al.* (1994) explained this finding in terms of the idea that taxonomically strong exemplars like Apple compete more strongly when subjects are trying to retrieve Pear, thus they suffer more weakening.

A key prediction of the competitive learning hypothesis is that, if a non-target (competing) memory *wins* the competition, it should be strengthened, not weakened. A retrieval-induced forgetting study conducted by Johnson and Anderson (2004) provides some support for this view. In the Johnson and Anderson study, subjects were asked to practice retrieving the subordinate meaning of a homograph (e.g. given the cue 'prune', subjects were asked to retrieve the non-dominant verb meaning, 'trim', instead of the dominant noun meaning, 'fruit'). Johnson and Anderson found that, in some conditions, practicing retrieval of the subordinate meaning led to strengthening of the dominant meaning (for a similar result, see Shivde & Anderson, 2001). To explain this finding, Johnson and Anderson argued that (initially) the dominant meaning is so strong that subjects inadvertently recall it when trying to recall the subordinate meaning; since the dominant meaning wins the competition on these trials, it undergoes strengthening instead of weakening.

Another phenomenon that can potentially be explained in terms of competitor weakening is *negative priming* (e.g. Tipper, 1985; Fox, 1995). In a typical negative priming experiment, subjects are given stimulus displays consisting of two stimuli, a *target* stimulus and a *competitor* stimulus. Subjects are instructed to attend to the target stimulus and to ignore the competitor stimulus (e.g. the experiment might be set up such that the target stimulus is always tinted red, and subjects are asked to attend to the red stimulus). The key manipulation is that stimuli that serve as competitors on one trial sometimes appear as the target stimulus on later trials. Negative priming studies have found that, relative to stimuli that are being presented for the first time, subjects are faster to respond to stimuli that were previously attended and slower to respond to stimuli that were previously ignored (Tipper, 1985).

The basic pattern of negative priming results fits nicely with the competitive learning theory outlined above: Target items win the competition, so they are strengthened. Competitor items receive some support from the stimulus display (but not enough to win the competition) so they are weakened.[4] The competitive learning account may also provide a way of explaining variance in the size of the negative priming effect. For example, Fox (1994) found that reducing the spacing between the target and competitor stimuli significantly increased the magnitude of the resulting negative priming effect. Moving the competitor closer to the target should make it compete more strongly; according to the competitive learning account, this increase in competition should lead to greater suppression. Grison and Strayer (2001) found that degrading the perceptual quality of the competitor reduced the negative priming effect, supporting the idea that weaker competitors are suppressed less (see also Fox, 1998; Strayer & Grison, 1999 for additional relevant findings). There is also evidence that, if the competitor becomes strong enough to win the competition, facilitation occurs instead of suppression. For example, Fuentes, Humphreys, Agis, Carmona, and Catena (1998) found that unifying the competitor and the target into a single visual object (a manipulation thought to increase processing of the competitor) caused the otherwise significant negative priming effect to reverse and become a significant positive priming effect.

The goal of our negative priming research is to provide more direct evidence in support of the competitive learning theory. Instead of making assumptions about competitor activation in a particular condition, we can use a pattern classifier (applied to EEG data) to directly measure target and competitor activation on a trial-by-trial basis, and then use these activation values to predict subsequent reaction times to the competitor. If the competitor activates strongly (i.e. the competitor happens to 'win' on that trial), we expect to see positive priming. If the competitor activates weakly (i.e. the competitor is active, but 'loses' to the target), we expect to see negative priming. The above predictions make it clear that, according to the competitive learning theory, negative priming should only occur when competitor activation falls within a narrowly defined range; too much or too little competitor activation will reduce the weakening effect or even lead to strengthening. This situation may help to explain why negative priming effects tend to be small (on the order of 20 ms). Using the classifier to focus on the set of trials where competitor activation falls in the correct range (not too high or too low) may allow us to observe a much more robust negative priming effect.

---

[4] For additional discussion of the idea that negative priming effects are competition-dependent, see Tipper (2001), Houghton and Tipper (1994) and Gotts and Plaut (2005).

At present, this research is still ongoing and we are not yet in a position to make firm conclusions about the relationship between classifier activity and reaction time. Nonetheless, we think that our design for the study is instructive regarding the kinds of questions that one can address using MVPA (especially as applied to EEG), so we describe it below.

Negative priming experiment design

Our negative priming paradigm resembles the paradigm that we used in the preliminary classification study (described above). Subjects perform a delayed-match-to-sample task using face, house, shoe, and chair stimuli. However, in this version, each display contains two items: a *target* item (tinted red) overlaid on top of a *competitor* item (presented in greyscale) from a different category (e.g. a shoe overlaid on top of a face; see Figure 17.4D). Subjects are asked to make their match judgments based on the target item and to ignore the competitor item. Since the target and the competitor are from different categories, we can use the classifier to derive separate readouts of target and competitor activation (e.g. if the target is a shoe and the competitor is a face, we can use the classifier's readout of 'shoe' as a proxy for target activation, and we can use the classifier's readout of 'face' as a proxy for competitor activation). We then use these readouts of competitor and target activation to predict reaction time when the competitor stimulus used on this trial (e.g. the face) subsequently re-appears as a target.

Here, as in the other two case studies, we use the general approach of training on stable cognitive states and generalizing to situations where cognitive states are more variable. We reasoned that target stimuli would elicit stronger and more stable representations than competitor stimuli. As such, our analysis procedure involves training the classifier to recognize the category of the target stimulus, and then using the classifier (trained on a subset of trials) to measure the activity of the target category and the competitor category on other trials.

This analysis procedure assumes that classifiers trained to detect the target category can also detect the competitor category. Preliminary results support this view. Figure 17.4E plots (for a single subject) the average classifier output associated with the target category, the competitor category, and the two other categories not being presented on a given trial. Classifier output for the target and competitor categories was well above the level of classifier output associated with the two other categories. This finding (which was consistently present across subjects) suggests that we will be able to derive separate readouts of target and competitor activation for our negative priming study.[5]

---

[5] The results shown in Figure 17.4E are from a version of the experiment where we trained the classifier on single-image stimuli (i.e. where no competitor was present) and then applied the classifier to superimposed target-competitor images. The overall pattern of results is the same when we train the classifier to recognize the target category from superimposed target-competitor images, and then we apply the classifier to other superimposed target-competitor images.

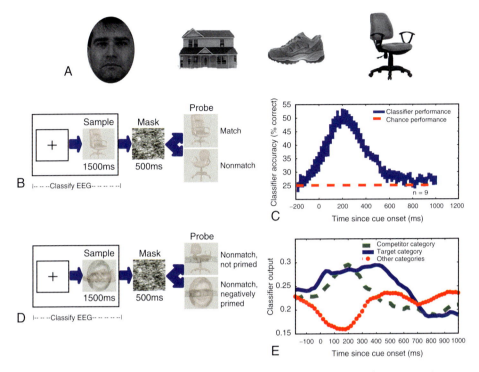

Figure 17.4 Illustration of stimuli and tasks used for EEG classification along with representative results. (A) Our studies used four categories of images: Faces, Houses, Shoes, and Chairs. (B) Illustration of the delayed-match-to-sample task used to present images to subjects. Only the EEG collected during the presentation of the sample stimulus was used to train and test the classifiers. (C) Average classifier generalization accuracy over nine subjects. The error bars indicate the standard error of the mean (across subjects). Classification rapidly increased to its peak accuracy value by approximately 200 ms and then dropped back down to chance by 600 ms (the fact that accuracy was above chance at t = 0 is an artefact of the wavelet decomposition procedure). (D) Illustration of the negative priming task. Subjects perform a delayed-match-to-sample task; they are told to focus exclusively on red images (targets) and to ignore superimposed black and white objects (competitors). On approximately 15% of trials, subjects are required to respond to the object they just ignored (e.g. the bottom example shows a trial where subjects ignore a face and then have to respond to the face). (E) Classifier output from a single representative subject for the negative priming task, showing the average activation of the target (to-be-attended) category and the competitor (to-be-ignored) category. The graph shows that both the target and competitor categories were more active, on average, than categories that were not present on screen.

Implications and perspectives on MVPA

In this paper, we presented three case studies of how MVPA can be used to test theories. In all three cases, the theory being tested could be described as an if-then rule:

- Case study 1: If *study-phase brain activity is reinstated at test*, then subjects will be more likely to recall additional studied details.

- Case study 2: If *subjects use recollection*, then subjects will be less likely to falsely recognize similar lures.

- Case study 3: If *the competing representation activates but then loses the competition*, then competitor weakening will occur (leading to a negative priming effect).

Testing these theories using MVPA involves a three-step process:

- First, we train the classifier to predict the cognitive state(s) of interest, using data from a part of the experiment where subjects' cognitive state is relatively well-controlled.

- Next, using data from a different part of the experiment (where subjects' cognitive state is less well controlled), we use the classifier to track the comings and goings of the cognitive states of interest.

- Finally, we plug these classifier estimates into theories (the if-then statements above) to generate behavioural predictions.

Effectively, this procedure is a form of bootstrapping: There are always going to be some situations where we have a relatively good understanding of what subjects are thinking, and other situations where we have a relatively poor understanding of what subjects are thinking. The goal of the multi-step procedure outlined above is to leverage our good understanding of subjects' cognitive state in one situation in order to gain insight into another (more murky) situation.

One of the key ideas motivating this approach is that the mapping between experimental conditions and cognitive states can be noisy: For example, we discussed in *Case Study 3* how it is very difficult to ensure that competitor activation falls within the range that is predicted to yield negative priming (i.e. not too high and not too low). By directly measuring the cognitive state of interest, we can soak up some of this within-condition variance that would otherwise be attributed to error. Another key benefit of MVPA is that it allows us to *covertly* measure cognitive variables of interest in situations where overtly asking about these variables might affect their strategies (e.g. asking subjects to directly report their use of recollection in *Case Study 2* might make them more likely to use recollection).

It is also worth discussing how our approach relates to concept of *reverse inference* (Poldrack, 2006). In the 2006 paper, Poldrack cautions against inferring that a cognitive process is present based on activation of a particular brain region. The problem with reverse inference is that a brain region might be activated by multiple different cognitive processes (other than the one of interest), making it impossible to ascertain which of these cognitive processes is causing the activation. To be clear, our MVPA analyses are a form of reverse inference. However, there are two properties of MVPA that mitigate the usual concerns about reverse inference. First, the patterns of activity that are detected by the classifier in MVPA are much more specific: While it is possible for a particular voxel to be involved in multiple disparate cognitive processes, the odds that a particular multi-voxel pattern will also be involved in very different kinds of cognitive processes are correspondingly lower (although perhaps not zero, depending on the pattern). The second, more important point is that we can obtain independent validation for our claims about the cognitive 'significance' of a particular brain pattern by measuring whether the presence/absence of that pattern predicts subjects' behaviour (in a manner consistent with our theory).

Brain-mapping with MVPA

Most of the MVPA examples in this paper have focused on using MVPA to track cognitive states, without much discussion of the specific neural instantiation of these states. However, as discussed at the end of *Case Study 2*, MVPA can also serve as a powerful tool for mapping cognitive functions onto brain structures, with strengths and weaknesses that are complementary to standard brain-mapping approaches. As discussed by Norman *et al.* (2006b), MVPA is not ideally suited to characterizing the roles of individual voxels; if your goal is to determine whether a particular voxel, on its own, contributes to a particular cognitive state, the best approach is to run a univariate analysis that focuses on that voxel. The chief advantage of MVPA, with regard to brain mapping, is that it can be used to sensitively assess whether a particular set of voxels (in aggregate) contains information about the cognitive states of interest (Kriegeskorte *et al.*, 2006).

The future of MVPA

At this point in time, we are still at a very early stage in the development of MVPA methods. While individual-trial classifier performance is above chance in the examples described here, our ability to decode a subject's 'instantaneous cognitive state' is still very far from 100% accurate. We typically need to look at data from a large number of trials in order to establish a link between classifier output and behaviour. Also, there are limits on the kinds of cognitive states that can be resolved with extant MVPA methods. The Polyn *et al.* (2005) study described in *Case Study 1* constitutes a 'best case scenario' for tracking cognitive states over time, insofar as Polyn *et al.* (2005) intentionally chose cognitive states (thinking about faces, locations, and objects) with highly discriminable neural substrates. As we increase the similarity of the cognitive states that are being studied, it stands to reason that our ability to track those states (at a fine time scale) should decrease accordingly.

Over time, we expect that improvements in imaging hardware and data analysis methods will boost the signal-to-noise ratio in MVPA analyses. Initial results from studies that have applied MVPA to high-resolution fMRI data are very promising (e.g. Sayres, Ress, & Grill-Spector, 2006). Also, better signal processing should help: There are several important properties of the fMRI signal relating to spatial structure (i.e. nearby voxels tend to represent similar things) and temporal structure (i.e. nearby time points tend to show similar patterns of activation) that are not routinely factored into MVPA analyses. Also, we expect that different cognitive states will fluctuate over time at different rates, and will vary in how they are instantiated in the brain (e.g. some cognitive states will have more localized neural substrates and other cognitive states will have more distributed neural substrates). As a general principle, giving the classifier better 'priors' about what a particular cognitive state should look like in the brain (and how it should vary over time) should improve the classifier's ability to track that cognitive state. Finally, one of the main factors limiting classifier performance in extant MVPA studies is lack of training data; there is only so much data that one can collect from a single subject in a single experiment. As such, classifier performance stands to benefit tremendously if we can develop ways of leveraging data from multiple subjects to constrain classifier estimates for a particular subject. For example, even though the 'shoe' brain pattern might vary from subject to subject, it might be possible to use multi-subject data to develop better priors on how the 'shoe' pattern might manifest itself in any one subject's brain.

Tracking parameters

While the technical developments listed above are important, it is easy to get caught up in trying to optimize classifier performance and then lose track of the main question addressed in this paper, namely: 'How can MVPA be used to test theories of memory?'. The framework presented in this paper (where MVPA is used to test the validity of 'if-then' statements relating cognitive states and outcomes) is a useful start. However, this 'if-then' way of framing theories does not come close to capturing the nuance and complexity of extant computational models of memory. These models contain numerous parameters and state variables and make precise quantitative predictions about how behaviour should vary as a function of these factors (see Norman, Detre, & Polyn, 2008 and Raaijmakers, 2005 for reviews of extant computational models of memory).

   In principle, it should be possible to extend the approach described in this paper in order to directly 'read out' the parameters of quantitative models based on brain activity. We can scan subjects in situations where (according to the theory) the parameter is likely to be high, and situations where (according to the theory) the parameter is likely to be low. Then, we can train the classifier to discriminate between brain states associated with high and low values of this parameter. Once we have trained classifiers to read out values associated with key parameters of the model, we can track the values of multiple parameters and plug these values back into the model to generate quantitative predictions about subjects' behaviour.

Conclusions

Cognitive neuroscience theories, at their core, are about how the brain represents and processes information. One can translate these predictions about information processing into predictions about the overall level of activation in a particular brain region; this approach has been highly productive (as described in other contributions to this volume). However, fine-grained information about the subject's cognitive state gets lost in this translation process (insofar as two meaningfully different representational states can result in the same overall amount of activity). The main benefit of MVPA is that it allows us to skip this translation step and directly test predictions about the information that should be present in the subject's brain at a particular point in time, and how this relates to behaviour. MVPA has a long way to go before it fully delivers on this promise, but the potential payoff is extremely high: By eliminating the need to translate model predictions into predictions about overall activity, MVPA promises to provide a much more transparent and 'higher-bandwidth' interface between theories and brain data.[6]

Acknowledgements

This research was supported by NIH grants R01MH069456 and P50MH062196 awarded to KAN and NIH NRSA grant F31MH077649 awarded to ELN. The authors would also like to thank James Haxby and members of the Princeton Neuroimaging Analysis Methods research group for helping us to develop these ideas.

References

Anderson, M. C. (2003). Rethinking interference theory: Executive control and the mechanisms of forgetting. *Journal of Memory and Language*, 49, 415–445.

Anderson, M. C., Bjork, R. A., & Bjork, E. L. (1994). Remembering can cause forgetting: Retrieval dynamics in long-term memory. *Journal of Experimental Psychology: Learning, Memory, and Cognition, 5*, 1063–1087.

Bartlett, F. C. (1932). *Remembering: A Study in Experimental and Social Psychology*. Cambridge: Cambridge University Press.

Calhoun, V. D., Adali, T., Pearlson, G. D., & Pekar, J. J. (2001). Spatial and temporal independent component analysis of functional MRI data containing a pair of task-related waveforms. *Human Brain Mapping, 13*, 43–53.

Carlson, T. A., Schrater, P., & He, S. (2003). Patterns of activity in the categorical representations of objects. *Journal of Cognitive Neuroscience, 15*, 704–717.

Cox, D. D. & Savoy, R. L. (2003). Functional magnetic resonance imaging (fMRI) "brain reading": detecting and classifying distributed patterns of fMRI activity in human visual cortex. *Neuroimage, 19*(2 Pt1), 261–70.

Curran, T. (2000). Brain potentials of recollection and familiarity. *Memory and Cognition, 28*, 923.

Fox, E. (1994). Interference and negative priming from ignored distractors: The role of selection difficulty. *Perception & Psychophysics, 56*(5), 565–574.

Fox, E. (1995). Negative priming from ignored distractors in visual selection. *Psychonomic Bulletin and Review, 2*, 145–173.

Fox, E. (1998). Perceptual grouping and visual selective attention. *Perception & Psychophysics, 60*(6), 1004–1021.

Frankel, H. C., Robison, S. G., & Norman, K. A. (2006). fMRI correlates of retrieval orientation: Tracking contextual reinstatement using pattern classification. Program No. 365.14. *2006 Neuroscience Meeting Planner*. Atlanta, GA: Society for Neuroscience. Online.

Friston, K. & Buchel, C. (2003). Functional connectivity. In R. Frackowiak, K. Friston, C. Frith, R. Dolan, K. Friston, C. Price, S. Zeki, J. Ashburner, & W. Penny (Eds), *Human Brain Function* (2nd Edn). Academic Press.

Fuentes, L. J., Humphreys, G. W., Agis, I. F., Carmona, E., & Catena, A. (1998). Object-based perceptual grouping affects negative priming. *Journal of Experimental Psychology: Human Perception and Performance, 24*(2), 664–672.

---

[6] The Matlab scripts that we use to run MVPA analyses are available for public download at http://www.csbmb.princeton.edu/mvpa.

Friston, K. J., Harrison, L., & Penny, W. (2003). Dynamic causal modelling. *Neuroimage, 19*, 1273–1302.

Gotts, S. J. & Plaut, D. C. (2005). Neural mechanisms underlying positive and negative repetition priming. *Journal of Cognitive Neuroscience, 17*(Suppl.), 189.

Grison, S. & Strayer, D. L. (2001). Negative priming and perceptual fluency: more than what meets the eye. *Perception & Psychophysics, 63*(6), 1063–1071.

Gronlund, S. D. & Ratcliff, R. (1989). Time course of item and associative information: Implications for global memory models. *Journal of Experimental Psychology: Learning, Memory, and Cognition, 15*, 846–858.

Gruppuso, V., Lindsay, D. S., & Kelley, C. M. (1997). The process-dissociation procedure and similarity: Defining and estimating recollection and familiarity in recognition memory. *Journal of Experimental Psychology: Learning*, Memory, and Cognition, 23, 259.

Hanson, S. J., Matsuka, T., & Haxby, J. V. (2004). Combinatorial codes in ventral temporal lobe for object recognition: Haxby (2001) revisited: is there a "face" area? *Neuroimage, 23*, 156–166.

Haxby, J. V., Gobbini, M. I., Furey, M. L., Ishai, A., Schouten, J. L., & Pietrini, P. (2001). Distributed and overlapping representations of faces and objects in ventral temporal cortex. *Science, 293*, 2425–2429.

Haynes, J.-D. & Rees, G. (2005a). Predicting the orientation of invisible stimuli from activity in human primary visual cortex. *Nature Neuroscience, 8*, 686–691.

Haynes, J.-D. & Rees, G. (2005b). Predicting the stream of consciousness from activity in human visual cortex. *Current Biology, 15*(14), 1301–1307.

Haynes, J.-D. & Rees, G. (2006). Decoding mental states from brain activity in humans. *Nature Reviews. Neuroscience, 7*(7), 523–534.

Haynes, J.-D., Sakai, K., Rees, G., Gilbert, S., Frith, C., & Passingham, R. E. (2007). Reading hidden intentions in the human brain. *Current Biology, 17*(4), 323–328.

Henson, R. (2005). What can functional neuroimaging tell the experimental psychologist?. *The Quarterly Journal of Experimental Psychology A, 58*(2), 193–233.

Hintzman, D. L. & Curran, T. (1994). Retrieval dynamics of recognition and frequency judgments: Evidence for separate processes of familiarity and recall. *Journal of Memory and Language, 33*, 1–18.

Hintzman, D. L., Curran, T., & Oppy, B. (1992). Effects of similarity and repetition on memory: Registration without learning. *Journal of Experimental Psychology: Learning, Memory, and Cognition, 18*, 667–680.

Huk. A. C. & Shadlen, M. N. (2005). Neural activity in macaque parietal cortex reflects temporal integration of visual motion signals during perceptual decision making. *Journal of Neuroscience, 25*(45), 10420–10436.

Houghton, G. & Tipper, S. P. (1994). A model of inhibitory mechanisms in selective attention. In D. Dagenbach & T. H. Carr (Eds), *Inhibitory Processes in Attention, Memory, and Language* (pp. 53–112). San Diego, CA: Academic Press.

Itier, R. J. & Taylor, M. J. (2004). N170 or N1? Spatiotemporal differences between object and face processing using ERPs. *Cerebral Cortex, 14*(2), 132–142.

Jacoby, L. L., Yonelinas, A. P., & Jennings, J. M. (1997). The relation between conscious and unconscious (automatic) influences: A declaration of independence. In J. D. Cohen & J. W. Schooler (Eds), *Scientific Approaches to Consciousness* (pp. 13–47). Mahwah, NJ: Lawrence Erlbaum Associates.

Jeffreys, D. A. (1989). A face-responsive potential recorded from the human scalp. *Experimental Brain Research, 78*(1), 193–202.

Johnson, S. K. & Anderson, M. C. (2004). The role of inhibitory control in forgetting semantic knowledge. *Psychological Science, 15*(7), 448–453.

Kahn, I., Davachi, L., & Wagner, A. D. (2004). Functional-neuroanatomic correlates of recollection: Implications for models of recognition memory. *Journal of Neuroscience*, 24, 4172–4180.

Kamitani, Y. & Tong, F. (2005). Decoding the visual and subjective contents of the human brain. *Nature Neuroscience*, 8, 679–85.

Kamitani, Y. & Tong, F. (2006). Decoding seen and attended motion directions from activity in the human visual cortex. *Current Biology*, 16(11), 1096–1102.

Kriegeskorte, N., Goebel, R., & Bandettini, P. (2006). Information-based functional brain mapping. *Proceedings of the National Academy of Sciences*, 103(10), 3863–3868.

LaConte, S., Anderson, J., Muley, S., Ashe, J., Frutiger, S., Rehm, K., Hansen, L. K., Yacoub, E., Hu, X., Rottenberg, D., & Strother, S. (2003). The evaluation of preprocessing choices in single-subject BOLD fMRI using NPAIRS performance metrics. *Neuroimage*, 18(1), 10–27.

LaConte, S., Strother, S., Cherkassky, V., Anderson, J., & Hu, X. (2005). Support vector machines for temporal classification of block design fMRI data. *Neuroimage*, 26(2), 317–329.

Malmberg, K. J. & Xu, J. (2007). On the flexibility and fallibility of associative memory. *Memory and Cognition*, 35(3), 545–556.

McIntosh, A. R., Bookstein, F. L., Haxby, J. V., & Grady, C. L. (1996). Spatial pattern analysis of functional brain images using partial least squares. *Neuroimage*, 3(3 Pt 1), 143–157.

McIntosh, A. R. & Lobaugh, N. J. (2004). Partial least squares analysis of neuroimaging data: applications and advances. *Neuroimage*, 23, S250–S263.

Mitchell, T. M., Hutchinson, R., Niculescu, R. S., Pereira, F., Wang, X., Just, M., & Newman, S. (2004). Learning to decode cognitive states from brain images. *Machine Learning*, 5, 145–175.

Mourao-Miranda, J., Bokde, A. L., Born, C., Hampel, H., & Stetter, M. (2005). Classifying brain states and determining the discriminating activation patterns: Support vector machine on functional MRI data. *Neuroimage*, 28(4), 980–995.

Muller-Putz, G. R., Scherer, R., Pfurtscheller, G., & Rupp, R. (2005). EEG-based neuroprosthesis control: a step towards clinical practice. *Neuroscience Letters*, 382, 169–174.

Newman, E. L. & Norman, K. A. (2006). Tracking the sub-trial dynamics of cognitive competition. Program No. 365.2. *2006 Neuroscience Meeting Planner*. Atlanta, GA: Society for Neuroscience. Online.

Norman, K. A. (2002). Differential effects of list strength on recollection and familiarity. *Journal of Experimental Psychology: Learning*, Memory, and Cognition, 28(6), 1083–1094.

Norman, K. A., Detre, G. J., & Polyn, S. M. (2008). Computational models of episodic memory. In R. Sun (Ed.), *The Cambridge Handbook of Computational Psychology*. New York: Cambridge University Press.

Norman, K. A., Newman, E. L., & Detre, G. J. (2007). A neural network model of retrieval-induced forgetting. *Psychological Review*, 114(4), 887–953.

Norman, K. A., Newman, E. L., Detre, G. J., & Polyn, S. M. (2006a). How inhibitory oscillations can train neural networks and punish competitors. *Neural Computation*, 18(7), 1577–1610.

Norman, K. A. & O'Reilly, R. C. (2003). Modeling hippocampal and neocortical contributions to recognition memory: A complementary-learning-systems approach. *Psychological Review*, 104, 611–646.

Norman, K. A., Polyn, S. M., Detre, G. J., & Haxby, J. V. (2006b). Beyond mind-reading: Multi-voxel pattern analysis of fMRI data. *Trends in Cognitive Science*, 10(9), 424–430.

Nyberg, L., Habib, R., & Tulving, E. (2000). Reactivation of encoding-related brain activity during memory retrieval. *Proceedings of the National Academy of Sciences*, 97, 11120.

O'Toole, A. J., Jiang, F., Abdi, H., & Haxby, J. V. (2005). Partially distributed representations of objects and faces in ventral temporal cortex. *Journal of Cognitive Neuroscience*, 17, 580–590.

Parra, L., Alvina, C., Tang, A., Pearlmutter, B., Yeung, N., Osman, A., & Sajda, P. (2002). Linear spatial integration for single-trial detection in encephalography. *Neuroimage, 17*, 223–230.

Peters, B. O., Pfurtscheller, G., & Flyvbjerb, H. (1998). Mining multi-channel EEG for its information content: an ANN-based method for a brain-computer interface. *Neural Networks, 11*, 1429–1433.

Philiastides, M. G., Ratcliff, R., & Sajda, P. (2006). Neural representation of task difficulty and decision making during perceptual categorization: a timing diagram. *Journal of Neuroscience, 26*(35), 8965–8975.

Philiastides, M. G. & Sajda, P. (2006). Temporal characterization of the neural correlates of perceptual decision making in the human brain. *Cerebral Cortex, 16*, 509–518.

Ploran, E. J., Nelson, S. M., Velanova, K., Donaldson, D. I., Petersen, S. E., & Wheeler, M. E. (2007). Evidence accumulation and the moment of recognition: Dissociating perceptual recognition processes using fMRI. *Journal of Neuroscience, 27*(44), 11912–11924.

Poldrack, R. A. (2006). Can cognitive processes be inferred from neuroimaging data?. *Trends in Cognitive Science, 10*(2), 59–63.

Polyn, S. M., Natu, V. S., Cohen, J. D., & Norman, K. A. (2005). Category-specific cortical activity precedes recall during memory search. *Science, 310*(5756), 1963–1966.

Quamme, J. R. & Norman, K. A. (2006). Using fMRI pattern classification of recollection and familiarity to predict false alarms in recognition memory. Program No. 365.6. *2006 Neuroscience Meeting Planner*. Atlanta, GA: Society for Neuroscience. Online.

Quamme, J. R., Weiss, D. J., & Norman, K. A. (2007, November). Pattern classification of fMRI retrieval states in recognition memory. *Poster presented at the 48th Annual Meeting of the Psychonomic Society, Long Beach, CA.*

Raaijmakers, J. G. W. (2005). Modeling implicit and explicit memory. In C. Izawa, & N. Ohta (Eds), *Human Learning and Memory: Advances in Theory and Application* (pp. 85–105). Mahwah, NJ: Erlbaum.

Ratcliff, R., Clark, S., & Shiffrin, R. M. (1990). The list strength effect: I. *Data and discussion. Journal of Experimental Psychology: Learning, Memory, and Cognition, 16*, 163–178.

Reder, L. M., Nhouyvanisvong, A., Schunn, C. D., Ayers, M. S., Angstadt, P., & Hiraki, K. A. (2000). A mechanistic account of the mirror effect for word frequency: A computational model of remember-know judgments in a continuous recognition paradigm. *Journal of Experimental Psychology: Learning, Memory, and Cognition, 26*, 294–320.

Rotello, C. M. & Heit, E. (1999). Two-process models of recognition memory: Evidence for recall-to-reject. *Journal of Memory and Language, 40*, 432.

Sayres, R., Ress, D., & Grill-Spector, K. (2006). Identifying distributed object representations in human extrastriate cortex. In Y. Weiss, B. Scholkopf, & J. Platt (Eds), *Advances in Neural Information Processing Systems 18* (pp. 1169–1176). Cambridge, MA: MIT Press.

Shadlen, M. N. & Newsome, W. T. (2001). Neural basis of a perceptual decision in the parietal cortex (area LIP) of the rhesus monkey. *Journal of Neurophysiology, 86*, 1916–1936.

Shivde, G. & Anderson, M. C. (2001). The role of inhibition in meaning selection: Insights from retrieval-induced forgetting. In D. S. Gorfein (Ed.), *On the Consequences of Meaning Selection: Perspectives on Resolving Lexical Ambiguity* (pp. 175–190). Washington, DC: American Psychological Association.

Smith, A. P. R., Henson, R. N. A., Dolan, R. J., & Rugg, M. D. (2004). fMRI correlates of the episodic retrieval of emotional contexts. *NeuroImage, 22*, 868–878.

Spiridon, M. & Kanwisher, N. (2002). How distributed is visual category information in human occipito-temporal cortex? An fMRI study. *Neuron, 35*(6), 1157–1165.

Strother, S., La Conte, S., Hansen, L., Anderson, J., Zhang, J., Pulapura, S., & Rottenberg, D. (2004). Optimizing the fMRI data-processing pipeline using prediction and reproducibility performance metrics: I. a preliminary group analysis. *Neuroimage, 23*(Suppl 1), S196–S1207.

Strayer, D. L. & Grison, S. (1999). Negative identity priming is contingent on stimulus repetition. *Journal of Experimental Psychology: Human Perception and Performance, 25*(1), 24–38.

Tipper, S. P. (1985). The negative priming effect: inhibitory priming by ignored objects. *The Quarterly Journal of Experimental Psychology A, 37*(4), 571–590.

Tipper, S. P. (2001). Does negative priming reflect inhibitory mechanisms? A review and integration of conflicting views. *The Quarterly Journal of Experimental Psychology A, 54*(2), 321–343.

Tipper, S. P., Bourque, T. A., Anderson, S. H., & Brehaut, J. C. (1989). Mechanisms of attention: a developmental study. *Journal of Experimental Child Psychology, 48*(3), 353–378.

Tsao, D. Y., Freiwald, W. A., Knutsen, T. A., Mandeville, J. B., & Tootell, R. B. (2003). Faces and objects in macaque cerebral cortex. *Nature Neuroscience, 6*(9), 989–995.

Tulving, E. & Thompson, D. (1973). Encoding specificity and retrieval processes in episodic memory. *Psychological Review, 80*, 352–373.

Vallabhaineni, A. & He, B. (2004). Motor imagery task classification for brain computer interface applications using spatiotemporal principle component analysis. *Neurological Research, 26*, 282–287.

Wagner, A. D., Shannon, B. J., Kahn, I., & Buckner, R. L. (2005). Parietal lobe contributions to episodic memory retrieval. *Trends in Cognitive Sciences, 9*, 445–453.

Wang, T., Deng, J., & He, B. (2004). Classifying EEG-based motor imagery tasks by means of time-frequency synthesized spatial patterns. *Clinical Neurophysiology, 115*, 2744–2753.

Wheeler, M. E. & Buckner, R. L. (2003). Functional dissociation among components of remembering: control, perceived oldness, and content. *Journal of Neuroscience, 23*, 3869–3880.

Wheeler, M. E., Petersen, S. E., & Buckner, R. L. (2000). Memory's echo: Vivid remembering reactivates sensory-specific cortex. *Proceedings of the National Academy of Sciences, 97*, 11125.

Wixted, J. T. & Stretch, V. (2004). In defense of the signal detection interpretation of remember/know judgments. *Psychonomic Bulletin and Review, 11*, 616–641.

Yonelinas, A. P. (2002). The nature of recollection and familiarity: A review of 30 years of research. *Journal of Memory and Language, 46*, 441–517.

Chapter 18

Imaging emotional influences on learning and memory

Kevin S. LaBar

Introduction

Like most other aspects of cognition, learning and memory systems evolved to help organisms solve the problems of survival and thus should be exquisitely tuned to the motivational and emotional consequences of behaviour. Psychologists have largely treated emotion and memory as separate topics of inquiry, with few theories of how these functions of the mind are intertwined. Neurobiological studies of non-human animals have provided more detailed accounts by which specific neural substrates, hormonal actions and putative psychological constructs contribute to emotional learning. Although animal studies are unparalleled in their precision in revealing neural mechanisms, they cannot account for aspects of emotional or mnemonic processing that are (arguably) uniquely human.

In this regard, neuroimaging studies of the human brain have much to offer researchers of emotional memory. However, it is important to keep in mind the scope of the questions that can be addressed by neuroimaging techniques. Schooler and Eich (2000) argued that there are two central questions that dominate the field of emotional memory: *Does emotion enhance or diminish the strength of memory for an event?* and *Are special mechanisms required to account for the effect(s) of emotion on memory?* Because emotions may influence not only accuracy but also other memory features, I would advocate for adding a third question to this list: *Does emotion alter the phenomenological (subjective) experience of memory for an event?* The question of *mechanism* is where well-designed neuroimaging studies can be particularly influential to psychological theory – by characterizing the neural interactions between emotion- and memory-processing regions of the brain and by relating neural activity with both indices of emotion (including physiological measures and self-report) and indices of memory (including performance measures and phenomenology). Owing to the inherently correlational nature of neuroimaging research, it is important to provide converging evidence with other approaches, particularly those that examine the perturbations of neural function in neurologic and psychiatric patients, by administering pharmacological agents, or via transcranial magnetic stimulation (to the extent possible in the brain regions implicated by the imaging findings). This chapter will briefly summarize relevant psychological and neurobiological theories and then illustrate how neuroimaging research has validated and extended the animal models and has led to new insights into mechanisms of emotional memory in humans.

Psychological theories of emotion and emotional memory

When approaching experimental studies of emotional memory, it is first necessary to decide which aspects of emotion and which aspects of memory will be the focus of investigation. This issue presents a challenge not only because of the scope of the two fields, but also because there is still no universally accepted theory for how emotions or memory functions are organized behaviourally or in the brain (let alone how they interact with each other). Psychological theories of emotion are comprised of three major classes (Ellsworth & Scherer, 2003). Categorical theories, derived primarily from evolutionary psychology, posit that each emotion is associated with a distinct mental representation and that some basic emotions, such as fear, are shared with other animals whereas complex social emotions, such as guilt, are unique to humans. According to this perspective, researchers should investigate emotional effects on memory by studying each emotion separately. Dimensional theories, derived primarily from social/personality and motivational psychology, posit that emotions are organized along a small number of fundamental dimensions (such as arousal and valence, approach and avoidance, or positive and negative affect) that intersect to create either circumplex or vector models. According to this perspective, researchers should investigate emotional effects on memory by systematically varying each emotion dimension. Finally, appraisal theories, derived primarily from cognitive psychology, posit that emotions are organized according to specific appraisal criteria that are used to evaluate emotional stimuli and situations. For instance, one may evaluate an emotional scenario according to its novelty value, pleasantness, goal significance and coping potential. Each emotion engenders the application of each appraisal criterion to a greater or lesser extent. According to this perspective, researchers should investigate emotional effects on memory by studying how each appraisal criterion affects memory. It is not yet clear which of these three theoretical perspectives most accurately characterizes the organization of affective space, as behavioural studies have provided some support for each one.

Psychological theories of memory only occasionally make direct reference to the role of emotion. Perhaps the best known attempt to account for emotional effects on memory is Gordon Bower's *spreading activation model* of mood and memory (Bower, 1981). According to Bower, each mood state is associated with particular nodes in the brain that represent basic emotional categories. Events that share the emotions affiliated with the mood state become linked to these nodes. When a given mood state is experienced, the emotion nodes associated with it become activated, and this activation spreads automatically to related memories and concepts according to the strength of the association between them and the particular emotion node. Moreover, emotion nodes that are not connected to the current mood state are inhibited such that the summation of activity across the nodes yields a net activation signature of the current mood. The associative network architecture of this theory accounts for *mood-congruent* memory effects since events and memories that are causally linked to the current mood state become activated automatically. The theory also accounts for *mood-dependent* memory in that the match between moods at encoding and retrieval benefits performance – an example of the encoding specificity principle (Tulving & Thomson, 1973).

Behavioural studies have shown that this theory only holds up under some circumstances (Bower & Forgas, 2000). In particular, mood effects on memory are most consistent when the moods induced are strong, when free recall rather than recognition memory is used as the dependent measure, and when the material is self-relevant. Although Bower did not specify particular brain substrates for the nodes in the network, his theory relies on a categorical representation of emotions in the brain, which is not well-established (Barrett, 2006). There are surprisingly few neuroimaging studies of mood effects on memory (Lewis *et al.*, 2005). Thus, neuroimaging has not been particularly impactful in understanding how the sustained processing of long-lasting mood states alters memory processes. This is clearly an important area for future research. Instead, most neuroimaging studies to date have examined the mnemonic impact of stimuli that induce transient changes in emotion. These studies have tested and extended neurobiological models of memory derived primarily from studies of non-human animals and human patients with circumscribed brain lesions.

Neurobiological models: Memory systems and memory modulation

Larry Squire's taxonomy of memory systems (Squire, 1986) specifically considers emotion within the domain of conditioned learning. According to this framework, the conditioning of emotional responses is a form of non-declarative (non-conscious) memory that requires the integrity of the amygdala. In a typical conditioning paradigm, a relatively innocuous stimulus (the conditioned stimulus or CS) is presented prior to an innately arousing unconditioned stimulus (the unconditioned stimulus or US). Once the predictive nature of the CS–US relationship is learned, the organism responds to the CS with physiological and behavioural responses that indicate that the emotional meaning of the CS has changed (appetitive responses to a CS predicting a rewarding US, and aversive responses to a CS predicting a noxious US). Damage to the amygdala across a variety of species impairs such learning, which is measured by a reduction in the magnitude of emotional responses elicited by the CS (LaBar & LeDoux, 2006). Most evidence in support of Squire's model has been derived from studies using noxious USs, which are called *fear conditioning* paradigms. Although the term 'fear' is used here, it is sometimes unclear if pure fear is being measured, especially for the relatively mild USs (such as loud noises) commonly used in humans for ethical reasons. Because few studies directly compare appetitive and aversive forms of conditioning, the available evidence could be interpreted according to either a categorical perspective of emotion (a learning effect specific to the emotion fear) or a dimensional perspective (a more general effect of high physiological arousal on learning).

While Squire's model concerns the role of the amygdala in conditioned behaviour, a broader role for the amygdala in emotional memory, including declarative forms of memory, has been proposed by James McGaugh in his *memory modulation hypothesis* (McGaugh, 2004). Derived initially from pharmacologic and lesion studies of rodents using avoidance-learning paradigms, this hypothesis states that the basolateral amygdala mediates the memory-modulating effects of adrenal stress hormones and other neurotransmitters on processing in other brain systems that contribute to memory acquisition and consolidation. These effects are exerted through both peripheral and central mechanisms, including feedback of circulating cortisol (corticosterone in rodents) and noradrenaline on central receptor sites in the amygdala, hippocampus, and neocortex. McGaugh hypothesizes further that these effects are specific to the encoding/consolidation stages of memory, they are triggered by situations of high arousal (supporting a dimensional approach to emotion), and that multiple forms of memory are impacted, depending on the processing taking place in the efferent targets of the amygdala's projections.

Imaging emotional influences

Fear conditioning

Neuroimaging studies have helped to elucidate the amygdala's key contributions to conditioned fear learning in humans. Several insights have been gained from neuroimaging techniques that have been difficult to ascertain using other research methods. First, imaging studies have provided anatomical specification of the contributions of adjacent medial temporal lobe (MTL) structures to task performance. In humans, selective organic damage to the amygdala is extremely rare, and neuropsychological studies of fear conditioning have almost always included patients whose damage included other MTL structures (Bechara *et al.*, 1995; LaBar *et al.*, 1995; Phelps *et al.*, 1998; Peper *et al.*, 2001; Hamann *et al.*, 2002). The spatial resolution of fMRI has clearly delineated that the amygdala and subjacent periamygdaloid cortex is involved in simple forms of conditioned fear acquisition (Buchel *et al.*, 1998; LaBar *et al.*, 1998; Morris *et al.*, 2001; Knight *et al.*, 2004; Morris & Dolan, 2004). In contrast, the hippocampus is involved only when the task is more complex. For instance, during *trace conditioning* a period of time separates the offset of the CS and the onset of the US, and hippocampal activity is thought to facilitate interval and/or response timing or to help maintain the CS representation on-line during the trace interval (Buchel *et al.*, 1999; Knight *et al.*, 2004). Because there is controversy over whether declarative knowledge is critical for fear conditioning in humans (LaBar & Disterhoft, 1998; Lovibond & Shanks, 2002), the neuroimaging evidence, in conjunction with studies of amnesic patients with selective hippocampal damage (Bechara *et al.*, 1995; LaBar & Phelps, 2005), have supported Squire's taxonomy by demonstrating a partial independence of neural systems supporting declarative knowledge and simple forms of conditioning.

In addition, neuroimaging studies have provided insights into the temporal dynamics underlying the amygdala's involvement in fear conditioning. Because amygdala-lesioned patients do not acquire conditioned fear, it has not been possible to determine how its involvement changes over the course of training or whether it contributes to the suppression (extinction) of fear behaviour. Some regions of the amygdala play a particularly key role early in training, when the CS–US contingency is initially learned (Buchel *et al.*, 1998, 1999; LaBar *et al.*, 1998; Morris *et al.*, 2001). These results suggest that a key driving force for amygdala elicitation is a change in the emotional salience of a stimulus. This interpretation is corroborated by studies of fear extinction, in which the reinforcer is removed and the previously feared CS is now associated with safety. During extinction training, amygdala activity transiently returns and is modified by interactions with the medial prefrontal cortex (PFC) and anterior cingulate, which are thought to provide a top-down signal for fear suppression (LaBar *et al.*, 1998; Morris & Dolan, 2004; Phelps *et al.*, 2004). Acquisition training-related amygdala activity correlates strongly with physiological indices of fear (skin conductance responses, SCRs) both within subjects (on a trial-by-trial basis) and between subjects (averaged across trials), implicating a tight coupling of central and peripheral indices of emotional learning (Figure. 18.1) (Furmark *et al.*, 1997; Buchel *et al.*, 1998; LaBar *et al.*, 1998; Cheng *et al.*, 2003).

Functional connectivity studies have further shown how the amygdala interacts with other brain regions during the processing of fear-conditioned stimuli. Morris and colleagues (1998) reported that conditioning-induced changes in auditory cortex responses to tone CSs were correlated with activity in the amygdala, basal forebrain and orbitofrontal cortex, implicating a conditioning-induced coupling of emotional and sensory processing. Moreover, functional connectivity analyses have helped to elucidate how the amygdala interacts with other brain regions as a function of awareness of the conditioning episode. Morris and colleagues (1999) compared functional connectivity maps to angry faces that had been conditioned either subliminally or supraliminally to an aversive noise US. In the subliminal case, CS-evoked responses in the amygdala showed greater functional connectivity with subcortical regions, including the pulvinar and superior colliculus, whereas in the supraliminal case there was greater connectivity with cortical regions. The relative reliance of conditioning processes on subcortical versus cortical routes of information processing has been widely debated in the field, particularly with reference to extrapolating rodent models to the human brain. These data illustrate how functional imaging studies can contribute to such debates using clever experimental manipulations combined with sophisticated statistical analyses of whole-brain imaging data sets.

Finally, alterations in fear-conditioning circuitry have begun to be investigated in neuropsychiatric disorders. A PET study of women suffering from posttraumatic stress disorder (PTSD) due to childhood sexual abuse found enhanced amygdala responses during acquisition of fear conditioning and reduced responses in the anterior cingulate during extinction training (Bremner *et al.*, 2005). This pattern suggests that PTSD is associated with an increased propensity to associate stimuli with aversive outcomes and an inability to engage regulatory circuits to dampen fear responses when they are no longer appropriate. In contrast, criminal psychopaths fail to engage the amygdala and associated frontolimbic structures during fear conditioning and correspondingly show blunted conditioned fear responses (Birbaumer *et al.*, 2005). Although preliminary, the clinical research highlights how models of emotional learning developed initially from the animal

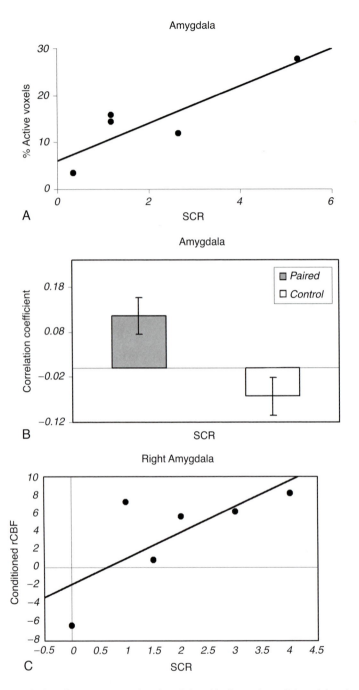

Figure 18.1 Correlations between central and peripheral indices of conditioned fear learning. Data pooled across three studies (A–C) show a consistent relationship between amygdala activation during fear acquisition and generation of conditioned skin conductance responses (SCR), a measure of sympathetic arousal. (A) and (C) report between-subjects correlations whereas (B) reports within-subjects correlations. (A) Adapted from LaBar et al. (1998); (B) Adapted from Cheng et al. (2003); and (C) Adapted from Furmark et al. (1997).

and human lesion literature can be adapted to imaging environments to understand how disease states impact the integrity of emotional learning circuits.

In sum, the available neuroimaging evidence has supported Squire's taxonomy of memory systems by revealing a role for the amygdala in the acquisition and extinction of conditioned fear. At the same time, the neuroimaging data have gone beyond the memory systems perspective to show how the amygdala's role changes during different training stages, how the amygdala interacts with other brain regions under different training regimens, including trace conditioning and subliminal forms of conditioning, and how the relevant circuitry is altered in patients suffering from mental illness. This line of work represents an excellent translational approach to the neuroscientific study of emotional memory using experimental paradigms that can be adapted across a variety of species and tested directly in clinical populations.

Explicit emotional memory encoding

For fear conditioning, it is widely believed that the computations that govern contingency learning occur primarily in the amygdala itself (Fanselow & LeDoux, 1999). In contrast, McGaugh's memory modulation hypothesis argues that the amygdala serves to modify memory processes occurring in other brain regions, rather than those that are intrinsic to intra-amygdala circuitry. Evidence from human neuroimaging studies have accumulated over the last decade to provide support for this additional role of the amygdala, largely by investigating activity in the amygdala and its interfaces with other MTL structures and the PFC during explicit memory encoding for emotional items and contexts (Figure 18.2).

Before reviewing this literature, it is important to identify criteria that must be met in order to provide full support for the memory modulation hypothesis. This hypothesis makes the following predictions: (1) stimuli that are high in emotional arousal will engage the amygdala relative to neutral stimuli; (2) there will be a selective retention advantage for emotionally arousing compared to neutral stimuli following an initial period of consolidation; (3) the magnitude of amygdala activity during (or immediately following) encoding will predict the magnitude of the behavioural retention advantage for emotionally arousing stimuli; (4) the amygdala will interact with memory-processing brain regions (including other MTL structures) during encoding; and (5) amygdala activity and its interactions with other structures will be greater for emotionally arousing stimuli that are subsequently remembered relative to those that are forgotten (the *difference-in-memory* or *Dm* effect, an index of *successful encoding* processes) (Paller & Wagner, 2002).

In the 1990's, PET studies using emotional film clips and pictures had provided some support for this hypothesis (Cahill *et al.*, 1996; Hamann *et al.*, 1999), but due to the relatively poor spatiotemporal resolution and the necessary use of blocked design protocols, it was impossible to establish Criteria 4 and 5 listed above. Using event-related fMRI, Canli and colleagues (2000) showed that the amygdala's response increases with self-reported arousal ratings for emotionally aversive pictures during encoding and that amygdala activity at encoding correlates with the strength of emotional memory across participants. Other studies have revealed gender differences in these emotional memory

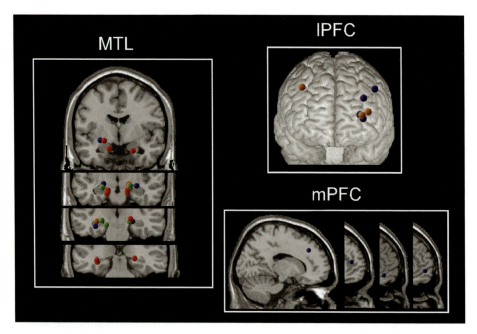

Figure 18.2 Encoding of emotional memories in the medial temporal lobes (MTL) and pre-frontal cortex (PFC). Data are pooled across 11 studies that showed emotional modulation of memory effects at encoding in the (A) amygdala, hippocampus, and surrounding cortices, and (B) medial and lateral PFC. Red indicates PET studies investigating correlations with subsequent memory performance; blue indicates event-related fMRI studies investigating correlations with subsequent memory performance; green indicates arousal-mediated Dm effects; yellow indicates valence-specific Dm effects. Only studies that reported peak spatial coordinates are included.

effects in that women exhibit a left-lateralized amygdala response and men exhibit a right-lateralized response (Cahill *et al.*, 2001, 2004; Canli *et al.*, 2002). The reasons for these gender differences are not yet understood (Cahill, 2006). Nonetheless, with regard to the memory modulation hypothesis, none of these experiments examined interactions of the amygdala with other brain regions nor directly compared memory for remembered versus forgotten items (Dm effect).

Evidence in support of the last two criteria has been recently established. In a re-analysis of an earlier PET data set, Kilpatrick and Cahill (2003) used structural equation modeling to infer that the amygdala exerted a directional influence on activity in the parahippoc-ampal gyrus and ventrolateral PFC during the encoding of emotionally aversive film clips. These film clips were subsequently remembered better than neutral clips, and the amygdala activity at encoding predicted the retention advantage for the emotional clips across participants. However, this study did not establish whether the modeled neural interactions themselves predicted encoding success (Criterion 5). Richardson and colleagues took the investigation of regional interactions a step further in an fMRI study of neurologic patients with partial damage to the MTL (Richardson *et al.*, 2004). The degree of sclerosis in the hippocampus and amygdala was quantified for each patient and was compared to the fMRI activity during the encoding of emotionally aversive and neutral words that were later remembered (hits). Across individuals, the degree of left hippocampal pathology predicted memory for both emotional and neutral words but the degree of amygdala pathology only predicted memory for emotional words. The researchers then examined the impact of MTL pathology on fMRI activity at encoding that distinguished words later retrieved with a sense of recollection ('remember') from those later retrieved with a sense of familiarity ('know') (see further discussion of this distinction below). Interestingly, the extent of hippocampal pathology inversely correlated with amygdala activity for recollected emotional words and the extent of amygdala pathology inversely correlated with hippocampal activity for the same words. Severe unilateral hippocampal pathology further induced a shift in the amygdala activation towards the contralateral hemisphere. The amygdala-hippocampal interactions were not significant during the encoding of neutral hits, implicating an emotion-induced reciprocal coupling of these structures to support memory.

More direct evidence for an interaction between emotional arousal and encoding success was recently established using the subsequent memory paradigm to compare brain activity to remembered versus forgotten stimuli as a function of arousal and valence (Dolcos et al., 2004a, 2004b; Kensinger & Corkin, 2004; Sergerie et al., 2005). Dolcos and colleagues (2004) found Dm effects for high-arousal pictures (both positive and negative valence) in the amygdala, entorhinal cortex, anterior hippocampus, and PFC (dorsolateral, dorsomedial and anterior ventrolateral). Positively valent pictures induced additional Dm effects in the ventromedial PFC. All of these effects were significantly greater than the Dm effects observed in the same regions for neutral stimuli. However, Dm effects were greater for neutral pictures in more posterior sectors of the hippocampus and parahippocampal gyrus, implicating an anterior-to-posterior gradient of arousal-modulated successful encoding activity along the longitudinal axis of the MTL. Finally, greater functional connectivity among the amygdala, entorhinal cortex, and hippocampus was observed for emotional Dm activity than for neutral Dm activity, which demonstrates a memory success by emotional arousal interaction, as predicted by Criterion 5. Kensinger and Corkin (2004) found Dm effects for high-arousal negative words in the amygdala and hippocampus, and for low-arousal negative and neutral words in the posterior ventrolateral PFC and hippocampus. Left dorsolateral PFC regions also show arousal-enhanced subsequent memory effects for facial expressions (both happy and fearful) whereas midline and right PFC regions show a specific modulation of happy expression on subsequent memory (Sergerie et al., 2005). Collectively, these results reveal dissociable influences of arousal and valence on successful memory encoding operations, consistent with two-factor dimensional theories of emotion and in strong support of the memory modulation hypothesis.

Explicit emotional memory retrieval

The memory modulation hypothesis focuses on arousal-enhanced consolidation processes and does not posit a critical role for the amygdala in mediating emotional effects on memory retrieval. Initial PET and blocked-design fMRI studies had not reported amygdala activation during emotional memory retrieval (Taylor *et al.*, 1998; Dolan *et al.*, 2000; Tabert *et al.*, 2001). However, these studies suffered from the same methodological limitations as discussed above for memory encoding. Current neuroimaging research is showing that amygdala activity is associated with specific retrieval operations that involve similar interactions with memory-processing regions as during encoding. As reviewed in other chapters in this volume, memory retrieval can be subdivided into dissociable processes of *recollection* and *familiarity* (Yonelinas *et al.*, 1996). Behavioural studies indicate that emotional arousal specifically enhances the feeling of remembering associated with the rich contextual detail of recollection-based retrieval (Ochsner, 2000; Talarico *et al.*, 2004). Sharot and colleagues (Sharot *et al.*, 2004) first showed that amygdala activity during the retrieval of aversive pictures is associated with recollection processes. Because memory was tested soon after encoding, though, there was no behavioural retention advantage for emotional pictures relative to neutral ones, nor was there any emotional enhancement of recollection-based activity in other MTL regions. Dolcos and colleagues (2005) extended these findings by scanning participants one year after encoding positive, negative, and neutral pictures. In this study, emotionally arousing pictures (both positive and negative in valence) were remembered better than neutral ones, and this mnemonic advantage was driven entirely by recollection-based retrieval. Retrieval success was defined as the difference in brain activity for remembered than forgotten items, and emotional arousal enhanced retrieval success activity and elicited greater functional connectivity in the amygdala, entorhinal cortex, and hippocampus. Furthermore, the arousal effects were greater for recollection than familiarity-based retrieval success in the amygdala and hippocampus, consistent with the behavioural retention advantage. These findings mirror those obtained in the MTL for successful encoding of emotional memories one year earlier (Dolcos *et al.*, 2004b) and further indicate relative specializations within MTL structures for specific retrieval processes.

An alternative approach to the neuroimaging of emotional memory retrieval is to examine the retrieval of emotional contextual information that is associated with neutral stimuli. Although this approach investigates memory for emotional contexts rather than emotional items, one advantage is that brain activation is not confounded by emotional effects on perceptual processing of the retrieval cue (since only neutral cues are presented at test). Studies of emotional item memory can circumvent this potential problem by comparing remembered versus forgotten emotional stimuli, in which case the main effect of emotion on retrieval cue perception is subtracted out (Dolcos *et al.*, 2005). Nonetheless, inferences drawn across emotional item and emotional context retrieval studies can contribute to the general theoretical debate regarding the specialized processing for these two forms of memory.

The MTL has been implicated in emotional context memory, but the specific activation pattern has varied widely across studies. Maratos and colleagues (2001) reported greater amygdala and hippocampal activity to correctly recognized neutral words (hits) embedded in negative sentence contexts compared to neutral sentence contexts. No effects were found in the MTL for neutral words encoded in positive sentence contexts. This study, though, did not report a retention advantage for emotional contextual encoding compared to neutral contextual encoding. In contrast, Erk and colleagues (2005) found that correctly recognized neutral words encoded in positive picture contexts elicited greater hippocampal activity than those that were forgotten. No effects were reported in the amygdala, and there was no MTL activity for correctly recognized words encoded in negative picture contexts. This study did not find a behavioural retention advantage for the positive encoding manipulation; however, no neutral control condition was included in the experimental design, so the main effect of arousal could not be established.

In a series of studies, Smith and colleagues examined the recognition of neutral objects that had been encoded into emotional or neutral picture contexts (Smith *et al.*, 2004, 2005, 2006). Their first study showed that objects encoded into positive contexts were recognized better than those encoded into negative or neutral contexts, and the hippocampus discriminated positive context hits from neutral context hits whereas the amygdala discriminated all emotional context hits from neutral context hits. Their follow-up study looked more specifically at accuracy in retrieving the source of the object (whether the associated context was positive, negative, or neutral in valence). Here they found that both positive and negative sources were recognized better than neutral sources. This behavioural finding was reflected in a memory X emotion interaction in the left amygdala (hits > misses), although the right amygdala and parahippocampal gyrus showed the opposite interaction (misses > hits). In the third study in the series, context memory for objects was assessed while participants made either *emotional discrimination* source judgements (negative vs. neutral picture contexts) or *people discrimination* source judgements (presence vs. absence of a person in the picture context). Negative sources improved both item and source memory, and this mnemonic advantage was reflected in the amygdala irrespective of the source task. The amygdala, parahippocampal gyrus and hippocampus showed an additional task effect, with greater overall activity and greater functional coupling during the emotional discrimination task than the person discrimination task.

Finally, Fenker and colleagues (2005) found that activity in the amygdala, hippocampus, and fusiform gyrus during retrieval of neutral words previously associated with face contexts was greater during recollection than familiarity. However, the recollection effect was only enhanced by facial expression (fearful > neutral) in the parahippocampal gyrus. Although these initial studies all point to a role for the MTL in emotional context retrieval, the specific pattern of behavioural and fMRI results are difficult to assimilate. To facilitate comparisons, this line of neuroimaging research could benefit by using a common dependent measure of memory (e.g. source hits vs. source misses) and by quantifying the arousal levels associated with the context manipulations. Different context manipulations (e.g. faces vs. scenes) are likely to yield different levels of emotional engagement, and under conditions of low arousal, amygdala-lesioned patients show intact benefits of emotional encoding contexts on memory for neutral words (Phelps *et al.*, 1997, 1998).

In sum, the amygdala and adjacent MTL memory structures (among other regions) participate in the retrieval of emotional item and emotional context memory. Because these regions also contribute to emotional memory encoding, it has been argued that these findings may simply reflect the emotional encoding of the retrieval act. That is, the activity may represent the re-encoding of the material into a long-term memory trace rather than reflecting retrieval processes *per se*. While this alternate explanation is challenging to reconcile, there are several observations in the existing data that may argue against it. First, there are some differences in the peak activation foci and/or lateralization of the activation patterns at encoding and retrieval which would argue against a strict re-encoding hypothesis. Second, the engagement of the amygdala and hippocampus is greater for some retrieval operations (recollection) than others (familiarity), which would not be predicted according to an encoding-of-retrieval account. Third, context memory effects are less robust in the amygdala during encoding (Kensinger & Schacter, 2006) than during retrieval, implicating an asymmetry according to the stage of memory processing. Lastly, MTL modulation is often seen for emotional contextual retrieval when no emotional information is presented at test. Additional evidence in support of MTL contributions to subjective aspects of remembering as well as details regarding its timing during the act of recollection have been elucidated in studies of autobiographical memory retrieval, as described next.

Memory phenomenology and retrieval of emotional autobiographical events

Recalling episodes from the personal past is one of the most effective ways to elicit changes in emotional and mood states. The sense of reliving and sensory vividness that accompany autobiographical memories are strongly intertwined with emotional intensity (Reisberg *et al.*, 1988; Talarico *et al.*, 2004). Several facets of autobiographical memory paradigms have clear advantages over laboratory-based assessments of emotional memory, including that (1) remote memories (years- to decades-old) can be investigated; (2) the memories have individually tailored personal significance and strong emotional salience; (3) the memories are complex enough to interrogate their experiential qualities (perceptual detail, narrative coherence, etc.); and (4) it usually takes time to select, re-assemble, and re-experience an autobiographical event from a generic retrieval cue, which enables a crude assessment of the spatiotemporal brain dynamics that take place during different stages of remembering. At the same time, autobiographical memory investigations are difficult to adapt for neuroimaging environments due to the lack of an appropriate control condition for subtractive methodology, the uncertainty in determining when and how the memory reconstruction process unfolds, the lack of verification of the accuracy of the memory, and the wide inter-subject and inter-item variability in encoding mechanisms, amount of rehearsal, and specificity of the memories (except in the case of staged events; see Cabeza *et al.*, 2004).

Hans Markowitch has proposed that the connections between the right ventrolateral PFC and MTL are especially critical for autobiographical memory retrieval, since patients with damage to the uncinate fasciculus that connects these regions often have a marked retrograde amnesia (Markowitsch, 1995). Neuroimaging studies of autobiographical memory have largely confirmed the involvement of the ventral and dorsal PFC, MTL, and other regions, including occipital-parietal areas involved in mental imagery (Maguire, 2001).

Moreover, there is greater functional connectivity between the right ventrolateral PFC, amygdala, and hippocampus during autobiographical memory retrieval than during semantic memory retrieval, in direct support of Markowitch's hypothesis (Greenberg *et al.*, 2005).

Some fMRI studies have investigated how activities in components of the autobiographical memory network vary according to the emotional qualities of the memory. Piefke and colleagues (2003) compared the valence of autobiographical memories and found positivity biases in the orbitofrontal cortex, temporal pole, and MTL, whereas negativity biases were found in the middle temporal gyrus. Other studies have reported correlations between amygdala and hippocampal activity during autobiographical retrieval and ratings of emotional intensity (Addis *et al.*, 2004; Daselaar *et al.*, 2008) (but see Maguire & Frith, 2003). Daselaar and colleagues (2008) further showed that two phenomenologically related features of autobiographical memory – emotional intensity and reliving – are dissociated spatially and temporally in the brain. This study capitalized on the protracted time course of retrieval when memories are probed using the Crovitz technique, in which participants are shown generic cue words (e.g. 'picnic') and are asked to generate a unique autobiographical event associated with it. Because it took 12 s on average to generate a full-blown memory, activity was divided into an early access/ reconstruction component and a later reexperiencing/elaboration component. Results showed that access-phase activity in the amygdala, hippocampus and somatosensory cortex predicted later emotional intensity judgements made after the memory was fully formed; in contrast, elaboration-phase activity in the ventral PFC, cingulate, and extrastriate cortex predicted the degree of reliving (Figure 18.3). In this way, the imaging data have made unique contributions to the field by revealing how subjective aspects of remembering are differentially processed in the brain and by characterizing the stage of retrieval at which those features of the memory are predominantly coded, even for features that are closely related and difficult to disentangle behaviourally. Furthermore, the early MTL modulation by emotional arousal implicates a function in the memory selection, reconstruction and/or reinstatement of the bodily state rather than a subsequent reflection on the event's significance after it has already been recovered.

Conclusions

Neuroimaging studies have made seminal contributions to advance an understanding of the biobehavioural mechanisms underlying emotional influences on learning and memory functions. These studies have been primarily focused on evaluating memory theories developed from studies of non-human animals and brain-lesioned patients. Neuroimaging studies have provided empirical evidence for Squire's taxonomy of memory systems by revealing the contributions of the amygdala to conditioned fear learning. In parallel, other studies have provided evidence for McGaugh's memory modulation hypothesis by demonstrating how the amygdala interacts with other memory-processing regions to consolidate arousing events into long-term storage. At the same time, the findings have extended these models to provide novel insights into the roles of the MTL and PFC in the

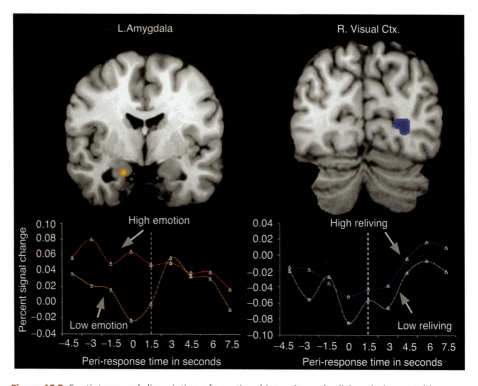

Figure 18.3 Spatiotemporal dissociation of emotional intensity and reliving during autobiographical memory retrieval. Participants indicated with a button press when a specific personal memory to a generic retrieval word cue was formed. According to the button press response on each trial (mean = 12.3 s), activity on each 30-second trial was divided into an early access/reconstruction phase and a late elaboration/re-experiencing phase. (A) Activity in the amygdala during the early phase predicted estimates of emotional intensity provided at the end of each trial. (B) Activity in the extrastriate cortex during the late phase predicted estimates of reliving provided at the end of each trial. From Daselaar *et al.* (2008).

extinction of conditioned fear memories and in the retrieval of emotional memories, including those concerning autobiographical events. Support for dimensional theories of emotion has emerged by determining how brain activity correlates with arousal and valence indices, which have different effects on memory, in convergence with data from brain-lesioned patients (LaBar, 2003, 2007; LaBar & Cabeza, 2006). Future work can make better contact with psychological theory by systematically investigating mood effects on memory and by directly testing categorical and component process theories of emotion.

Acknowledgements

Supported by NSF CAREER award 0239614 and NIH grant R01 AG023123. The author wishes to thank Steve Green for assistance with creating the figures.

References

Addis, D. R., Moscovitch, M., Crawley, A. P., & McAndrews, M. P. (2004). Recollective qualities modulate hippocampal activation during autobiographical memory retrieval. *Hippocampus*, *14*, 752–762.

Barrett, L. F. (2006). Are emotions natural kinds? *Perspectives on Psychological Science*, *1*, 28–58.

Bechara, A., Tranel, D., Damasio, H., Adolphs, R., Rockland, C., & Damasio, A. R. (1995). Double dissociation of conditioning and declarative knowledge relative to the amygdala and hippocampus in humans. *Science*, *269*, 1115–1118.

Birbaumer, N., Veit, R., Lotze, M., Erb, M., Hermann, C., Grodd, W., & Flor, H. (2005). Deficient fear conditioning in psychopathy: a functional magnetic resonance imaging study. *Arch Gen Psychiatry*, *62*, 799–805.

Bower, G. H. (1981). Mood and memory. *American Psychology*, *36*, 129–148.

Bower, G. H. & Forgas, J. P. (2000). Affect, memory, and social cognition. In: E. Eich, J. F. Kihlstrom, G. H. Bower, J. P. Forgas, & P. M. Niedenthal (Eds), *Cognition and Emotion*. New York, Oxford University Press.

Bremner, J. D., Vermetten, E. E., Schmahl, C. C., Vaccarino, V. V., Vythilingam, M. M., Afzal, N. N., Grillon, C. C., & Charney, D. S. (2005). Positron emission tomographic imaging of neural correlates of a fear acquisition and extinction paradigm in women with childhood sexual-abuse-related post-traumatic stress disorder. *Psychological Medicine*, *35*, 791.

Buchel, C., Dolan, R. J., Armony, J. L., & Friston, K. J. (1999). Amygdala-hippocampal involvement in human aversive trace conditioning revealed through event-related functional magnetic resonance imaging. *Journal of Neuroscience*, *19*, 10869–10876.

Buchel, C., Morris, J., Dolan, R. J., & Friston, K. J. (1998). Brain systems mediating aversive conditioning: an event-related fMRI study. *Neuron*, *20*, 947–957.

Cabeza, R., Prince, S. E., Daselaar, S. M., Greenberg, D. L., Budde, M., Dolcos, F., LaBar, K. S., & Rubin, D. C. (2004). Brain activity during episodic retrieval of autobiographical and laboratory events: an fMRI study using a novel photo paradigm. *Journal of Cognitive Neuroscience*, *16*, 1583–1594.

Cahill, L. (2006). Why sex matters for neuroscience. *Nature Reviews Neuroscience*, *7*(6), 477–484.

Cahill, L., Haier, R. J., Fallon, J., Alkire, M. T., Tang, C., Keator, D., Wu, J., & McGaugh, J. L. (1996). Amygdala activity at encoding correlated with long-term, free recall of emotional information. *Proceedings of the National Academy Science in the United States of America*, *93*, 8016–8021.

Cahill, L., Haier, R. J., White, N. S., Fallon, J., Kilpatrick, L., Lawrence, C., Potkin, S. G., & Alkire, M. T. (2001). Sex-related difference in amygdala activity during emotionally influenced memory storage. *Neurobiology of Learning and Memory*, *75*, 1–9.

Cahill, L., Uncapher, M., Kilpatrick, L., Alkire, M. T., & Turner, J. (2004). Sex-related hemispheric lateralization of amygdala function in emotionally influenced memory: an FMRI investigation. *Learning and Memory*, *11*, 261–266.

Canli, T., Desmond, J. E., Zhao, Z., & Gabrieli, J. D. (2002). Sex differences in the neural basis of emotional memories. *Proceedings of the National Academy of Science in the United States of America*, *99*, 10789–10794.

Canli, T., Zhao, Z., Brewer, J., Gabrieli, J. D., & Cahill, L. (2000). Event-related activation in the human amygdala associates with later memory for individual emotional experience. *Journal of Neuroscience*, *20*, RC99.

Cheng, D. T., Knight, D. C., Smith, C. N., Stein, E. A., & Helmstetter, F. J. (2003). Functional MRI of human amygdala activity during Pavlovian fear conditioning: stimulus processing versus response expression. *Behavioral Neuroscience*, *117*, 3–10.

Daselaar, S. M., Rice, H. J., Greenberg, D. L., Cabeza, R., LaBar, K. S., & Rubin, D. C. (2008). The spatiotemporal dynamics of autobiographical memory: Neural correlates of recall, emotional intensity, and reliving. *Cerebral Cortex*, *18*, 217–229.

Dolan, R. J., Lane, R., Chua, P., & Fletcher, P. (2000). Dissociable temporal lobe activations during emotional episodic memory retrieval. *NeuroImage, 11*, 203–209.

Dolcos, F., LaBar, K., & Cabeza, R. (2004a). Dissociable effects of arousal and valence on prefrontal activity indexing emotional evauation and subsequent memory: an event-related fMRI study. *NeuroImage, 23*, 64–74.

Dolcos, F., LaBar, K. S., & Cabeza, R. (2004b). Interaction between the amygdala and the medial temporal lobe memory system predicts better memory for emotional events. *Neuron, 42*, 855–863.

Dolcos, F., LaBar, K. S., & Cabeza, R. (2005). Remembering one year later: role of the amygdala and the medial temporal lobe memory system in retrieving emotional memories. *Proceedings of the National Academy of Science in the United States of America, 102*, 2626–2631.

Ellsworth, P. C. & Scherer, K. R. (2003). Appraisal processes in emotion. In: R. J. Davidson, K. R. Scherer, & H. H. Goldsmith (Eds), *Handbook of Affective Sciences*. New York, Oxford University Press.

Erk, S., Martin, S., & Walter, H. (2005). Emotional context during encoding of neutral items modulates brain activation not only during encoding but also during recognition. *NeuroImage, 26*, 829.

Fanselow, M. S. & LeDoux, J. E. (1999). Why we think plasticity underlying Pavlovian fear conditioning occurs in the basolateral amygdala. *Neuron, 23*, 229–232.

Fenker, D. B., Schott, B. H., Richardson-Klavehn, A., Heinze, H. J., & Duzel, E. (2005). Recapitulating emotional context: activity of amygdala, hippocampus and fusiform cortex during recollection and familiarity. *The European Journal of Neuroscience, 21*, 1993–1999.

Furmark, T., Fischer, H., Wik, G., Larsson, M., & Fredrikson, M. (1997). The amygdala and individual differences in human fear conditioning. *Neuroreport, 8*, 3957–3960.

Greenberg, D. L., Rice, H. J., Cooper, J. J., Cabeza, R., Rubin, D. C., & LaBar, K. S. (2005). Co-activation of the amygdala, hippocampus and inferior frontal gyrus during autobiographical memory retrieval. *Neuropsychologia, 43*, 659–674.

Hamann, S., Monarch, E. S., & Goldstein, F. C. (2002). Impaired fear conditioning in Alzheimer's disease. *Neuropsychologia, 40*, 1187–1195.

Hamann, S. B., Ely, T. D., Grafton, S. T., & Kilts, C. D. (1999). Amygdala activity related to enhanced memory for pleasant and aversive stimuli. *Nature Neuroscience, 2*, 289–293.

Kensinger, E. A. & Corkin, S. (2004). Two routes to emotional memory: distinct neural processes for valence and arousal. *Proceedings of the National Academy of Science in the United States of America, 101*, 3310–3315.

Kensinger, E. A. & Schacter, D. L. (2006). Amygdala activity is associated with the successful encoding of item, but not source, information for positive and negative stimuli. *Journal of Neuroscience, 26*, 2564–2570.

Kilpatrick, L. & Cahill, L. (2003). Amygdala modulation of parahippocampal and frontal regions during emotionally influenced memory storage. *NeuroImage, 20*, 2091–2099.

Knight, D. C., Cheng, D. T., Smith, C. N., Stein, E. A., & Helmstetter, F. J. (2004). Neural substrates mediating human delay and trace fear conditioning. *Journal of Neuroscience, 24*, 218–228.

LaBar, K. S., LeDoux, J. E., Spencer, D. D., & Phelps, E. A. (1995). Impaired fear conditioning following unilateral temporal lobectomy in humans. *The Journal of Neuroscience, 15*, 6846.

LaBar, K. S. (2003). Emotional memory functions of the human amygdala. *Current Neurology and Neuroscience Reports, 3*, 363–364.

LaBar, K. S. (2007). Beyond fear: Emotional memory mechanisms in the human brain. *Current Directions in Psychological Science, 16*, 173–177.

LaBar, K. S. & Disterhoft, J. F. (1998). Conditioning, awareness, and the hippocampus. *Hippocampus, 8*, 620–626.

LaBar, K. S., Gatenby, J. C., Gore, J. C., Ledoux, J. E., & Phelps, E. A. (1998). Human amygdala activation during conditioned fear acquisition and extinction: a mixed-trial fMRI study. *Neuron*, *20*, 937–945.

LaBar, K. S. & LeDoux, J. E. (2006). Fear and anxiety pathways. In: S. Moldin & J. L. Rubenstein (Eds), *Understanding Autism: From Basic Neuroscience to Treatment*. Boca Raton, FL: CRC Press.

LaBar, K. S. & Cabeza, R. R. (2006). Cognitive neuroscience of emotional memory. *Nature Reviews. Neuroscience*, *7*, 54.

LaBar, K. S. & Phelps, E. A. (2005). Reinstatement of conditioned fear in humans is context dependent and impaired in amnesia. *Behavioral Neuroscience*, *119*, 677.

Lewis, P. A., Critchley, H. D., Smith, A. P., & Dolan, R. J. (2005). Brain mechanisms for mood congruent memory facilitation. *NeuroImage*, *25*, 1214.

Lovibond, P. F. & Shanks, D. R. (2002). The role of awareness in Pavlovian conditioning: empirical evidence and theoretical implications. *Journal of Experimental Psychology. Animal Behavior Processes*, *28*, 3–26.

Maguire, E. A. (2001). Neuroimaging studies of autobiographical event memory. *Philosophical Transactions of the oyal Society of London. Series B*, *356*, 1441–1451.

Maguire, E. A. & Frith, C. D. (2003). Lateral asymmetry in the hippocampal response to the remoteness of autobiographical memories. *Journal of Neuroscience*, *23*, 5302–5307.

Maratos, E. J., Dolan, R. J., Morris, J. S., Henson, R. N., & Rugg, M. D. (2001). Neural activity associated with episodic memory for emotional context. *Neuropsychologia*, *39*, 910.

Markowitsch, H. J. (1995). Which brain regions are critically involved in the retrieval of old episodic memory? *Brain Reseach. Brain Research Reviews*, *21*, 117–127.

McGaugh, J. L. (2004). The amygdala modulates the consolidation of memories of emotionally arousing experiences. *Annual Review of Neuroscience*, *27*, 1–28.

Morris, J. S., Buchel, C., & Dolan, R. J. (2001). Parallel neural responses in amygdala subregions and sensory cortex during implicit fear conditioning. *NeuroImage*, *13*, 1044–1052.

Morris, J. S. & Dolan, R. J. (2004). Dissociable amygdala and orbitofrontal responses during reversal fear conditioning. *NeuroImage*, *22*, 372–380.

Morris, J. S., Friston, K. J., & Dolan, R. J. (1998). Experience-dependent modulation of tonotopic neural responses in human auditory cortex. *Proceedings of the Royal Society of London B: Biological Sciences*, *265*, 649–657.

Morris, J. S., Ohman, A., & Dolan, R. J. (1999). A subcortical pathway to the right amygdala mediating "unseen" fear. *Proceedings of the National Academy of Sciences USA*, *96*, 1680–1685.

Ochsner, K. N. (2000). Are affective events richly recollected or simply familiar? The experience and process of recognizing feelings past. *Journal of Experimental Psychology. General*, *129*, 242–261.

Paller, K. A. & Wagner, A. D. (2002). Observing the transformation of experience into memory. *Trends in Cognitive Science*, *6*, 93–102.

Peper, M., Karcher, S., Wohlfarth, R., Reinshagen, G., & LeDoux, J. E. (2001). Aversive learning in patients with unilateral lesions of the amygdala and hippocampus. *Biological Psychology*, *58*, 1–23.

Phelps, E. A., LaBar, K. S., Anderson, A. K., O'Connor, K. J., Fulbright, R. K., & Spencer, D. D. (1998). Specifying the contributions of the human amygdala to emotional memory: A case study. *Neurocase*, *4*, 527–540.

Phelps, E. A., LaBar, K. S., & Spencer, D. D. (1997). Memory for emotional words following unilateral temporal lobectomy. *Brain Cognition*, *35*, 85–109.

Phelps, E. A., Delgado, M. R., Nearing, K. I., & Ledoux, J. E. (2004). Extinction learning in humans: role of the amygdala and vmPFC. *Neuron*, *43*, 897.

Piefke, M., Weiss, P. H., Zilles, K., Markowitsch, H. J., & Fink, G. R. (2003). Differential remoteness and emotional tone modulate the neural correlates of autobiographical memory. *Brain*, *126*, 650–668.

Reisberg, D., Heuer, F., McLean, J., & O'Shaughnessy, M. (1988). The quantity, not the quality, of affect predicts memory vividness. *Bulletin of the Psychonomic Society*, *26*, 100–103.

Richardson, M. P., Strange, B. A., & Dolan, R. J. (2004). Encoding of emotional memories depends on amygdala and hippocampus and their interactions. *Nature Neuroscience*, *7*, 278–285.

Schooler, J. W. & Eich, E. (2000). Memory for emotional events. In: E. Tulving & F. I. M. Craik (Eds), *The Oxford Handbook of Memory*. New York, Oxford University Press.

Sergerie, K., Lepage, M., & Armony, J. L. (2005). A face to remember: emotional expression modulates prefrontal activity during memory formation. *NeuroImage*, *24*, 580–585.

Sharot, T., Delgado, M. R., & Phelps, E. A. (2004). How emotion enhances the feeling of remembering. *Nature Neuroscience*, *7*, 1376–1380.

Smith, P. R., Henson, N. A., Dolan, J. & Rugg, D. (2004). fMRI correlates of the episodic retrieval of emotional contexts. *NeuroImage*, *22*, 868.

Smith, P. R., Stephan, K. E., Rugg, M. D., & Dolan, J. (2006). Task and content modulate amygdala-hippocampal connectivity in emotional retrieval. *Neuron*, *49*, 631.

Smith, P. R., Henson, N. A., Rugg, D., & Dolan, J. (2005). Modulation of retrieval processing reflects accuracy of emotional source memory. *Learning & Memory*, *12*, 472–479.

Squire, L. R. (1986). Mechanisms of memory. *Science*, *232*, 1612–1619.

Tabert, M. H., Borod, J. C., Tang, C. Y., Lange, G., Wei, T. C., Johnson, R., Nusbaum, A. O., & Buchsbaum, M. S. (2001). Differential amygdala activation during emotional decision and recognition memory tasks using unpleasant words: an fMRI study. *Neuropsychologia*, *39*, 556–573.

Talarico, J. M., LaBar, K. S., & Rubin, D. C. (2004). Emotional intensity predicts autobiographical memory experience. *Memory and Cognition*, *32*, 1118–1132.

Taylor, S. F., Liberzon, I., Fig, L. M., Decker, L. R., Minoshima, S., & Koeppe, R. A. (1998). The effect of emotional content on visual recognition memory: a PET activation study. *NeuroImage*, *8*, 188–197.

Tulving, E. & Thomson, D. M. (1973). Encoding specificity and retrieval processes in episodic memory. *Psychological Review*, *80*, 352–373.

Yonelinas, A. P., Dobbins, I., Szymanski, M. D., Dhaliwal, H. S., & King, L. (1996). Signal-detection, threshold, and dual-process models of recognition memory: ROCs and conscious recollection. *Consciousness and Cognition*, *5*, 418–441.

Chapter 19

Developing theories that bridge mind and brain: Some thoughts of a cognitive psychologist

Andrew P. Yonelinas

The current volume presents numerous examples of neuroimaging studies that have advanced our understanding of the processes and representations underlying human memory. These studies can be described as reflecting three general approaches: (a) *exploratory* studies where the goal is to reveal which brain regions or neural networks are involved in a given task or cognitive process; (b) *validation* studies in which findings from other research domains such as animal learning studies or neuropsychological studies are confirmed or disconfirmed in healthy human subjects; and (c) *hyothetico-deductive* studies in which *a priori* predictions of existing theories are empirically tested. These categories are not mutually exclusive, and in fact, most neuroimaging studies exhibit characteristics of more than one of these types. However, in assessing the contribution of imaging studies to the science of memory, I think it is useful to separately consider the importance of each of these different approaches.

The exploratory approach would appear to be the least common nowadays, if one can take the current set of neuroimaging papers as being representative of the field as a whole. This was not the case a decade-and-a-half ago when functional neuroimaging was in its infancy. As a cognitive psychologist who is more comfortable with theories of memory than neuroanatomy, I am quite happy to see the move towards more theoretically driven studies. Nonetheless, I do appreciate that in the early days of any new methodology, an exploratory approach is perhaps quite appropriate, as the empirical landscape is largely unknown and one does not want to overlook important new findings simply because they are not theoretically predicted. As an illustration, I think that the initial disappointment in the early 90's at not finding hippocampal activity associated with episodic memory was countered by the finding of robust prefrontal involvement during episodic encoding and retrieval (e.g. Tulving *et al.*, 1994; Kapur *et al.*, 1994; Shallice *et al.*, 1994). This work was, to a great extent, responsible for the re-awakening of many memory researchers to the involvement of frontally mediated executive control processes in memory encoding and retrieval.

Validation studies appear to be quite common in the neuroimaging literature these days. These studies attempt to validate findings from other research domains, such as neurophysiological studies of rats and nonhuman primates as well as human neuropsychological studies. Although validation studies may not appear to be the most exciting sorts of science, the importance of these studies should not be underestimated. For example, although it may have seemed quite clear from animal experiments and studies of human amnesic patients that the hippocampus played a critical role in supporting episodic memory, verifying that this region was involved in episodic memory in healthy human subjects was of the utmost importance. That is, with animal studies there is always the concern that the behavioural tasks are not measuring episodic memory, or that the brain/function relationships might be somewhat different across species (e.g. Tulving, 2001). In addition, with human lesion studies there are important concerns about lesion localization, and the possibility that neural plasticity may confound the interpretation of those results (e.g. Rorden & Karnath, 2004). It is important to remember that scientific facts are never discovered in single experiments, or even in single experimental paradigms, but rather they emerge when a wide array of methods and paradigms lead to a convergent set of conclusions (Garner, Hake, & Eriksen, 1956). If all neuroimaging research ever accomplished was to verify findings for physiological and neuropsychological studies, this alone would be a momentous step forward.

Hypothetico-deductive studies are of course the types of studies that we all tend to strive for, and this appears be as true of today's imaging studies as it is for behavioural studies of memory. In some cases, this approach involves testing *a prior* predictions of an existing theory. In these cases, we strive for predictions that are counterintuitive, or at least that are not entirely obvious. Determining how obvious a prediction is, however, is to some extent open to debate, however, in some cases, we have the luxury of being able to identify two theories that are sufficiently well specified to make *conflicting* predictions, and thus studies can be designed to pit the two against each other.

It is sometimes suggested that neuroimaging studies do not contribute much to psychological theories because those theories do not actually say *anything* testable about the brain (e.g. Coltheart, 2006; Page, 2006). This argument seems to be rooted in a form of radical functionalism that assumes that mental functions are independent of brain structures. However, the science of memory is perhaps one of the best examples of an area in which studies of the brain, such as those using neuroimaging methods, are well matched to the current psychological theories because those theories have long aimed to integrate both brain and behaviour. One classical example is the debate about whether the memory engram is localized or distributed across the cortex (e.g. Lashley, 1950; Scoville & Milner, 1957). Other critical theoretical debates include whether memory reflects a single system or a set of multiple partially independent memory systems or components (Tulving, 2002; Atkinson & Juola, 1974), whether the medial temporal lobes are critical for encoding or retrieval (Cermak & Reale, 1978; Huppert & Peircy, 1976), and whether episodic memories are consolidated/transferred from the hippocampus to the cortex (Squire, Cohen, & Nadel, 1984; Nadel & Moscovitch, 1997). Another recent example, is reflected in the current debates about the neural substrates of recollection and familiarity. One class of recognition models has assumed that the hippocampus and perirhinal cortex are preferentially involved in recollection and familiarity-based memory (Aggleton & Brown, 1999;

Eichenbaum, Otto, & Cohen, 1994; Norman & O'Reilly, 2002; Yonelinas *et al.*, 2002), whereas another class has suggested that both regions are equally involved in both processes (Squire, 1994). A review of the neuroimaging literature shows that the evidence strongly favours the former set of theories, and these results are in good agreement with results from animal studies as well as human neuropsychological studies (for review, see Eichenbaum, Yonelinas, & Ranganath, 2007). In all of these theoretical debates, neuroimaging studies have had much to contribute.

Nonetheless, not all memory theories make predictions that can be addressed by neuroimaging methods. This issue is not unique to neuroimaging methods of course. For example, many memory theories have focused on recognition accuracy and have not said much about response time (e.g. most signal detection theories of recognition). Thus, there are cases in which it is impossible to directly contrast some models because the domains for which they are applicable simply do not overlap. So, a purely behavioural model may make no predictions about the brain at all. Ultimately, we strive for theories that can account for both the brain and behaviour. However, unfortunately, I do not think that we are near that stage in the science of memory. At least not quite yet. At best, we can look to see that the theories we use to account for results from different research domains are at least compatible with one another. In addition, if we have two models that can account equally well for the behavioural data, but one of them can also account for key aspects of the neuroimaging data, then the latter model is of course to be preferred.

The papers in this section include some compelling illustrations of each of the three types of studies I discussed earlier. For example, Patrick Khader and Frank Rosler integrate recent imaging and electrophysiological work with earlier neuropsychological and behavioural studies that indicate that there are material-specific cortical networks that are systematically activated during long term memory retrieval and that these overlap considerably with those activated during perception and working memory of those stimuli. The results are consistent with models that have postulated that long-term memory traces are encoded as connectivity changes within modality-specific brain regions, and that retrieval involves the re-instantiation of activation within these regions. They include in this, a number of their own recent studies looking at long-term representations using a new 'fan paradigm' that provides some strong evidence for this hypothesis. This work seems to combine the validation and hypothetico-deductive approaches, and it represents a nice example of how imaging methods can be used to address an issue that is quite difficult to address with pure cognitive/behavioural studies, or even with traditional neuropsychological studies.

Alumit Ishai reports on studies examining memory for pictorial materials, and presents some compelling evidence that visual imagery involves content-related activation within the same brain regions that are activated during perception. This work can also be viewed as reflecting a validation approach. However, in addition she points out that cognitive theories often focus on simple binary oppositions, and argues that the imaging literature on visual imagery and recognition memory have indicated that these processes are mediated by a distributed cortical network. She argues that these results demand an integrative theory of human memory that has to account for this wide spread of patterns of activation and for the dynamics and effective connectivity within cortical networks. So at some level, these imaging results also present a more direct challenge to our current theories of memory.

Kevin LaBar provides a host of good examples of how imaging results have validated, challenged, and extended theories of emotion and memory. For example, he provides evidence that imaging studies have been useful in contrasting the theory that the amydala is involved in conditioned behaviour, with the notion that it plays a broader role in memory modulation. In addition, these studies have verify the amydala's key role in conditioning, and have extended lesion work in illustrating the contributions of adjacent temporal lobe regions such as the periamygdaloid context and the hippocampus in different forms of conditioning – issues that would be difficult to ascertain using other research methods. He also describes work providing new insights into the temporal dynamics underlying the amydala's involvement in fear conditioning.

Finally, Ken Norman, Joel Quamme, and Ehren Newman describe multivariate methods for tracking cognitive states using multi-voxel pattern analysis (MVPA) whereby a pattern classifier is applied to multi-voxel patterns of brain activity and is training to detect the spatially distributed neural correlates of a specific cognitive state. The method is shown to be useful in testing the contextual reinstatement hypothesis of memory search. That is, if a subject's cognitive state at test matches the general properties of their cognitive state at study, then specific details should come to mind. They present results that indicate that category-specific patterns of brain activity associated with studying faces, locations, and objects start to emerge just before recall of specific items from that category during a free recall test. In addition, the method is shown to be useful in testing whether recollection and familiarity based retrieval orientation effects can be identified. Their results show that it is possible to use MVPA to tract the extent to which recollection is contributing to performance. In monitoring such mental states this method provides information that might not be available using invasive methods such as having the subjects report on when they are in that state – a process that may disrupt the mental state. Thus, this method in particular has enormous potential to address issues that are difficult to address with typical cognitive paradigms.

In closing, I will take this opportunity to briefly, but shamelessly, plug a recent behavioural study that I was involved with, because I think it is somewhat unique in showing how neuroimaging studies can influence memory theories and how they can motive novel behavioural research. The study was motivated by a consideration of several neuroimaging studies that have indicated that encoding activity in the hippocampus is associated with accurate source recognition (i.e. what colour was the word presented in?), whereas activity in the perirhinal cortex is associated with familiarity-based recognition and relatively insensitive to source memory accuracy (for a review, see Eichenbaum, Yonelinas, & Ranganath, 2007). In contrast, one recent study reported that perirhinal activity during encoding was associated with accurate source memory performance (Staresina & Davachi, 2006). The latter study was unique, however, in that it required subjects to link the item to the source colour by imagining the object in that source colour (i.e. how plausible is it that this object would be in this particular colour?). Based on an examination of that study, Rachel Diana hypothesized that when source information is encoded as a feature of a relevant item representation (i.e. 'unitized' see Yonelinas *et al.,* 1999) familiarity may support source recognition. That is, the source colour was no longer an arbitrary aspect of the studied item, rather it was treated as an integral part of the encoded item. To test this she conducted a series of behavioural source recognition experiments examining receiver operating characteristics and response deadline performance (Diana, Yonelinas, & Ranganath, 2008). These studies indicated that familiarity did in fact contributed to accurate source recognition to a greater degree following a source encoding task that encouraged unitization, as compared to a source encoding task that did not encourage unitization.

These behavioural results were motivated by a careful examination of the neuroimaging literature, and they showed us something that is counter to what many current theories of recognition memory lead us to expect. That is, they showed that familiarity is *not* limited to supporting item recognition judgements, but rather that under just the right conditions, familiarity can support accurate source memory judgements. I hope that as more cognitive psychologists carefully think about neuroimaging results we begin to see more behavioural studies that are motivated by the type of neuroimaging studies described in the current book.

References

Aggleton, J. P. & Brown, M. W. (1999). Episodic memory, amnesia, and the hippocampal-anterior thalamic axis. *Behavioral and Brain Sciences, 22*(3), 425–444.

Atkinson, R. C. & Juola, J. F. (1974). Search and decision processes in recognition memory. In D. H. Krantz, R. C. Atkinson, R. D. Luce, & P. Suppes (Eds), *Contemporary Developments in Mathematical Psychology (Vol.1): Learning, Memory & Thinking.* (pp. 242–293). San Francisco: Freeman.

Cermak, L. S. & Reale, L. (1978). Depth of processing and retention of words by alcoholic Korsakoff patients. *Journal of Experimental Psychology, 4*(2), 65–174.

Coltheart, M. (2006). What has functional neuroimaging told us about the mind (so far)? *Cortex, 42*(3):323–331.

Diana, R. A., Yonelinas, A. P., & Ranganath, C. (2008). The effects of unitization on familiarity-based source memory: Testing a behavioral prediction derived from neuroimaging data. *Journal of Experimental Psychology: Learning Memory and Cognition, 34*(1), 730–740.

Garner, W. R., Hake, H. W., & Eriksen, C. W. (1956). Operationalism and the concept of perception. *Psychological Review, 63,* 149–159.

Eichenbaum, H., Otto, T., & Cohen, N. (1994). Two functional components of the hippocampal memory system. *Behavioral and Brain Sciences, 17,* 449–518.

Eichenbaum, H., Yonelinas, A. P., & Ranganath, C. (2007). The medial temporal lobe and recognition memory. *Annual Review of Neuroscience, 30,* 123–152.

Huppert, F. & Piercy, M. (1976). Recognition memory in amnesic patients: Effects of temporal context and familiarity of material. *Cortex, 12,* 3–20.

Lashley K. (1950). In search of the engram. *Symposium for the Society for Experimental Biology* (Vol 4). New York: Cambridge Univeristy Press.

Nadel, L. & Moscovitch, M. (1997). Memory consolidation, retrograde amnesia and the hippocampal complex. *Current Opinion in Neurobiology, 7,* 217–227.

O'Reilly, R. C. & Norman, K. A. (2002). Hippocampal and neocortical contributions to memory: advances in the complementary learning systems framework. *Trends in Cognitive Sciences, 1,* 505–510.

Page, M. P. (2006). What can't functional neuroimaging tell the cognitive psychologist? *Cortex, 42*(3), 428–443.

Rorden, C. & Karnath, H. (2004). Using human brain lesions to infer function: a relic from a past era in the fMRI age? *Nature Reviews Neuroscience, 5,* 812–819.

Shallice, T., Fletcher, P., Frith C. D., Grasby, P., Frackowiak, R. S., & Dolan, R. J. (1994) Brain regions associated with acquisition and retrieval of verbal episodic memory. *Nature, 14;368*(6472), 633–635.

Squire, L. R. (1994). Declarative and nondeclarative memory: Multiple brain systems supporting learning and memory. In E. Daniel L. Schacter, & E. Endel Tulving (Eds), *Memory systems 1994.* (pp. 203–231). Cambridge, MA, US.

Squire, L. R., Cohen, N. J., & Nadel, R. E., (1984). The medial temporal region and memory consolidation: a new hypothesis. In H. Weingartner & E. Parker (Eds), *Memory Consolidation.* Hillsdale, NJ: Lawrence Erlbaum Associates.

Staresina, B. P. & Davachi, L. (2006). Differential encoding mechanisms for subsequent associative recognition and free recall. *Journal of Neuroscience, 20;26*(38), 9836.

Tulving E. (2002). Episodic memory: from mind to brain. *Annual Review of Psychology, 53,* 1–25.

Tulving E. (2001). Episodic memory and common sense: how far apart? *Philosophical Transactions of the Royal Society of London. Series B, Biological Sciences, 356*(1413), 1505–1515.

Tulving, E., Kapur, S., Markowitsch, H. J., Craik, F. I., Habib, R., & Houle S. (1994). Neuroanatomical correlates of retrieval in episodic memory: auditory sentence recognition. *Proceedings of the National Academy of Science in the United States of America, 15;91*(6), 2012–2015.

Kapur, S., Craik, F. I., Tulving, E., Wilson, A. A., Houle, S., & Brown, G. M. (1994) Neuroanatomical correlates of encoding in episodic memory: levels of processing effect. *Proceedings of the National Academy of Science in the United States of America, 91*(6), 2008–2011.

Scoville, W. B. & Milner, B. (1957). Loss of recent memory after bilateral hippocampal lesions. *Journal of Neurology, Neurosurgery and Psychiatry, 20*(1), 11–21.

Yonelinas, A. P., Kroll, N. E. A., Dobbins, I. G., & Soltani, M. (1999). Recognition memory for faces: When familiarity supports associative recognition judgments. *Psychonomic Bulletin and Review, 6,* 654–661.

Yonelinas, A. P., Kroll, N. E., Quamme, J. R., Lazzara, M. M., Sauve, M. J., Widaman, K. F., & Knight, R. T. (2002). Effects of extensive temporal lobe damage or mild hypoxia on recollection and familiarity. *Nature Neuroscience, 5*(11), 1236–1241.

Part 5

Control processes during encoding and retrieval

Chapter 20

Episodic memory storage and retrieval: Insights from electrophysiological measures

Axel Mecklinger and Theodor Jäger

Introduction: Dual-process models of recognition memory

Recognition memory refers to the ability of becoming aware that a particular item or information has been encountered in a previous episode. The present chapter will deal with this form of episodic memory by considering theoretical assumptions about its basic cognitive mechanisms. Furthermore, it will be demonstrated how electrophysiological measures of human brain activity have promoted our understanding of the neurocognitive processes involved in recognition memory and by this have supported models of episodic memory.

A fundamental question in contemporary memory research is whether a single type of memory can account for recognition memory performance or whether recognition memory involves more than a single memory process. While the latter class of models (i.e. dual process models) emphasize on empirical dissociations that cannot be accounted for by the view that recognition memory involves just one type of memory, opponents of the former view argue that some dissociations can more simply be interpreted in terms of strong and weak memories (Squire, Wixted, & Clark 2007).

The core assumption of a variety of dual-process models is that recognizing can be based on two distinct phenomenal experiences: *Familiarity*-based recognition occurs when someone has a feeling of 'knowing' an item from somewhere, but cannot recall any further information on the episodic context during which the item was originally experienced. By contrast, if *recollection*-based recognition occurs, then such contextual information (e.g. the spatio-temporal context of the episode) can be retrieved. This distinction of familiarity and recollection as two basic and distinguishable sub-processes underlying our ability to recognize previously encountered information has been established in formal dual-process models of recognition memory (e.g. Aggleton & Brown, 1999, 2006; Jacoby, 1991; Mandler, 1980; Quamme, Yonelinas, & Kroll, 2006; Tulving, 1985; Yonelinas, 2001, 2002; but see Hirshman & Master, 1997; Slotnick & Dodson, 2005, for different views). To date, a considerable body of evidence has been obtained in the support of proposals of the dual-process account (see Aggleton & Brown, 2006; Yonelinas, 2002, for reviews).

The central characteristics of familiarity and recollection as described by formal dual-process models are the following (see Yonelinas, 2002): Familiarity is assumed to reflect a fast-acting, relatively automatic, and item-specific memory process. Some models propose that information supporting familiarity is of continuously varying strength, whereby the familiarity of 'old' (i.e. studied) and 'new' (i.e. unstudied) items form overlapping Gaussian distributions (Yonelinas, 1997). By contrast, recollection is considered as somewhat slower and more effortful/elaborate memory process that can establish links between arbitrary information (e.g. items and contextual information). Some models assume that information supporting recollection has a threshold-like character, resulting in the retrieval of items with high confidence if they exceed a certain threshold, or producing retrieval failures if items fall below the threshold above which recollection can occur.

After establishing the basic functional characteristics of familiarity and recollection, the question arises how the contributions of these two processes can be estimated in a recognition memory task at hand. Several techniques and operational definitions have been proposed to derive behavioural estimates of familiarity and recollection from observed parameters of performance through the application of model equations (see Quamme et al., 2006; Yonelinas, 2002, for reviews). The most important of these techniques involve the process-dissociation procedure (Jacoby, 1991), the remember/know procedure (Tulving, 1985), and the receiver operating characteristics (ROC) procedure (Yonelinas, 1997). It is worth noting that the derivation of estimates by using these techniques relies on specific model constraints, such as the assumption that familiarity and recollection operate independently (Rugg & Yonelinas, 2003).

Familiarity and recollection have been found to be distinguishable on a physiological basis, as they seem to rely on partially non-overlapping neuronal networks. The medial temporal lobe is essential for declarative long-term memory in general, but within this structure the hippocampal formation is assumed to play a significant role for recollection. In the surrounding parahippocampal region comprising the entorhinal, perirhinal, and parahippocampal cortices, the anterior part centered on the perirhinal cortex seems to be the generator of familiarity signals (Aggleton & Brown, 2006). In the following, the source of familiarity information will be referred to as anterior medial temporal lobe cortex (MTLC). A considerable number of neuroimaging and animal studies supports the hypothesis that familiarity and recollection critically rely on the hippocampus and anterior MTLC, respectively (e.g. Gonsalves, Kahn, Curran, Norman, & Wagner, 2005; Grill-Spector, Henson, & Martin, 2006; Henson, Cansino, Herron, Robb, & Rugg, 2003; Li, Miller, & Desimone, 1993; Montaldi, Spencer, Roberts, & Mayes, 2006). Recently, lateral and medial prefrontal and parietal regions have also been found to be differently activated by familiarity and recollection (Yonelinas, Otten, Shaw, & Rugg, 2005). Rather than reflecting functions that are specific for familiarity and recollection, these prefrontal and parietal regions may reflect processes supporting memory retrieval or processes that act downstream from the computation of familiarity and recollection signals, such as the monitoring or verification of retrieved information or the focusing of attention to retrieved information (Wagner, Shannon, Kahn, & Bucker, 2005).

Further support for the neuroanatomical dissociation of familiarity and recollection is provided by neuropsychological case studies, revealing that brain lesions including the hippocampus and surrounding MTLC disrupt both recollection and familiarity, whereas selective hippocampal damage appears to disrupt recollection while leaving familiarity relatively intact (e.g. Holdstock, Mayes, Gong, Roberts, & Kapur, 2005; Mayes, Holdstock, Isaac, Hunkin, & Roberts, 2002; Mecklinger, Cramon, & Matthes-von Cramon, 1998; Yonelinas *et al.*, 2002; see Quamme *et al.*, 2006, for a review). Conversely, recent neuropsychological case studies and animal studies found evidence for both recollection and familiarity signals in the hippocampus (Squire *et al.*, 2007; Wais, Wixted, Hopkins, & Squire, 2006).

In an attempt to formalize and model the neurocognitive mechanisms underlying familiarity and recollection, Norman and O'Reilly (2003) have put forth an integrative neural-network model of recognition memory. In this intriguing model, the physiological properties of the hippocampus and surrounding anterior MTLC structures are taken as constraints for computational principles. The hippocampal formation with its sparse level of neural firing is proposed to be critical for recollection because it can establish associations between non-overlapping, arbitrarily paired items that are themselves represented in anterior MTLC. Specifically, the hippocampus creates pattern-separated representations of to-be-associated items in region CA3 that are linked to each other and to a copy of the anterior MTLC input pattern via region CA1. At test, the hippocampus enables pattern-completion and retrieves the complete studied pattern in response to a partial cue. However, note that this recollection mechanism may break down when the overlap between to-be-associated information is too high, since pattern-separated representations cannot be established in this case (Schacter, Norman, & Koutstaal, 1998).

By contrast, consistent with findings of neuroimaging and animal studies, Norman and O'Reilly (2003) assume that familiarity judgements are supported by the anterior MTLC on the basis of the relative sharpness of item representations. During learning, a sharpening process results in a smaller number of anterior MTLC neurons that are specifically tuned to represent a particular stimulus whereas other neurons are inhibited, which decreases total anterior MTLC activity in response to a familiar relative to a novel item and enables familiarity-based recognition judgements (*cf.* Grill-Spector *et al.*, 2006). Furthermore, the anterior MTLC is suggested to assign overlapping representations to similar stimuli, which enables the extraction of shared structures of items and statistical regularities of the environment. An important feature of the model is that the same anterior MTLC structures are involved in both extracting and representing stimulus features and computing familiarity signals.

In sum, considerable evidences from behavioural, neuroimaging, animal, and neuropsychological studies support the distinction between familiarity and recollection as two basic and qualitatively distinct mechanisms underlying our ability to recognize previously encountered information. With regard to their neural substrates, recollection is assumed to critically rely on the functional integrity of the hippocampus, whereas familiarity seems to be generated independently by the adjacent cortical regions (i.e. anterior MTLC). Prefrontal and parietal regions that are frequently found to be activated in recognition memory tasks are presumably not specifically tied to computing recollection and familiarity signals, but may be engaged as a consequence of memory retrieval, like the monitoring and evaluation of retrieved information, or the top-down control for computing familiarity and recollection signals.

Electrophysiological correlates of recognition memory

In the later part of the chapter, we will present a selective overview of studies suggesting that familiarity and recollection can be mapped onto distinct aspects of event-related brain potentials (ERPs) recorded during the retrieval phase of recognition memory tasks. The basic logic of the ERP approach is that if familiarity and recollection are distinct cognitive processes, they should also have qualitatively distinct ERP correlates. Qualitatively distinct ERP signatures imply that dissociable neural populations have been activated by the respective experimental manipulations. Our goal is to demonstrate that electrophysiological measures are helpful in advancing psychological theories on recognition memory beyond implications derived from behavioural, neuroimaging, animal, or neuropsychological studies and, therefore, can contribute to the validation of contemporary models of episodic memory. In this section, we will mainly refer to ERP findings obtained from *item* recognition memory, whereas the next section will be devoted to *associative* recognition memory. The former tasks involve distinguishing between old and new single items; the latter require retrieving particular pairings of items; e.g. pairs of test stimuli presented identically during encoding have to be distinguished from pairs of studied items that were recombined from study to test.

ERPs are computed by averaging portions of the electroencephalogram (EEG) that are related to cognitive processes elicited by particular events, such as items that are to be judged as 'old' or 'new'. Thus, ERPs reflect changes in scalp-recorded electrophysiological brain activity and the amplitudes, latencies, and topographical distributions of ERP components or effects can be tied to ongoing cognitive processes. The most important virtue of this technique (beyond other techniques such as fMRI or PET) is its excellent temporal resolution (in the domain of milliseconds) with which functionally relevant brain processes can be monitored. Hence, the temporal onset of retrieval-related processes (such as familiarity or recollection) as revealed by ERPs can be compared to other signs of retrieval-related brain activity, as for example single-unit recordings in the monkey's brain (Xiang & Brown, 2004). Another virtue of analysing ERP correlates of familiarity and recollection is that these measures reflect functionally relevant brain activity in predefined experimental conditions and by this rely to a fewer extent on explicit model assumptions or model equations as the behavioural measures mentioned above.

A related approach in the electrophysiological research of human memory focuses on oscillatory behaviour of neuronal systems. While EEG frequency analyses have stimulated discussions about the neurogenesis of ERP components (Makeig *et al.*, 2002), at present measures of oscillatory brain activity as compared to ERPs still lack functional sensitivity to discriminate between experimental manipulations, and only few studies have so far used EEG spectral parameters to explicitly address theories on recognition memory (Klimesch *et al.*, 2005; Mecklinger, Johansson, Parra, & Hanslmayr, 2007). However, recent developments in signal-processing techniques have improved the signal-to-noise ratio of oscillatory brain activity as well as its functional precision, so that these measures together with ERP measures will definitely enhance our understanding of the neural processes underlying memory processes in the near future.

In anticipating the main finding of ERP studies, we would like to point out that familiarity and recollection seem to be associated with dissociable electrophysiological correlates. Specifically, familiarity is reflected in more positive going ERP deflections for studied compared to non-studied items, with a maximum difference over frontal electrodes, approximately between 300 and 500 ms poststimulus. This effect has been termed the *mid-frontal old/new effect*. By contrast, recollection is associated with a somewhat later occurring ERP effect, namely more positive going waveforms for studied compared to non-studied items between *ca.* 400 and 800 ms poststimulus. This ERP difference is termed the *parietal old/new effect* and has its maximum over (left) parietal electrodes (for reviews see Allan, Wilding, & Rugg, 1998; Curran, Tepe, & Piatt, 2006b; Friedman & Johnson, 2000; Mecklinger, 2000; Rugg & Curran, 2007; Wilding & Herron, 2006).

Which empirical findings support the proposal that these two spatio-temporally dissociable ERP effects are specifically related to familiarity and recollection, respectively? For instance, Smith (1993) showed that the amplitude of the mid-frontal old/new effect was the same regardless of whether items have been consciously recollected or only engendered a feeling of familiarity, whereas the parietal old/new effect was enhanced when participants reported conscious recollection (see Düzel *et al.*, 1997, for similar results). In line with behavioural studies and with the assumption that recollection is a more elaborate, effortful process than familiarity, Rugg *et al.* (1998) demonstrated that the mid-frontal old/new effect is insensitive to depth of processing effects (e.g. deep vs. shallow encoding), whereas the parietal effect is substantially stronger for deeply relative to shallowly encoded items.

Curran (2000) revealed that the mid-frontal old/new effect was similar for studied words and plurality-reversed lure words that were judged as 'old', whereas the parietal old/new effect discriminated between studied and plurality-reversed words (see also Curran & Cleary, 2003). Nessler, Mecklinger, and Penney (2001 found that the mid-frontal old/new effect was similar for true recognition of words and false recognition of semantically related but unstudied words, whereas the parietal old/new effect was greater for true than for false recognition. The findings of these studies are consistent with the proposal that false recognition of (semantically or perceptually) related lures occurs in cases of high familiarity and that, depending on task characteristics, familiarity is derived either from perceptual or conceptual similarity between study and test items. The observation that the mid-frontal effect declined when the retention interval is increased from study to test, whereas the parietal effect is not affected by this manipulation (Nessler & Mecklinger, 2003), is consistent with models of recognition memory assuming that familiarity declines more rapidly than recollection (Yonelinas, 2002).

Düzel, Vargha-Khadem, Heinze, and Mishkin (2001) studied the amnesic patient Jon, who suffers from early and isolated hippocampal injury with apparently intact surrounding medial and lateral temporal cortices. In line with the view that recollection but not familiarity presupposes the integrity of the hippocampus, Jon shows a relatively preserved mid-frontal old/new effect, but a substantially diminished parietal old/new effect. Even though the above-mentioned study did not apply adequate operational definitions of familiarity and recollection, the results support the view of dissociable neural correlates of recognition memory sub-processes. Similar results are reported by Tendolkar *et al.* (1999) for 10 patients with reduced hippocampal volume due to Alzheimer's disease. In a source memory recognition task, the patients only exhibited the mid-frontal but not the parietal old/new effect that was present in healthy controls.

Curran (2004) demonstrated that dividing attention during encoding reduces the parietal, but not the mid-frontal old/new effect. This finding supports the assumption that familiarity operates more automatically than recollection. Consistent with results that the amnestic drug midazolam impairs behavioural estimates of recollection more so than those of familiarity, Curran, DeBuse, Woroch, and Hirshman (2006a) showed that the drug selectively diminished the parietal old/new effect compared to a saline control condition, whereas the mid-frontal old/new effect was unaffected.

Using two different categories of 'old' responses by which participants could indicate either partial or full retrieval of the study episode, Vilberg, Moosavi, and Rugg (2006) showed that the parietal old/new effect is greater when participants can recollect larger amounts of information, whereas the mid-frontal old/new effect is insensitive to the amount of information recollected. Woodruff, Hayama, and Rugg (2006) found that single words engendering feelings of familiarity in the absence of recollection elicited a mid-frontal but no parietal ERP old/new effect. The former effect also varied with the strength of the familiarity signal, operationally defined as the confidence with which an 'old' response was given. By contrast, words that were reported to be accompanied by recollection of specific contextual details elicited an additional parietal old/new effect that was not modulated by familiarity. The findings of these two studies indicate that the mid-frontal old/new effect varies as a function of familiarity strength, whereas the parietal old/new effect is specific for recollection. The assumption that familiarity reflects a strength-like signal and that 'old' decisions are made when familiarity exceeds a response criterion also implies that familiarity should contribute to 'old' decisions to a larger extent when a conservative rather than a liberal response criterion is selected. In support of this assumption, Azimian-Faridani and Wilding (2006) showed that under a conservative response criterion, the waveforms in the 300–500 ms time interval to hits and correct rejections at frontal recordings were more positive going than under a liberal response criterion.

In a recent series of experiments conducted in our lab, we further tested the functional characteristics of the ERP correlates of familiarity and recollection using morphed faces as stimulus materials. An interesting feature of the morphing procedure is that each face can be continuously transformed in any other face (see Jäger, Seiler, & Mecklinger, 2005). This allows examining the impact of even subtle changes in face similarity between study

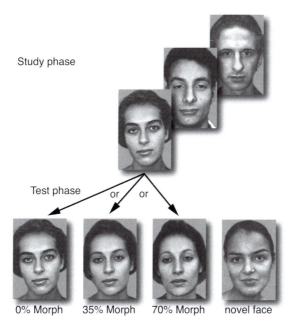

Study phase

Test phase or or

0% Morph   35% Morph   70% Morph   novel face

Figure 20.1 Illustration of the study and the test phase of Kipp *et al.* (2006).

and test. In one study (Kipp, Jäger, & Mecklinger, 2006), 16 participants performed an item recognition task for face stimuli. The key experimental manipulation was that the test phase included old faces and faces that, though physically different from study faces, preserved person identity from study to test (see Figure 20.1 for illustration): As revealed by a pilot rating study, 35% morphed faces were still perceived as representing the *same* person as the parent (i.e. 0% morphed) face, although the faces could reliably be discriminated on a physical level (Jäger *et al.*, 2005). By contrast, 70% morphed face stimuli were typically judged to depict *different* persons as the parent faces. Participants were required to respond 'old' whenever they recognized a *person* that was memorized during the study phase (i.e. 0% and 35% morphed faces) and to respond 'new' when they encounter a person previously unseen (i.e. 70% morphed and new faces).[1]

We hypothesized that repeated faces (i.e. 0% morphed faces), should elicit typical mid-frontal and parietal old/new effects, as recognition of such faces can be based on familiarity and/or recollection. By contrast, for 35% morphed faces correctly classified as 'old', we expected high levels of familiarity, as slightly morphed faces share strong similarities (and highly overlapping anterior MTLC representations) with faces that were actually studied. As these faces did not appear in the study phase, no recollection of the study context and by this no parietal old/new effect was expected. For 70% morphed faces

---

[1] After old/new decisions participants were also required to make physical judgments about whether or not the face stimuli judged as 'old' were physically identical to the memorized face stimuli. However, there were too few trials to allow separate ERP analyses for trials with correct or incorrect physical judgements, respectively.

judged as 'new', we expected no reliable mid-frontal or parietal old/new effects, as these face stimuli did not share physical or identity features with the studied 0% morphed faces.

Behavioural results revealed high hit rates for repeated faces (90% 'old' responses) and 35% morphed faces (79% 'old' responses). In addition, the majority of the 70% morphed faces were rejected as 'new' persons (75% 'new' responses) and participants were accurate in rejecting completely novel face stimuli (84% 'new' responses).

As can be seen in the middle row of Figure 20.2, we obtained a broad old/new effect with a maximum at mid-frontal (i.e. Fz) electrodes between 400 and 600 ms poststimulus. The topographical map for this mid-frontal old/new effect reflects the contrast between repeated faces and the average of 70% morphed and novel faces. Moreover, results shown in the lower row of Figure 20.2 revealed a left parietal old/new effect (i.e. P5) between 600 and 800 ms for old faces but not for 35% morphed faces. The topographical map for this parietal old/new effect reflects the contrast between repeated and 35% morphed faces.

In line with our expectations, these data indicate that both familiarity and recollection contributed to item recognition judgements for repeated face stimuli, as revealed by the presence of mid-frontal and left parietal old/new effects. As both effects were differentially modulated by morphing degree, the following conclusions are warranted: Repeated faces and 35% morphed faces that preserved face identity could be judged as 'old' because they were accompanied by feelings of familiarity, as reflected by the presence of a mid-frontal old/new effect. Note that we initially expected the 35% morphed faces to elicit equal familiarity levels as repeated faces, because we did not expect familiarity signals to be diagnostic or sensitive for such subtle perceptual modifications. However, the results revealed a graded mid-frontal old/new effect for 35% morphed compared to repeated faces.[2] Together with the higher hit rate for repeated than for 35% morphed faces, the finding of a graded frontal old/new effect is consistent with the view that familiarity relies on a continuously distributed strength-like memory process, whereby 'old' responses are given when memory strength exceeds a certain criterion. Interpreting this finding in terms of the strength models of familiarity with overlapping distributions of 'old' and 'new' items (Yonelinas, 1997), it appears that the familiarity distribution of 35% morphed faces, as compared to the distribution of repeated faces, is somewhat shifted towards the distribution of novel faces. However, a substantial proportion of both distributions (i.e. those of 35% morphed and repeated faces) seem to exceed the response criterion to the right and thus lead to correct 'old' judgements (Quamme, 2004; Yonelinas, 1997, 2001). Graded mid-frontal old/new effects have also been reported in experiments that systematically varied study-test similarity by presenting mirror-reversed versions of studied objects at test (Groh-Bordin, Zimmer, & Mecklinger, 2005) or by varying the study

---

[2] The mid-frontal old/new effect (captured at electrode Fz) was reliable for repeated and for 35% morphed faces [$ts(15) > 4.13$, $ps < 0.001$], but not for 70% morphed faces [$t(15) = 0.93$, $p = 0.365$], and mean amplitudes were significantly greater for repeated compared to 35% morphed faces [$t(15) = 2.67$, $p < 0.05$]. By contrast, the left parietal old/new effect (captured at electrode P5) was only elicited by repeated faces [$t(15) = 2.91$, $p < 0.05$], but not by 35% or 70% morphed faces [$ts(15) < 0.50$].

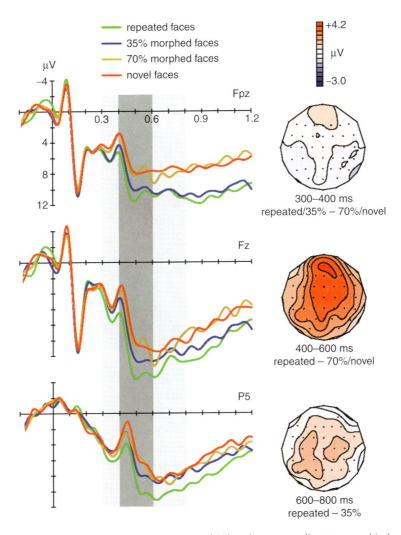

Figure 20.2 ERPs (shown at electrodes Fpz, Fz, and P5) and corresponding topographical maps of Kipp *et al.* (2006). The three time windows used to capture the anterior-frontal (300–400 ms), the mid-frontal (400–600 ms), and the left parietal (600–800 ms) old/new effects are shaded.

modality (spoken words/objects) of visually tested objects (Mecklinger, 2006). Taken together, these studies provide strong support for the view that the information supporting familiarity-based recognition is a continuously varying strength-like signal.

By contrast, a parietal old/new effect was exclusively elicited by identically repeated faces. The absence of a parietal old/new effect for 35% morphed faces is consistent with the view that recollection relies on a threshold process, by which only repeated items exceed a response threshold, whereas for 35% morphed faces though generating strong feelings of familiarity, no episodic information was actually recollected. It also seems that the 35% morphed faces represent insufficient retrieval cues for the elicitation of (immediate) recollections about the *parent* faces that were initially memorized.

Interestingly, as shown in the upper row of Figure 20.2, our study revealed an additional early (300–400 ms) ERP effect at fronto-polar recordings sites (i.e. Fpz). This effect discriminated faces classified as 'old' (i.e. repeated and 35% morphed faces) from faces receiving a 'new' response (i.e. 70% morphed and novel faces).[3] The topographical map for this anterior-frontal old/new effect between 300 and 400 ms reflects the contrast between the average of repeated and 35% morphed faces and the average of 70% morphed and novel faces. ERP old/new effects with similar anterior-frontal distributions and even earlier onset latencies (at around 200 ms) have been reported in a variety of recent studies (Curran & Dien, 2003; Ecker, Zimmer, Groh-Bordin, & Mecklinger, in press; Jäger, Mecklinger, & Kipp, 2006; Tsivilis, Otten, & Rugg, 2001). Early repetition effects are often found when short or even zero lag repetition intervals are used (Penney, Mecklinger, & Nessler, 2001; Rugg & Nieto-Vegas, 1999). With longer intervals as in the present study, these effects seem to be modality-specific. Even though a functional account of these early fronto-polar ERP effects is still missing and it is unclear to what extent they reflect implicit priming mechanisms or are more exclusively related to explicit memory tasks (see Curran & Dien, 2003, for a discussion), it is conceivable that they are associated with differential novelty processing and/or priming processes that contribute to intentional and explicit memory retrieval. Further studies will be required to elucidate in more detail how these early effects are functionally related to the mid-frontal and parietal old/new effects, i.e. the putative correlates of familiarity and recollection.

Taken together, our study revealed that the mid-frontal and the parietal old/new effect respond differentially to subtle perceptual manipulations, indicating that slightly altered faces elicit feelings of familiarity in the absence of recollection of episodic information. A real-life example of such experiences may be a situation in which we encounter a person after several years. Owing to advanced biological age and other changes, the appearance of the person may have altered to some degree. In this situation, we may very likely have feelings of 'knowing' the person from somewhere, but may not immediately recall specific information such as the person's name or the circumstances in which we were dealing with the person.

In concluding this section on ERP correlates of item recognition memory, our selective review of ERP investigations carried out in different laboratories with different stimulus materials and experimental setups indicates that the mid-frontal and the parietal old/new effect can indeed be associated with familiarity and recollection, respectively. From the converse point of view, it also seems clear that ERP studies can be helpful for constraining and verifying psychological theories. For instance, the dissociation of the two old/new effects and their corresponding characteristics strongly suggests the existence of two functionally distinct mechanisms underlying recognition memory, as proposed by formal dual-process models. A neural dissociation of familiarity and recollection is also strong evidence against single-process models of recognition memory and enables inferences on

---

[3] The anterior-frontal old/new effect (captured at electrode Fpz) between 300 and 400 ms was reliable for repeated and 35% morphed faces [$ts(15) > 2.16$, $ps < 0.05$], with no difference between the two [$t(15) = 0.51$].

the neurocomputational mechanisms of distinct neural populations contributing to our ability to recognize previously encountered information.

Electrophysiological correlates of associative recognition memory

This section will focus on associative (rather than item) recognition memory. As the starting point of the following discussion, we want to point to the fact that the dual-process account makes relatively strong claims about the underlying mechanisms of item vs. associative recognition memory (Yonelinas, 2001, 2002). Specifically, both familiarity and recollection are assumed to support item recognition judgements, as stimuli can be judged 'old' if participants recollect information about the study episode or if an item is sufficiently familiar. By contrast, only recollection but not familiarity is assumed to support associative recognition judgements, as individual stimuli are equally familiar in both intact and recombined pairs and thus familiarity cannot be diagnostic to distinguish between them. Therefore, accepting intact or rejecting recombined pairs is thought to require recollection for the particular pairings of stimuli. The theoretical assumption that familiarity cannot support associative recognition memory arises from the view that familiarity reflects neural activation of single items (Yonelinas, 2002) that are represented in anterior MTLC (Norman & O'Reilly, 2003). From the assumption that the hippocampus but not the anterior MTLC is able to encode and retrieve associations between arbitrarily paired items, it follows that hippocampal recollection is imperatively needed for the retrieval of such associations.

The hypothesis about the differential contributions of familiarity and recollection to tests of item and associative recognition memory is consistent with a number of findings. First, whereas item recognition typically elicits both, a mid-frontal and a parietal old/new effect, associative recognition memory is found to trigger a parietal old/new effect only (Donaldson & Rugg, 1998, 1999). Second, ROCs are typically curvilinear and asymmetrical along the diagonal for item recognition, but relatively linear for associative recognition memory tasks (Yonelinas, 1997). These shapes reflect contributions of continuously varying familiarity signals and threshold-like recollection to item recognition, but isolated contributions of recollection to associative recognition memory. Third, amnesic patients with impairments in recollection due to hippocampal lesions but spared familiarity often show no or only small deficits in item recognition, but substantial impairments in associative recognition memory (e.g. Holdstock *et al.*, 2005; Mayes *et al.*, 2004). Finally, speeded old/new judgements (thought to mainly reflect familiarity) provide accurate item recognition but unreliable associative recognition performance (Hintzman, Caulton, & Levitin, 1998).

Although these findings on the first glance fit in well with theoretical assumptions on the neurocomputational bases of familiarity and recollection, the claim that familiarity cannot support the retrieval of associations is not without counterarguments and controversially discussed (see Aggleton & Brown, 2006; Mecklinger, 2006; Yonelinas, 2002). Specifically, the current debate concerns the potential circumstances under which familiarity can support associative recognition judgements. One hypothesis formulated by Yonelinas and colleagues (Yonelinas, Kroll, Dobbins, & Soltani, 1999; see also Quamme, 2004; Quamme, Yonelinas, & Norman, 2007) and adopted and extended by other authors (Giovanello, Keane, & Verfaellie, 2006; Jäger et al., 2006; Rhodes & Donaldson, 2007) posits that familiarity can contribute to associative recognition memory given that the to-be-associated stimuli are encoded as a coherent whole and form a bound or 'unitized' representation. *Unitization* refers to conditions in which two or more previously separate items are strengthened with experience and become represented as a single unit (Hayes-Roth, 1977; Cesaro, 1985; Graf & Schacter, 1989). By this, unitary structures – other than associative structures – can be perceived and remembered as one entity, i.e. they result in unitary memory traces (e.g. facial features that are bound together to form a single face). This idea, hereinafter referred to as the *unitization hypothesis* (Quamme, 2004), suggests that associations can be retrieved independently from hippocampal recollection given that the associations are unitized within the anterior MTLC. This may be possible when to-be-associated items are perceived as a coherent entity, like pairs of items that frequently co-occur and thus share strong pre-experimental associations (e.g. word-pairs such as *sea-food* or *traffic-jam*; Giovanello et al., 2006; Quamme, 2004; Rhodes & Donaldson, 2007), or when unrelated items are encoded as if they referred to a single object (Quamme, 2004; Quamme et al., 2007).

The view that associative memories differ in the degree to which their components can be unitized and therefore can create memory representations that support either familiarity or recollection has also recently been postulated by Mayes, Montaldi, and Migo (2007; see also Mayes et al., 2004). In addition to unitized (intra-item) associations (e.g. the entity of a face), the model assumes that also within-domain associations composed of similar but not unitized items (e.g. two faces or a table and a chair) can be supported by familiarity. Empirical evidence for this view comes from a single amnesic patient (Y.R.), who shows selective hippocampal atrophy. She demonstrates selective impairments in associative recognition for between-domain associations, but sparing of unitized and within-domain associations. The intact performance for within-domain associations has been taken to reflect that familiarity can support associative recognition even in the absence of unitization (the implications of this view will be discussed later).

One source of evidence for the assumption that unitization can create familiarity-supporting memory representations comes from studies that used strongly pre-experimentally integrated items. Opitz and Cornell (2006) required participants to memorize four words in each study trial (e.g. *oasis, camel, chair, desert*, etc.). In two encoding conditions, participants either indicated which word did not fit in the associative context of the other three words (the associative condition) or indicated which of the four words denoted the smallest object (the relational condition). The objective behind this manipulation was that only the associative condition should promote the encoding of pre-existing semantic associations between words. During the test phase, studied words of both conditions and new words were presented as retrieval cues. Results revealed a mid-frontal old/new effect in the associative but not in the relational condition. As the mid-frontal old/new effect in the associative condition was enhanced for those words for which the complete word triplet was retrieved, the results argue against the view that enhanced memory strength for words encoded in the associative condition (i.e. item memory) may have contributed to the differences in the mid-frontal old/new effect. Rather, the results are consistent with the view that activation of pre-existing semantic relationships during encoding can create familiarity-supporting memory representations.

In another recent ERP study, Greve, van Rossum, and Donaldson (2007) found a mid-frontal old/new effect for word-pairs that had to be discriminated from recombined and new word-pairs only when the word-pairs were semantically related, again supporting the view that pre-existing semantic knowledge can be used to form unitized memory representations that support familiarity-based recognition.

However, in contrast to these findings, Rhodes and Donaldson (2007) did *not* find that familiarity supports associative recognition judgements for solely semantically related word-pairs (e.g. *prince-duke*). Rather, the results specifically supported the unitization hypothesis, as a mid-frontal old/new effect was elicited for word-pairs sharing a strong association and were rated as having the most unitized representation (e.g. *traffic-jam*, *glow-worm*, etc.). The effect was absent for purely semantic pairings (e.g. *cereal-bread*). However, an objection against the 'unitization-supports-familiarity' interpretation in the latter two studies could be that rather than contrasting same and rearranged pairings – a common practice in associative recognition memory research – the authors compared same pairings with new pairings, such that contributions of differential memory strength of single words to the mid-frontal old/new effect cannot be excluded.

Another approach for testing the validity of the unitization hypothesis is to use arbitrarily paired items and to manipulate unitization by study manipulations that either encourages or discourages forming a single entity. Rather than relying on pre-experimental knowledge, this approach bears the advantage that it allows to directly examine whether unitization effects on familiarity-based recognition can be initiated by the type of process- ing engaged at encoding. By this, it enables investigating the learning mechanisms and the kind of memory representations they generate. Using unrelated word-pairs as study materials, Quamme *et al.* (2007) examined the impact of encoding processing on associa- tive recognition memory. Word-pairs were either studied as separate parts of sentences or as newly learned compounds. Amnesic patients, who had previously demonstrated impaired recollection and spared familiarity, showed a memory advantage in the compound (unitization) condition over the sentence condition. When testing conditions were changed to restrict responses to familiarity, the same advantage of unitization at study was found for normal controls.

In a recent ERP study, we investigated the unitization hypothesis in more detail (Jäger *et al.*, 2006). Using an associative recognition memory task for face-pairs, we aimed to examine the circumstances under which face parts are unitized in a way that they form familiarity-supporting memory representations. In one condition, participants memorized pairs of sequentially presented face stimuli depicting two different persons (the *inter-item* condition). During a subsequent test phase, participants initially had to judge a *single test face* as 'old' or 'new'. Thereafter, for correctly identified old faces, a forced-choice judgement was required in which participants had to indicate which of two studied faces presented side by side was initially paired with the single test face during the study phase, by this probing memory for the association of the two study faces.

On the basis of the dual-process account, and consistent with previous findings on associative recognition memory (Donaldson & Rugg, 1998, 1999; Yonelinas, 1997), we expected performance in the inter-item condition to mainly rely on recollection, as the binding and retrieval of arbitrarily paired faces is proposed to strongly depend on hippocampal recollection, whereas anterior MTLC familiarity cannot be diagnostic for such associative judgements (Norman & O'Reilly, 2003; Quamme, 2004). In other words, we expected a strong parietal but no mid-frontal old/new effect in this condition. This effect should also be larger for hits followed by correct relative to incorrect associative (i.e. forced-choice) judgements.

In a second condition (the *intra-item* condition), in which participants also memorized pairs of physically different faces, the faces were rated to depict the same person to a high degree. The face stimuli were again created by a morphing software (Jäger *et al.*, 2005). The face-pairs of this condition consisted of either 35% plus 0% or 100% plus 70% morphed faces drawn from the same morph-continua, but presented in separate study trials. By this, it was possible to present 35% morphed faces as single test faces in the test phase, and their 0% and 70% morphed versions for the forced-choice judgements. Notably, as the 0% and 70% morphed faces were equally distant in morphing degree from the 35% faces, forced-choice judgements could not be made solely on the basis of differences in face similarity, but instead required retrieving associative memory representations established during encoding.

Our hypotheses regarding the intra-item condition were as follows: As to-be-associated face stimuli contained highly overlapping features and could be bound together in a way that they are perceived as a single person, encoding of such face-pairs and their features presumably engages unitization processes in anterior MTLC. These unitized representations may involve enhanced activation of the two images' overlapping features and reduced activation of non-overlapping ones (a process termed 'sharpening'; Norman & O'Reilly, 2003) and should thus support familiarity-based recognition. We expected a reliable mid-frontal old/new effect during old/new judgements of faces that should be larger for correct than for incorrect associative (forced-choice) judgements. By contrast, recollection may not be capable of supporting associations in the intra-item condition, as recollection is suggested to break down when the overlap between to-be-associated information is too high, because pattern-separated representations cannot be established in this case (Schacter *et al.*, 1998). In consequence, an attenuated or at least significantly smaller parietal old/new effect was expected compared to the inter-item condition in which recollection is assumed to play the most critical role.

Performance (old/new discrimination and associative judgements) was better in the intra-item condition than in the inter-item condition. As can be seen in Figure 20.3, in the *intra-item* condition there was a mid-frontal old/new effect between 300 and 400 ms post-stimulus (see electrode Fz). Consistent with our hypothesis that unitization of face features across both faces forms familiarity-supporting associative memory representations, this

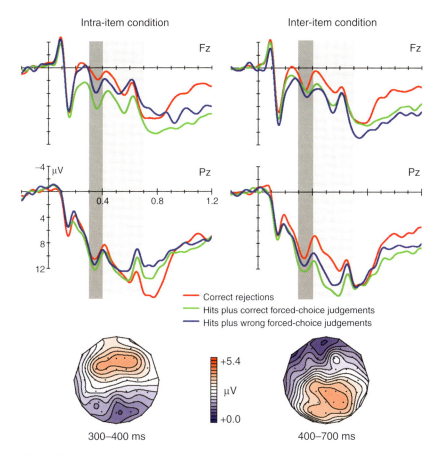

Figure 20.3 ERPs (shown at electrodes Fz and Pz) and corresponding topographical maps of Jäger *et al.* (2006). The two time windows used to capture the mid-frontal (300–400 ms) and the parietal (400–700 ms) old/new effects are shaded. Topographical maps reflect the difference between hits plus correct forced-choice judgements and correct rejections. ERPs and the topographical map on the left-hand side show the mid-frontal old/new effect obtained in the intra-item condition; ERPs and the topographical map on the right-hand side show the parietal old/new effect obtained in the inter-item condition. This is a modified version of a figure presented by Jäger *et al.* (2006).

mid-frontal old/new effect was significantly greater for hits followed by correct relative to incorrect associative judgements. By contrast, no parietal old/new effect (measured between 400 and 700 ms) was apparent in this condition (see electrode Pz). Conversely, in the *inter-item* condition, there was no reliable mid-frontal old/new effect. However, a pronounced parietal old/new effect emerged between 400 and 700 ms, which, confirming our predictions, was significantly larger for hits followed by correct relative to incorrect associative judgements.

To summarize, we obtained a double dissociation of the ERP correlates of familiarity and recollection. The mid-frontal old/new effect was significantly larger in the intra-item condition compared to the inter-item condition, whereas the parietal old/new effect was significantly larger in the inter-item condition compared to the intra-item condition. Notably, confirming the view that both effects reflect associative recognition memory, the mid-frontal and the parietal old/new effect discriminated correct from incorrect associative judgements. Consistent with our hypotheses, familiarity supported associative recognition judgements given that the to-be-associated stimuli were unitizable, i.e. in the intra-item condition, whereas recollection seemed to break down in this condition, presumably because the overlap between to-be-associated stimuli was too high. Conversely, in the inter-item condition associative recognition memory was supported by recollection, whereas similarly to previous studies familiarity did not seem to contribute to recognition judgements at all, presumably because familiarity is not diagnostic for distinguishing between correct and incorrect arbitrary face-pairings. Moreover, the finding of two spatio-temporally and functionally dissociable ERP old/new effects strongly supports dual- (rather than single-) process models of recognition memory.

Notably, the absence of a mid-frontal old/new effect in the inter-item condition, in which the association of two very similar items (i.e. two faces) had to be memorized, sheds some light on the limits of unitization mechanisms and the formation of familiarity-supporting memory representations. Unitization processes seem to rely on an entity-creating framework (the layout of a face or a semantic concept) into which items can be integrated. This view is also supported by a recent animal study on memory consolidation, showing that the presence of an associative schema (i.e. a fixed spatial arrangement) into which new information (i.e. flavours) can be encoded, allows the consolidation of new memory traces even after one trial learning in hippocampal-lesioned animals (Tse *et al.*, 2007).

It has also been argued that objective criteria for unitization have to be established (see Ceraso, 1985, for a proposal) and that inferring unitization from the presence of familiarity-based recognition bears the risk of circularity (Mayes *et al.*, 2007). The pre-experimental ratings of facial and personal identity for the morphed faces in the present study or the unitization ratings employed for word-pairs (Rhodes & Donaldson, 2007) in our view would meet such criteria for objective measures of unitization. The view expressed by the unitization account, namely that items to be recognized may combine with other items to higher order units with emergent properties was not only at the heart of the work of early Gestalt psychology (Ceraso, 1985). It is also of central relevance in other and broader models of knowledge representation (Hayes-Roth, 1977). From a memory retrieval point of view, an important and interesting feature of unitized representations is that they allow 'redintegration', a process by which a whole memory representation can be reinstated by a partial cue (Horowitz & Prytulak, 1969). Such a process is less likely for associative structures, where a partial cue usually leads to the retrieval of parts of a memory trace.

To summarize, extending the classically held view that associative memory relies on recollection without benefiting from familiarity, recent studies suggest that associative memories differ in the degree to which their components can be bound by anterior MTLC or hippocampal structures, respectively. Items that can be unitized and represented as a single entity can form memory representations that support familiarity-based recognition, whereas arbitrary or even similar components that cannot be bound together to form an entity form recollection-supporting memories. Anterior MTLC structures centered on the perirhinal cortex and the hippocampus by means of their neurocomputational mechanism can be considered as the most likely neural substrates for the two forms of associative memories.

Pre-experimentally unitized associations (e.g. *traffic-jam*) and associations that were unitized by encoding instructions can form familiarity-supporting memory representations. This view not only implies that processes engaged during encoding play an important role for unitization, it also raises the question whether pre-experimental and long-term unitization processes that lead to semantic knowledge structures and unitization induced by an encoding trial rely on the same or on distinct neurocomputational mechanisms. In terms of the Norman and O'Reilly (2003) model, one may speculate that semantic knowledge may have arisen from long-term sharpening. In other words, the repeated exposure to specific item combinations may have enhanced the binding of these items and reduced the binding to others, resulting in lower neural responsiveness in anterior MTLC. A critical role of anterior MTLC structures for semantic processing is also demonstrated by intracranial recordings (Fernandez, Klaver, Fell, Grunwald, & Elger, 2002; Meyer *et al.*, 2005). By this, items that were unitized (by means of a sharpening mechanism) into a single entity by encoding processes (single trial learning) as well as semantically related items (long-term learning) are interconnected in anterior MTLC, which enables associative retrieval independent from the hippocampus in both cases.

Within the discussion of the contributions of familiarity and recollection to associative recognition memory, it is worth referring to a somewhat related line of research examining the sensitivity of familiarity for *contextual influences*. While some situations may require familiarity-based recognition of unitized associations, such as encountering a person after a long time, other real world situations, like seeing an object in many different contexts, require familiarity to be item-specific and acontextual. Some findings of ERP studies indeed indicate that familiarity is sensitive for influences of contextual information, by this challenging the common assumption that familiarity represents an acontextual, item-specific form of recognition memory that should not be influenced by contextual information. Specifically, Tsivilis *et al.* (2001) reported that during item recognition the mid-frontal old/new effect was attenuated when to-be-judged objects were superimposed on novel, but irrelevant backgrounds. Using the same paradigm, Piatt, Curran, Collins and Woroch (reported in Curran *et al.*, 2006b) found that the mid-frontal old/new effect was more pronounced when object-background pairings were the same as in the study phase than when they were rearranged into novel pairings of studied objects and studied backgrounds.

However, in a recent study by Ecker *et al.* (2007), these contextual influences on the mid-frontal old/new effect disappeared when participants were specifically instructed to prevent directing attention to the (task-irrelevant) backgrounds and to focus attention exclusively on the objects when judging their old/new status. In light of these findings, it is reasonable to assume that previously found context effects on item familiarity are mediated by attentional and/or perceptual factors (e.g. attention directed towards backgrounds or impoverished figure-ground segmentation). This is consistent with the theoretical view that familiarity subserves genuinely acontextual forms of recognition memory. Depending on the situational characteristics, features of an episode may either be bound and retrieved as a coherent entity or attentional processes may render some features more salient and prevent contextual influences on familiarity-based recognition.

Conclusions: open issues and directions for future research

Although many studies have started to unravel the neurocognitive processes underlying our ability to recognize previously encountered information and have added to the converging evidence on the putative ERP correlates of familiarity and recollection, there are many open and timely questions that may be addressed in future (ERP) studies.

A first avenue for further ERP research may be to critically examine theoretical assumptions on the functional characteristics of familiarity and recollection. Findings from ERP studies generally agree with the assumption that familiarity is available earlier than recollection (Mecklinger, 2000) or that familiarity operates more automatically than recollection (Curran, 2004). However, other model assumptions have not been extensively tested, such as the view that familiarity and recollection represent *independent* memory processes. Note that this assumption may be hard (if not impossible) to test in behavioural studies, because the most important techniques for estimating familiarity and recollection *a priori* rely on the independence assumption. Also, the independence assumption would predict that certain brain lesions should lead to a loss of recollection and a sparing of familiarity, whereas other lesions should produce the opposite pattern. However, such a double dissociation is hard to find in clinical populations. Even though lesions restricted to the hippocampus in most cases remove the recollection component while sparing familiarity, the opposite pattern is very rarely found. Lesions restricted to the anterior MTLC region while sparing the hippocampus are not only hard to find (but see Bowles *et al.*, 2007 for an example). As the parahippocampal region is the main input zone for the hippocampus, lesions to this area should also disconnect the hippocampus from surrounding areas and by this attenuate recollection (Aggleton & Brown, 2006).

By contrast, ERP measures are not constrained by model assumptions, do not rely on the size and location of brain lesions, and can easily be recorded from non-clinical populations. By this, ERPs may be well-suited for testing the independence assumption. Indeed, findings of ERP studies seem to confirm that familiarity and recollection can occur independently, as in some conditions a mid-frontal but no parietal old/new effect is observed (Curran *et al.*, 2006a; Düzel *et al.*, 2001; Jäger *et al.*, 2006; Woodruff *et al.*, 2006), whereas in other conditions the parietal old/new effect is exclusively elicited (Donaldson & Rugg, 1998, 1999; Jäger *et al.*, 2006; Opitz & Cornell, 2006; Rhodes & Donaldson, 2007; Yovel & Paller, 2004). Moreover, double dissociations between the mid-frontal and the parietal old/new effects have recently been demonstrated within the same experimental setup (Jäger *et al.*, 2006; Woodruff *et al.*, 2006). These findings indicate that familiarity and recollection operate independently, with their relative contributions presumably relying on specific demands of the task at hand. A situation in which a retrieval cue elicits recollection without familiarity may be intuitively hard to imagine. Why should an episode that we retrieve in great detail not also be familiar? From the independence assumption, however, it follows that recollection can either co-occur or take place independently from familiarity. Recollection without familiarity may, for example, be a direct consequence of the computational mechanisms underlying both forms of remembering. How exactly features or items processed in anterior MTLC converge to form a familiarity-supporting memory representation is still unclear. However, the independence assumption together with empirical findings suggests that hippocampus-based recollection should become more and more relevant the less unitization of information occurs in anterior MTLC. This view also implies that specific task instructions, e.g. the specificity with which information has to be retrieved upon presentation of a retrieval cue, such as discriminating old from equally familiar recombined pairs of items, may also promote recollection-based memories without engaging familiarity. Future studies will be required that more specifically address the issue under which conditions familiarity and recollection operate independently.

Another interesting issue is whether familiarity and recollection can be elicited automatically, even if a task does not explicitly entail the retrieval of previous episodes (e.g. in implicit memory tasks). From a real-world view, one may expect that feelings of familiarity or recollective experiences do not depend on the prerequisite that one's cognitive system is explicitly prepared for treating stimuli as episodic retrieval cues, a state termed *retrieval mode* (Wilding & Herron, 2006). From the theoretical view, familiarity is considered to occur relatively automatically, but recollection is supposed to involve more effortful operations. From this it follows that familiarity signals should not depend on top down processes that set up retrieval modes. However, a recent study by Groh-Bordin *et al.* (2005) examining ERP correlates of explicit and implicit memory suggests that familiarity signals may indeed depend on the adaptation of a retrieval mode. Findings revealed a mid-frontal and a parietal old/new effect in the explicit memory task in which participants had to make old/new judgements about visually presented objects. By contrast, neither of these ERP effects was apparent in an implicit memory task in which participants had to make living/non-living judgements about novel and repeated objects. Rather, a late occipitoparietal repetition effect was found that could be topographically dissociated from the parietal old/new effect in the explicit task. These finding suggests that neither familiarity nor recollection signals are elicited in implicit memory tasks in which the brain is not set up for treating external events as episodic retrieval cues, but are rather contingent upon the adoption of a retrieval mode in order to be initiated. Hence, familiarity does not seem to be automatic in such a sense that it can occur even in tasks in which no reference to previous occurrences of stimuli is made.

A hint towards the role of top-down processes during memory retrieval comes from single-unit recordings in monkeys. Neuronal responses signaling stimulus familiarity in a serial recognition task were found in the medial and ventral prefrontal cortex (Xiang & Brown, 2004). Interestingly, these responses had about the same onset latencies (200–300 ms) as the scalp recorded mid-frontal old/new effect and were considerably longer than the earliest neuronal responses to familiarity in the inferior temporal lobes (Li *et al.*, 1993). This implies that prefrontal activation cannot be the source of anterior MTLC responses to familiarity, whereas later portions of anterior MTLC responses might well be modulated by PFC responses. Taken together, these data suggest that familiarity is triggered early and automatically by appropriate sensory input to anterior MTLC, but only if the brain is prepared to treat this input as cues for episodic retrieval, familiarity-based recognition occurs. Otherwise, as in implicit memory tests, these early discharges may initiate other processes and facilitate performance, but do not lead to the formation of familiarity-supporting memory representations. Another important implication of the above-mentioned single-unit studies is that medial and ventral prefrontal regions together with anterior MTLC regions may be involved in the generation of the scalp-recorded mid-frontal old/new effect. Further studies are warranted that examine the role of top-down processes in initiating and guiding memory retrieval processes and the computation of familiarity and recollection signals as well as the neural networks generating the scalp recorded old/new effects.

Although there is substantial evidence linking a mid-frontal and a parietal old/new effect to familiarity and recollection, respectively, there are also findings challenging this proposal (see Curran *et al.*, 2006b, for a discussion). For instance, Finnigan, Humphreys, Dennis, and Geffen (2002 found an early 300–500 ms old/new effect (over left parietal electrodes) that was linked to memory strength, by this resembling the concept of familiarity. However, a later 500–800 ms parietal old/new effect typically associated with recollection was taken to reflect the accuracy or confidence of memory decisions rather than recollection. Another account of the mid-frontal old/new effect is provided by Paller and colleagues. In one of their studies (Yovel & Paller, 2004) participants had to learn associations between unfamiliar faces and occupations. Familiarity-based recognition was inferred when participants recognized faces without retrieving any further information such as their associated occupations. By contrast, recollection-based recognition was assumed when participants could also recall occupations or other contextual information. Yovel and Paller (2004) found that recollection- and familiarity-based recognition were both associated with positive-going ERPs at parietal sites, revealing only a quantitative but no qualitative (e.g. topographical or temporal) difference between the two types of recognition responses. Hence, these findings suggest that recollective and familiarity-based recognition are mediated by the same neural network. On the basis of this study and other findings, Paller and colleagues propose that the mid-frontal old/new effect reflects conceptual priming rather than familiarity. (see Paller, Voss, & Boehm, 2007, for a review).

However, several lines of evidence argue against the view that the mid-frontal old/new effect reflects conceptual priming. First, a replication of the Yovel and Paller (2004) study with a different set of face stimuli revealed a reliable mid-frontal old/new effect for (familiar) faces retrieved without their associated occupations (Curran & Hancock, 2007). Second, arguing against the conceptual priming account of the mid-frontal old/new effect, a variety of studies using non-conceptual stimuli, like meaningless geometrical shapes (Curran, Tanaka, & Weiskopf, 2002; Groh-Bordin, Zimmer, & Ecker, 2006) or unfamiliar faces (Nessler, Mecklinger, & Penney 2005; Johansson, Mecklinger, & Treese, 2004) found the effect. Finally, the mid-frontal old/new effect is modulated by variables affecting recognition memory, like the adaptation of a response criterion (Azimian-Faridani & Wilding, 2006), signal strength (Woodruff *et al.*, 2006), or study-test similarity (Curran, 2000; Nessler *et al.*, 2001). These modulations are difficult to account for by the view that the mid-frontal old/new effect is a reflection of conceptual priming.

Another issue to be further addressed is the question about the circumstances under which familiarity contributes to associative recognition memory (Aggleton & Brown, 2006; Mayes *et al.*, 2007). As outlined in this chapter, there is growing evidence for the unitization hypothesis, i.e. the assumption that familiarity can support associative recognition judgements given that items or features are unitized into single entities. Also, using encoding conditions that encourage holistic processing, unitization seems to be possible for arbitrary items. However, findings of whether familiarity also supports associative retrieval of pre-experimentally unitized (semantic) associations have been somewhat mixed and deserve further investigation. With regard to the unitization view, future studies may specifically tackle the boundary conditions under which unitization can take place. Do items that are unitizable have some particular characteristics, such as being perceptually highly overlapping or being encodable in entity-creating frameworks? What are the encoding conditions that allow unitization of completely arbitrary items? Can unitization also occur for pairs of items of different modalities or is unitization constrained to visual stimuli represented in close proximity within anterior MTLC? As the anterior MTLC receives input from polymodal association cortices (Suzuki, 1996), the formation of unitized memory representations should not be limited to the visual modality.

In conclusion, although behavioural, animal, neuropsychological, neuroimaging, and electrophysiological studies have disclosed exciting findings on the puzzle about the cognitive processes underlying our ability to recognize previously encountered information, many issues remain to be resolved and provide the basis for questions addressed in future studies on recognition memory.

References

Aggleton, J. P. & Brown, M. W. (1999). Episodic memory, amnesia, and the hippocampal-anterior thalamic axis. *Behavioral and Brain Sciences, 22*, 425–489.

Aggleton, J. P. & Brown, M. W. (2006). Interleaving brain systems for episodic and recognition memory. *Trends in Cognitive Sciences, 10*, 455–463.

Allan, K., Wilding, E. L., & Rugg, M. D. (1998). Electrophysiological evidence for dissociable processes contributing to recollection. *Acta Psychologica, 98*, 231–252.

Azimian-Faridani, N. & Wilding, E. L. (2006). The influence of criterion shifts on electrophysiological correlates of recognition memory. *Journal of Cognitive Neuroscience. 18*, 107–108.

Bowles, B., Crupi, C., Mirsattari, S. M., Pigott, S. Parrent, A. G., Pruessner, J. C., Yonelinas, A. P. & Köhler, S. (2007). Impaired familiarity with preserved recollection after anterior temporal-lobe resection that spares the hippocampus. *PNAS, 104–41*, 16382–16387.

Ceraso, J. (1985). Unit formation in perception and memory. *The Psychology of Learning and Motivation, 19*, 179–210.

Curran, T. (2000). Brain potentials of recollection and familiarity. *Memory & Cognition, 28*, 923–938.

Curran, T. (2004). Effects of attention and confidence on the hypothesized ERP correlates of recollection and familiarity. *Neuropsychologia, 42*, 1088–1106.

Curran, T. & Cleary, A. M. (2003). Using ERPs to dissociate recollection from familiarity in picture recognition. *Cognitive Brain Research, 15*, 191–205.

Curran, T., DeBuse, C., Woroch, B., & Hirshman, E. (2006a). Combined pharmacological and electrophysiological dissociation of familiarity and recollection. *Journal of Neuroscience, 26*, 1979–1985.

Curran, T. & Dien, J. (2003). Differentiating amodal familiarity from modality-specific memory processes: An ERP study. *Psychophysiology, 40*, 979–988.

Curran, T. & Hancock, J. (2007). The FN400 indexes familiarity-based recognition of faces. *NeuroImage, 36*, 464–471.

Curran, T., Tanaka, J. W., Weiskopf, D. M. (2002). An electrophysiological comparison of visual categorization and recognition memory. *Cognitive, Affective & Behavioral Neuroscience, 2–1*, 1–18.

Curran, T., Tepe, K., & Piatt, C. (2006b). Event-related potential explorations of dual processes in recognition memory. In H. D. Zimmer, A. Mecklinger, & U. Lindenberger (Eds), *Handbook of Binding and Memory: Perspectives from Cognitive Neuroscience* (pp. 467–492). Oxford: Oxford University Press.

Donaldson, D. I. & Rugg, M. D. (1998). Recognition memory for new associations: Electrophysiological evidence for the role of recollection. *Neuropsychologia, 36*, 377–395.

Donaldson, D. I. & Rugg, M. D. (1999). Event-related potential studies of associative recognition and recall: Electrophysiological evidence for context dependent retrieval processes. *Cognitive Brain Research, 8*, 1–16.

Düzel, E., Vargha-Khadem, F., Heinze, H. -J., & Mishkin, M. (2001). Brain activity evidence for recognition without recollection after early hippocampal damage. *PNAS, 98*, 8101–8106.

Düzel, E., Yonelinas, A. P., Mangun, G. R., Heinze, H. -J., & Tulving, E. (1997). Event-related brain potential correlates of two states of conscious awareness in memory. *PNAS, 94*, 5973–5978.

Ecker, U. K. H., Zimmer, H. D., Groh-Bordin, C., & Mecklinger, A. (2007). Context effects on familiarity are familiarity effects of context - An electrophysiological study. *International Journal of Psychophysiology, 64*, 146–156.

Fernandez, G., Klaver, P., Fell, J., Grunwald, T., & Elger, C. (2002). Human declarative memory formation: Segregating rhinal and hippocampal contributions. *Hippocampus, 12*, 514–519.

Finnigan, S., Humphreys, M. S., Dennis, S., & Geffen, G. (2002). ERP 'old/new' effects: Memory strength and decisional factor(s). *Neuropsychologia, 40*, 2288–2304.

Friedman, D. & Johnson, R. Jr. (2000). Event-related potential (ERP) studies of memory encoding and retrieval: A selective review. *Microscopy Research and Technique, 51*, 6–28.

Giovanello, K. S., Keane, M. M., & Verfaellie, M. (2006). The contribution of familiarity to associative memory in amnesia. *Neuropsychologia, 44*, 1859–1865.

Gonsalves, B., Kahn, I., Curran, T., Norman, K. A., & Wagner, A. D. (2005). Memory strength and repetition suppression: Multimodal imaging of medial temporal cortical contributions to recognition. *Neuron, 47*, 751–761.

Graf, P. & Schacter, D. L. (1989). Unitization and grouping mediate dissociations in memory for new associations. *Journal of Experimental Psychology: Learning, Memory, and Cognition, 15*, 930–940.

Greve, A., van Rossum, M. C. W., & Donaldson, D. I. (2007). Investigating the functional interaction between semantic and episodic memory: Convergent behavioral and electrophysiological evidence for the role of familiarity. *NeuroImage, 34*, 801–814.

Grill-Spector, K., Henson, R., & Martin, A. (2006). Repetition and the brain: Neural models of stimulus-specific effects. *Trends in Cognitive Sciences*, *10*, 14–23.

Groh-Bordin, C., Zimmer, H. D., & Ecker, U. K. H. (2006). Has the butcher on the bus dyed his hair? When color changes modulate ERP correlates of familiarity and recollection. *NeuroImage*, *32*, 1879–1890.

Groh-Bordin, C., Zimmer, H. D., & Mecklinger, A. (2005). Feature binding in perceptual priming and in episodic object recognition: Evidence from event-related brain potentials. *Cognitive Brain Research*, *24*, 556–567.

Hayes-Roth, B. (1977). Evolution of cognitive structures and processes. *Psychological Review*, *84*, 260–278.

Henson, R. N. A., Cansino, S., Herron, J. E., Robb, W. G., & Rugg, M. D. (2003). A familiarity signal in human anterior medial temporal cortex? *Hippocampus*, *13*, 164–174.

Hintzman, D. L., Caulton, D. A., & Levitin, D. J. (1998). Retrieval dynamics in recognition and list discrimination: Further evidence of separate processes of familiarity and recall. *Memory & Cognition*, *26*, 449–462.

Hirshman, E. & Master, S. (1997). Modeling the conscious correlates of recognition memory: Reflections on the remember-know paradigm. *Memory & Cognition*, *25*, 345–351.

Holdstock, J. S., Mayes, A. R., Gong, Q. Y., Roberts, N., & Kapur, N. (2005). Item recognition is less impaired than recall and associative recognition in a patient with selective hippocampal damage. *Hippocampus*, *15*, 203–315.

Horowitz, L. M. & Prytulak, L. S. (1969). Redintegrative memory. *Psychological Review*, *76*, 519–531.

Jacoby, L. L. (1991). A process dissociation framework: Separating automatic from intentional uses of memory. *Journal of Memory and Language*, *30*, 513–541.

Jäger, T., Mecklinger, A., & Kipp, K. H. (2006). Intra- and inter-item associations doubly dissociate the electrophysiological correlates of familiarity and recollection. *Neuron*, *52*, 535–545.

Jäger, T., Seiler, K. H., & Mecklinger, A. (2005). Picture database of morphed faces (MoFa): Technical Report. *Psydok Online* (http://psydok.sulb.uni-saarland.de/volltexte/2005/505/).

Johansson, M., Mecklinger, A., & Treese, A. C. (2004). Recognition memory for emotional and neutral faces: An event-related potential study. *Journal of Cognitive Neuroscience.* *16*, 1840–1853

Kipp, K., Jäger, T., & Mecklinger, A. (2006). Intra- and inter-item binding in memory for morphed faces: An ERP investigation. *Journal of Cognitive Neuroscience (Supplement)*, *143*, 144–.

Klimesch, W., Hansmayr, S., Sauseng, P., Gruber, W., Brozinsky, C. J., Kroll, N. E. A., Yonelinas, A. P., & Doppelmayr, M. (2005). Oscillatory EEG correlates of episodic trace decay. *Cerebral Cortex*, *16*, 280–290.

Li, L., Miller, E. K., & Desimone, R. (1993). The representation of stimulus familiarity in anterior inferior temporal cortex. *Journal of Neurophysiology*, *69*, 1918–1929.

Mandler, G. (1980). Recognizing: The judgment of previous occurrence. *Psychological Review*, *87*, 252–271.

Mayes, A. R., Holdstock, J. S., Isaac, C. L., Hunkin, N. M., & Roberts, N. (2002). Relative sparing of item recognition memory in a patient with adult-onset damage limited to the hippocampus. *Hippocampus*, *12*, 325–340.

Mayes, A. R., Holdstock, J. S., Isaac, C. L., Montaldi, D., Grigor, J., Gummer, A., Cariga, P., Downes, J. J., Tsivilis, D., Gaffan, D., Gong, Q., & Norman, K. A. (2004). Associative recognition in a patient with selective hippocampal lesions and relatively normal item recognition. *Hippocampus*, *14*, 763–784.

Makeig, S., Westerfield, M., Jung, T. -P., Enghoff, S., Townsend, J., Courchesne, E., & Sejnowski, T. J. (2002). Dynamic brain sources of visual evoked responses. *Science*, *295*, 690–694.

Mayes, A., Montaldi, D., & Migo, E. (2007). Associative memory and the medial temporal lobes. *Trends in Cognitive Sciences, 11*, 127–135.

Mecklinger, A. (2000). Interfacing mind and brain: A neurocognitive model of recognition memory. *Psychophysiology, 37*, 565–582.

Mecklinger, A. (2006). Electrophysiological measures of familiarity memory. *Clinical EEG and Neuroscience, 37*, 292–299.

Mecklinger, A., Cramon, D. Y., & Matthes-von Cramon, G. (1998). Event-related potential evidence for a specific recognition memory deficit in adult survivors of cerebral hypoxia. *Brain, 121*, 1919–1935.

Mecklinger, A., Johansson, M., Parra, M., & Hanslmayr, S. (2007). Source-retrieval requirements influence late ERP memory effects. *Brain Research, 1172*, 110–123.

Meyer, P., Mecklinger, A., Grunwald, T., Fell, J., Elger, C. E., & Friederici, A. D. (2005). Language processing within the human medial temporal lobe. *Hippocampus, 15*, 451–459.

Montaldi, D., Spencer, T. J., Roberts, N., & Mayes, A. R. (2006). The neural systems that mediates familiarity memory. *Hippocampus, 16*, 504–520.

Nessler, D. & Mecklinger, A. (2003). ERP correlates of true and false recognition after different retention delays: stimulus and response related processes. *Psychophysiology, 40*, 1–14.

Nessler, D., Mecklinger, A., & Penney, T. B. (2001). Event related brain potentials and illusory memories: The effects of differential encoding. *Cognitive Brain Research, 10*, 283–301.

Nessler, D., Mecklinger, A., & Penney, T. B. (2005). Perceptual fluency, semantic familiarity, and recognition-related familiarity: An electrophysiological exploration. *Cognitive Brain Research, 22*, 265–288.

Norman, K. A. & O'Reilly, R. C. (2003). Modeling hippocampal and neocortical contribu.tions to recognition memory: A complementary-learning-systems approach. *Psychological Review, 110*, 611–646.

Opitz, B. & Cornell, S. (2006). Contribution of familiarity and recollection to associative recognition memory: Insights from event-related potentials. *Journal of Cognitive Neuroscience, 18*, 1595–1605.

Paller, K. A., Voss, J. L., & Boehm, S. G. (2007). Validating neural correlates of familiarity. *Trends in Cognitive Science, 11–6*, 243–250.

Penney, T. B., Mecklinger, A., & Nessler, D. (2001). Repetiton related ERP effects in a visual object target detection task. *Cognitive Brain Research, 10*, 239–250.

Quamme, J. R. (2004). *The role of unitization in the representation of associations in human memory.* Dissertation at University of California, Davis, USA.

Quamme, J. R., Yonelinas, A. P., & Kroll, N. E. A. (2006). Unpacking explicit memory: The contribution of recollection and familiarity. In H. D. Zimmer, A. Mecklinger, & U. Lindenberger (Eds), *Handbook of Binding and Memory: Perspectives from Cognitive Neuroscience* (pp. 445–466). Oxford: Oxford University Press.

Quamme, J. R., Yonelinas, A. P., & Norman, K. A. (2007). Effect of unitization on associative recognition in amnesia. *Hippocampus, 17*, 192–200.

Rhodes, S. M. & Donaldson, D. I. (2007). Electrophysiological evidence for the influence of unitization on the processes engaged during episodic retrieval: Enhancing familiarity based remembering. *Neuropsychologia, 45*, 412–424.

Rugg, M. D. & Curran, T. (2007). Event-related potentials and recognition memory. *Trends in Cognitive Sciences, 11*, 251–257.

Rugg, M. D. & Nieto-Vegas, M. (1999). Modality specific effects of immediate word repetition: Electrophysiological evidence. *NeuroReport, 1*, 2661–2664.

Rugg, M. D., Walla, P., Schloerscheidt, A. M., Fletcher, P. C., Frith, C. D., & Dolan, R. J. (1998). Neural correlates of depth of processing effects on recollection: Evidence from brain potentials and positron emission tomography. *Experimental Brain Research, 123*, 18–23.

Rugg, M. D. & Yonelinas, A. P. (2003). Human recognition memory: A cognitive neuroscience perspective. *Trends in Cognitive Sciences*, *7*, 313–319.

Schacter, D. L., Norman, K. A., & Koutstaal, W. (1998). The cognitive neuroscience of constructive memory. *Annual Review of Psychology*, *49*, 289–318.

Slotnick, S. D. & Dodson, C. S. (2005). Support for a continuous (single-process) model of recognition memory and source memory. *Memory & Cognition*, *33*, 151–170.

Smith, M. E. (1993). Neurophysiological manifestations of recollective experience during recognition memory judgments. *Journal of Cognitive Neuroscience*, *5*, 1–13.

Squire, L. R., Wixted, J. T., & Clark, R. E. (2007). Recognition memory and the medial temporal lobe: a new perspective. *Nature Reviews Neuroscience*, *8*, 872–883.

Suzuki, W. A. (1996). The anatomy, physiology and functions of the perirhinal cortex. *Current Opinion in Neurobiology*, *6*, 179–186.

Tendolkar, I., Schoenfeld, A., Golz, G., Fernandez, G., Kühl, K. P., Ferszt, R., & Heinze, H. -J. (1999). Neural correlates of recognition memory with and without recollection in patients with Alzheimer's disease and healthy controls. *Neuroscience Letters*, *263*, 45–48.

Tse, D., Langston, R. F., Kakeyama, M., Bethus, I., Sponner, P. A., Wood, E. R., Witter, M. P., & Morris, R. G. M. (2007). Schemas and memory consolidation. *Science, 316*, 76–82.

Tsivilis, D., Otten, L., & Rugg, M. D. (2001). Context effects on the neural correlates of recognition memory: An electrophysiological study. *Neuron, 31*, 497–505.

Tulving, E. (1985). Memory and consciousness. *Canadian Psychology, 26*, 1–12.

Vilberg, K. L., Moosavi, R. F., & Rugg, M. D. (2006). The relationship between electrophysiological correlates of recollection and amount of information retrieved. *Brain Research, 1122*, 161–170.

Wagner, A. D., Shannon, B. J., Kahn, I., & Buckner, R. L. (2005). Parietal lobe contributions to episodic memory retrieval. *Trends in Cognitive Sciences, 9*, 445–453.

Wais, P. E., Wixted, J. T., Hopkins, R. O., & Squire, L. R. (2006). The hippocampus supports both the recollection and familiarity components of recognition memory. *Neuron, 49*, 459–466.

Wilding, E. L. & Herron, J. E. (2006). Electrophysiological measures of episodic memory control and memory retrieval. *Clinical EEG and Neuroscience, 37*, 315–321.

Woodruff, C. C., Hayama, H. R., & Rugg, M. D. (2006). Electrophysiological dissociation of the neural correlates of recollection and familiarity. *Brain Research, 1100*, 125–135.

Yonelinas, A. P. (1997). Recognition memory ROCs for item and associative information: Evidence from a dual-process signal-detection model. *Memory & Cognition, 25*, 747–763.

Yonelinas, A. P. (2001). Components of episodic memory: The contribution of recollection and familiarity. *Philosophical Transactions of the Royal Society of London, Series B, 356*, 1636–1374.

Yonelinas, A. P. (2002). The nature of recollection and familiarity: A review of 30 years of research. *Journal of Memory and Language, 46*, 441–517.

Yonelinas, A. P., Kroll, N. E. A., Dobbins, I. G., & Soltani, M. (1999). Recognition memory for faces: When familiarity supports associative recognition judgments. *Psychonomic Bulletin & Review, 6*, 654–661.

Yonelinas, A. P., Kroll, N. E. A., Quamme, J. R., Lazzara, M. M., Sauve, M. J., Widaman, K. F., & Knight, R. T. (2002). Effects of extensive temporal lobe damage or mild hypoxia on recollection and familiarity. *Nature Neuroscience, 5*, 1236–1241.

Yonelinas, A. P., Otten, L. J., Shaw, K. N., & Rugg, M. D. (2005). Separating the brain regions involved in recollection and familiarity in recognition memory. *Journal of Neuroscience, 25*, 3002–3008.

Yovel, G. & Paller, K. A. (2004). The neural basis of the butcher-on-the-bus phenomenon: When a face seems familiar but is not remembered. *NeuroImage, 21*, 789–800.

Xiang, J. -Z. & Brown, M. W. (2004). Neuronal responses related to long-term recognition memory processes in prefrontal cortex. *Neuron, 42*, 817–829.

Chapter 21

Memory and the awareness of remembering

Ken A. Paller, Joel L. Voss and Carmen E. Westerberg

Introduction

Determining exactly how the operation of the brain leads to conscious experience is one of the Holy Grails of contemporary scientific research. Awareness is the core of our mental lives, and ultimately the one most highly valued component of our human biological make-up. Many of the complex mental functions that guide our day-to-day activities, including perception, imagination, problem solving, volitional action, attention, and autobiographical memory, cannot be explained fully without including conscious awareness in the explanation. Nonetheless, prospects for a thorough scientific understanding of consciousness often seem daunting.

To show how progress can be made in understanding consciousness, we focus here on the conscious experience of remembering. We propose that significant insights into consciousness can be gained by using neuroimaging to elucidate differences between conscious memory experiences and non-conscious memory experiences. We qualify this proposal by noting that methods for measuring human brain activity provide powerful tools but that the scientific investigation of consciousness must rely on a wider range of methods. The application of neuroimaging to the problems of memory and consciousness can be most fruitful when evidence is sought with reference to all four dimensions of the problem: cognitive, neural, behavioural, and subjective. This theoretical stance may appear to conflict with the goal inherent in the title of the conference that precipitated this book (*Neuroimaging and Psychological Theories of Human Memory*), that of establishing psychological theories – indeed, we propose that investigators should not seek pure psychological theories of memory. We must not settle for purely cognitive theories, purely behavioural theories, purely neural theories, or purely subjective theories of memory. All four dimensions are essential for understanding memory and consciousness. We thus envision a comprehensive scientific analysis of conscious phenomena like recollection, an approach that may bring us closer to specifying the essential ingredients that yield conscious experience and thus closer to solving long-standing mysteries about the human mind.

What is consciousness?

One challenge in building an appropriate framework for studying consciousness is providing a suitable operational definition. Philosophers and scientists have not yet settled on a unitary definition of consciousness, despite debate that can be traced back over two millennia to Greek philosophers in the West and Indian philosophers in the East. However, as noted by Farber and Churchland (1995), a final definition is not a prerequisite for today's scientific progress. Rather, preliminary definitions allow investigations to make useful progress and foster the simultaneous evolution of multiple theories and conceptualizations of consciousness.

Towards this end, Zeman (2002) provides a helpful framework that distinguishes three distinct meanings of the word *consciousness*. First, a person is said to be conscious in a clinical setting if they are awake, in the sense of not being in a coma, in a trance, or under general anesthesia. In this context, consciousness refers to a person's alertness or orientation to time and place. A second definition (which is the primary focus of discussion in the remainder of this chapter) emphasizes the subjective experience of a percept, a thought, a memory, an emotion, or some other mental content. In this sense, consciousness (or synonymously, awareness) has been referred to variously as primary memory, the spotlight of attention, the stream of consciousness, the working-memory buffer, or the running span of subjective experience. Zeman's final definition likens consciousness to the mind more generally, including volition and long-term intentions, such that ideas can be part of consciousness in this sense whether or not they are constantly at the forefront of thought. For example, a student can have the conscious goal of completing all the requirements for graduation without necessarily being aware of this intention every second of every day. The phrase *fully cognizant* could perhaps be substituted for this third meaning of *consciousness*.

In attempting to understand what it means to be conscious, Zeman (2002) also argues that it is helpful to consider the etiology of the word *conscious*. The English term evolved from the Latin word *conscius*, which means 'knowing with another'. This highlights the sharing of a dialogue between two entities, as in to share knowledge with others – or with one's self. Today we often use the closely related term *self-conscious* to refer to the instance when one has conceptualized one's own self and its place in the world. Interestingly, in some languages a single word is used to describe both *conscious* and *self-conscious*. The German word *Bewusstsein* and the Danish word *bevidsthed* are two such examples. It is also interesting to consider the Indian Sanskrit word *smṛti*, often translated as *mindfulness*, which is a concept closely related to consciousness in that it pertains to the quality of one's awareness of the present. But *smṛti* is also translated to mean memory of the past, which has been explained with reference to philosophical accounts portraying close connections between memory and mindfulness (Gyatso, 1992). Indeed, it may be essential for our understanding of memory to co-evolve with our understanding of consciousness.

How should we develop a scientific framework for examining subjective awareness? In most circumstances, science relies on the third-person perspective, where observations are objective and are available for verification by multiple observers. Subjective experiences do not easily conform to these notions but they are central to directly determining when and how consciousness is taking place. As others have also pointed out (e.g. Flanagan, 1992; Tulving, 1985), we argue that investigations should not avoid this important source of information, despite the difficulty of verifying reports of subjective experiences across different individuals. Introspective evidence is essential, in concert with converging cognitive, behavioural, and neural descriptions, for a complete understanding of consciousness.

The opposing alternative is to keep one's distance from introspection. Psychological research has occasionally adopted this approach, as in the strict emphasis on behavioural observations in Behaviourism. Today, closing the door on everything but behavioural observations is widely seen as detrimental to the development of suitable theories. Although the exclusionary approach in Behaviourism is unpopular, there are other attempts to close the door on certain types of evidence. Lamme (2006) advocated building theories of consciousness on neural evidence, specifically excluding introspective evidence. In contrast, some advocates of psychological or cognitive theories take the position that neural evidence is unimportant. We argue that all of these strategies are bound to come up short because they ignore essential aspects of the problem. Ignoring consciousness, or pretending that it does not exist (*cf.* James, 1904), is no solution. Indeed, if science is charged with explaining the world, then it would be inconsistent to ignore the first-person perspective, because it is a central aspect of our world. As Zeman (2002) observed, even science itself begins and ends with experience and thought. Our human consciousness, its limits and its vast potential, unavoidably colours all of our scientific observations and our attempts to gain understanding.

Cross-disciplinary perspectives are needed for developing explanations of mental functions. In our conceptualization, several different perspectives can be emphasized to different degrees, but all must be included. The pyramid in Figure 21.1 illustrates this idea with a pyramid created from four sides, each representing a different aspect of a comprehensive neurocognitive theory of a mental function. One such function to consider is that of

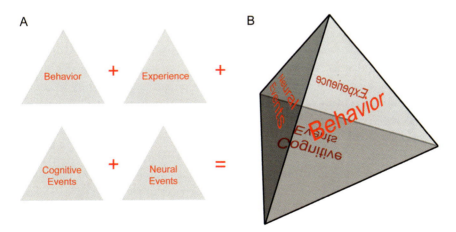

Figure 21.1 Scientific inquiry into mental function can be conceptualized using a pyramid metaphor. There are four sides, each corresponding to a different perspective on a mental function (A). The pyramid represents a comprehensive neurocognitive account of the mental function in question, which must include each of these four perspectives along with an explanation of how the four are related to each other (B).

consciously remembering a previously experienced episode. Building a theory to explain this function requires bringing together all four sides of the pyramid. The glue that connects all edges together can be thought of as the framework that binds together all four aspects into a cohesive theory. One side represents a behavioural phenomenon, which often can be the entry point for inquiry – we might wish to understand a particular behaviour, as in recalling and recognizing. Another side represents the neural events responsible for that behaviour. The third side represents a description of the cognitive representations and processes that underlie the behaviour, and the fourth side represents any subjective experience that accompanies the behaviour, directly available only to one observer. Although each side has a separate description (and sometimes a separate scientific discipline), a theoretical framework is needed to relate the four perspectives together. In a sense, then, the four sides must ultimately be conceived as part of the same whole.

This illustration also underscores the idea that a theoretical account entirely restricted to one side of the pyramid is inadequate. Although interesting scientific accounts can undoubtedly be generated from any one of the perspectives, ultimately such accounts are incomplete. Indeed, none of the perspectives is optional. The perspective from subjective experience, in particular, is essential for a full understanding of a mental function like recollection, as it is indeed a key part of the phenomenon that we wish to explain. Perhaps the most difficult challenge in understanding a mental function is to generate an account of how each of the four perspectives relates to the others, thus cementing the four sides together.

Conscious and non-conscious memory expressions

Memory phenomena are typically subdivided into two broad categories, and although different terms have been used by different investigators, there is a solid consensus that the two categories differ in the degree to which they involve awareness of remembering. *Declarative memory* refers to the ability to remember prior autobiographical episodes and complex facts, as assessed in recall and recognition tests (Squire, 1987). The ability to mentally reinstate facts and events from one's own past allows for the development and stability of a self-identity. These memories serve as a basis for an individual's 'life story'. Other types of memory that do not provide this potential accessibility to conscious reflection are collectively referred to as *non-declarative memory*. This large category includes memory phenomena that shape how one behaves in various situations and includes phenomena such as skills, habits, conditioning, and priming. The same basic distinction is carried by the terms *explicit memory* and *implicit memory*.

When a person expresses declarative memory behaviourally, he or she may also have *the conscious experience of remembering*, which we refer to using the term *recollection*, following Schacter (1989) and Tulving (1983). Recollection can occur either if memory retrieval was under intentional control or if retrieval was unintentional (i.e. incidental recollection). In contrast, there is no awareness of remembering when non-declarative memory is expressed unless declarative memory can be concomitantly expressed.

The ability to recollect an episode is mediated by two major steps: memory retrieval and metamemory inference. First, the combination of perceptual features that together make up a personally experienced episode must be retrieved. Successful retrieval depends on several processing stages, including initial encoding, storage, analysis of retrieval cues, control processes that enable strategic encoding and/or retrieval, search strategies, working memory for the contents of retrieval, and so on. Once a declarative memory is retrieved, a further inference must be made. A metamemory judgement, often based on recalling source- or context-specifying information, is necessary for one to come to the final realization: 'I remember…'. This realization is not an essential defining feature of declarative memory; the inference is often not at the focus of attention. However, it would generally be possible to overtly or covertly declare that memory retrieval has occurred. Thus, the 'conscious experience of remembering' goes one step beyond declarative memory retrieval *per se*, as it includes the concurrent awareness that the information retrieved is the direct result of previous memory storage.

How can we approach the difficulty of integrating subjective experience into an objective scientific account of recollection? Consider by contrast attempts at eliminative reductionism, which might focus inquiry on the neural events that support behavioural memory phenomena, such that subjective experience itself would ultimately be excluded (e.g. Churchland, 1995). Awareness would conceivably be accounted for entirely by the other perspectives, but this would not be inconceivable as a suitable outcome because the subjective experience is what we wish to explain, not something we can refute. Whereas a theoretical account of cognitive and neural events may appear to explain how a declarative memory is retrieved, to fully understand remembering a declarative memory, subjective experience cannot be disregarded.

At the other end, an elaborate introspective account of remembering can stand on its own, as it has in philosophical accounts of memory. But that by itself would also be unsatisfactory, given the scientific goal of understanding the relationships among the four perspectives.

Several technologies can allow us to observe brain activity associated with conscious and non-conscious memory phenomena in behaving human volunteers. Given that these methods provide images of brain activity, they can be referred to collectively as neuroimaging techniques, including functional magnetic resonance imaging (fMRI), electroencephalography (EEG), magnetoencephalography (MEG), near-infrared spectroscopy (NIRS), and so on. Whereas we emphasize observations on brain function here, some neuroimaging techniques can provide information concerning the structural integrity of the brain, also leading to important insights into the neural substrates of memory and consciousness. In order to maximize the usefulness of these neural observations, it is important to consider what is already known about human memory, the brain, and consciousness. Neuropsychological studies of patients with circumscribed amnesia have provided many relevant insights into declarative memory, its neural basis, and the nature of memory disorders. Likewise, careful behavioural analyses of memory and the ensuing cognitive models that have been developed also provide frameworks within which neuroimaging evidence can be interpreted. In investigations of memory, a wide range of techniques and methods of inquiry can thus contribute to theoretical advances.

To make progress towards achieving a scientific understanding of the relationship between behavioural, neural, cognitive and subjective aspects of recollection, it can be useful to start with behavioural observations, first striving for some consensus about how to measure the recall and recognition of facts and events. Using these behavioural measures, we can gather evidence on neural correlates of declarative memory performance and on correlations between brain dysfunction and memory deficits. With the combination of behavioural and neural observations, we can generate ideas about cognitive structures and processes that describe relevant information processing steps. We can then attempt to link the subjective experience of remembering with the cognitive and neural accounts of memory processing and the behavioural signs of memory retrieval. Further insights can be gleaned by contrasting these accounts of declarative memory with parallel accounts of other types of memory. In this way, we begin to see from each perspective what makes declarative memory distinctive.

Of course, there are also other scenarios for relating the four perspectives to each other. For example, valuable information can be obtained by starting from a neural perspective (e.g. asking how a specific neuroanatomical structure such as the hippocampus is associated with specific behavioural, subjective, and cognitive features).

Contrasting recollection with other memory expressions

Key insights into declarative memory have been achieved by contrasting it with other types of memory. Neuropsychological investigations have been particularly useful in this endeavour. Although recollection is impaired in individuals with amnesia due to circumscribed damage to the hippocampus and surrounding cortex, non-declarative memory, and in particular, priming – facilitated processing of a stimulus due to prior experience with that stimulus – is preserved in these individuals (Gabrieli, 1998; Schacter, 1987, 1996; Squire, 1987). A classic example of preserved memory function in amnesia is the story of Dr. Claparède's hidden pin (Claparède, 1911/1951; Kihlstrom, 1995). The doctor extended his hand to greet an amnesic patient, but the patient withdrew and refused to shake hands. At their previous meeting, Claparède had secretly placed a pin in his hand, pricking the patient and causing discomfort. Although the patient could not recollect this event, she did exhibit some memory for the meeting that influenced her behaviour in an implicit way.

Within declarative memory, a distinction has been made between *recollection* and *familiarity*. Familiarity involves an implied (if not explicit) acknowledgement that an event has been experienced before, but unlike recollection, familiarity does not include retrieval of contextual details of the initial learning episode or other source-specifying information. Rather, the current situation or stimulus seems familiar without specific knowledge of why it is familiar. A wealth of behavioural studies support the existence of these two distinct forms of declarative memory (see Yonelinas, 2002, for review), and neuropsychological evidence suggests that recollection and familiarity may to some extent be neurally dissociable. For example, recollective recognition was found to be disrupted and familiarity-driven recognition preserved in the prodromal stage of Alzheimer's disease known as amnestic mild cognitive impairment (Westerberg *et al.*, 2006). The earlier definition of *recollection* discussed above (awareness of remembering) is nearly the same as the definition of *recollection* within the recollection/familiarity framework, except that in the latter case, awareness must concern specific aspects of a prior episode beyond awareness of memory retrieval *per se*. There are thus two aspects to the formal meaning of 'awareness of remembering': (1) awareness that memory retrieval has occurred and (2) retrieval of specific memory features such as spatiotemporal context that identify a prior learning episode. The second will not occur without the first; a pure familiarity experience, however, would entail the first without the second.

Neuroimaging provides another way to contrast recollection with other memory phenomena without relying on neurological patients with memory impairments. Recent studies have investigated differences between recollection and implicit category learning (Reber, Gitelman, Parrish, & Mesulam, 2003), cognitive skill learning (Poldrack, Desmond, Glover, & Gabrieli, 1998), visual search facilitation (Miller *et al.*, 2006), and so on. These sorts of contrasts have provided many insights into these memory distinctions. Here, we will focus on neuroimaging studies that have examined differences between recollection and priming.

First, it is important to consider the theoretical constructs that have been developed thus far concerning declarative and non-declarative memory (Figure 21.2). Declarative memory is exhibited through the recall and recognition of facts and events. Neural characterizations typically appeal to neocortical networks that become linked together via cross-cortical storage mechanisms initiated by the hippocampus (e.g. Paller, 1997, 2002). Cognitive models often describe declarative memories as composed of information fragments that are linked together by virtue of encoding processes that yield relational

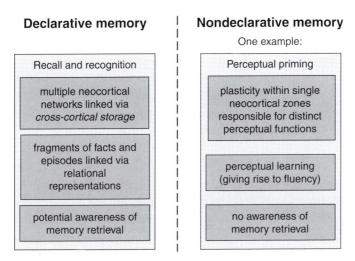

Figure 21.2 Theoretical features of declarative and non-declarative memory, including behavioural, neural, cognitive, and subjective perspectives. Note that other examples of non-declarative memory may differ from perceptual priming.

representations (e.g. Shimamura, 2002: Eichenbaum & Cohen, 2001). As discussed above, the retrieval of a declarative memory is often accompanied by the awareness of memory retrieval.

Perceptual priming is a type of non-declarative memory that is exhibited through speeded or more accurate responses to a stimulus due to prior experience with that stimulus, and based on altered processing of perceptual features of the stimulus. Relevant neural plasticity may be confined to isolated neocortical zones responsible for distinct perceptual functions (Paller, 1997). At a cognitive level, these changes may be defined as perceptual learning or perceptual fluency.

Within each of these categories of declarative and non-declarative memory, there are multiple memory phenomena that can be described in terms of the behaviour exhibited and the subjective experience that accompanies each behaviour. In declarative memory, a recollective report consists of remembering a prior episode with sufficient detail to recall the source of the memory. A pure familiarity experience occurs when an episode is familiar, but without knowledge of the source of the memory (Mandler, 1980). Within non-declarative memory, perceptual priming consists of facilitated perceptual processing without any necessary awareness of the relation between the facilitation and a prior learning episode. Similarly, conceptual priming is exhibited by facilitated conceptual processing without any necessary awareness of the relation between the facilitation and a prior learning episode.

According to this taxonomy, familiarity and priming clearly lie on different sides of the declarative/non-declarative distinction. There is widespread agreement that familiarity and priming are behaviourally distinct phenomena, but there is continuing controversy over the extent to which they share common neurocognitive mechanisms. Indeed, it has been suggested that familiarity and conceptual priming are behavioural manifestations of the same underlying processes (Whittlesea, 1993; Wolk et al., 2004, 2005; Yonelinas, 2002). Such speculations are of great importance because they strike at the heart of the border between declarative and non-declarative memory and have implications for understanding what is unique about memories accompanied by subjective awareness. Is this border permeable, or is its whole construction possibly misguided? We argue that additional neural evidence may be useful, and perhaps necessary, to sort out how to conceptualize the border areas of the declarative/non-declarative distinction and how to precisely classify the memory phenomena on either side.

Isolating neural correlates of recollection

It is important to build up a neural perspective on recollection to complement the cognitive, behavioural, and phenomenological descriptions. Towards this end, neural correlates of recollection have been extensively studied using event-related potentials (ERPs), which are time-locked signals extracted from EEG recordings from electrodes placed on the scalp. In the ERP literature, the most consistently reported finding during recognition is that positive potentials to old items are greater than those to new items from approximately 400–800 ms. These effects are typically evident at many scalp locations and show a maximal difference over midline or left parietal locations. The amplitude of these differences generally increases with increasing memory strength, as assessed using behavioural indices such as recognition confidence. Potentials elicited by recognized items (hits) tend to be larger compared to potentials elicited by old items that are forgotten (misses) and compared to potentials to new items that are correctly identified (correct rejections).

Early investigations of these old/new ERP effects endorsed a variety of hypotheses concerning their functional significance, including associations with memory strength (Johnson, Pfefferbaum, & Kopell, 1985), relative familiarity (Rugg, 1990), contextual retrieval (Smith & Halgren, 1989), and processes that do not contribute to recognition judgements (Rugg & Nagy, 1989). Despite the early lack of consensus about the meaning of these ERPs, many researchers speculated that the effects included modulation of two ERP components: N400 potentials and P300 potentials (e.g. Halgren & Smith, 1987).

One investigation that convincingly associated ERPs with recollection utilized a levels-of-processing manipulation at study (Paller & Kutas, 1992). Behavioural results showed that this manipulation influenced recall and recognition performance, with superior memory following semantic encoding that required visual imagery ('deep' encoding) than following encoding that focused attention on letter information ('shallow' encoding). In contrast, the same level of priming was observed on an implicit memory test of word identification for both encoding tasks. ERPs recorded during the implicit memory test were compared across the two encoding conditions, and corresponding differences were interpreted as ERP correlates of recollection. This ERP difference based on type of encoding began at a latency of 500 ms and was only present for words that were successfully identified in the test phase (all words were difficult to identify because of their brief duration and backward masking). Unlike typical old/new ERP effects, this effect could not be attributed to differences in perceptual priming because perceptual priming was equivalent for the two encoding conditions (conceptual priming was not measured, but is considered below). Furthermore, post-experiment debriefing indicated that during the word-identification test subjects noticed previously encoded words, even though this was irrelevant to their task. In other words, subjects were cognizant during the word-identification test of seeing words from the prior context of the study phase earlier in the experiment. The authors thus inferred that incidental recollection took place during the test phase, particularly when word meaning had been encoded deeply, and that ERPs were sensitive to the differential processing associated with recollection.

Subsequent studies using the same design strategy have substantiated the association between ERPs and recollection and extended the results to the use of other encoding tasks and memory tests (Paller, Kutas, & McIsaac, 1995), stimulus modalities (Gonsalves & Paller, 2000), and stimulus classes (e.g. faces; Paller *et al.*, 1999). Other studies using quite different designs have also reported late parietal ERPs related to recollection. For example, in *remember/know* paradigms in which *remember* responses are thought to reflect recollection and *know* responses are thought to reflect familiarity, larger late parietal ERPs have been consistently associated with *remember* responses (e.g. Curran, 2004;

Düzel *et al.*, 1997; Smith, 1993). Similarly, correct source judgements, which presumably require recollection, elicit larger late parietal ERPs than do incorrect source judgements (Senkfor & Van Petten, 1998; Trott *et al.*, 1999; Wilding & Rugg, 1996). These late parietal ERPs can thus be taken as signals of the successful retrieval of episodic memories linked with conscious remembering (see Friedman & Johnson, 2000; Voss & Paller, 2008; for reviews).

Results from memory-disordered patients have also confirmed associations between successful episodic retrieval and late positive ERPs. Amnesic patients exhibit impaired conscious recognition as well as reduced or absent late positive amplitudes (Olichney *et al.*, 2000, 2006). In addition, administration of benzodiazepine drugs to healthy subjects prior to encoding creates a temporary state of amnesia such that both subsequent recollection and concomitant late parietal potentials are severely disrupted (e.g. Curran *et al.*, 2006). Taken together, evidence from a variety of experimental paradigms converges on the conclusion that recollective expressions of memory reliably occur with a particular ERP signature (Figure 21.3).

Neural comparisons between recollection and perceptual priming

Neural perspectives on recollection can be valuable for a comprehensive understanding of recollection as well as for delineating how recollection differs from non-conscious forms of memory. In either case it is essential that these neural measures accurately reflect the memory phenomena in question. This has been a pervasive problem in the field because multiple memory processes can be operative at the same time. For example, automatic processing that supports perceptual and conceptual priming may occur during recognition tests, even if behavioural measures of priming are not obtained, and this processing can potentially be reflected in neural measures interpreted as neural markers of recognition (Paller, Voss, & Boehm, 2007). In the prior section we considered ways to obtain neural correlates of recollection while minimizing possible contamination from priming. We emphasized contamination from perceptual priming, and we will consider conceptual priming in the next section.

Likewise, the possibility of contamination must also be considered when the research focus is on implicit memory. Experiments undertaken to isolate neural correlates of priming must allocate proper attention to possible contamination from declarative memory. Such contamination is problematic in many priming tests because of the tendency for subjects to recognize repeated stimuli or recall prior episodes in addition to following instructions for the priming test.

To isolate ERP correlates of perceptual priming, Paller and colleagues (2003) used a paradigm in which faces were minimally encoded such that perceptual priming occurred in the absence of recognition. Subjects viewed each face for 100 ms at a central location while one of two subtly different yellow crosses was simultaneously shown unpredictably in one of four quadrants 1.8° from fixation. While maintaining central fixation, subjects attempted to identify which one of the two yellow crosses was present, and further stimulus processing was disrupted via backward masking. Subsequently, yes-no recognition

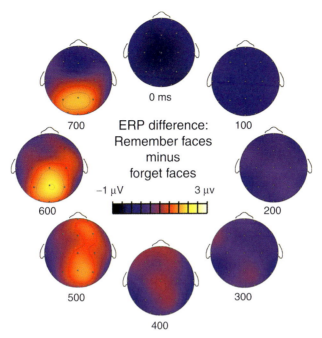

Figure 21.3 Neural correlates of conscious recollection. Subjects encoded faces either with the intention to remember them (remember faces) or to forget them (forget faces). Each remember face was accompanied by a short biographical vignette. All faces and vignettes were presented three times, a procedure which yielded very strong memory for the remember faces. ERPs were recorded during a test phase that included the remember faces, the forget faces, and new faces. Subjects detected occasional target faces (faces that appeared twice in immediate succession) in addition to having the opportunity to rehearse their memories for the remember faces and associated information. Subjects were told to engage in this rehearsal because a memory test for this information would be given afterwards. Indeed, subjects were highly accurate when asked at the end of the experiment to recall the biographical information when cued by the corresponding remember face. Also, recognition of individual faces was superior for remember compared to forget faces, whereas perceptual priming did not differ between the two conditions. ERPs from the test phase were computed and measured over consecutive 100-ms intervals following face onset. Progressive topographic maps were computed for the differences between ERPs to remember faces and ERPs to forget faces. Each map represents the head as if viewed from above, with different potential amplitudes indicated by the colour scale. Whereas ERP differences were minimal in the first few hundred ms, subsequent positive difference potentials were larger for remember faces than for forget faces. These late positive potentials were thus taken to index recollective processing uncontaminated by perceptual priming. Data are from Paller, Bozic, Ranganath, Grabowecky, and Yamada (1999).

memory for these minimally processed faces was not significantly better than chance, and forced-choice recognition was only slightly above chance. Reliable perceptual priming for these faces, however, was observed on two implicit memory tests. Therefore, ERPs elicited by these faces could conceivably reflect neural events responsible for perceptual priming, whereas contributions from recognition processes would be negligible (the number of faces endorsed as old was virtually the same for these faces and for new faces). Furthermore, a contribution from recognition to ERPs in this condition is inconsistent with the finding that they did not resemble reduced versions of ERPs associated with above-chance recognition. Indeed, a high level of recognition was found for one condition in the same experiment with faces presented at study for a longer duration and without disruptive perifoveal visual discriminations or backward masking. ERPs elicited when these faces appeared in the test phase presumably reflected conscious memory and could be directly compared with ERPs associated with perceptual priming (Figure 21.4).

Neural correlates of recognition included late positive potentials closely resembling potentials associated with face-cued recollection in other experiments (Paller *et al.*, 1999; Yovel & Paller, 2004), whereas perceptual priming was associated with a relative ERP negativity over anterior sites from approximately 200–400 ms after face onset. These results indicate that spatiotemporally distinct ERPs of opposite polarities are associated with conscious remembering and perceptual priming. This pattern of results was replicated in a second experiment in which ERP recordings were made during an implicit memory test such that priming was concurrently observed (Paller *et al.*, 2003, Experiment 2). Such findings complement neuroanatomical dissociations in amnesic patients, and are consistent with the hypothesis that implicit access to memory is supported by

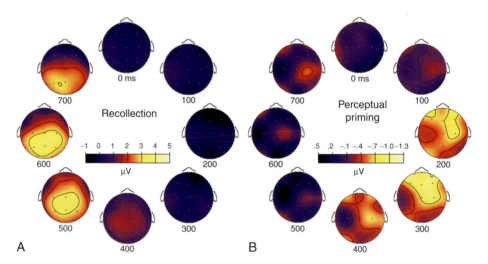

Figure 21.4 Neural correlates of recollection and perceptual priming with faces. ERP differences between remembered faces and new faces are displayed in (A). The inference that this contrast specifically concerns recollection is further supported by similarities to results from prior analyses of face recollection (e.g. Paller *et al.*, 1999; as shown in Figure 21.3) as well as to results from ERP contrasts based on a variation of the remember/know paradigm used to directly compare recollection and familiarity with faces (Yovel & Paller, 2004). ERP differences between primed-but-not-remembered faces and new faces are displayed in B. Differences were averaged over consecutive 100-ms intervals starting at the latency indicated underneath each topographic map (same format as in Figure 21.3). Light colours in the colour scale indicate positive differences in (A) and negative differences in (B). Figure adapted from Paller *et al.* (2003).

neural processing that is qualitatively distinct from that supporting conscious access to memory.

Another way to examine possible neural distinctions between recollection and perceptual priming is to consider ERPs to unrecognized but studied test items, because these ERPs could reflect implicit memory in the absence of recollection. In one study, recognized test items elicited late parietal ERPs (similar to those described in the prior section) whereas all studied test items (including both recognized and unrecognized items) elicited earlier parietal ERPs (300–500 ms). These results were interpreted as distinct neural correlates for recollection and perceptual priming, respectively (Rugg *et al.*, 1998). However, the reasoning that priming occurs for unrecognized items in the absence of a behavioural manifestation of priming is incomplete and potentially misleading. Methods that make use of concomitant behavioural indices of priming are thus preferable.

Differences between declarative and non-declarative memory have also been examined by contrasting neural correlates of encoding associated with subsequent recollection and subsequent perceptual priming. Schott and colleagues (2002) accomplished this by using deep versus shallow encoding conditions, followed by an ingenious two-stage procedure to assess memory. Following word encoding, three-letter word stems were presented in an explicit memory test (cued recall), but subjects were encouraged to guess if they could not remember a studied word so that priming might also occur. After each stem was completed, subjects indicated using strict criteria whether they recognized the word from the encoding phase. Encoding trials were categorized as showing priming if the subject produced the word at the completion stage but failed to endorse it as an old word (i.e. priming-without-recognition). Trials were categorized as remembered when the correct response was made at both stages, and as forgotten if not produced at the completion stage. This method provides behavioural indications of both explicit retrieval and priming, and is thus preferable to methods that merely assume that priming transpires for all repeated stimuli. Subsequent-memory analyses thus revealed an electrophysiological Difference based on subsequent memory (*Dm*), as assessed in the stem-completion priming test, that took the form of a relative ERP negativity over central and fronto-central locations approximately 200–400 ms after word onset (resembling ERP correlates of perceptual priming identified during memory testing, Paller *et al.*, 2003). Furthermore, Dm for priming was distinct from ERP differences between deep vs. shallow encoding as well as from Dm for recognition, which both included relatively positive potentials at later intervals with different topographies. Collectively, these results (along with those from a follow-up study using fMRI, Schott *et al.*, 2006) constitute critical first steps in characterizing the neurocognitive relationship between expressions of declarative memory and expressions of perceptual implicit memory.

Conscious familiarity and non-conscious conceptual priming

Another form of priming known as *conceptual priming* can occur whenever concepts are repeated. Note that the same concept can be engendered by perceptually identical or perceptually quite different stimuli. Behavioural measures of conceptual priming are similar to those of perceptual priming in that they can be produced in the absence of awareness of memory retrieval and typically take the form of faster or more accurate responses to certain stimuli. These altered behavioural responses are thought to reflect facilitated processing of stimulus meaning, beyond processing of the basic physical features of a stimulus. Although the functional implications of conceptual priming are unclear, this type of priming may be allied with short-term mnemonic operations that are preserved in amnesic patients, as in their normal language comprehension.

Because the neural processing that supports conceptual priming can occur whenever concepts are repeated, regardless of whether a behavioural test of conceptual priming is provided, it is possible that neural activity associated with conceptual priming occurs incidentally during tests of recognition memory for meaningful stimuli. A widely cited hypothesis is that frontal N400 potentials at retrieval index the form of declarative memory referred to as familiarity (Curran, Tepe, & Piatt, 2006; Rugg & Curran, 2007). However, similar potentials are intact in amnesic patients (Olichney et al., 2000), raising the possibility that frontal N400s do not reflect declarative memory but instead reflect a form of memory that is not disrupted in amnesia. Olichney and colleagues (2000) proposed that preserved conceptual priming in amnesic patients could be reflected by these preserved ERP differences. It is thus possible that frontal N400 potentials do not index familiarity but instead reflect conceptual priming that occurs concurrently with explicit memory, as argued by Paller and colleagues (2007). Further work is needed to disentangle these two memory functions.

In two recent studies that directly examined this issue, celebrity faces were used to elicit neural correlates of conceptual priming and explicit memory (Voss & Paller, 2006; Voss, Reber, Mesulam, Parrish, & Paller, 2007). Conceptual priming was manipulated by presenting associated biographical information in conjunction with half of the celebrity faces. Later, electrophysiological recordings were obtained while subjects rapidly discriminated celebrity faces from other faces. Evidence for conceptual priming consisted of faster and more accurate responses to the faces previously presented with biographical information compared to responses to the other celebrity faces, even though all the celebrity faces had been viewed an equivalent number of times. Electrophysiological responses were obtained during the famous/non-famous discrimination test, and were characterized as a function of conceptual priming and also as a function of explicit memory ratings obtained in a final phase of the experiment (Voss & Paller, 2006). Conceptual priming was strongly associated with frontal N400 potentials (Figure 21.5) whereas explicit memory again was linked with late positive potentials at posterior locations. Furthermore, fMRI measures collected using a similar design revealed left inferior prefrontal cortex repetition suppression effects for conceptual priming and right parietal cortex repetition enhancement effects for familiarity (Voss et al., 2007).

These results attest to the likelihood that neural activity related to conceptual implicit memory is commonly produced in experiments designed to focus on declarative memory, no matter what technique of neuroimaging is used. Furthermore, the hypothesis that frontal N400 potentials are unique neural signatures of familiarity must be called into question, because it might partially (or entirely) reflect the operation of implicit memory (Paller et al., 2007). Much work will be needed to accurately elucidate the neural

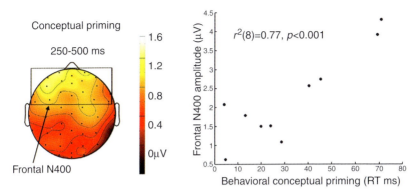

Figure 21.5 Neural correlates of conceptual priming. ERPs to famous faces were recorded while subjects discriminated between famous and non-famous faces. ERPs to famous faces that had previously been presented with corresponding biographical information (primed faces) were contrasted with ERPs to famous faces previously presented without corresponding information (unprimed faces). Conceptual priming was found in the form of faster and more accurate behavioural responses for primed compared to unprimed faces. The difference between ERPs from these two conditions was computed at each electrode location and is shown as a topographic map (left). Frontal differences in the interval from 250–500 ms were interpreted as ERP correlates of conceptual priming. Across individuals, the magnitude of these frontal N400 ERP differences (quantified in each subject at the electrode exhibiting the greatest ERP difference) was found to correlate with the magnitude of conceptual priming indexed behaviourally (right). Figure adapted from Voss and Paller (2006) and Paller *et al.* (2007).

substrates of these memory processes, but doing so is critical for understanding the neural substrates of familiarity and of priming. This approach highlights the necessity of employing experimental manipulations and multiple behavioural/phenomenological measures that can allow for valid associations between neuroimaging measures and memory functions, such that this information can be used to build an accurate characterization of the brain processes that support memory performance.

Consciousness and memory

Starting with general considerations about how to approach the scientific investigation of conscious memory phenomena, we have explored various practical and theoretical issues in memory research and arrived at several recommendations. These recommendations can be summarized as follows.

Memory phenomena like recollection should be investigated with sufficient attention given to each of the four critical perspectives displayed on the pyramid in Figure 21.1: *Behavioural*, *Neural*, *Cognitive*, and *Subjective*. A comprehensive analysis of such phenomena cannot neglect any of these perspectives, but rather must be devoted to understanding each of them as well as the relationships among them.

A fruitful avenue for investigating conscious memory phenomena is to contrast them with other memory phenomena that do not entail the same subjective experiences (e.g. perceptual and conceptual priming).

In studying specific memory phenomena and their neural characteristics, special attention is required to avoid cross-contamination, whereby neurocognitive processing responsible for one type of memory can occur during a paradigm designed to examine another type of memory. Various steps can be taken to minimize the possibility that behavioural and neural measures of one type of memory are not contaminated by another type of memory, and converging approaches can be used to validate such measures.

Notwithstanding the benefits of studying distinct memory functions by characterizing each in isolation, there are also drawbacks. These memory phenomena do not normally occur in a void, but rather, we usually engage combinations of multiple memory functions and other cognitive functions. Moreover, many memory phenomena in everyday experience, and even some laboratory memory phenomena, may not fit cleanly within the categories of declarative/non-declarative, recollection/familiarity, perceptual/conceptual, and so on. Also, some complex types of associative priming and conditioning seem to have many characteristics in common with declarative memory, and thus are not so unambiguously categorized. Yet, as argued by Tulving and Schacter, systematic classification of each form of memory is essential to fully understand memory processes and mechanisms, as '...facts discovered about one form of memory need not hold for other forms' (Tulving & Schacter, 1990, p. 305).

In addition to characterizing each form of memory in isolation, a complete understanding may not be fully realized without considering how these phenomena are related to each other and come to fruition in the context of the larger neurocognitive picture. A multiplicity of distinct memory processes likely contributes to everyday memory behaviour.

A common mode in science is to isolate one phenomenon for study by removing, or holding constant, various other factors. By these means, the one phenomenon can be understood, and we often understand it in contradistinction to other phenomena. The scientific enterprise has been very productive in deriving knowledge of the world of external phenomena with this strategy. In analyses of the mind, the same approach has also been very effective. Yet, limitations of these methods should be explicitly acknowledged. It is possible that in some cases we may have mistakenly subdivided phenomena in the wrong way, in which case we have failed *to carve nature at her joints*. Furthermore, even when we succeed in finding the appropriate divisions so as to carve exactly at each joint, we may still do violence by this carving. That is, the divisions that allow us to identify and study distinct phenomena can introduce some distortion. We must zero in and identify the parts to achieve any understanding, but we may neglect aspects of the whole that are out of focus when only analyzing the parts.

Conscious phenomena certainly provide prime examples of the limitations of carving nature at her joints, as we can lose sight of the many factors that come together to produce conscious experience, not just in the individual's brain activity but in social, cultural, and other influences that have accrued through an individual's development and shaped the kinds of thoughts he or she experiences. Although carving is essential, the carving per se introduces distortion – isolating one type of mental event for study may obscure the place of an individual's mental operations in a larger context. However, after taking the pieces apart in our analyses, we can attempt to remedy this situation by putting the parts back together in a way that calls attention to the interdependence among them.

We have argued that consciousness should feature prominently in scientific analyses of declarative memory, such that first-person perspectives remain essential elements of our analyses (echoing the earlier argument by Tulving, 1985). Many concepts in memory research are inexorably tied to consciousness, including the distinction between declarative and non-declarative memory. Any systematic theory of human memory must thus take consciousness into account. Behavioural descriptions of different memory functions are just a starting point. To go beyond merely acknowledging these different types of memory, further research is needed to clarify each more completely, respecting the four sides of the pyramid.

Beyond the confines of memory research, countless theories about the neural substrates of conscious experience have been proposed. In summarizing some of these theories, Zeman (2002) noted that many of them appeal to a *neural dialogue* of sorts (e.g. Crick & Koch, 2003; Edelman, 1992; Weiskrantz, 1997; Zeki & Bartels, 1999). This theoretical feature harkens back to the notion of consciousness as a sharing of information with oneself – but in this case among different networks of neurons in one's brain. To connect this notion to theories of memory, it may be that declarative memories can engender the conscious experience of remembering by virtue of the confluence of multiple cortical networks that are inherent in the concept of *cross-cortical storage* (Paller, 1997). These separate networks, each responsible for a distinct type of information, will each represent separate features of the declarative memory. For an episode experienced years ago, the features might include a particular spatial lay-out and location, certain visual objects and people present, information from multiple sensory modalities, emotional colouring, connections to events that came before as well as to related events that followed, and so on. Models of declarative memory generally posit that these distinct features or fragments must become linked together for enduring memory storage to be successful. Retrieval, rehearsal, and consolidation would thus entail synchronous activation across dispersed cortical networks – and this synchronous cross-cortical activity may be of the same type necessary for conscious experience more generally. The possibilities that such networks are linked through thalamo-cortical interactions, cortico-cortical interactions and/or gamma-frequency synchrony remain to be clarified.

We still wonder how people can possibly accomplish the extraordinary feat of bringing to mind an event from their past and consciously re-experiencing it in a way that approximates mental time-travel. Although this is a formidable scientific challenge, many methodologies are currently available to broaden our behavioural, cognitive, neural, and subjective perspectives on this question. Research on this question makes contact with a variety of theories in cognitive neuroscience, covering topics such as strategic memory search, retrieval evaluation, working memory, metamemory, and attention. Neuroimaging – and contemporary cognitive neuroscience more generally – has accrued an extensive empirical base with increasingly elaborate neurocognitive conceptualizations on many fronts.

Considering the progress made thus far, there is reason to be optimistic that further explorations of declarative memory will produce new advances in our scientific understanding of the first-person experience of remembering.

Acknowledgements

We thank the conference organizers for inviting us to address the topic of memory and consciousness. Research support is gratefully acknowledged from the United States National Science Foundation (BCS 0518800) and National Institutes of Health (R01 NS34639, P30 AG13854, F32 MH073247, T32 NS047987, and T32 AG20506).

References

Churchland, P. M. (1995). *The Engine of Reason, the Seat of the Soul*. Cambridge, MA: MIT Press.

Claparedè, E. (1951). Recognition and 'me-ness.' In D. Rapaport (Ed.), *Organization and Pathology of Thought* (pp. 58–75). New York: Columbia University Press. (Reprinted from *Archives de Psychologie*, 1911, *11*, 79–90).

Crick, F. & Koch, C. (2003). A framework for consciousness. *Nature Neuroscience, 6*, 119–126.

Curran T. (2004). Effects of attention and confidence on the hypothesized ERP correlates of recollection and familiarity. *Neuropsychologia, 42*, 1088–1106.

Curran T., DeBuse C., Woroch B., & Hirshman, E. (2006). Combined pharmacological and electrophysiological dissociation of familiarity and recollection. *Journal of Neuroscience, 26*, 1979–1985.

Curran, T., Tepe, K. L., & Piatt, C. (2006). ERP explorations of dual processes in recognition memory. In H. D. Zimmer, A. Mecklinger, & U. Lindenberger (Eds), *Binding in Human Memory: A Neurocognitive Approach* (pp. 467–492). Oxford: Oxford University Press.

Düzel, E., Yonelinas, A. P., Mangun, G. R., Heinze, H. -J., & Tulving E. (1997). Event-related potential correlates of two states of conscious awareness in memory. *Proceedings of the National Academy of Sciences of the United States of America, 94*, 5973–5978.

Edelman, G. M. (1992). *Bright Air, Brilliant Fire: On the Matter of the Mind*. New York: Basic Books.

Eichenbaum, H. & Cohen, N. J. (2001). *From Conditioning to Conscious Recollection: Memory Systems of the Brain*. Oxford: Oxford University Press.

Farber, I. & Churchland, P. S. (1995). Consciousness and the neurosciences: Philosophical and theoretical issues. In M. S. Gazzaniga (Ed.), *The Cognitive Neurosciences*. Cambridge: MIT Press.

Flanagan, O. (1992). *Consciousness Reconsidered*. Cambridge, MA: MIT Press.

Friedman, D. & Johnson, R. (2000). Event-related potential (ERP) studies of memory encoding and retrieval: A selective review. *Microscopy Research and Technique, 51*, 6–28.

Gabrieli, J. D. (1998). Cognitive neuroscience of human memory. *Annual Review of Psychology, 49*, 87–115.

Gonsalves, B. & Paller, K. A. (2000). Brain potentials associated with recollective processing of spoken words. *Memory & Cognition, 28*, 321–330.

Gyatso, J. (1992). *In the Mirror of Memory: Reflections on Mindfulness and Remembrance in Indian and Tibetan Buddhism*. Albany, NY: State University of New York Press.

Halgren, E. & Smith, M. E. (1987). Cognitive evoked potentials as modulatory processes in human memory formation and retrieval. *Human Neurobiology, 6*, 129–139.

James, W. (1904). Does 'consciousness' exist? *Journal of Philosophy, Psychology, and Scientific Methods, 1*, 477–491.

Johnson, R., Pfefferbaum, A., & Kopell, B. S. (1985). P300 and long-term memory: Latency predicts recognition performance. *Psychophysiology, 22,* 497–507.

Kihlstrom, J. H. (1995). Memory and consciousness: An appreciation of Claparedè and recognition et moiitè. *Consciousness & Cognition, 4,* 379–386.

Lamme, V. A. F. (2006). Towards a true neural stance on consciousness. *Trends in Cognitive Sciences, 10,* 494–501.

Mandler, G. (1980). Recognizing: The judgment of previous occurrence. *Psychological Review, 87,* 252–271.

Miller, B. B., Reber, P. J., Gitelman, D. R., Parrish, T. B., Cohen, N. J., & Paller, K. A. (2006). Different brain mechanisms support implicit versus explicit learning in a visual search task. Poster presented at the 13th annual meeting of the Cognitive Neuroscience Society, San Francisco, CA. *Journal of Cognitive Neuroscience, 18* (Suppl.), 133. Available online at: http://www.cogneurosociety.org/content/meeting.

Olichney, J. M., Van Petten, C., Paller, K. A., Salmon, D. P., Iragui, V. J., & Kutas, M. (2000). Word repetition in amnesia: Electrophysiological measures of impaired and spared memory. *Brain, 123,* 1948–1963.

Olichney, J. M., Iragui, V. J., Salmon, D. P., Riggins, B. R., Morris, S. K., & Kutas, M. (2006). Absent event-related potential (ERP) word repetition effects in mild Alzheimer's disease. *Clinical Neurophysiology, 117,* 1319–1330.

Paller, K. A. (1997). Consolidating dispersed neocortical memories: The missing link in amnesia. *Memory, 5,* 73–88.

Paller, K. A. (2002). Cross-cortical consolidation as the core defect in amnesia: Prospects for hypothesis-testing with neuropsychology and neuroimaging. In: L. R. Squire and D. L. Schacter (Eds), *The Neuropsychology of Memory,* 3rd edn (pp. 73–87). New York: Guilford Press.

Paller, K. A., Bozic, V. S., Ranganath, C., Grabowecky, M., & Yamada, S. (1999). Brain waves following remembered faces index conscious recollection. *Cognitive Brain Research, 7,* 519–531.

Paller, K. A., Hutson, C. A., Miller, B. B., & Boehm, S. G. (2003). Neural manifestations of memory with and without awareness. *Neuron, 38,* 507–516.

Paller, K. A. & Kutas, M. (1992). Brain potentials during memory retrieval provide neurophysiological support for the distinction between conscious recollection and priming. *Journal of Cognitive Neuroscience, 4,* 375–391.

Paller, K. A., Kutas, M., & McIsaac, H. K. (1995). Monitoring conscious recollection via the electrical activity of the brain. *Psychological Science, 6,* 107–111.

Paller, K. A., Voss, J. L., & Boehm, S. G. (2007). Validating neural correlates of familiarity. *Trends in Cognitive Sciences, 11,* 243–250.

Poldrack, R. A., Desmond, J. E., Glover, G. H., & Gabrieli, J. D. (1998). The neural basis of visual skill learning: an fMRI study of mirror reading. *Cerebral Cortex, 8,* 1–10.

Reber, P. J., Gitelman, D. R., Parrish, T. B., & Mesulam, M.-M. (2003). Dissociating explicit and implicit category knowledge with fMRI. *Journal of Cognitive Neuroscience, 15,* 574–583.

Rugg, M. D. (1990). Event-related brain potentials and recognition memory for low- and high-frequency words. *Memory & Cognition, 18,* 367–379.

Rugg, M. D. & Curran, T. (2007). Event-related potentials and recognition memory. *Trends in Cognitive Sciences, 11,* 251–257.

Rugg, M. D. & Nagy, M. E. (1989). Event-related potentials and recognition memory for words. *Electroencepholography and Clinical Neurophysiology, 72,* 395–406.

Rugg, M. D., Mark, R. E., Walla, P., Schloerscheidt, A. M., Birch, C. S., & Allan, K. (1998). Dissociation of the neural correlates of implicit and explicit memory. *Nature, 392,* 595–598.

Schacter, D. L. (1987). Implicit memory: History and current status. *Journal of Experimental Psychology: Learning, Memory, and Cognition, 13,* 501–518.

Schacter, D. L. (1989). On the relation between memory and consciousness: Dissociable interactions and conscious experience. In H. L. Roediger III & F. I. M. Craik (Eds), *Varieties of Memory and Consciousness: Essays in Honour of Endel Tulving* (pp. 355–389). Hillsdale, NJ: Lawrence Erlbaum Associates.

Schacter, D. L. (1996). *Searching for Memory: The Brain, the Mind, and the Past.* New York: Basic Books.

Schott, B., Richardson-Klavehn, A., Heinze, H. J., & Düzel, E. (2002). Perceptual priming versus explicit memory: Dissociable neural correlates at encoding. *Journal of Cognitive Neuroscience, 14,* 578–592.

Schott, B. H., Richardson-Klavehn, A., Henson, R. N., Becker, C., Heinze, H. J., & Düzel, E. (2006). Neuroanatomical dissociation of encoding processes related to priming and explicit memory. *Journal of Neuroscience, 26,* 792–800.

Senkfor, A. J. & Van Petten C. (1998). Who said what? An event-related potential investigation of source and item memory. *Journal of Experimental Psychology: Learning, Memory, & Cognition, 24,* 1005–1025.

Shimamura, A. P. (2002). Relational binding theory and the role of consolidation in memory retrieval. In L. R. Squire & D. L. Schacter (Eds), *Neuropsychology of Memory,* 3rd edn (pp. 61–72). New York: The Guilford Press.

Smith, M. E. (1993). Neurophysiological manifestations of recollective experience during recognition memory judgments. *Journal of Cognitive Neuroscience, 5,* 1–13.

Smith, M. E., & Halgren, E. (1989). Dissociation of recognition memory components following temporal lobe lesions. *Journal of Experimental Psychology: Learning, Memory, & Cognition, 15,* 50–60.

Squire, L. R. (1987). *Memory and Brain.* Oxford: Oxford University Press.

Trott, C. T., Friedman, D., Ritter, W., Fabiani, M., & Snodgrass, J. G. (1999). Episodic memory and priming for temporal source: Event-related potentials reveal age-related differences in prefrontal functioning. *Psychology of Aging, 14,* 390–413.

Tulving, E. (1983). *Elements of Episodic Memory.* Oxford: The Clarendon Press.

Tulving, E. (1985). Memory and consciousness. *Canadian Psychology, 26,* 1–12.

Tulving, E. & Schacter, D. L. (1990). Priming and human memory systems. *Science, 247,* 301–306.

Voss, J. L. & Paller, K. A. (2006). Fluent conceptual processing and explicit memory for faces are electrophysiologically distinct. *Journal of Neuroscience, 18,* 926–933.

Voss, J. L. & Paller, K. A. (2008). Neural substrates of remembering: Electroencephalographic studies. In J. H. Byrne (Ed.), *Learning and Memory – A Comprehensive Reference.* Elsevier Press.

Voss, J. L., Reber, P. J., Mesulam, M.-M., Parrish, T. B., & Paller, K. A. (2007). Familiarity and conceptual priming engage distinct cortical networks. *Cerebral Cortex, Advance Access published online on December 1, 2007,* doi:10.1093/cercor/bhm200.

Weiskrantz, L. (1997). *Consciousness Lost and Found: A Neuropsychological Exploration.* Oxford: Oxford University Press.

Westerberg, C. E., Paller, K. A., Weintraub, S., Mesulam, M.-M, Holdstock, J. S., Mayes, A. R., & Reber, P. J. (2006). When memory does not fail: Familiarity-based recognition in mild cognitive impairment and Alzheimer's disease. *Neuropsychology, 20,* 193–205.

Whittlesea, B. W. A. (1993). Illusions of familiarity. *Journal of Experimental Psychology: Learning, Memory, & Cognition, 19,* 1235–1253.

Wilding, E. L. & Rugg, M. D. (1996). An event-related potential study of recognition memory with and without retrieval of source. *Brain, 119,* 889–905.

Wolk, D. A., Schacter, D. L., Berman, A. R., Holcomb, P. J., Daffner, K. R., & Budson, A. E. (2004). An electrophysiological investigation of the relationship between conceptual fluency and familiarity. *Neuroscience Letters, 369,* 150–155.

Wolk, D. A., Schacter, D. L., Berman, A. R., Holcomb, P. J., Daffner, K. R., & Budson, A. E. (2005). Patients with mild Alzheimer's disease attribute conceptual fluency to prior experience. *Neuropsychologia, 43,* 1662–1672.

Yonelinas, A. P. (2002). The nature of recollection and familiarity: A review of 30 years of research. *Journal of Memory and Language, 46,* 441–517.

Yovel, G. & Paller, K. A. (2004). The neural basis of the butcher-on-the-bus phenomenon: When a face seems familiar but is not remembered. *Neuroimage, 21,* 789–800.

Zeki, S. & Bartels, A. (1999). Toward a theory of visual consciousness. *Consciousness and Cognition, 8,* 225–259.

Zeman, A. (2002). *Consciousness: A User's Guide.* New Haven, CT: Yale University Press.

Chapter 22

Constraints on cognitive theory from neuroimaging studies of source memory

Jon S. Simons

Introduction

When making the decision that the joke you have just been told is one you have heard before, you may recollect a number of details about the context in which the joke was previously encountered. These details may relate to where and when the joke was heard, who told it, and who else was present. For example, you might remember that you heard it before during a best man speech at a wedding last summer, or you might remember that in fact it was you who previously told the joke (and perhaps the person who told it just now stole the joke from you). Additionally, you may remember some of your thoughts and reactions at the time of previously encountering the joke: For example, as is often the case when the author of the present chapter tells a joke, that it was not particularly funny.

Characterizing source memory and related functions

A number of cognitive theories have been proposed to describe the processes involved in retrieving these different kinds of contextual detail. *Source monitoring* theory proposes that there is a set of decision processes that are involved in making attributions about the origins of previously encountered information, and that a subset of these processes (termed *reality monitoring* processes) support the ability to discriminate information that was generated by internal cognitive functions such as thought and imagination from information that was derived from the outside world by perceptual processes (Johnson & Raye, 1981; Johnson, Hashtroudi, & Lindsay, 1993). Another line of research has focused on characterizing the functionally distinct, largely sequentially operating processing stages supporting recollection, including the specification of retrieval cues and criteria for success, and the monitoring and evaluation of retrieved information against the specified verification criteria (Tulving, 1983; Burgess & Shallice, 1996; Schacter, Norman, & Koutstaal, 1998; Rugg, 2006). A further area of interest relates to whether the act of remembering events from the past might share common processing characteristics with other cognitive functions (Tulving, 1983; D'Argembeau & Van der Linden, 2004; Buckner & Carroll, 2007; Schacter & Addis, 2007), such as thinking about events that might occur in the future (prospective memory; McDaniel & Einstein, 1992; Ellis, 1996) and attending to the mental states of oneself and other agents (mentalizing; Frith & Frith, 2003).

At present, no single cognitive theory that I am aware of encompasses all of these issues, but individually, these areas of investigation have received a great deal of attention from cognitive psychologists, who have explored the effects of experimental manipulations on behavioural measures such as accuracy and reaction time, and have provided numerous insights into the operating characteristics of remembering (Mandler, 1980; Tulving, 1983; Ratcliff, Van Zandt, & McKoon, 1995; Clark & Gronlund, 1996; Kelley & Wixted, 2001; Yonelinas, 2002; Rotello, Macmillan, & Reeder, 2004). Further constraints on theorizing have been obtained from the study of older adults as well as patients with brain lesions and other disorders affecting cognitive function. Such neuropsychological studies, often employing dissociation logic (Shallice, 1988), have provided support for a number of key conceptual distinctions such as the separation of source recollection and item recognition, general source attribution processes and those supporting reality monitoring, and cue specification and post-retrieval monitoring processes. Typically, these studies have highlighted the prefrontal cortex (PFC) as one of the critical structures for accurate recollection (Janowsky, Shimamura, & Squire, 1989; Schacter, Kaszniak, Kihlstrom, & Valdiserri, 1991; McDaniel & Einstein, 1992; Burgess & Shallice, 1996; Henkel, Johnson, & De Leonardis, 1998; Glisky, Rubin, & Davidson, 2001; Simons *et al.*, 2002; Duarte, Ranganath, & Knight, 2005).

Using neuroimaging data to constrain cognitive theory

In recent years, an increasingly important contribution has been made by studies using functional neuroimaging techniques such as functional magnetic resonance imaging (fMRI). Such techniques offer high spatial resolution, sufficient temporal resolution to permit some (albeit limited) separation of sequentially occurring processes, and the ability to document activity patterns in networks of connected regions distributed across the whole brain (Fletcher & Henson, 2001; Simons & Spiers, 2003). This is not, of course, to say that imaging has become the only tool to be used in seeking to understand recollection. Many fundamental insights continue to be obtained without going anywhere near a scanner. Furthermore, good neuroimaging experiments tend to be those that are closely guided and constrained by cognitive theory, preferably seeking convergence with neuropsychological evidence relating to the necessity of activated brain regions.

When undertaken well, neuroimaging studies can produce data that may be thought of as another dependent variable for distinguishing between competing cognitive theories and generating hypotheses for further investigation (Henson, 2005). In particular, inferences based on significant *region-by-condition interactions* in patterns of brain activity can be considered analogous to the dissociation logic used in neuropsychology (Shallice, 2003; Henson, 2005, 2006). Another formalized strategy is the *reverse inference*, analogous to probabilistic association logic, according to which activity in the same specific brain region for two different tasks implies that both tasks must share one or more cognitive processes (Poldrack, 2006). The reverse inference relies for its usefulness on the anatomical specificity that can be obtained from neuroimaging but is not so readily available in neuropsychological studies. By adopting one or both of these inferential strategies, it is possible for researchers to use neuroimaging data to constrain their cognitive theories, either by introducing further distinctions to a conceptualized cognitive system on the basis of observed dissociations in activity, or by expanding the scope of a cognitive model as a result of a reverse inference to include processes which may not have been predicted *a priori*.

In the last decade or so, a growing number of memory researchers have designed theoretically motivated functional neuroimaging experiments constrained by cognitive theory and neuropsychological data. The results of these studies have, in a number of cases, been interpreted on the basis of region-by-condition interactions and/or reverse inferences, providing additional insights into the functional organization of memory processes. Many of these developments, for example relating to important roles played by regions of the medial temporal lobe, are discussed in other chapters in the present volume. In this chapter, I describe some of the insights that have impacted on our conceptual understanding of source recollection, focusing on the areas of investigation outlined earlier: internally and externally generated context; pre- and post-retrieval processing stages; and commonalities between recollection, prospective memory, and mentalizing. These insights center on anterior PFC, a region for which accruing evidence suggests an important role in central cognitive control processes that are relevant to each of these functions. I go on to outline a cognitive hypothesis of these control processes and their operating principles, a hypothesis that has primarily been developed and constrained on the basis of deductive inferences drawn from functional neuroimaging data.

Recollection of internally vs. externally generated context

Functional neuroimaging studies of source memory, consistent with the neuropsychological literature, have supported the distinction made by cognitive theories between source recollection and item recognition. Early neuroimaging studies also echoed lesion evidence emphasizing the importance of PFC regions in the recollection of source information (Nyberg *et al.*, 1996; Nolde, Johnson, & D'Esposito, 1998; Rugg, Fletcher, Chua, & Dolan, 1999; Henson, Shallice, & Dolan, 1999; Ranganath, Johnson, & D'Esposito, 2000). Source-related activation was consistently observed in ventrolateral (Brodmann Area [BA] 45/47) and dorsolateral (BA 9/46) PFC, and was also reported in some studies (but not universally) in anterior PFC (approximating BA 10). Roles were ascribed for the ventrolateral region in the specification of retrieval cues (Dobbins, Foley, Schacter, & Wagner, 2002), and for dorsolateral PFC in the post-retrieval monitoring of recovered information (Rugg *et al.*, 1999; Henson *et al.*, 1999) (see next section for more on this).

Understanding the role in source memory played by anterior PFC has been less straightforward. This may be partly because of a long-running debate in the recognition memory literature over whether activation in this region during old/new recognition reflected the cognitive state (or 'retrieval mode') an individual was in prior to remembering (Nyberg *et al.*, 1995), the particular aspects of mnemonic information to which attention was directed ('retrieval orientation') (Rugg & Wilding, 2000), the amount of cognitive resources ('retrieval effort') expended during a retrieval attempt (Schacter, Alpert, Savage, Rauch, & Albert, 1996), or the level of accuracy ('retrieval success') achieved in recovering the sought-after information (Rugg, Fletcher, Frith, Frackowiak, & Dolan, 1996). Another reason that the involvement of anterior PFC in source memory may have been difficult to characterize was that whereas a number of neuroimaging experiments reported activation in this region during the recollection of source details (Rugg et al., 1999; Ranganath et al., 2000; Dobbins et al., 2002; Kahn, Davachi, & Wagner, 2004), other equally well-conducted, apparently very similar studies failed to identify activation in this region (Nyberg et al., 1996; Henson et al., 1999; Suzuki et al., 2002).

It is always problematic to attempt a theoretical explanation that can account for null results. The lack of anterior PFC activation in the three studies cited above could be attributable to lack of experimental power or to susceptibility distortion in the fMRI signal due to the proximity of anterior PFC to the sinus area. However, a potentially more theoretically interesting account, which would require testing in a within-subjects experiment, is that the types of context used in all the previous studies tended to differ according to whether, at the time of encoding, they were derived from the outside world (e.g. when or where an event occurred) or were generated internally (e.g. one's thoughts about the event). The experiments that had tested recollection of which of two encoding tasks had been undertaken by participants with each target stimulus all observed significant activation in anterior PFC (Rugg et al., 1999; Dobbins et al., 2002; Kahn et al., 2004). However, studies that had focused on perceptual contextual features, such as the position or size on the monitor screen in which target stimuli had been studied, produced inconsistent results in anterior PFC with some reporting significant activation (Ranganath et al., 2000; Cansino, Maquet, Dolan, & Rugg, 2002) and others not (Nyberg et al., 1996; Henson et al., 1999; Suzuki et al., 2002). If anterior PFC were sensitive to the internal/external nature of recollection decisions, this would support the 'reality monitoring' processing distinction made by cognitive theories of source memory between recollection of the cognitive operations engaged by participants in carrying out a study task versus recollecting perceptual details derived from the outside world relating to the study episode (Johnson & Raye, 1981; Johnson et al., 1993).

A number of recent studies have investigated whether neuroimaging evidence can be found to support the existence of reality monitoring processes, by manipulating within subjects the recollection of internally and externally generated source details. The emerging consensus from these studies is that anterior PFC is among the brain regions sensitive to reality monitoring distinctions, consistently exhibiting differential activation during the retrieval of aspects of context that were internally generated vs. perceptually derived at the time of encoding (Simons, Owen, Fletcher, & Burgess, 2005; Simons, Gilbert, Owen, Fletcher, & Burgess, 2005; Dobbins & Wagner, 2005; Simons, Davis, Gilbert, Frith, & Burgess, 2006; Vinogradov et al., 2006; Kensinger & Schacter, 2006; Simons, Henson, Gilbert, & Fletcher, 2008). For example, Simons, Owen et al. (2005) directly contrasted recollection of the encoding task carried out during initial presentation of stimuli with recollection of where on the monitor screen the stimuli had been presented. They observed a significant region-by-condition interaction within anterior PFC, with lateral regions associated with recollection of both task and position details, and a medial anterior region exhibiting significantly greater activation during recollection of encoding task than of stimulus position. Similar lateral-medial anterior dissociations have since been observed in a number of subsequent studies, with the lateral region activated consistently during all source conditions tested, and the medial region sensitive to reality monitoring manipulations (Simons, Gilbert *et al.*, 2005; Dobbins & Wagner, 2005; Simons *et al.*, 2008).

As shown in Figure 22.1, medial anterior PFC has been shown to exhibit differential activation during recollection of the encoding task undertaken contrasted with remembering where on the screen (Simons, Owen *et al.*, 2005) or when in time (Simons, Gilbert *et al.*, 2005) stimuli were presented, or remembering their size on the screen (Dobbins & Wagner, 2005). The same region is involved in remembering whether verbal phrases were previously presented in full on the screen (e.g. 'bacon and eggs'), or whether a word was missing which participants had to imagine (e.g. 'bacon and ?') in order to complete the phrase themselves (Simons, Davis *et al.*, 2006; Vinogradov *et al.*, 2006). Likewise, medial anterior PFC is differentially engaged during recollection of whether an object was previously seen or imagined by participants (Kensinger & Schacter, 2006). Finally, medial anterior PFC has been shown to be associated with remembering whether oneself or another person previously performed a particular operation on stimuli (Simons *et al.*, 2008). The sensitivity of this region to reality monitoring distinctions is apparent regardless of whether words, faces, or objects are being remembered (Simons, Owen *et al.*, 2005; Simons, Gilbert *et al.*, 2005; Dobbins & Wagner, 2005; Kensinger & Schacter, 2006), suggesting that the effect is independent of stimulus type. Moreover, medial anterior activation has been observed irrespective of whether the 'internal' or 'external' condition is associated with lower recollection accuracy and longer reaction times or vice versa, or whether such behavioural factors are matched between conditions (Simons, Owen *et al.*, 2005; Simons, Gilbert *et al.*, 2005), suggesting that an account in terms of differential task difficulty is unlikely to be sufficient.

Distinct processing stages of source recollection

A number of cognitive theories of retrieval have proposed that there are functionally distinct processing stages involved in retrieving a stored representation from memory (Tulving, 1983; Burgess & Shallice, 1996; Schacter *et al.*, 1998; Rugg, 2006). These processing stages, illustrated in Figure 22.2, are considered to operate in a largely sequential, iterative fashion, beginning with the retrieval orientation stage of specifying retrieval cues and criteria for success on the basis of the task instructions and presented target stimulus. Once these pre-retrieval specification processes have been completed, a goal-directed search of mnemonic representations can be undertaken seeking concordance between the retrieval cue and stored information. If the search was sufficiently well-specified, potential target memories will be identified and their associated stored representations reactivated and maintained online in working memory. The retrieved information will be monitored and evaluated against the specified verification criteria and, if the criteria for

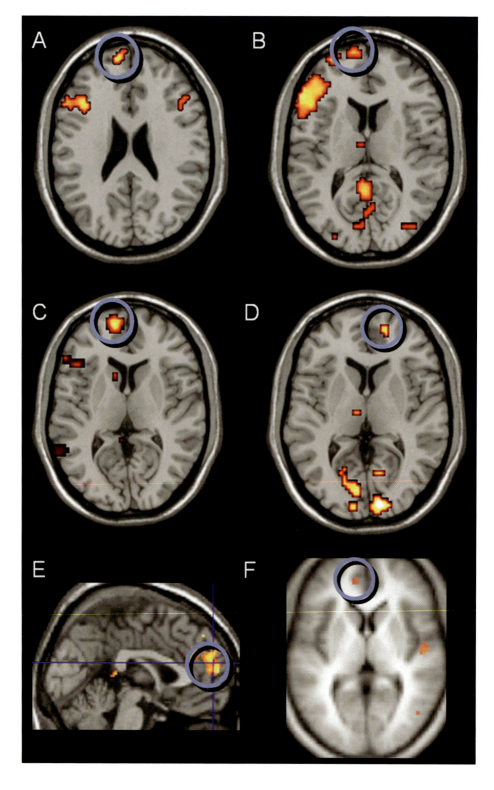

successful retrieval are satisfied, an appropriate behavioural response can be made. Alternatively, if the retrieved mnemonic information is insufficient or incorrect, the retrieval cues and verification criteria can be modified and further retrieval searches attempted.

Because it can be difficult in neuropsychological studies of memory dysfunction to establish which of the processing stages may be impaired in any one individual (Fletcher & Henson, 2001), much of the information on whether separable brain regions might support each of these stages of retrieval comes from functional neuroimaging. Such studies have highlighted that different areas of PFC may support pre-retrieval and post-retrieval cognitive control processes. For example, Dobbins *et al.* (2002) identified a region of ventrolateral PFC which was activated during both semantic processing and source recollection tasks, but not during item recognition. On the basis of this pattern of activation, the authors interpreted the likely function of this region in recollection as reflecting the controlled semantic analysis necessary for the specification of effective retrieval cues. This region was differentiated from a more posterior region of ventrolateral PFC, which showed significant activity across semantic processing, source recollection, and item recognition tasks, consistent with previous suggestions of a role in lexical/ phonological maintenance in working memory (Poldrack *et al.*, 1999; Smith & Jonides, 1999).

The post-retrieval stage of monitoring recovered information against pre-specified verification criteria has also been examined in a number of neuroimaging experiments, with evidence suggesting the involvement of dorsolateral PFC regions (Fletcher, Shallice, Frith, Frackowiak, & Dolan, 1998; Henson *et al.*, 1999; Rugg *et al.*, 1999; Henson, Rugg, & Shallice, 2000). For example, Henson *et al.* (2000) operationalized monitoring by contrasting situations in which participants expressed low confidence in their memory with situations in which they were highly confident, observing activation in right dorsolateral PFC. Similar results implicating dorsolateral PFC were also found when the higher monitoring demands of a source recollection task were contrasted with item recognition, considered to rely more on judgements of familiarity (Henson *et al.*, 1999; Rugg *et al.*, 1999). However, as described in the previous section, some studies contrasting source

---

Figure 22.1 Examples of the consistent sensitivity exhibited by medial anterior PFC to the recollection of source details that were internally generated vs. external-derived during encoding. (A) Remembering encoding task vs. remembering stimulus position (adapted from Simons, Owen *et al.*, 2005, with permission from Elsevier). (B) Remembering encoding task vs. remembering time of presentation (reprinted from Duncan *et al.*, 2005, with permission from Oxford University Press). (C) Remembering encoding task vs. remembering stimulus size (Dobbins & Wagner, 2005, kindly provided by Ian Dobbins). (D) Remembering the perceived/imagined status of a word vs. remembering its position (adapted from Simons, Davis *et al.*, 2006, with permission from Elsevier). (E) Remembering whether a word was imagined vs. remembering whether it was perceived (adapted from Vinogradov *et al.*, 2006, with permission from Elsevier). (F) Remembering whether an object was imagined vs. perceived (Kensinger & Schacter, 2006, kindly provided by Elizabeth Kensinger).

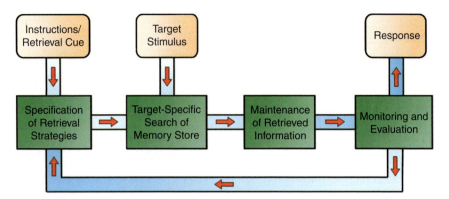

Figure 22.2 Diagram illustrating the sequential, iterative processing stages considered to be involved in recollection. Retrieval cues and verification criteria are specified, and a goal-directed search of the memory store undertaken. Information that has been retrieved from memory is maintained in working memory while being monitored and evaluated against the pre-specified verification criteria. If the criteria for successful retrieval are met, a behavioural response can be implemented. Alternatively, retrieval strategies can be modified and subsequent searches of memory undertaken.

recollection with item recognition also observed activation in anterior PFC (Rugg *et al.*, 1999; Ranganath *et al.*, 2000; Dobbins *et al.*, 2002), which further investigation suggested may be determined by the 'internal' vs. 'external' nature of the source detail being recollected (Simons, Owen *et al.*, 2005; Dobbins & Wagner, 2005). An unresolved question is which stage(s) of the retrieval process might be subserved by anterior PFC.

We have recently attempted to address this issue by teasing apart whether anterior PFC might show differential activity associated with pre- or post-retrieval processes. Focusing first on evidence for a role in pre-retrieval processes such as retrieval orientation and/or cue specification, we designed a source memory test phase in which each trial began with an instruction specifying which of two different source details were to be recollected on that trial, presented prior to the onset of a previously-studied target stimulus. We hypothesized that retrieval orientation processes might be expected to be recruited when the retrieval instruction was presented, continuing to be engaged on presentation of the target stimulus and as the retrieval search ensued. In one experiment (Simons, Gilbert *et al.*, 2005), a manipulation was employed whereby a recollection instruction was either followed by a target stimulus (which would provoke a retrieval search) or followed by a control stimulus (in which case a retrieval search would not be undertaken). Any activation that was observed in both conditions could be considered to reflect processes occurring prior to the inception of a retrieval search. A conjunction contrast, identifying regions of significant activation common to both search and no-search conditions, revealed significant activation in left lateral anterior PFC, as well as in the ventrolateral region attributed to cue specification by Dobbins *et al.* (2002).

This result was replicated in a subsequent study in which the onsets of the retrieval instruction and the target stimulus were separated by a randomly varying number of seconds (similar to the method used by Sakai & Passingham, 2003). Activity associated specifically with the retrieval instruction rather than the target stimulus was seen in the same region of left lateral anterior PFC as in the previous study (Simons *et al.*, 2008). Similar findings were also reported by Dobbins and Han (2006), although the lateral anterior PFC region they implicated in pre-retrieval processes was located on the right, perhaps reflecting the use of pictorial stimuli in that study (although stimulus-specific asymmetries in anterior PFC have not been noted previously; Simons, Owen *et al.*, 2005; Simons, Gilbert *et al.*, 2005). In all three studies examining retrieval orientation processes, no significant pre-retrieval activity was observed in medial anterior PFC; moreover, significant region-by-condition interactions in the studies from Simons *et al.* confirmed the specific nature of the lateral anterior PFC role in these processes.

Turning to post-retrieval monitoring processes, we hypothesized that even if the retrieval process does iterate, post-retrieval monitoring should typically occur later in time than pre-retrieval cue specification. Therefore, regions that subserve such post-retrieval processes may be those that are associated with source recollection, but in which activity peaks significantly later than that in retrieval orientation-related regions. As shown in Figure 22.3, when the time-courses of lateral and medial anterior PFC regions involved in source recollection were extracted, the peak of activity in the medial region occurred significantly later than that in the lateral region associated with pre-retrieval processes (Simons, Gilbert *et al.*, 2005). This latency difference did not merely reflect possible differences in vasculature between regions, because there was no difference in latency between lateral and medial anterior PFC regions associated with performance during a semantic retrieval baseline condition. Instead, this result suggests that medial anterior PFC contributes to a later stage of retrieval than cue specification, such as post-retrieval monitoring.

The suggestion that medial anterior PFC is involved in a late stage of retrieval is not direct evidence for a role in monitoring specifically. However, the proposed association with post-retrieval monitoring was given additional support by recent evidence of task-dependent differences in functional connectivity between medial anterior PFC and right dorsolateral PFC during source recollection (Simons *et al.*, 2008). As noted above, numerous studies have linked dorsolateral PFC with post-retrieval monitoring processes (Fletcher *et al.*, 1998; Henson *et al.*, 1999; Rugg *et al.*, 1999; Henson *et al.*, 2000). When activity in medial anterior PFC was entered into a psychophysiological interaction analysis, the region of the brain to show the most significant task-specific covariation in activity was right dorsolateral PFC (Simons *et al.*, 2008). This connectivity pattern indicates that, during source recollection, medial anterior PFC may modulate activity in right dorsolateral PFC during the monitoring of retrieved contextual information.

Commonalities between recollection, prospective memory, and mentalizing

One of the cardinal features of episodic memory is the concept of 'mental time-travel' (Tulving, 1983), the idea that the act of remembering involves projecting oneself to a different time to

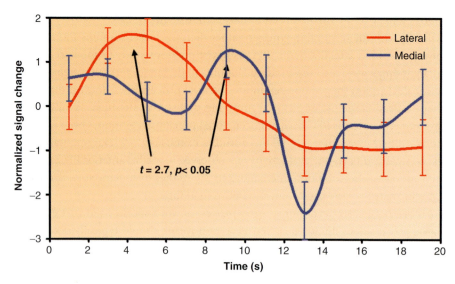

Figure 22.3 Time-course analysis suggesting that lateral (in red) and medial (in blue) anterior PFC are involved in temporally-distinct stages of the recollection process (Simons, Gilbert *et al.*, 2005, used with permission). Further investigation identified the role of lateral anterior PFC as relating to pre-retrieval cue specification, with activity linked to the onset of retrieval instructions irrespective of whether a retrieval search occurred. By contrast, evidence suggested that medial anterior PFC may subserve a later, perhaps post-retrieval stage of processing, with activity peaking significantly after lateral anterior PFC and exhibiting task-dependent differences in functional connectivity with right dorsolateral PFC, previously linked to post-retrieval monitoring operations. Error bars denote standard errors.

recollect details of a previous experience. Other cognitive functions share this character-istic of mentally projecting oneself into another time or place (Tulving, 1983; D'Argembeau & Van der Linden, 2004; Buckner & Carroll, 2007; Schacter & Addis, 2007). For example, prospective memory involves thinking about the future, considering events that might occur or keeping in mind intentions to act (McDaniel & Einstein, 1992; Ellis, 1996). In addition, forming a theory of mind, or mentalizing, involves considering a situation from another person's perspective, in essence projecting oneself into that person's mind (Frith & Frith, 2003; Saxe, Carey, & Kanwisher, 2004). In recent years, evidence has accumu-lated to suggest that the cognitive functions of recollection, prospective memory, and mentalizing may share neural substrates, as well as common processes. Damage to regions of PFC has been associated with source recollection deficits (Janowsky *et al.*, 1989; Simons *et al.*, 2002; Duarte *et al.*, 2005), with impairment to prospective memory (Burgess, Veitch, de Lacy Costello, & Shallice, 2000), and with difficulties on reasoning tasks requir-ing a theory of mind (Stone, Baron-Cohen, & Knight, 1998; Stuss, Gallup, & Alexander, 2001; although see Bird, Castelli, Malik, Frith, & Husain, 2004).

One region that has been suggested to be particularly critical is the medial area of PFC, and reverse inference evidence from functional neuroimaging substantiates the view that this area plays an important role. The consistent, reproducible involvement of medial anterior PFC in source recollection has already been discussed in this chapter. A number of studies have implicated a very similar region in performance of prospective memory tasks (see Figure 22.4), with activity being seen when participants undertake a cognitive task while maintaining a delayed intention to act in the future (at a particular time in the future or when a particular cue event occurs) (Okuda *et al.*, 1998; Burgess, Quayle, & Frith, 2001; Burgess, Scott, & Frith, 2003; Simons, Schölvinck, Gilbert, Frith, & Burgess, 2006). In a recent study, we examined just how critical this region is to prospective memory by manipulating both the salience of the cue event signaling that the intended action should be performed, and the complexity of the intention to be retrieved (drawing on distinctions made in the cognitive literature by McDaniel & Einstein, 1992). Despite significant effects of these manipulations on behavioural performance, strikingly similar patterns of activation were observed in anterior PFC (Simons, Schölvinck *et al.*, 2006).

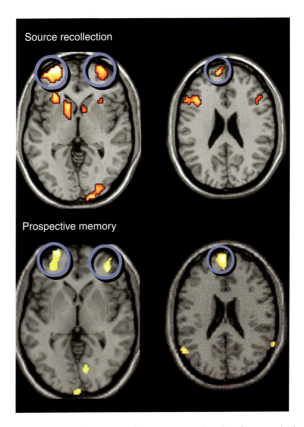

Figure 22.4 Anterior PFC regions important for source recollection (e.g. retrieving details of the encoding task undertaken when stimuli were previously encountered) closely resemble those involved in prospective memory (e.g. retrieving a delayed intention to act when a particular target stimulus is presented). Figures adapted from Simons, Owen *et al.* (2005) and Burgess *et al.* (2003), with permission from Elsevier.

These activations closely resembled those linked to source recollection, attesting to the importance of this region for both cognitive functions.

A related line of research has involved directly contrasting activity associated with recalling events from the past versus imagining events in the future (Okuda *et al.*, 2003; Addis, Wong, & Schacter, 2007; Szpunar, Watson, & McDermott, 2007). For example, Okuda *et al.* (2003) scanned participants while they were talking about events that had occurred in the past or would occur in the future. Activation common to both conditions was observed in medial anterior PFC, among other areas. Similar results were observed recently by Addis *et al.* (2007) and Szpunar *et al.* (2007), who presented participants with cue words and asked them to recall a past event or imagine an event in the future related to each word. These investigators endeavoured to control phenomenological characteristics of the target recollections such as level of detail, personal significance, and specificity in time, factors on which narrative accounts of past and future events often differ (D'Argembeau & Van der Linden, 2004). Just as in the study by Okuda *et al.*, striking commonalities were observed by Addis *et al.* and Szpunar *et al.* in medial anterior PFC across the elaboration of past and future events. Together, the results of these studies provide within-subject evidence confirming that the processes supported by medial anterior PFC are central to both recollection and prospective memory.

Another cognitive function that has been suggested (e.g. Buckner & Carroll, 2007) to require similar processes of self-projection is 'mentalizing', the ability to understand and represent another individual's perspective (Frith & Frith, 2003; Saxe *et al.*, 2004; Amodio & Frith, 2006). This ability is considered to involve the utilization of a theory of mind, the mental projection of oneself into another individual's mind to understand what that individual thinks or believes about the world (Premack & Woodruff, 1978). Much research has concentrated on the development of theory of mind in children (Frith & Frith, 2003), but in recent years neuroimaging studies have characterized the neural substrates of mentalizing. These studies have consistently observed medial PFC activation during such tasks as inferring the emotional states of oneself and others (Ochsner *et al.*, 2004), evaluating personality traits relating to the self or other people (Kelley *et al.*, 2002; Macrae, Moran, Heatherton, Banfield, & Kelley, 2004), and interpreting, on the basis of stories or cartoons, the beliefs or intentions held by other people (Fletcher *et al.*, 1995; Brunet, Sarfati, Hardy-Bayle, & Decety, 2000).

Although neuroimaging studies of mentalizing have typically reported activation in medial anterior PFC, the precise locus of activity has often been more caudal than the area linked with source recollection and prospective memory (Gilbert, Spengler *et al.*, 2006; see also Gilbert *et al.*, 2007). One account for this variation could be that source and prospective memory tasks usually relate solely to one's own personal experience, projecting oneself to a different time from the present, whereas mentalizing tasks often require judgements to be made from the perspective of another person, projecting oneself into that person's mind. In a recent study (Simons *et al.*, 2008), we attempted to test this hypothesis by contrasting a form of source recollection previously linked with the more rostral region of medial anterior PFC ('Did I previously perceive or imagine that stimulus?') with a form that might require consideration of another person's perspective ('Did I or the experimenter previously perform the encoding task with that stimulus?'). The sole activation difference between the two kinds of judgement lay in greater activity in medial anterior PFC when recollecting whether the participant or the experimenter had carried out an operation during prior encoding as compared to recollecting whether an item had been perceived or imagined. Critically, this activation was located in a relatively caudal region of medial anterior PFC, with a coordinate on the rostro-caudal axis that was significantly closer to the anterior commissure origin than the coordinates from previous source recollection and prospective memory studies. This relatively caudal activation associated with recollection requiring consideration of one's own and another person's perspective lay instead in the center of the distribution of mentalizing-related anterior PFC activations reported in a recent meta-analysis (Gilbert, Spengler *et al.*, 2006).

From neuroimaging findings to cognitive hypothesis

The neuroimaging findings reviewed in this chapter have converged to suggest that regions of anterior PFC support processes that: (a) are central to source recollection, and in particular reality monitoring, discriminating information that was generated by internal cognitive functions from information perceived from the outside world; (b) make distinct contributions to pre-retrieval cue specification and post-retrieval monitoring operations; and (c) are common to functions such as prospective memory and mentalizing, in addition to source recollection. These findings, some of which are based on region-by-condition interactions and some on reverse inference, are difficult to fit into any single extant account of source recollection. Instead, they have contributed to the formulation of a new cognitive hypothesis of the general processing operations supported by anterior PFC, characterized as an information processing gateway (see Figure 22.5) that serves to bias attention between stimulus-oriented and stimulus-independent thoughts (Burgess, Simons, Dumontheil, & Gilbert, 2005). This hypothesis is based almost entirely on inferences drawn from neuroimaging data, as patients with focal lesions selectively affecting anterior PFC are extremely rare and the region is structurally very different in even the closest non-human primates (Semendeferi, Armstrong, Schleicher, Zilles, & Van Hoesen, 2001).

According to the 'gateway' hypothesis, source memory relies on the differential allocation of attention between internally represented mnemonic information and the currently-perceived stimuli that provoke its retrieval (Simons, Gilbert *et al.*, 2005). Taken one stage further, the hypothesis provides an account for reality monitoring in terms of sensitivity to the internal versus external nature of the original source of stored mnemonic representations (e.g. internally generated imaginings versus externally derived perceptions). The available evidence indicates that activity in medial anterior PFC is consistently greater during recollection of internally-generated than externally-derived source details (Simons, Owen *et al.*, 2005; Simons, Gilbert *et al.*, 2005; Dobbins & Wagner, 2005; Simons, Davis *et al.*, 2006; Vinogradov *et al.*, 2006; Kensinger & Schacter, 2006). Intriguingly, the dominance in activity for processing of information that was previously

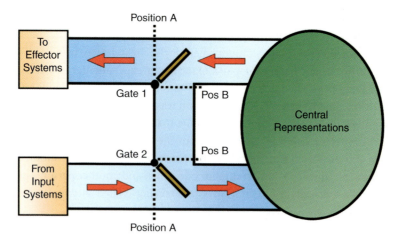

Figure 22.5 Diagram illustrating the Gateway Hypothesis, describing a cognitive control system, supported by anterior PFC, that biases attention between stimulus-oriented and stimulus-independent thought (adapted from Burgess *et al.*, 2005, with permission from Oxford University Press). Adjustment of gates 1 and 2 to position A will favour stimulus-independent thought, whereas if both gates are at position B, attention is oriented towards interacting with external stimuli. Different configurations of the gates are proposed to account for empirical observations of sensitivity to internally and externally generated context; distinctions between pre- and post-retrieval processing stages; and commonalities between recollection, prospective memory, and mentalizing. See main text for details.

internally generated is typically inverted during tasks that require the processing of *currently* perceived or imagined stimuli. For example, Gilbert *et al.* (2005) observed greater activation in medial anterior PFC when participants performed tasks on the basis of visually-presented stimuli than when they performed the same tasks 'in their heads' (see also Janata *et al.*, 2002; Small *et al.*, 2003; Gilbert, Simons, Frith, & Burgess, 2006). Although the reasons for the polarity reversal in processing of remembered and current information are not yet fully understood, taken together the results do suggest a general, low-level set of processes that are responsible for discriminating between internally and externally generated information.

   A full account of the proposed operating characteristics of the gateway hypothesis are beyond the scope of this chapter (readers may refer to Burgess *et al.*, 2005, for further details). However, the general cognitive control function of biasing attention between internally generated thoughts and stimulus-oriented perceptions is likely recruited to the benefit of a number of the processing stages of recollection (Simons, Gilbert *et al.*, 2005; Simons *et al.*, 2008). For example, pre-retrieval operations may involve the transformation of a visually presented retrieval instruction specifying the type of recollection required on an upcoming trial from an externally derived perceptual representation into stimulus-independent task parameters that orient attention towards particular contextual details, and generate, select, and initiate retrieval strategies and verification criteria. Stimulus-oriented processing of a presented target stimulus, about which details of previous

exposure context are to be retrieved, can operate to direct searches of the internal mnemonic store, from which matching stored representations can be evaluated against the
specified verification criteria. If the retrieved information does not meet the criteria for a
response, further stimulus-oriented processing may be used to identify other properties
of the presented stimulus as a basis for modifying the retrieval strategies and criteria for
further searches to be undertaken. Alternatively, if the criteria for successful retrieval are
met, an appropriate behavioural response can be output through effector systems.

An account in terms of a processing 'gateway' can also be applied to other cognitive
functions that have been hypothesized to share functional properties with source recollection, such as prospective memory and mentalizing. Prospective memory can be considered to involve the biasing of attention between stimulus-oriented processing of the
cognitive task being undertaken and stimulus-independent processing of the delayed
intention to act (Burgess et al., 2003; Burgess et al., 2005; Simons, Schölvinck et al., 2006).
During performance of the ongoing cognitive task, attention must be oriented towards
the task stimuli both so satisfactory behavioural performance can be maintained, and so
that a prospective memory cue stimulus can be detected when it is presented. Once the
cue is identified, attention must be disengaged from the external stimuli and oriented
towards internal representations so that the relevant intention can be retrieved from
memory and the specified action effected. Similarly, mentalizing can be conceived as
involving the disengagement of attention from the external world in favour of stimulus-
independent processing to generate a representation of the world that simulates the perspective that may be held by another person (Amodio & Frith, 2006; Buckner & Carroll,
2007). Generating such a representation may involve both stimulus-oriented processing
of the current behaviour of that person in relation to other salient people and/or objects
in the world, as well as stimulus-independent processing of any prior experience that may
be available of that person (or, indeed, of oneself) in related previous circumstances, in
order to construct a sufficiently detailed representation of what the person's beliefs,
motives, and intentions are likely to be that their future behaviour can be predicted.

It should be noted that the gateway hypothesis is at present considered very much to be
a work in progress. There are still a number of areas that are poorly understood. For
example, further work is required to establish the dynamics by which the processing of
previously experienced and currently perceived internally and externally generated information appears to differ. One possible means of investigating this issue might be by
examining activity associated with recollecting source details about stimuli that, in the
test phase, are being imagined by participants rather than being presented externally. In
addition, it has yet to be established whether precisely the same processes are involved in
the prospective functions of maintaining a delayed intention to act and imagining an
event that might occur in the future. Future studies can investigate whether the same
regions of anterior PFC are involved in both forms of projection into the future. Moreover,
our understanding of the processes that may be common to source recollection, prospective memory, and mentalizing is somewhat vague and underspecified. These processes
require more detailed exposition, and future studies should be undertaken to identify

other, as yet unconsidered, cognitive functions that may also rely on these common processes. Such studies will need to consider the means by which attending to stimulus-oriented and stimulus-independent information might contribute to an account of other cognitive functions (e.g. mentalizing processes as a component of source recollection), as well as seeking to understand the roles in these control processes played by other brain regions that almost certainly interact with anterior PFC, such as the medial temporal lobe (Simons & Spiers, 2003).

Finally, the hypothesis makes predictions about the manner in which cognitive functions such as source memory might break down in neurological or psychiatric disorders. For example, it has not so far been shown in the same patients that focal anterior PFC lesions impair performance on reality monitoring, prospective memory, and mentalizing tasks, as would be predicted if all of these functions rely on attentional switching between stimulus-oriented and stimulus-independent processing. Furthermore, reduced ability to distinguish information perceived in the outside world from imagined information might be one explanation for the hallucinations and delusions often seen in schizophrenia (Frith, 1992; Johnson & Raye, 2000). We have some evidence that tentatively supports such an account (Simons, Davis et al., 2006; Simons et al., 2008), but the relationship between reality monitoring deficits and psychotic phenomena, or indeed between impairments to recollection, prospective memory, and mentalizing, remain to be fully tested.

Conclusions

I have tried in this chapter to describe a number of neuroimaging studies of source memory and related functions, conducted in our laboratory and by other investigators, that have been motivated and constrained by cognitive theories and which have, in turn, informed the development of a new cognitive theory, the gateway hypothesis. This hypothesis, which has been shaped considerably by neuroimaging data, can account for empirical observations such as differential sensitivity of medial anterior PFC to the recollection of source details that were previously internally generated or externally derived; the distinct contribution made by lateral and medial anterior PFC towards pre- and post-retrieval stages of the retrieval process; and the common involvement of medial anterior PFC regions in prospective memory and mentalizing, as well as source recollection. Hopefully, these studies provide just one example of how neuroimaging results can inform cognitive theories of memory. If neuroimaging studies are designed with the primary aim of testing predictions derived from cognitive theories, and inferences about the resulting patterns of brain activity are based on significant region-by-condition interactions or probabilistic designations of cognitive processes to specific brain regions, there seems no reason why neuroimaging should be considered as anything other than one more form of evidence for adjudicating between competing psychological theories. Presumably, most investigators would agree that the ultimate aim of our scientific discipline is to provide the fullest possible understanding of how we remember. In which case, seeking convergent evidence from all available experimental techniques can only take us further towards that goal.

Acknowledgements

I am very grateful to Paul Fletcher, Sam Gilbert, and Dan Schacter for valuable comments and discussion, and to Ian Dobbins, Elizabeth Kensinger, and Sophia Vinogradov for providing images for use in Figure 22.1. Preparation of this chapter was supported by the Wellcome Trust.

References

Addis, D. R., Wong, A. T., & Schacter, D. L. (2007). Remembering the past and imagining the future: Common and distinct neural substrates during event construction and elaboration. *Neuropsychologia*, *45*, 1363–1377.

Amodio, D. M. & Frith, C. D. (2006). Meeting of minds: The medial frontal cortex and social cognition. *Nature Reviews Neuroscience*, *7*, 268–277.

Bird, C. M., Castelli, F., Malik, O., Frith, U., & Husain, M. (2004). The impact of extensive medial frontal lobe damage on 'Theory of Mind' and cognition. *Brain*, *127*, 914–928.

Brunet, E., Sarfati, Y., Hardy-Bayle, M. C., & Decety, J. (2000). A PET investigation of the attribution of intentions with a nonverbal task. *NeuroImage*, *11*, 157–166.

Buckner, R. L. & Carroll, D. C. (2007). Self-projection and the brain. *Trends in Cognitive Sciences*, *11*, 49–57.

Burgess, P. W., Quayle, A., & Frith, C. D. (2001). Brain regions involved in prospective memory as determined by positron emission tomography. *Neuropsychologia*, *39*, 545–555.

Burgess, P. W., Scott, S. K., & Frith, C. D. (2003). The role of the rostral frontal cortex (area 10) in prospective memory: A lateral versus medial dissociation. *Neuropsychologia*, *41*, 906–918.

Burgess, P. W. & Shallice, T. (1996). Confabulation and the control of recollection. *Memory*, *4*, 359–411.

Burgess, P. W., Simons, J. S., Dumontheil, I., & Gilbert, S. J. (2005). The gateway hypothesis of rostral prefrontal cortex (area 10) function. In: J. Duncan, L. Phillips, & P. McLeod (Eds), *Measuring the Mind: Speed, Control, and Age* (pp. 217–248). Oxford: Oxford University Press.

Burgess, P. W., Veitch, E., de Lacy Costello, A., & Shallice, T. (2000). The cognitive and neuroanatomical correlates of multitasking. *Neuropsychologia*, *38*, 848–863.

Cansino, S., Maquet, P., Dolan, R. J., & Rugg, M. D. (2002). Brain activity underlying encoding and retrieval of source memory. *Cerebral Cortex*, *12*, 1048–1056.

Clark, S. E. & Gronlund, S. D. (1996). Global matching models of recognition memory: How the models match the data. *Psychonomic Bulletin and Review*, *3*, 37–60.

D'Argembeau, A. & Van der Linden, M. (2004). Phenomenal characteristics associated with projecting oneself back into the past and forwards into the future: Influence of valence and temporal distance. *Consciousness and Cognition*, *13*, 844–858.

Dobbins, I. G., Foley, H., Schacter, D. L., & Wagner, A. D. (2002). Executive control during episodic retrieval: Multiple prefrontal processes subserve source memory. *Neuron*, *35*, 989–996.

Dobbins, I. G. & Han, S. (2006). Cue- versus probe-dependent prefrontal cortex activity during contextual remembering. *Journal of Cognitive Neuroscience*, *18*, 1439–1452.

Dobbins, I. G. & Wagner, A. D. (2005). Domain-general and domain-sensitive prefrontal mechanisms for recollecting events and detecting novelty. *Cerebral Cortex*, *15*, 1768–1778.

Duarte, A., Ranganath, C., & Knight, R. T. (2005). Effects of unilateral prefrontal lesions on familiarity, recollection, and source memory. *Journal of Neuroscience*, *25*, 8333–8337.

Ellis, J. (1996). Prospective memory or the realization of delayed intentions: A conceptual framework for research. In: M. Brandimonte, G. O. Einstein, & M. A. McDaniel (Eds), *Prospective Memory: Theory and Applications*. Mahwah, NJ: Lawrence Erlbaum Associates.

Fletcher, P. C., Happe, F., Frith, U., Baker, S. C., Dolan, R. J., Frackowiak, R. S. J., *et al.* (1995). Other minds in the brain: A functional imaging study of "theory of mind" in story comprehension. *Cognition, 57,* 109–128.

Fletcher, P. C. & Henson, R. N. A. (2001). Frontal lobes and human memory: Insights from functional neuroimaging. *Brain, 124,* 849–881.

Fletcher, P. C., Shallice, T., Frith, C. D., Frackowiak, R. S. J., & Dolan, R. J. (1998). The functional roles of prefrontal cortex in episodic memory: II. *Retrieval. Brain, 121,* 1249–1256.

Frith, C. D. (1992). *The Cognitive Neuropsychology of Schizophrenia.* Hove: Lawrence Erlbaum.

Frith, U. & Frith, C. D. (2003). Development and neurophysiology of mentalizing. *Philosophical Transactions of the Royal Society of London Series B: Biological Sciences, 358,* 459–473.

Gilbert, S. J., Frith, C. D., & Burgess, P. W. (2005). Involvement of rostral prefrontal cortex in selection between stimulus-oriented and stimulus-independent thought. *European Journal of Neuroscience, 21,* 1423–1431.

Gilbert, S. J., Simons, J. S., Frith, C. D., & Burgess, P. W. (2006). Performance-related activity in medial rostral prefrontal cortex (area 10) during low-demand tasks. *Journal of Experimental Psychology: Human Perception and Performance, 32,* 45–58.

Gilbert, S. J., Spengler, S., Simons, J. S., Steele, J. D., Lawrie, S. M., Frith, C. D., *et al.* (2006). Functional specialization within rostral prefrontal cortex (area 10): A meta-analysis. *Journal of Cognitive Neuroscience, 18,* 932–948.

Gilbert, S. J., Williamson, I., Dumontheil, I., Simons, J. S., Frith, C. D., & Burgess, P. W. (2007). Distinct regions of medial rostral prefrontal cortex supporting social and nonsocial functions. *Social Cognitive and Affective Neuroscience, 2,* 217–226.

Glisky, E. L., Rubin, S. R., & Davidson, P. S. R. (2001). Source memory in older adults: An encoding or retrieval problem?. *Journal of Experimental Psychology: Learning, Memory, and Cognition, 27,* 1131–1146.

Henkel, L. A., Johnson, M. K., & De Leonardis, D. M. (1998). Aging and source monitoring: Cognitive processes and neuropsychological correlates. *Journal of Experimental Psychology: General, 127,* 251–268.

Henson, R. (2005). What can functional neuroimaging tell the experimental psychologist? *Quarterly Journal of Experimental Psychology, 58A,* 193–233.

Henson, R. (2006). Forward inference using functional neuroimaging: dissociations versus associations. *Trends in Cognitive Sciences, 10,* 64–69.

Henson, R. N. A., Rugg, M. D., & Shallice, T. (2000). Confidence in recognition memory for words: Dissociating right prefrontal roles in episodic retrieval. *Journal of Cognitive Neuroscience, 12,* 913–923.

Henson, R. N. A., Shallice, T., & Dolan, R. J. (1999). Right prefrontal cortex and episodic memory retrieval: A functional MRI test of the monitoring hypothesis. *Brain, 122,* 1367–1381.

Janata, P., Birk, J. L., Van Horn, J. D., Leman, M., Tillman, B., & Bharucha, J. J. (2002). The cortical topography of tonal structures underlying Western music. *Science, 298,* 2167–2170.

Janowsky, J. S., Shimamura, A. P., & Squire, L. R. (1989). Source memory impairment in patients with frontal lobe lesions. *Neuropsychologia, 27,* 1043–1056.

Johnson, M. K., Hashtroudi, S., & Lindsay, D. S. (1993). Source monitoring. *Psychological Bulletin, 114,* 3–28.

Johnson, M. K. & Raye, C. L. (1981). Reality monitoring. *Psychological Review, 88,* 67–85.

Johnson, M. K. & Raye, C. L. (2000). Cognitive and brain mechanisms of false memories and beliefs. In: D. L. Schacter & E. Scarry (Eds), *Memory, Brain, and Belief* (pp. 35–86). Cambridge, MA: Harvard University Press.

Kahn, I., Davachi, L., & Wagner, A. D. (2004). Functional-neuroanatomic correlates of recollection: Implications for models of recognition memory. *Journal of Neuroscience, 24*, 4172–4180.

Kelley, R. & Wixted, J. T. (2001). On the nature of associative information in recognition memory. *Journal of Experimental Psychology: Learning, Memory, and Cognition, 27*, 701–722.

Kelley, W. M., Macrae, C. N., Wyland, C. L., Caglar, S., Inati, S., & Heatherton, T. F. (2002). Finding the self? An event-related fMRI study. *Journal of Cognitive Neuroscience, 14*, 785–794.

Kensinger, E. A. & Schacter, D. L. (2006). Neural processes underlying memory attribution on a reality-monitoring task. *Cerebral Cortex, 16*, 1126–1133.

Macrae, C. N., Moran, J. M., Heatherton, T. F., Banfield, J. F., & Kelley, W. M. (2004). Medial prefrontal activity predicts memory for self. *Cerebral Cortex, 14*, 647–654.

Mandler, G. (1980). Recognizing: The judgment of previous occurrence. *Psychological Review, 87*, 252–271.

McDaniel, M. A. & Einstein, G. O. (1992). Aging and prospective memory: Basic findings and practical applications. In: T. E. Scruggs & M. A. Mastropieri (Eds), *Advances in Learning and Behavioral Disabilities* (pp. 87–105). Greenwich, CT: JAI Press.

Nolde, S. F., Johnson, M. K., & D'Esposito, M. (1998). Left prefrontal activation during episodic remembering: An event-related fMRI study. *NeuroReport, 9*, 3509–3514.

Nyberg, L., McIntosh, A. R., Cabeza, R., Habib, R., Houle, S., & Tulving, E. (1996). General and specific brain regions involved in encoding and retrieval of events: What, where, and when. *Proceedings of the National Academy of Sciences USA, 93*, 11280–11285.

Nyberg, L., Tulving, E., Habib, R., Nilsson, L. G., Kapur, S., Houle, S., et al. (1995). Functional brain maps of retrieval mode and recovery of episodic information. *NeuroReport, 7*, 249–252.

Ochsner, K. N., Knierim, K., Ludlow, D. H., Hanelin, J., Ramachandran, T., Glover, G., et al. (2004). Reflecting upon feelings: An fMRI study of neural systems supporting the attribution of emotion to self and other. *Journal of Cognitive Neuroscience, 16*, 1746–1772.

Okuda, J., Fujii, T., Ohtake, H., Tsukiura, T., Tanji, K., Suzuki, K., et al. (2003). Thinking of the future and past: The roles of the frontal pole and the medial temporal lobes. *NeuroImage, 19*, 1369–1380.

Okuda, J., Fujii, T., Yamadori, A., Kawashima, R., Tsukiura, T., Fukatsu, R., et al. (1998). Participation of the prefrontal cortices in prospective memory: Evidence from a PET study in humans. *Neuroscience Letters, 253*, 127–130.

Poldrack, R. A. (2006). Can cognitive processes be inferred from neuroimaging data? *Trends in Cognitive Sciences, 10*, 59–63.

Poldrack, R. A., Wagner, A. D., Prull, M. W., Desmond, J. E., Glover, G. H., & Gabrieli, J. D. E. (1999). Functional specialization for semantic and phonological processing in the left inferior frontal cortex. *NeuroImage, 10*, 15–35.

Premack, D. & Woodruff, G. (1978). Chimpanzee problem solving: A test for comprehension. *Science, 202*, 532–535.

Ranganath, C., Johnson, M. K., & D'Esposito, M. (2000). Left anterior prefrontal activation increases with demands to recall specific perceptual information. *Journal of Neuroscience, 20:RC108*, 1–5.

Ratcliff, R., Van Zandt, T., & McKoon, G. (1995). Process dissociation, single-process theories, and recognition memory. *Journal of Experimental Psychology: General, 124*, 352–374.

Rotello, C. M., Macmillan, N. A., & Reeder, J. A. (2004). Sum-difference theory of remembering and knowing: A two-dimensional signal-detection model. *Psychological Review, 111*, 588–616.

Rugg, M. D. (2006). Retrieval processing in human memory: Electrophysiological and fMRI evidence. In: M. S. Gazzaniga (Ed.), *The Cognitive Neurosciences*.

Rugg, M. D., Fletcher, P. C., Chua, P. M. L., & Dolan, R. J. (1999). The role of the prefrontal cortex in recognition memory and memory for source: An fMRI study. *NeuroImage, 10*, 520–529.

Rugg, M. D., Fletcher, P. C., Frith, C. D., Frackowiak, R. S. J., & Dolan, R. J. (1996). Differential activation of the prefrontal cortex in successful and unsuccessful memory retrieval. *Brain, 119,* 2073–2083.

Rugg, M. D. & Wilding, E. L. (2000). Retrieval processing and episodic memory. *Trends in Cognitive Sciences, 4,* 108–115.

Sakai, K. & Passingham, R. E. (2003). Prefrontal interactions reflect future task operations. *Nature Neuroscience, 6,* 75–81.

Saxe, R., Carey, S., & Kanwisher, N. (2004). Understanding other minds: Linking developmental psychology and functional neuroimaging. *Annual Review of Psychology, 55,* 87–124.

Schacter, D. L. & Addis, D. R. (2007). The cognitive neuroscience of constructive memory: Remembering the past and imagining the future. *Philosophical Transactions of the Royal Society of London Series B: Biological Sciences, 362,* 773–786.

Schacter, D. L., Alpert, N. M., Savage, C. R., Rauch, S. L., & Albert, M. S. (1996). Conscious recollection and the human hippocampal formation: Evidence from positron emission tomography. *Proceedings of the National Academy of Sciences USA, 93,* 321–325.

Schacter, D. L., Kaszniak, A. W., Kihlstrom, J. F., & Valdiserri, M. (1991). The relation between source memory and aging. *Psychology and Aging, 6,* 559–568.

Schacter, D. L., Norman, K. A., & Koutstaal, W. (1998). The cognitive neuroscience of constructive memory. *Annual Review of Psychology, 49,* 289–318.

Semendeferi, K., Armstrong, E., Schleicher, A., Zilles, K., & Van Hoesen, G. W. (2001). Prefrontal cortex in humans and apes: A comparative study of area 10. *American Journal of Physical Anthropology, 114,* 224–241.

Shallice, T. (1988). From neuropsychology to mental structure. Cambridge: Cambridge University Press.

Shallice, T. (2003). Functional imaging and neuropsychology findings: How can they be linked? *NeuroImage, 20,* S146–S154.

Simons, J. S., Davis, S. W., Gilbert, S. J., Frith, C. D., & Burgess, P. W. (2006). Discriminating imagined from perceived information engages brain areas implicated in schizophrenia. *NeuroImage, 32,* 696–703.

Simons, J. S., Gilbert, S. J., Owen, A. M., Fletcher, P. C., & Burgess, P. W. (2005). Distinct roles for lateral and medial anterior prefrontal cortex in contextual recollection. *Journal of Neurophysiology, 94,* 813–820.

Simons, J. S., Henson, R. N. A., Gilbert, S. J., & Fletcher, P. C. (2008). Separable forms of reality monitoring supported by anterior prefrontal cortex. *Journal of Cognitive Neuroscience, 20,* 447–457.

Simons, J. S., Owen, A. M., Fletcher, P. C., & Burgess, P. W. (2005). Anterior prefrontal cortex and the recollection of contextual information. *Neuropsychologia, 43,* 1774–1783.

Simons, J. S., Schölvinck, M. L., Gilbert, S. J., Frith, C. D., & Burgess, P. W. (2006). Differential components of prospective memory? Evidence from fMRI. *Neuropsychologia, 44,* 1388–1397.

Simons, J. S. & Spiers, H. J. (2003). Prefrontal and medial temporal lobe interactions in long-term memory. *Nature Reviews Neuroscience, 4,* 637–648.

Simons, J. S., Verfaellie, M., Galton, C. J., Miller, B. L., Hodges, J. R., & Graham, K. S. (2002). Recollection-based memory in frontotemporal dementia: Implications for theories of long-term memory. *Brain, 125,* 2523–2536.

Small, D. M., Gitelman, D. R., Gregory, M. D., Nobre, A. C., Parrish, T. B., & Mesulam, M. M. (2003). The posterior cingulate and medial prefrontal cortex mediate the anticipatory allocation of spatial attention. *NeuroImage, 18,* 633–641.

Smith, E. E. & Jonides, J. (1999). Storage and executive processes in the frontal lobes. *Science, 283,* 1657–1661.

Stone, V. E., Baron-Cohen, S., & Knight, R. T. (1998). Frontal lobe contributions to theory of mind. *Journal of Cognitive Neuroscience, 10*, 640–656.

Stuss, D. T., Gallup, G. G., & Alexander, M. P. (2001). The frontal lobes are necessary for 'theory of mind'. *Brain, 124*, 279–286.

Suzuki, M., Fujii, T., Tsukiura, T., Okuda, J., Umetsu, A., Nagasaka, T., *et al.* (2002). Neural basis of temporal context memory: A functional MRI study. *NeuroImage, 17*, 1790–1796.

Szpunar, K. K., Watson, J. M., & McDermott, K. B. (2007). Neural substrates of envisioning the future. *Proceedings of the National Academy of Sciences USA, 104*, 642–647.

Tulving, E. (1983). *Elements of Episodic Memory*. Oxford, UK: Clarendon Press.

Vinogradov, S., Luks, T. L., Simpson, G. V., Schulman, B. J., Glenn, S., & Wong, A. E. (2006). Brain activation patterns during memory of cognitive agency. *NeuroImage, 31*, 896–905.

Yonelinas, A. P. (2002). The nature of recollection and familiarity: A review of 30 years of research. *Journal of Memory and Language, 46*, 441–517.

Chapter 23

Oscillatory and haemodynamic medial temporal responses preceding stimulus onset modulate episodic memory

Emrah Düzel and Sebastian Guderian

Introduction

Episodic memory allows us to vividly remember events unfolding around us (Tulving, 1985). A hallmark of episodic memory is that different types of information about events such as time, location, and context, can be encoded and later remembered as memory contents that belong together. The medial temporal lobes (MTL), particularly the hippocampi, are thought to play a key role in both the integration of the various aspects of events during episodic memory formation, as well as the reinstatement of their corresponding representations during episodic retrieval (Mishkin, Suzuki, Gadian, & Vargha-Khadem, 1997; Nyberg *et al.*, 2000). Much of the research on MTL function has been devoted to the mechanisms that underlie the processing of episodes as they are encoded or retrieved. It is widely assumed that the hippocampi play a key role in orchestrating dynamic interactions between distributed neocortical areas during mnemonic processing of stimulus-information (McClelland, McNaughton, & O'Reilly, 1995; Rolls, 1996; Treves & Rolls, 1994). Within this framework, the widespread interconnections of parahippocampal and rhinal cortices provide the anatomical basis for the medial temporal lobes to act as convergence zones and associative integrators for information from many unimodal and multimodal cortical association areas (Eichenbaum, Schoenbaum, Young, & Bunsey, 1996; Lavenex, Suzuki, & Amaral, 2002, 2004; Murray & Bussey, 1999).

In this chapter we will extend this traditional stimulus-processing view of MTL function by showing that MTL-activity modulates memory formation not only in response to an event, but already plays a role in establishing optimal encoding states prior to the onset of events. We will present evidence for such prestimulus states using magnetoencephalographic measures of theta (3-8 Hz) oscillations generated in the MTL (Guderian, Schott, Richardson-Klavehn, & Duzel, in press). These oscillatory properties of MTL function will be complemented by fMRI data (Wittmann, Bunzeck, Dolan, & Duzel, 2007) showing hippocampal activation related to the anticipation of novel stimuli and evidence that such anticipation is associated with improved long-term memory formation. Although it is not yet clear how the oscillatory and haemodynamic prestimulus responses of the MTL are related to each other, the available evidence suggest that the contribution of the medial temporal lobes to episodic memory extends beyond mere stimulus-processing and involves also preparatory or anticipatory and motivational mechanisms that are instantiated prior to stimulus onset.

Theta oscillations and memory

Before presenting our findings regarding MTL-prestimulus oscillatory dynamics, we will first review some recent findings implicating theta oscillations in memory processes within and beyond the MTL. We argue that theta oscillations in these brain regions play a role in the integration of distributed cortical information during mnemonic processing. Recent studies in animals (Jones & Wilson, 2005; Lee, Simpson, Logothetis, & Rainer, 2005; Lisman & Otmakhova, 2001; Mehta, Lee, & Wilson, 2002) and humans (Duzel, Neufang, & Heinze, 2005; Guderian & Duzel, 2005; Klimesch et al., 2001; Neufang, Heinze, & Duzel, 2006; Tesche & Karhu, 2000) ranging from the cellular to the systemic level have provided important insights into the role of theta oscillations for synaptic plasticity, information coding and cognitive functioning. Neural oscillations in general have been viewed as providing a clocking mechanism that can shape and coordinate the firing of neural populations (Jones & Wilson, 2005; Singer, 1999; Varela, Lachaux, Rodriguez, & Martinerie, 2001; Jacobs, Kahana, Ekstrom & Fried, 2007). Direct evidence for a role of theta oscillations in coordinating distant brain regions comes from recent animal studies. Research in rodents demonstrated that neurons in the medial prefrontal cortex show phasic firing locked to the hippocampal theta rhythm when navigation through a T-maze requires the maintenance of a goal and target location in working memory (Jones & Wilson, 2005). In this study, approximately 40% of units in the medial prefrontal cortex (mPFC) were phase-locked to the hippocampal CA1 theta rhythm. CA1-mPFC entrainment was specific to 4- to 12-Hz and was evident at every level examined, including individual pairs of co-active neurons, theta phase-locking of neurons to theta local field potentials (LFPs), and hippocampal-prefrontal theta LFP coherence (Jones & Wilson, 2005). Monosynaptic projections from the hippocampus to the medial PFC are thought to be the anatomical and physiological foundations for such coherence between these two structures. There is no evidence for direct projections from mPFC back to the hippocampus, suggesting that the hippocampus drives mPFC firing rather than vice versa and compatible with this idea, mPFC peak activity lagged approximately behind the peak activity of hippocampal units (Jones & Wilson, 2005). This finding points to a possible organizing role for hippocampal theta-patterned output in hippocampal-neocortical synchronization (Jones & Wilson, 2005).

Such a patterning or organizing role for theta has recently also been observed during visual delay maintenance in the visual system of non-human primates (Lee et al., 2005). Single neurons in area V4 tend to fire at a particular phase of the theta rhythm, and spikes near the preferred theta phase showed a larger stimulus selectivity than other spikes (Lee et al., 2005). These findings extend earlier studies of theta frequency oscillations in relation to spatial navigation and hippocampal coding of an animal's location within a place field (Huxter, Burgess, & O'Keefe, 2003; O'Keefe & Conway, 1978;

O'Keefe & Recce, 1993) to a more general role of theta oscillations in modulating distributed cortical processing.

In humans, invasive recordings in patients with pharmacoresistant epilepsy have shown a role of neocortical theta oscillations during spatial navigation (Caplan *et al.*, 2003; Kahana, Seelig, & Madsen, 2001), working memory (Raghavachari *et al.*, 2006) and episodic memory encoding (Sederberg, Kahana, Howard, Donner, & Madsen, 2003; Sederberg *et al.*, 2007; Rizzuto, Madsen, Bromfield, Schulze-Bonhage, & Kahana, 2006). Evidence for a role of theta oscillations in synchronizing distributed brain areas comes from studies investigating recollection of personal events (Guderian & Duzel, 2005; Neufang *et al.*, 2006). A large number of studies suggest that recollection is critically dependent on the hippocampus (Brown & Aggleton, 2001; Duzel, Vargha-Khadem, Heinze, & Mishkin, 2001; Fortin, Wright, & Eichenbaum, 2004; Mishkin, Vargha-Khadem, & Gadian, 1998; Vargha-Khadem *et al.*, 1997; Yonelinas *et al.*, 2002) while it is less clear whether this is also the case for familiarity (Squire, Stark, & Clark, 2004). During recollection, theta oscillations might mediate a dynamic link between hippocampal and neocortical areas, thereby allowing a reinstatement of retrieved information in distributed neocortical assemblies, as has been postulated by several computational models of hippocampus-dependent memory (e.g. Marr, 1971; McClelland *et al.*, 1995; Rolls, 2000a, 2000b; Treves & Rolls, 1994). Using MEG, we recently showed that theta oscillations were higher in amplitude during recollection than during familiarity (Guderian & Duzel, 2005). These theta oscillations were induced in nature, meaning that they showed considerable phase variability from trial to trial. By calculating phase differences between sensor pairs at each time point of each trial we were able to extract the field distribution of coherent theta oscillations and used this information to localize brain sources of synchronized theta-generators giving rise to the oscillations. The results suggested that recollection is associated with an induced activity increase in a distributed synchronous theta network including prefrontal, mediotemporal, and visual areas. These findings are compatible with the notion that theta oscillations are related to the integration of distributed cortical representations with mediotemporal processing during recollection.

Prestimulus medial temporal theta-states of encoding

Besides their putative role in stimulus-processing, MTL theta oscillations can modulate memory formation in animals even prior to the onset of a stimulus. It has been shown that there is enhanced learning in classical conditioning depending on the theta-state preceding stimulus onset (Griffin, Asaka, Darling, & Berry, 2004; Seager, Johnson, Chabot, Asaka, & Berry, 2002). These findings complement other recent observations that perception of a stimulus can be influenced by pre-stimulus brain activity (Linkenkaer-Hansen, Nikulin, Palva, Ilmoniemi, & Palva, 2004; Super, van der Togt, Spekreijse, & Lamme, 2003) and raise the possibility that the brain state immediately preceding an event could affect stimulus processing and later episodic memory. Although a number of electrophysiological (e.g. Paller, Kutas, & Mayes, 1987; B. Schott, Richardson-Klavehn, Heinze, & Duzel, 2002) and haemodynamic studies (e.g. Brewer, Zhao, Desmond, Glover, & Gabrieli, 1998; Otten, Henson, & Rugg, 2002; B. H. Schott, Richardson-Klavehn *et al.*, 2006;

Wagner *et al.*, 1998) have shown that the ability to recollect an event and its spatio-temporal context is associated with specific patterns of brain activity during the time the event is originally experienced, these studies have not investigated to what extent oscillatory dynamics in the prestimulus time window modulate this relationship.

To examine whether pre-stimulus theta-states predict episodic encoding success, we obtained whole-head magnetoencephalographic (MEG) recordings from 24 healthy young adults while they performed either semantic (pleasantness-rating, deep processing) or phonemic (syllable-counting, shallow processing) judgements on lists of visually presented words. After a delay, each list was followed by a free recall test. Theta oscillations before and after word onsets at study were quantified using single-trial wavelet transformations separately for words that were later recalled and later forgotten. Figure 23.1 (left column) shows that, as word onset approached, there was an increase in theta amplitude at left anterior temporal sensors for later recalled words (solid line) but not for later forgotten words (dashed line), leading to significant differences in amplitude starting at about −200 ms. We henceforth term this difference the pre-stimulus DM (difference due to later memory) effect (Paller, McCarthy, & Wood, 1988). Source analysis located these theta oscillations as well as the prestimulus DM-effect to the MTL (Figure 23.1, right column). In the post-stimulus time-window there was a stronger amplitude decrease for later recalled relative to later forgotten words from 550 to 1000 ms at right occipitotemporal sensors (henceforth termed the late DM effect). We investigated the relationship between the pre-stimulus and late DM effects by calculating the across-participants correlation between theta amplitude differences (later recalled minus later forgotten) in the pre-stimulus (−200 ms to 0 ms) and late (600 ms to 900 ms) time windows. The correlation was a trend for a negative correlation ($R = -0.39$; $p = 0.062$; two-tailed). Both DM effects were not significantly dependent on the levels of processing (LOP, deep, or shallow) at encoding. That is, separating the theta amplitudes by LOP revealed that theta amplitude was specifically modulated by encoding success rather than being influenced by the particular encoding-task demands (Figure 23.1, middle column).

Thus, increased MTL theta oscillatory amplitude predicted successful memory for items even before they were presented. The pre-stimulus DM effect was not significantly different during deep versus shallow study processing, suggesting that it did not reflect a qualitative difference in cognitive processing and could hence be interpreted as a mere extension of the well-known LOP effect of encoding (Craik & Lockhart, 1972) to the pre-stimulus time window. Moreover, differences in arousal or attention prior to the onset of later recalled versus later forgotten words should result in differences in behavioural RTs during the study tasks, but we found no such differences.

If pre-stimulus theta amplitude is indeed associated with successful encoding, the recall rate in individual participants should increase as a function of increased pre-stimulus theta amplitude. To investigate this possibility, we separated the trials during encoding for each participant into five equally sized bins of increasing theta amplitude. We then sorted the trials in every bin (or theta rank) according to their behavioural status (i.e. recalled vs. forgotten and deep vs. shallow). Thus, we were able to analyse the recall rate in individual participants as a function of LOP and five levels of pre-stimulus

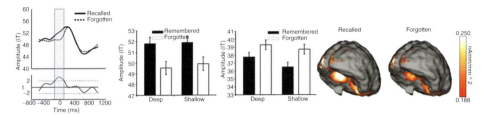

Figure 23.1 Left: Subsequently recalled (solid lines) and forgotten (dashed lines) stimuli differ in theta-amplitude even before stimulus onset (data from left fronto-temporal MEG sensors, t-values indicate significant theta-amplitude differences between recalled and forgotten words, stimulus onset at 0 ms). Left histogram: This prestimulus effect is independent of whether subjects had to prepare for a deep (semantic decision) or a shallow (phonemic decision) study task for the upcoming stimulus (middle histogram in figure). Right histogram: In the post-stimulus time-window there was a stronger amplitude decrease for later recalled relative to later forgotten words from 550 to 1000 ms at right occipitotemporal sensors. Source analyses (right brain outlines) indicate that the difference in prestimulus theta-amplitude was generated in the medial temporal lobe.

theta amplitude. A two-way ANOVA on recall rates with the factors LOP (deep vs. shallow) and theta rank (levels 1–5) showed both a main effect of LOP $[F(1,23) = 27.4; p < 0.001]$ and theta rank $[F(3.1,71.1) = 50.6; p < 0.001]$. The lack of a significant interaction $[F(2.7,62.6) = 0.6; p > 0.65]$ suggests that encoding success is modulated independently by the level of cognitive processing and the theta amplitude prior to stimulus onset. We fitted a first order polynomial to the recall rates as a function of theta rank for each subject and tested whether the resulting slope was significantly different from zero across participants. The result was significant $(t(23) = 11.45, p < 0.001)$, indicating that recall rate increased as a function of increasing theta amplitude. Remarkably, in all 24 participants the slope was greater than zero and the highest theta rank was associated with a higher recall rate than the lowest theta rank. We also tested whether reaction times during study changed as a function of theta rank, which would suggest that theta amplitude before stimulus onset could exert its effect on encoding through general arousal or attentional mechanisms. We again fitted a first order polynomial to the reaction times as a function of theta rank and found that the slopes were not significantly different from zero $(t(23) = -0.69, p > 0.45)$, indicating that the reaction times during study did not depend on pre-stimulus theta amplitude.

These findings across and within individuals indicate that the prestimulus theta effect was linked to a specific memory-related MTL state rather than to task-preparation and was unlikely to reflect fluctuations in arousal or attention. Taken together with the recent finding that pre-stimulus ERP slow-shifts correlate with encoding success (Otten, Quayle, Akram, Ditewig, & Rugg, 2006), these findings suggest that episodic memory encoding can be enhanced by two different and potentially independent pre-stimulus phenomena. One is a slow shift related to a semantic preparatory task set and contributes to improving encoding of words processed deeply (Otten *et al.*, 2006). The other is a theta modulation and is related to a task-independent brain state that improves encoding irrespective of whether words are processed deeply or shallowly. Both phenomena independently provide important evidence for the operation of item-independent encoding processes. As noted by Otten *et al.* (2006), whereas post-stimulus effects may be attributable to variation between to-be-remembered items in some characteristic that influences their later memorability, such as distinctiveness, no such hypothesis can be entertained for effects that occur prior to stimulus presentation. It should be noted, however, that because the number of 'shallow, subsequently remembered' items is usually smaller than the number of 'deep, subsequently remembered' items, the differences between our data the finding of Otten *et al.* (2006) may just be due to ERP slow shifts being less sensitive than MEG frequency decomposition. Also, it is unclear what the neural generators of the prestimulus effects in the Otten *et al.* (2006) study were and we therefore cannot fully rule out the possibility that both studies report different manifestations of the same regional phenomenon.

The fact that subjects recalled more items in the deep condition in the absence of an amplitude difference of the prestimulus theta effect between deep and shallow study conditions suggests that the prestimulus theta effect occurred more frequently in the deep task than in the shallow task but had the same neural generator and amplitude in both conditions. Figure 23.2 illustrates this scenario. Hence, it seems plausible that the prestimulus theta state is more frequent under the influence of expectancies related to meaningful stimulus processing. In the following section, we will report functional imaging data showing activation of the hippocampus in anticipation of a novel stimulus and will discuss how the sets of results may be related to each other.

Anticipation of novelty recruits hippocampus and substantia nigra/VTA while promoting recollection

Recent models of hippocampus-dependent memory formation emphasize a functional relationship between novelty detection in the hippocampus and enhancement of hippocampal plasticity by novelty-induced dopaminergic modulation arising from the SN/VTA (Lisman & Grace, 2005). Indeed, single-neuron recordings in animals and recent functional magnetic resonance imaging (fMRI) studies in humans provide convergent evidence that the SN/VTA midbrain region is activated not only by reward (Schultz, 1998)

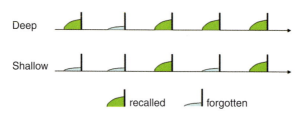

Figure 23.2 A model to illustrate the relationship between prestimulus theta-states and level-of-processing. The outcome illustrated in Figure 23.1 can be explained if theta-states favourable for successful episodic encoding are more frequent under deep as compared to shallow processing task instructions while their overall amplitude and topography remain the same under both task conditions.

but also by novel stimuli even in the absence of reinforcement (Bunzeck & Duzel, 2006; B. H. Schott et al., 2004; Schultz, 1998). The hippocampus is believed to provide the major input for a novelty signal in SN/VTA (Lisman & Grace, 2005). Dopamine released by SN/VTA neurons, in turn, is critical for stabilizing and maintaining long-term potentiation (LTP) and long-term depression (LTD) in hippocampal region CA1 (Frey & Morris, 1998; Sajikumar & Frey, 2004; Lemon & Manahan-Vaughan, 2006). FMRI data have shown that joint SN/VTA and hippocampal activation is associated with successful long-term memory formation (B. H. Schott, Seidenbecher et al., 2006) and reward-related improvement in novel stimulus encoding (Adcock, Thangavel, Whitfield-Gabrieli, Knutson, & Gabrieli, 2005; Wittmann et al., 2005).

The functional-anatomical overlap of reward and novelty processing in the SN/VTA raises the possibility that mesolimbic novelty-processing shows a similar anticipatory response to predicted novelty as it does to predicted reward (Schultz, 1998). We investigated anticipatory responses to novel and familiar stimuli in an fMRI paradigm modeled upon reward anticipation procedures (Wittmann et al., 2007). Participants engaged in 12 sessions of 5.7 min duration, each containing 40 trials of 4.5–12 s length. During each trial, participants saw a yellow or blue square (1500 ms) indicating with 75% accuracy whether the following picture would be familiar or novel. After a variable delay (0–4.5 s), a picture from the predicted category was shown in 75% of the trials, and a picture from the unpredicted category, novel following a familiarity cue and familiar following a novelty cue, was shown in 25% of the trials (1500 ms). Both categories were shown equally often. Participants indicated with a fast button press (right or left index or middle finger) whether the picture was from the familiar category or not. A fixation phase of variable duration followed (1.5-4.5 s). The cue colours associated with each picture category were counterbalanced across participants, as well as the responding hand and the assignment of the fingers to the categories.

Thus, coloured squares served as cues that predicted subsequent presentation of novel or previously familiarized images of scenes. As the fMRI experiment required a large number of trials, we also conducted a purely behavioural version in which trial numbers were more optimal to assess how episodic memory performance was affected by anticipation of novelty using a remember/know paradigm (Tulving, 1985). Behaviourally, cue validity was associated with a significant effect on subjects' reaction times during discrimination of novel and familiar stimuli (correct responses to validly cued stimuli were faster than correct responses following invalid cues), showing that cues predicting novel or familiar events were processed by subjects (Wittmann et al., 2007). FMRI analysis revealed that cues predicting novel images elicited significantly higher SN/VTA and hippocampus activation than cues predicting familiar stimuli (Figure 23.3). Once predicted, novelty itself (comparison of expected novel and expected familiar pictures) elicited a hippocampal response but not a SN/VTA response. These data show that the SN/VTA is activated during the anticipation of novel events. This finding is compatible with the view that SN/VTA might signal the prediction of an upcoming novel event. The fact that it does not respond to the predicted novel stimulus, on the other hand, suggests that it also computes a prediction error: a correctly predicted novel stimulus does not cause a prediction error and hence there is no SN/VTA response to the predicted novelty (while an

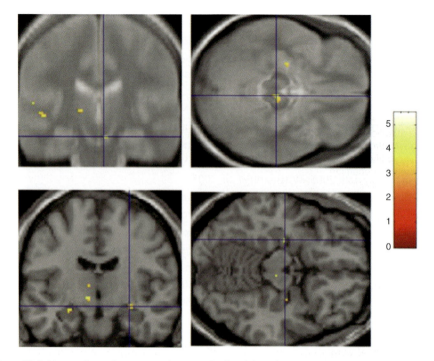

Figure 23.3 Haemodynamic response increase in the right substantia nigra/VTA and in bilateral hippocampi for cues predicting novel pictures as compared to cues predicting familiar pictures. Statistical threshold for all contrasts: $p < 0.005$, uncorrected. Minimal cluster size: 5 voxels.

unpredicted novel stimulus does cause a prediction error and this was accompanied by SN/VTA activation). In contrast, hippocampal activation reflected both anticipation and actual subsequent novelty.

The activation of the hippocampus by novel stimuli per se is highly compatible with the so-called VTA-hippocampal loop model, according to which hippocampal novelty signals to the SN/VTA result from an intrahippocampal comparison of stimulus information with stored associations (Lisman & Grace, 2005). According to this model (see Figure 23.4 for an illustration of the model), the hippocampal formation computes an early novelty signal and this signal is conveyed through the subiculum, the nucleus accumbens and through inhibition of the ventral pallidum to the SN/VTA. The inhibition of the ventral pallidum results in a disinhibtion of the SN/VTA with the effect that more dopaminergic neurons enter a tonic firing mode and can therefore be transferred into a burst-firing mode through local integration of other, probably prefrontal, inputs. The resulting dopaminergic tonic/burst-firing leads to dopamine release in the hippocampus which is critical for hippocampal long-term plasticity and may also modify hippocampal responses to novelty. Hippocampal activation in response to novelty-predicting cues, on the other hand, can not be explained by this model, because there is no novel stimulus that could elicit a hippocampal signal to the SN/VTA. We suggest that a dopaminergic

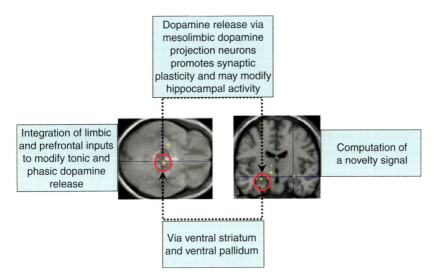

Figure 23.4 Schematic illustration of how the hippocampal formation and the SN/VTA may interact.

prediction signal contributes to hippocampal activation via dopaminergic input to the hippocampus (Jay, 2003). Indeed, previous results indicate that several brain areas outside the mesolimbic system show differential anticipatory responses in reward paradigms. A recent example is the demonstration of such responses in primary visual cortex V1 (Shuler & Bear, 2006). These responses are hypothesized to be modulated through dopaminergic neurotransmission. A similar mechanism could apply to the processing of novelty. Irrespective of whether the dopaminergic midbrain modulates the hippocampus or vice versa, co-activation of the hippocampus and SN/VTA could be associated with increased dopaminergic input to the hippocampus during anticipation. This, in turn, could induce a state that enhances learning for upcoming novel stimuli, a model that is computationally feasible (Blumenfeld, Preminger, Sagi, & Tsodyks, 2006). In keeping with the idea that pre-activation of hippocampus during anticipation facilitates learning, the behavioural data show that expected novel pictures engendered a higher remember/know response difference than unexpected novel pictures when memory was tested one day later.

We recently reported that memory for reward-predicting stimuli was also associated with a higher remember/know ratio as compared to stimuli that predicted the absence of reward (Wittmann *et al.*, 2005), and this memory improvement was associated with increased SN/VTA and hippocampal activation in response to reward-predicting stimuli at the time of encoding. Our current results extend these findings to incorporate an SN/VTA contribution to the enhancement of hippocampus dependent memory that is established by the earliest predictor of novelty. We suggest that together, the SN/VTA and the hippocampal response to anticipated novelty are part of a motivationally relevant learning signal to explore an environment (Bunzeck & Duzel, 2006).

Conclusions

Computational models of reward processing (Kakade & Dayan, 2002) are compatible with the notion that the functional and anatomical overlap between reward and novelty processing in the SN/VTA might well serve to motivate exploratory behaviour. Novelty may motivate exploration in the search for potential rewards (act as a so-called exploration bonus), enabling organisms to find new food sources and facilitate encoding the episodic, contextual, and spatial circumstances of their potential discovery. From this vantage point, novelty serves as a motivational learning signal that enhances hippocampus-dependent episodic memory formation.

Conceptualizing novelty as an exploration bonus that enhances episodic memory formation through energizing exploration opens an interesting perspective on encoding that we have tried to highlight in the current chapter. In our view, this motivational regulation of hippocampus-dependent memory is called into play not just by stimulus novelty but if additionally information about the stimulus can be integrated into preexisting knowledge or schemas. In this sense, meaningful processing of a novel stimulus is a more potent hippocampal learning signal than a perceptually shallow processing of a novel stimulus. The prospect that an upcoming novel stimulus will be processed meaningfully, in relation to existing knowledge, makes the anticipation of that novel stimulus a motivationally important in the sense of an exploration bonus. From this perspective, psychological theories of successful encoding, such as the levels of processing framework (Craik & Lockhardt, 1972), could be extended to bridge the gap between their emphasis on post-stimulus processes and these neuromodulatory mechanisms enacted in the prestimulus time window. By the same token, we suggest that the fields of reinforcement learning and declarative memory, which over the last decades have generated largely separate literatures, are moving closer.

We presented evidence that induced theta oscillations not only play a role in the synchronizing of distributed neural activations with medial temporal lobe regions (Guderian & Duzel, 2005; Rolls, 1996) during recollection, but also modulate encoding in a state-dependent manner even prior to stimulus onset (Guderian et al., in press). Such a prestimulus theta-state is more likely if participants are cued to process the anticipated stimulus meaningfully (Guderian et al., in revision). It is currently unknown how prestimulus theta effects in the MTL could be linked to anticipatory SN/VTA activation and any related increase in mesolimbic dopamine release. Given that hippocampal theta oscillations are closely linked to cholinergic neurotransmission (Buzsaki, 2002; Hasselmo, Hay, Ilyn, & Gorchetchnikov, 2002) and cholinergic septo-hippocampal projection neurons receive substantial dopaminergic input from the midbrain (Smiley, Subramanian, & Mesulam, 1999) it seems plausible that the dopaminergic midbrain, the cholinergic septum, and the MTL act together during the anticipation of novelty and its meaningful processing. Consistently, activation of D1/5 receptors in the medial septum can lead to an increase in the number of theta bursts (whereas injection of atropine, a cholinergic antagonist, consistently disrupts theta burst pattern; Fitch, Sahr, Eastwood, Zhou, & Yang, 2006). This supports the idea that SN/VTA activation (and consequent dopamine D1/5 stimulation through increased dopamine-release) may indirectly regulate theta rhythm in the hippocampus (Fitch et al., 2006). FMRI studies of activity in basal forebrain regions housing cholinergic neurons is complicated by technical issues related to susceptibility artifacts (Weiskopf, Hutton, Josephs, Turner, & Deichmann, 2007) and our functional imaging protocol in the fMRI study of novelty anticipation (Wittmann *et al.*, 2007) was not optimized for this brain region. We therefore cannot exclude the possibility that the anticipation of novelty is also associated with activation of the basal forebrain areas known to include cholinergic populations that can modulate septo-hippocampal theta more directly. Ultimately, understanding the relationship between dopaminergic/cholinergic neuromodulation, theta-dynamics, and hippocampal activity will require combining multimodal imaging with pharmacological approaches.

Our finding that MTL theta state predicts later memory, before to-be-remembered information is even perceived, suggests that memory might be improved by timing stimulus presentation to optimal theta states. A potential application of our finding might be that individuals could learn to optimize their MTL theta state via neurofeedback. This possibility is supported by the finding that deep study processing led to enhanced encoding while leaving the magnitude of the MTL theta state associated with successful encoding unchanged. This suggests that, while being specifically related to encoding, MTL theta can be manipulated by non-mnemonic cognitive control processes that could be trained using neurofeedback. In fact, some of these concepts regarding anticipatory activity and its utility for neurofeedback to boost memory and learning have been advanced decades ago (Bauer, & Nirnberger, 1981; Bauer, & Nirnberger, 1981) and we believe physiological and psychological understanding of declarative memory processing has sufficiently advanced to reformulate them.

Future methodological directions in multimodal imaging

The presence of prestimulus effects poses a caveat for studies of functional imaging of episodic memory. It is currently unclear, to what extent functional imaging data on the contribution of the MTL to stimulus-encoding actually reflect prestimulus states related to anticipation and motivation in addition to stimulus-processing *per se*. From a methodological point of view, it seems important to try to disentangle the prestimulus modulation of MTL activity from memory processing of stimulus-information (for a related argument also see Otten *et al.*, 2006). The fMRI findings discussed above (Wittmann *et al.*, 2007) suggest that this is possible using suitable experimental procedures.

Our data also suggest that one common element linking prestimulus mechanisms of memory and stimulus-related memory processing is neuromodulation. We believe that there is a realistic perspective of bridging animal models of neuromodulation of MTL structures and human physiology of memory formation through multimodal imaging in combination with pharmacology. We argue that combining haemodynamic and structural imaging of brain regions that are known to house dopaminergic and cholinergic neurons (e.g. SN/VTA and basal forebrain) with electromagnetic studies of oscillatory dynamics holds the promise to promote our understanding on how MTL processes are modulated by salience, valence, anticipation, predictions and motivation. One of the questions that remain to be answered in this context is whether the haemodynamic responses of neuromodulatory brain structures are correlated with transmitter release in target regions. Such questions can be addressed by combining fMRI studies with positron emission tomography (PET) studies of transmitter release in within-subject designs. Indeed, there is evidence form such an approach that the fMRI SN/VTA activation to reward prediction is correlated with dopamine-release in the nucleus accumbens (a major target region of SN/VTA neurons) as measured with 11C-raclopride PET (Schott, Minuzzi, Krebs, Elmenhorst, Lang, Winz, Seidenbecher, Coenen, Heinze, Zilles, Düzel, Bauer, in press). We therefore propose that despite being inherently indirect, combining fMRI of neuromodulatory brain regions with electromagnetic studies of oscillatory dynamics will be a fruitful methodological approach to advance memory research in humans.

Acknowledgements

Supported by grants from the Deutsche Forschungsgemeinschaft (KFG 167 'Kognitive Kontrolle von Gedaechtnis', TP1 and TP3), the Helmholtz Society, the Volkswagen Foundation, BMBFT (CAI), and The Wellcome Trust. We thank Michael Scholz for assistance with data analysis and Maja Fremuth for assistance with data acquisition.

References

Adcock, R. A., Thangavel, A., Whitfield-Gabrieli, S., Knutson, B., & Gabrieli, J. D. (2006). Reward-motivated learning: mesolimbic activation precedes memory formation. *Neuron, 50*(3), 507–517.

Bauer, H. & Nirnberger, G. (1981). Concept identification as a function of preceding negative or positive spontaneous shifts in slow brain potentials. *Psychophysiology, 18*, 466–469.

Bauer, H. & Nirnberger, G. (1980). Paired associated learning with feedback of DC potential shifts of the cerebral cortex. *Archiv Für Psychologie, 132*, 237–239.

Blumenfeld, B., Preminger, S., Sagi, D., & Tsodyks, M. (2006). Dynamics of memory representations in networks with novelty-facilitated synaptic plasticity. *Neuron, 52*(2), 383–394.

Brewer, J. B., Zhao, Z., Desmond, J. E., Glover, G. H., & Gabrieli, J. D. E. (1998). Making Memories: Brain Activity that Predicts How Well Visual Experience Will Be Remembered. *Science, 281*, 1185–1187.

Brown, M. & Aggleton, J. P. (2001). Recognition memory: What are the roles of the perirhinal cortex and the hippocampus. *Nature Reviews Neuroscience, 2*, 51–61.

Bunzeck, N. & Duzel, E. (2006). Absolute stimulus-novelty is coded by the human substantia nigra/VTA. *Neuron, 3*, 369–379.

Bunzeck, N., Schutze, H., Stallforth, S., Kaufmann, J., Duzel, S., Heinze, H. J., *et al.* (2008). Mesolimbic novelty processing in older adults. *Cerebral Cortex, 17*(12), 1992–2002.

Buzsaki, G. (2002). Theta oscillations in the hippocampus. *Neuron, 33*(3), 325–340.

Caplan, J. B., Madsen, J. R., Schulze-Bonhage, A., Aschenbrenner-Scheibe, R., Newman, E. L., & Kahana, M. J. (2003). Human theta oscillations related to sensorimotor integration and spatial learning. *Journal of Neuroscience, 23*(11), 4726–4736.

Craik, F. I. & Lockhart, R. S. (1972). Levels of processing: A framework for memory research. *Journal of Verbal Learning & Verbal Behavior, 11*(6), 671–684.

Duzel, E., Neufang, M., & Heinze, H. J. (2005). The Oscillatory Dynamics of Recognition Memory and its Relationship to Event-related Responses. *Cerebral Cortex, 15*(12), 1992–2002.

Duzel, E., Vargha-Khadem, F., Heinze, H. J., & Mishkin, M. (2001). Brain activity evidence for recognition without recollection after early hippocampal damage. *Proceedings of the National Academy of Science of the United States of America, 98*, 8101–8106.

Eichenbaum, H., Schoenbaum, G., Young, B., & Bunsey, M. (1996). Functional organization of the hippocampal memory system. *Proceedings of the National Academy of Science of the United States of America, 93*(24), 13500–13507.

Fitch, T. E., Sahr, R. N., Eastwood, B. J., Zhou, F. C., & Yang, C. R. (2006). Dopamine D1/5 receptor modulation of firing rate and bidirectional theta burst firing in medial septal/vertical limb of diagonal band neurons in vivo. *Journal of Neurophysiology, 95*(5), 2808–2820.

Fortin, N. J., Wright, S. P., & Eichenbaum, H. (2004). Recollection-like memory retrieval in rats is dependent on the hippocampus. *Nature, 431*(7005), 188–191.

Frey, U. & Morris, R. G. (1998). Synaptic tagging: implications for late maintenance of hippocampal long-term potentiation. *Trends in Neuroscience, 21*(5), 181–188.

Griffin, A. L., Asaka, Y., Darling, R. D., & Berry, S. D. (2004). Theta-contingent trial presentation accelerates learning rate and enhances hippocampal plasticity during trace eyeblink conditioning. *Behavioral Neuroscience, 118*(2), 403–411.

Guderian, S. & Duzel, E. (2005). Induced theta oscillations mediate large-scale synchrony with mediotemporal areas during recollection in humans. *Hippocampus, 15*(7), 901–912.

Guderian, S., Schott, B., Richardson-Klavehn, A., & Duzel, E. (in press). Medial temporal theta state before an event predicts episodic encoding success in humans. *PNAS.*

Hasselmo, M. E. & Wyble, B. P. (1997). Free recall and recognition in a network model of the hippocampus: Simulating effects of scopolamine on human memory function. *Behav Brain Res, 89*(1–2), 1–34.

Hasselmo, M. E., Hay, J., Ilyn, M., & Gorchetchnikov, A. (2002). Neuromodulation, theta rhythm and rat spatial navigation. *Neural Networks, 15*(4–6), 689–707.

Huxter, J., Burgess, N., & O'Keefe, J. (2003). Independent rate and temporal coding in hippocampal pyramidal cells. *Nature, 425*(6960), 828–832.

Jay, T. M. (2003). Dopamine: a potential substrate for synaptic plasticity and memory mechanisms. *Progress in Neurobiology, 69*(6), 375–390.

Jacobs, J., Kahana, M. J., Ekstrom, A. D., & Fried, I. (2007). Brain oscillations control timing of single-neuron activity in humans. *Journal of Neuroscience, 27*(14), 3839–3844.

Jones, M. W. & Wilson, M. A. (2005). Theta rhythms coordinate hippocampal-prefrontal interactions in a spatial memory task. *PLoS Biology, 3*(12), e402.

Kahana, M. J., Seelig, D., & Madsen, J. R. (2001). Theta returns. *Current Opinion in Neurobiology, 11*(6), 739–744.

Kakade, S. & Dayan, P. (2002). Dopamine: generalization and bonuses. *Neural Networks, 15*(4–6), 549–559.

Klimesch, W., Doppelmayr, M., Stadler, W., Pollhuber, D., Sauseng, P., & Rohm, D. (2001). Episodic retrieval is reflected by a process specific increase in human electroencephalographic theta activity. *Neuroscience Letters, 302*(1), 49–52.

Lavenex, P., Suzuki, W. A., & Amaral, D. G. (2002). Perirhinal and parahippocampal cortices of the macaque monkey: projections to the neocortex. *The Journal of Comparative Neurology, 447*(4), 394–420.

Lavenex, P., Suzuki, W. A., & Amaral, D. G. (2004). Perirhinal and parahippocampal cortices of the macaque monkey: Intrinsic projections and interconnections. *The Journal of Comparative Neurology, 472*(3), 371–394.

Lee, H., Simpson, G. V., Logothetis, N. K., & Rainer, G. (2005). Phase locking of single neuron activity to theta oscillations during working memory in monkey extrastriate visual cortex. *Neuron, 45*(1), 147–156.

Lemon, N. & Manahan-Vaughan, D. (2006). Dopamine D1/D5 receptors gate the acquisition of novel information through hippocampal long-term potentiation and long-term depression. *Journal of Neuroscience, 26*(29), 7723–7729.

Linkenkaer-Hansen, K., Nikulin, V. V., Palva, S., Ilmoniemi, R. J., & Palva, J. M. (2004). Prestimulus oscillations enhance psychophysical performance in humans. *Journal of Neuroscience, 24*(45), 10186–10190.

Lisman, J. E. & Grace, A. A. (2005). The Hippocampal-VTA Loop: Controlling the Entry of Information into Long-Term Memory. *Neuron, 46*(5), 703–713.

Lisman, J. E. & Otmakhova, N. A. (2001). Storage, recall, and novelty detection of sequences by the hippocampus: elaborating on the SOCRATIC model to account for normal and aberrant effects of dopamine. *Hippocampus, 11*(5), 551–568.

Marr, D. (1971). Simple memory: a theory for archicortex. *Philosophical Transactions of the Royal Society of London. Series B, Biological Sciences, 262*(841), 23–81.

McClelland, J. L., McNaughton, B. L., & O'Reilly, R. C. (1995). Why there are complementary learning systems in the hippocampus and neocortex: insights from the successes and failures of connectionist models of learning and memory. *Psychological Review, 102*(3), 419–457.

Mehta, M. R., Lee, A. K., & Wilson, M. A. (2002). Role of experience and oscillations in transforming a rate code into a temporal code. *Nature, 417*(6890), 741–746.

Mishkin, M., Suzuki, W. A., Gadian, D. G., & Vargha-Khadem, F. (1997). Hierarchical organization of cognitive memory. *Philosophical Transactions of the Royal Society of London. Series B, Biological Sciences, 352*(1360), 1461–1467.

Mishkin, M., Vargha-Khadem, F., & Gadian, D. G. (1998). Amnesia and the organization of the hippocampal system. *Hippocampus, 8*(3), 212–216.

Murray, E. A. & Bussey, T. J. (1999). Perceptual-mnemonic functions of the perirhinal cortex. *Trends in Cognitive Sciences, 3*(4), 142–151.

Neufang, M., Heinze, H. J., & Duzel, E. (2006). Electromagnetic correlates of recognition memory processes. *Clinical EEG and Neuroscience, 37*(4), 300–308.

Nyberg, L., Persson, J., Habib, R., Tulving, E., McIntosh, A. R., Cabeza, R., *et al.* (2000). Large scale neurocognitive networks underlying episodic memory. *Journal of Cognitive Neuroscience, 12*(1), 163–173.

O'Keefe, J. & Conway, D. H. (1978). Hippocampal place units in the freely moving rat: why they fire where they fire. *Experimental Brain Research, 31*(4), 573–590.

O'Keefe, J. & Recce, M. L. (1993). Phase relationship between hippocampal place units and the EEG theta rhythm. *Hippocampus, 3*(3), 317–330.

Otten, L. J., Henson, R. N., & Rugg, M. D. (2002). State-related and item-related neural correlates of successful memory encoding. *Nature Neuroscience, 5*(12), 1339–1344.

Otten, L. J., Quayle, A. H., Akram, S., Ditewig, T. A., & Rugg, M. D. (2006). Brain activity before an event predicts later recollection. *Nature Neuroscience, 9*(4), 489–491.

Paller, K. A., Kutas, M., & Mayes, A. R. (1987). Neural correlates of encoding in an incidental learning paradigm. *Electroencephalography & Clinical Neurophysiology, 67*(4), 360–371.

Paller, K. A., McCarthy, G., & Wood, C. C. (1988). ERPs predictive of subsequent recall and recognition performance. Special Issue: Event related potential investigations of cognition. *Biological Psychology, 26*(1–3), 269–276.

Raghavachari, S., Lisman, J. E., Tully, M., Madsen, J. R., Bromfield, E. B., & Kahana, M. J. (2006). Theta oscillations in human cortex during a working-memory task: evidence for local generators. *Journal of Neurophysiology, 95*(3), 1630–1638.

Rizzuto, D. S., Madsen, J. R., Bromfield, E. B., Schulze-Bonhage, A., & Kahana, M. J. (2006). Human neocortical oscillations exhibit theta phase differences between encoding and retrieval. *Neuroimage, 31*(3), 1352–1358.

Rolls, E. T. (1996). A theory of hippocampal function in memory. *Hippocampus*, *6*(6), 601–620.

Rolls, E. T. (2000a). Hippocampo-cortical and cortico-cortical backprojections. *Hippocampus*, *10*(4), 380–388.

Rolls, E. T. (2000b). Memory systems in the brain. *Annual Review of Psychology*, *51*, 599–630.

Sajikumar, S. & Frey, J. U. (2004). Late-associativity, synaptic tagging, and the role of dopamine during LTP and LTD. *Neurobiology of Learning and Memory*, *82*(1), 12–25.

Schott, B. H., Minuzzi, L., Krebs, M., Elmenhorst, D., Lang, M., Winz, O., Seidenbecher, C. I., Coenen, H., Heinze, H. J., Zilles, K., Düzel, E., Bauer, A. (in press). Mesolimbic fMRI activations during reward anticipation correlate with reward-related ventral striatal dopamine release. *Journal of Neuroscience*.

Schott, B., Richardson-Klavehn, A., Heinze, H. J., & Duzel, E. (2002). Perceptual priming versus explicit memory: dissociable neural correlates at encoding. *Journal of Cognitive Neuroscience*, *14*(4), 578–592.

Schott, B. H., Richardson-Klavehn, A., Henson, R. N., Becker, C., Heinze, H. J., & Duzel, E. (2006). Neuroanatomical dissociation of encoding processes related to priming and explicit memory. *Journal of Neuroscience*, *26*(3), 792–800.

Schott, B. H., Seidenbecher, C. I., Fenker, D. B., Lauer, C. J., Bunzeck, N., Bernstein, H. G., *et al.* (2006). The dopaminergic midbrain participates in human episodic memory formation: evidence from genetic imaging. *Journal of Neuroscience*, *26*(5), 1407–1417.

Schott, B. H., Sellner, D. B., Lauer, C. J., Habib, R., Frey, J. U., Guderian, S., *et al.* (2004). Activation of midbrain structures by associative novelty and the formation of explicit memory in humans. *Learning and Memory*, *11*(4), 383–387.

Schultz, W. (1998). Predictive reward signal of dopamine neurons. *Journal of Neurophysiology*, *80*(1), 1–27.

Seager, M. A., Johnson, L. D., Chabot, E. S., Asaka, Y., & Berry, S. D. (2002). Oscillatory brain states and learning: Impact of hippocampal theta-contingent training. *Proceedings of the National Academy of Science of the United States of America*, *99*(3), 1616–1620.

Sederberg, P. B., Kahana, M. J., Howard, M. W., Donner, E. J., & Madsen, J. R. (2003). Theta and gamma oscillations during encoding predict subsequent recall. *Journal of Neuroscience*, *23*(34), 10809–10814.

Sederberg, P. B., Schulze-Bonhage, A., Madsen, J. R., Bromfield, E. B., McCarthy, D. C., Brandt, A., *et al.* (2007). Hippocampal and neocortical gamma oscillations predict memory formation in humans. *Cerebral Cortex*, *17*(5), 1190–1196.

Shuler, M. G. & Bear, M. F. (2006). Reward timing in the primary visual cortex. *Science*, *311*(5767), 1606–1609.

Singer, W. (1999). Neuronal synchrony: a versatile code for the definition of relations? *Neuron*, *24*(1), 49–65, 111–125.

Smiley, J. F., Subramanian, M., & Mesulam, M. M. (1999). Monoaminergic-cholinergic interactions in the primate basal forebrain. *Neuroscience*, *93*(3), 817–829.

Squire, L. R., Stark, C. E., & Clark, R. E. (2004). The medial temporal lobe. *Annual Review of Neuroscience*, *27*, 279–306.

Super, H., van der Togt, C., Spekreijse, H., & Lamme, V. A. (2003). Internal state of monkey primary visual cortex (V1) predicts figure-ground perception. *Journal of Neuroscience*, *23*(8), 3407–3414.

Tesche, C. D. & Karhu, J. (2000). Theta oscillations index human hippocampal activation during a working memory task. *Proceedings of the National Academy of Science of the United States of America*, *97*(2), 919–924.

Treves, A. & Rolls, E. T. (1994). Computational analysis of the role of the hippocampus in memory. *Hippocampus*, *4*(3), 374–391.

Tulving, E. (1985). Memory and consciousness. *Canadian Psychology*, *26*(1), 1–12.

Varela, F., Lachaux, J. P., Rodriguez, E., & Martinerie, J. (2001). The brainweb: phase synchronization and large-scale integration. *Nature Reviews Neuroscience, 2*(4), 229–239.

Vargha-Khadem, F., Gadian, D. G., Watkins, K. E., Connelly, A., Van Paesschen, W., & Mishkin, M. (1997). Differential Effects of Early Hippocampal Pathology on Episodic and Semantic Memory. *Science, 277*(5324), 376–380.

Wagner, A. D., Schacter, D. L., Rotte, M., Koutstaal, W., Maril, A., Dale, A. M., *et al.* (1998). Building Memories: Remembering and Forgetting of Verbal Experiences as Predicted by Brain Activity. *Science, 281*, 1188–1191.

Weiskopf, N., Hutton, C., Josephs, O., Turner, R., & Deichmann, R. (2007). Optimized EPI for fMRI studies of the orbitofrontal cortex: compensation of susceptibility-induced gradients in the readout direction. *Magma, 20*(1), 39–49.

Wittmann, B. C., Bunzeck, N., Dolan, R., & Duzel, E. (2007). Anticipation of novelty recruits reward system and hippocampus while promoting recollection. *NeuroImage. 38*, 194–202.

Wittmann, B. C., Schott, B. H., Guderian, S., Frey, J. U., Heinze, H. J., & Duzel, E. (2005). Reward-related FMRI activation of dopaminergic midbrain is associated with enhanced hippocampus-dependent long-term memory formation. *Neuron, 45*(3), 459–467.

Yonelinas, A. P., Kroll, N. E., Quamme, J. R., Lazzara, M. M., Sauve, M. J., Widaman, K. F., *et al.* (2002). Effects of extensive temporal lobe damage or mild hypoxia on recollection and familiarity. *Nature Neuroscience, 5*(11), 1236–1241.

Chapter 24

Functional neuroimaging and cognitive theory

Michael D. Rugg

Introduction

The theme of the present volume – the role of functional neuroimaging[1] in developing and adjudicating between cognitive theories of memory – refers to a somewhat controversial application of functional neuroimaging data. It is widely agreed (though see Uttal, 2001) that measures of task- or item-related brain activity are informative about the neural systems involved in cognition and behaviour, an application of functional neuroimaging that is well-exemplified by Duzel and Guderian (this volume). More controversial however is the idea that measures of brain activity can also be used to inform theorizing at a purely psychological (or 'functional') level of explanation (e.g. Fodor, 1999; Coltheart, 2006; Harley, 2004ab). In the present chapter, I briefly outline some of the issues associated with efforts to use measures of brain activity to illuminate functional models of memory. Previous discussions covering some of the same ground can be found in Henson (2005), Rugg and Coles (1995), and Rugg (1999).

As is outlined in the chapter by Simons (this volume; see Henson, 2005, for a more detailed exposition) there are two principal ways in which neuroimaging data can be employed to inform functional models of cognition, at least in principle. First, the data can be treated in the same way as a behavioural measure, the idea being to use task- or condition-related dissociations in brain activity (rather than, say, accuracy or response time) to dissociate functionally distinct cognitive processes. A second way of using neuroimaging data to draw functional conclusions is through the use of 'reverse inference' (what Henson (2005) refers to as 'structure-to-function' inferences). In this case, the neural correlate of a given cognitive operation is assumed to be sufficiently reliable and specific that its presence can serve as a marker for the engagement of the operation.

In what follows, I briefly discuss issues surrounding these two ways of applying neuroimaging data to the investigation of memory at the functional level. Each of these discussions takes as it starting point the description of the relevant application by Simons (this volume).

---

[1] In the present context functional neuroimaging refers to both haemodynamic (fMRI, PET) and electrophysiological (EEG, MEG) measures of brain activity.

Neural dissociations

As argued by Simons, 'if undertaken properly' statistically significant interactions between experimental condition, measures of brain activity, and brain region can be interpreted as evidence that the experimental conditions engaged functionally distinct cognitive operations, using a logic analogous to that employed to interpret task dissociations in neuropsychology (Shallice, 1988). Examples of this approach include the fMRI data reported by Simons (this volume) demonstrating a dissociation between lateral and medial anterior prefrontal activity and retrieval of perceptual versus conceptual contextual attributes, and the ERP studies reported by Mecklinger and Jager (this volume) in which the scalp topography of ERP 'old/new effects' varies according to whether recognition memory is supported by recollection or familiarity. The first of these findings is interpreted as evidence for a functional distinction between retrieval of stimulus-derived and stimulus-independent context. The second finding is held to support dual-process models of recognition memory (where recollection and familiarity are held to be functionally distinct forms of memory) over single-process models (in which the two forms of recognition are argued to fall along a single continuum of memory 'strength').

Along with Simons (this volume) I believe that the dissociative logic outlined above is potentially a powerful method for identifying functionally distinct cognitive operations and, as such, has much to offer the development of cognitive models of memory. That said, some caveats and qualifications are in order (see also Henson, 2005; Rugg & Coles, 1995; Rugg, 1999). Rather than rehearse all of these here, I focus on one issue that has arguably received less attention than it deserves.

The issue in question arises because of a disjunction between how cognitive operations and the representations on which they operate are usually conceived in experimental psychology and cognitive science, and how cognitive processes are implemented in the brain. At the psychological (functional) level a distinction is commonly drawn between a specific cognitive process, e.g. the computation of the familiarity of a recognition memory test item, and the nature of the information upon which the process acts. From this perspective it makes perfect sense to formulate a model of familiarity assessment that, computationally, operates identically regardless of the nature of the information that is being assessed (e.g. whether the information is verbal or pictorial). This separation between 'process' and 'representation' (or 'content') is unlikely to be generally honoured at the level of brain however; it has long been known that the representation of different classes of information – faces versus words, say – depends on anatomically dissociable cortical regions[2]. So while from a functional perspective we might conceive of a single, computationally homogeneous cognitive process as being 'fed' a variety of different inputs, in each case generating an appropriate output (e.g. familiarity levels of words or faces, depending on the input), from the perspective of the brain this scenario is highly

---

[2] This argument is unaffected by the eventual outcome of the debate whether different stimulus classes are strictly segregated at the cortical level, or are represented in a more distributed fashion across the cortical surface (cf. Haxby et al., 2001; Spiridon et al., 2006), so long as the *patterns* of activity elicited by various stimulus classes differ systematically.

implausible. Rather, as is made explicit in neurally-inspired connectionist cognitive models, the distinction between process and representation is difficult, if not impossible, to draw at the neural level. It follows that even if two experimental conditions engage formally the same cognitive operation(s), a neural dissociation will be obtained nonetheless if the operation(s) are acting on different, anatomically separated representations. Admittedly, this issue is in some ways already well-recognized, although it is arguable that its implications have not been fully appreciated. For example, to my knowledge no-one has ever suggested that condition-dependent differences in the lateralization of memory-related hippocampal activity (which can take the form of a 'classical' double-dissociation; Powell *et al.*, 2005) indicate that the left and right hippocampi support functionally distinct mnemonic processes. Rather, such findings are generally interpreted as evidence for the engagement of functionally equivalent cognitive processes operating on different classes of information [verbal (left hemisphere) vs. non-verbal (right hemisphere)].

This seemingly banal example of a case where a neural dissociation carries little theoretical weight (at least for an understanding of cognitive architecture) illustrates two points. First, and rather obviously, it demonstrates that the finding of a neural dissociation may be *necessary* for the claim of a functional dissociation but it is not *sufficient*; it is also necessary to rule out the alternative possibility that the neural dissociation arises because of differences in the informational content (representations) being operated upon. Second, the example illustrates the value of knowledge about the brain in the interpretation of neural dissociations. The reason why condition by laterality interactions in hippocampal activity are not taken as evidence for the engagement of functionally distinct cognitive operations is that we know first, that the left and right hippocampi are structurally (and hence very likely functionally) equivalent, and second, that the human brain is functionally lateralized. In a similar vein, it is unlikely anyone would view a neural dissociation between, say, retrieval-related activity elicited by faces and words as evidence for a theoretically interesting functional dissociation, given the more mundane possibilities that arise from the fact that these two classes of stimuli are represented in anatomically distinct cortical regions. On the other hand, few (although see Squire *et al.*, 2007) would disagree that findings of a dissociation between retrieval-related activity in perirhinal cortex and the hippocampus according to whether recognition is based on familiarity or recollection (e.g. Davachi *et al.*, 2003) suggest that these two classes of recognition judgement depend upon functionally distinct mnemonic processes. In this case, the interpretation of the findings in terms of a functional dissociation is supported by a large body of anatomical and behavioural neuroscience evidence suggesting that these structures are computationally distinct. A similar case can be made for other neural dissociations that involve structurally and computationally distinct brain regions, such as the dissociations that have been reported between performance-related hippocampal and striatal activity during the learning of a cognitive skill (Foerde *et al.*, 2006). And as a final example, the dissociations obtained in ERP studies of recognition memory between the 'mid-frontal' and 'left parietal' old new effects which, crucially, differ markedly in both their scalp topographies and time-courses (Mecklinger and Jager, this volume), are generally regarded as evidence that recognition test items engage dissociable cognitive operations (although disagreement remains about the functional roles of these processes (Paller *et al.*, this volume).

Difficulties in the interpretation of a neural dissociation are most likely to arise when there is a lack of relevant prior knowledge about the brain regions demonstrating the dissociation, or when the dissociation is relatively subtle in character. As an example, consider findings demonstrating that the locus along the left inferior gyrus of neural activity elicited by words depends on whether the task emphasizes semantic or phonological processing (Poldrack *et al.*, 1999). Whether this dissociation reflects differences in the computations supported by dorsal and ventral aspects of this region, as opposed to differences in the nature of the representations supported by these different cortical regions, remains a topic of vigorous debate (Badre & Wagner, 2007; Gold & Buckner, 2002; Snyder *et al.*, 2007). A similar ambiguity in the interpretation of task by region interactions can be found in Simons (this volume). He reviews evidence from his own and others' work demonstrating a dissociation between activity in medial and lateral anterior prefrontal cortex, and whether task-relevant contextual information was derived through an internal cognitive operation or from the environment. It is not obvious (to me at least) whether this dissociation should be interpreted as evidence that retrieval of these two classes of contextual information engages functionally distinct cognitive operations, or whether the two classes of information are represented in an anatomically segregated manner, but are acted on by functionally equivalent cognitive operations.

As many readers will be aware, the above two cases are examples of a wider, long-standing debate about whether task- and stimulus-based dissociations in prefrontal activity should be interpreted in terms of process or content (*cf.* Davachi *et al.*, 2004; Petrides, 2005). From the standpoint of efforts to understand the functions of the different subregions of the prefrontal cortex this debate is perfectly appropriate, and serves as an important stimulus for further research. But from the standpoint of a researcher interested specifically in functional models of cognition it is unclear how findings such as these – given the ambiguity of their interpretation – could be used in a rigorous way to arbitrate between competing functional models. To reiterate, a neural dissociation would seem to serve most convincingly as evidence of a functional dissociation when there is prior knowledge to suggest that the brain regions demonstrating the dissociation are computationally distinct.

Finally, it is worth noting that ambiguity in the interpretation of neural dissociations cuts both ways. There are circumstances where the theoretical relevance of these dissociations depends on the validity of a content- rather than a process-oriented interpretation. For example, it is widely held that episodic retrieval depends on the 'reinstatement' or 'recapitulation' of processing engaged during encoding (e.g. Norman & O'Reilly, 2003), leading to the prediction that the cortical correlates of episodic retrieval should be content-dependent. This finding has been reported in a number of studies (e.g. Johnson & Rugg, 2007; Kahn *et al.*, 2004; Wheeler & Buckner, 2000) and has been taken as evidence in favour of the prediction. The possibility that at least these some of these content-dependent dissociations may actually reflect the engagement of functionally distinct retrieval operations has received scant attention.

Reverse inference

Reverse inference is the term coined by Poldrack (2006) to refer to the practice of treating a pattern of brain activity, or even the activity in a single brain region, as a 'marker' for the engagement of a specific cognitive operation. Examples of reverse inference abound in the memory literature. To give just two from my own research, there is the use of the left parietal old/new ERP effect as a marker of successful recollection (Herron & Rugg, 2003), and the interpretation of encoding-related activity in the intra-parietal sulcus as evidence that memory for multiple features of a study item requires that those features were bound into a common perceptual representation at encoding (Uncapher *et al.*, 2006).

As elegantly discussed by Poldrack (2006), the validity of a reverse inference depends critically on the specificity of the relationship between a given pattern of brain activity and a given functional process or state. For the inference to hold, it is not enough that the engagement of the process is invariably associated with the pattern of activity in question, it is also necessary that *no other* process is associated with that activity pattern. At the level of single, anatomically circumscribed cortical regions this stipulation seems a tall order, in that it implies an exclusive, one-to-one mapping between a specific cognitive operation and a specific region[3]. More promising perhaps are efforts to associate a specific *pattern* of activity with the engagement of a single cognitive operation. Presumably, the more complex the pattern, the more likely it is to be associated with only one operation.

The use of reverse inference runs up against two other problematic issues. The first of these relates to the problem of determining when a particular pattern of brain activity is *not* present, thereby licensing the conclusion that the associated cognitive operation was not engaged. As is well recognized, considerable caution is required before accepting a null hypothesis, especially when the expected effect size, and therefore the power of the experiment, is not known (as is the case in most neuroimaging experiments). Hence, regardless of the specificity of the marker of a given cognitive operation, one would be ill-advised to rely on reverse inference in order to fractionate experimental conditions according to whether they did or did not engage that operation[4].

The second issue is also a measurement problem, broadly speaking. Put simply, how similar do two patterns of brain activity have to be before it is concluded that they signify the engagement of the same cognitive operation? Measurement noise alone guarantees that the two patterns will never be absolutely identical. Moreover, given the limitations of

---

[3] Note that this is a stronger requirement than what is needed to support the interpretation of a neural dissociation as evidence for a functional dissociation. This requires only that there is an *invariant* relationship between a given cognitive process and activity in a given region, not an *exclusive* relationship.

[4] This issue also constitutes a problem for the interpretation of neural dissociations. Consider a study in which a classical 'cross-over' double dissociation is found between two brain regions, such that condition A elicits more activity than condition B in region Y, while B elicits more activity than A in region Z. Is the interpretation of this finding dependent on whether or not the activity levels for condition B in region Y, and A in region Z, are significantly greater than baseline (where baseline refers to an appropriate control condition)?

spatial resolution of current methodologies, even if two patterns of activity were to appear identical, one could never establish that the identity extended to recruitment of the same neuronal populations at the level, say, of cortical columns. Indeed, in the absence of a theory of how cognitive processes are implemented in the brain, or what constitutes the 'grain size' of cortical functional specialization, what criteria should be used to decide when the patterns of neural activity elicited in two experiments or experimental conditions constitute a neural association rather than a dissociation? In the case of a single region, do we require that the overlap between conditions is total, partial, or merely that the same broad region is activated (the discussion of the role of medial anterior frontal cortex in recollection vs. 'mentalizing' in Simons (this volume) touches on this problem). And does it matter whether other regions are co-active with our region of interest? Furthermore, in the case of a pattern of activity distributed across multiple regions, do we require merely that the same regions are co-active, or impose the additional constraint that the relative levels of activity in each region are maintained across conditions?

By way of digression, it is worth noting that resolution of this last issue has important implications not only for the interpretation of fMRI findings, but also for dissociations in the scalp topographies of ERP effects (for examples of such dissociations, see Mecklinger & Jager, and Paller et al., both in this volume). Currently, it is commonplace for an interaction between experimental condition and scalp topography to be taken as evidence for a functional dissociation; indeed, topographical dissociations are sometimes even construed as evidence for the engagement of distinct neural populations (e.g. Leynes et al., 1998). As has been pointed out previously however (Rugg & Coles, 1995; Otten & Rugg, 2005; Urbach & Kutas, 2006), differences in ERP scalp topographies do not necessarily signify the engagement of different populations of neural generators; a shift in the relative activity levels of the members of a common generator population will also result in a different scalp topography. Thus, depending on one's theoretical notions about how cognitive processes are implemented in the brain (e.g. whether variations in the relative [or, for that matter, absolute] levels of activity in a common set of regions are functionally significant), an ERP topographical dissociation may or may not be indicative of a functional dissociation. This ambiguity in the interpretation of ERPs is largely eliminated if analysis is conducted at the level not of scalp topographical data, but of the underlying generators. In this case, analogously with fMRI, conclusions can be based on direct evidence about the loci of task- or condition-dependent modulation of neural activity. Unfortunately, robust, generally applicable methods for localizing the neural generators of scalp electromagnetic fields have yet to be developed.

The foregoing discussion of some of the problems surrounding reverse inference should not be taken as a wholesale prescription against the practice. Attempting to understand an existing data set by drawing parallels with prior findings is an inherent part of science, and is frequently the spur for the formulation of new hypotheses. Because of the limitations discussed above, however, reverse inference is only rarely likely to offer a compelling approach to *testing* hypotheses, as opposed to formulating them. In any case, it is arguable that when making a reverse inference, researchers should explicitly address the issues noted above, most notably, the criteria to be employed in determining when a pattern of brain activity is to be taken as a marker for a specific cognitive operation.

Concluding comments

There seems no reason in principle why task- or condition-related dissociations in neural activity should not be informative at the functional level. Importantly, the interpretation of a neural dissociation as evidence for a functional dissociation does not require the naïve assumption of a one-to-one mapping between specific cognitive processes and circumscribed brain regions. It does require however that there is an invariant relationship between engagement of a given process and activity in one or more regions. Moreover, since brain activity is influenced by both the nature of the process that is engaged, and the content on which the process operates, neural dissociations can be interpreted as functional dissociations only when a purely content-based account can be ruled out. This is easiest to do when the neural dissociation involves brain regions that are already known to support functionally distinct computations. Thus, even when the aim of a functional neuroimaging experiment is to inform theories framed in purely functional terms, interpretation of the findings will be facilitated, perhaps crucially, by relevant neurobiological information. In other words, even when employed in service of purely psychological questions, measures of brain activity are not best treated as 'just another dependent variable', with a status equivalent to behavioural indices such as reaction time or error rate (*cf*. Henson, 2005).

References

Badre, D. & Wagner, A. D. (2007). Left ventrolateral prefrontal cortex and the cognitive control of memory. *Neuropsychologia*, *45*, 2883–2901.

Coltheart, M. (2006). What has functional neuroimaging told us about the mind (so far). *Cortex*, *42*, 323–331.

Davachi, L, Mitchell, J. P., & Wagner, A. D. (2003). Multiple routes to memory: distinct medial temporal lobe processes build item and source memories. *Proceedings of the National Academy of Sciences USA*, *100*, 2157–2162.

Davachi, L., Romanski, L. M., Chafee, M. V., & Goldman-Rakic, P. S. (2004). Domain specificity in cognitive systems. In: M. S. Gazzaniga (Ed.), *The Cognitive Neurosciences III* (pp. 665–678). Cambridge MA: MIT Press.

Foerde, K, Knowlton, B. J., & Poldrack, R. A. (2006). Modulation of competing memory systems by distraction. *Proceedings of the National Academy of Sciences USA*, *103*, 11778–11783.

Fodor, J. (1999). Let your brain alone. *London Review of Books*. 30 September.

Gold, B. T. & Buckner, R. L. (2002). Common prefrontal regions coactivate with dissociable posterior regions during controlled semantic and phonological tasks. *Neuron*, *35*, 803–812.

Harley, T. A. (2004a). Does cognitive neuropsychology have a future?. *Cognitive Neuropsychology*, *21*, 3–16.

Harley, T. A. (2004b). Promises, promises. *Cognitive Neuropsychology*, *21*, 51–56.

Haxby, J. V., Gobbini, M. I., Furey, M. L., Ishai, A., Schouten, J. L., & Pietrini, P. (2001). Distributed and overlapping representations of faces and objects in ventral temporal cortex. *Science*, *293*, 2425–2430.

Henson, R. N. A. (2005). What can functional neuroimaging tell the experimental psychologist? *Quarterly Journal of Experimental Psychology*, *58A*, 193–233.

Herron, J. E. & Rugg, M. D. (2003). Strategic influences on recollection in the exclusion task: Electrophysiological evidence. *Psychonomic Bulletin and Review*, *10*, 703–710.

Johnson, J. D. & Rugg, M. D. (2007). Recollection and the reinstatement of encoding-related cortical activity. *Cerebral Cortex*, *17*, 2507–2515.

Kahn, I., Davachi, L., & Wagner, A. D. (2004). Functional-neuroanatomic correlates of recollection: implications for models of recognition memory. *Journal of Neuroscience*, *28*, 4172–4180.

Leynes, P. A., Allen, J. D., & Marsh, R. L. (1998). Topographic differences in CNV amplitude reflect different preparatory processes. *International Journal of Psychophysiology*, *31*, 33,44.

Norman, K. A. & O'Reilly, R. C. (2003). Modeling hippocampal and neocortical contributions to recognition memory: a complementary-learning systems approach. *Psychological Review*, *110*, 611–646.

Otten, L. J. & Rugg, M. D. (2005). Interpreting event-related brain potentials. In: T. C. Handy (Ed.), *Event Related Potentials*, Cambridge MA: MIT Press.

Petrides, M. (2005). Lateral prefrontal cortex: architectonic and functional organization. *Philosophical Transactions of the Royal Society of London B Biological Sciences*, *360*, 781–795.

Poldrack, R. A. (2006). Can cognitive processes be inferred from neuroimaging data? *Trends in Cognitive Sciences*, *10*, 59–63.

Poldrack, R. A., Wagner, A. D., Prull, M. W., Desmond, J. E., Glover, G. H., & Gabrieli, J. D. (1999). Functional specialization for semantic and phonological processing in the left inferior prefrontal cortex. *Neuroimage*, *10*, 15–35.

Powell H. W., Koepp M. J., Symms M. R., Boulby P. A., Salek-Haddadi A., Thompson P. J., Duncan J. S., & Richardson M. P. (2005). Material-specific lateralization of memory encoding in the medial temporal lobe: blocked versus event-related design. *Neuroimage*, *27*, 231–239.

Rugg, M. D. (1999). Functional neuroimaging in cognitive neuroscience. In: C. M. Brown & P. Hagoort (Eds), *The Neurocognition of Language* (pp. 16–36). Oxford: Oxford University Press.

Rugg, M. D. & Coles, M. G. H. (1995). The ERP and cognitive psychology: conceptual issues. In: M. D. Rugg & M. G. H. Coles (Eds), *Electrophysiology of Mind* (pp. 27–39). Oxford: Oxford University Press.

Shallice, T. (1988). From Neuropsychology to Mental Structure. Cambridge: Cambridge University Press.

Snyder, H. R., Feigenson, K., & Thompson-Schill, S. L. (2007). Prefrontal cortical response to conflict during semantic and phonological tasks. *Journal of Cognitive Neuroscience*, *19*, 761–775.

Spiridon, M., Fischl, B., & Kanwisher, N. (2006). Location and spatial profile of category-specific regions in human extrastriate cortex. *Human Brain Mapping*, *27*, 77–89.

Squire, L. R., Wixted, J. T., & Clark, R. E. (2007). Recognition memory and the medial temporal lobe: a new perspective. *Nature Reviews neuroscience*, *8*, 872–883.

Uncapher, M. R., Otten, L. J., & Rugg, M. D. (2006). Episodic encoding is more than the sum of its parts: an fMRI investigation of multifeatural contextual encoding. *Neuron*, *52*, 547–556.

Urbach, T. P. & Kutas, M. (2006). Interpreting event-related brain potential (ERP) distributions: implications of baseline potentials and variability with application to amplitude normalization by vector scaling. *Biological Psychology*, *72*, 333–343.

Uttal, W. R. (2001). *The new phrenology: The limits of localizing cognitive processes in the brain.* Cambridge, MA: MIT Press.

Wheeler, M. E., Petersen, S. E., & Buckner, R. L. (2000). Memory's echo: vivid remembering reactivates sensory-specific cortex. *Proceedings of the National Academy of Sciences USA*, *97*, 11125–11129.

Subject index

Name index

Abbott, L.F. 68, 76
Abdi, H. 300, 327
Aberg, C. 297
Abrahamsen, A. 132, 133, 157
Abrams, R.A. 279
Adali, T. 299, 325
Adam, M. 31, 40
Adams, C.M. 76
Adams, J.L. 62
Adcock, R.A. 433, 438
Addis, D.R. 114, 122, 123, 161, 244, 248, 343, 345, 405, 414, 416, 421, 424
Adolphs, R. 345
Adriany, G. 24
Aerts, J. 122, 124
Aertsen, A. 18, 23
Afzal, N. 345
Aggleton, J.P. 350, 353, 357, 358, 367, 374, 377, 429, 438
Agis, I.F. 319, 325
Aguirre, G.K. 186, 194, 241, 253, 257, 261, 266, 273, 277, 291, 294, 298
Akbudak, E. 277
Akram, S. 161, 431, 440
Albert, D. 27, 40
Albert, M.S. 408, 424
Albright, T.D. 285, 295
Alexander, G.E. 213, 224
Alexander, M.P. 414, 425
Alfonso-Reese, L.A. 106
Alivisatos, B. 176, 193
Alkire, M.T. 345
Allamano, N. 219, 224
Allan, K. 361, 377, 401
Allen, J.D. 450
Allison, T. 132, 161, 284, 296
Allman, J.M. 159
Alpert, N.M. 279, 408, 424
Alsop, D.C. 277
Alvarez, P. 170, 194, 232, 248
Alvino, C. 327
Amaral, D.G. 427, 439
Amodio, D.M. 416, 419, 421
Andersen, P. 24
Andersen, R.A. 285, 297
Anderson, A.K. 347
Anderson, A.W. 23, 176, 192, 239, 250, 292, 296
Anderson, J. 303, 327, 328
Anderson, J.A. 131, 133, 134, 138, 142, 143, 144, 152, 156
Anderson, J.R. 131, 132, 133, 142, 144, 145, 156, 286, 294
Anderson, M.C. 133, 134, 138, 139, 141, 144, 157, 159, 160, 316, 318, 325, 326, 328
Anderson, N.D. 277

Anderson, S.H. 329
Andrews, T.C. 212
Angstadt, P. 328
Anllo-Vento, L. 219, 224
Antuono, P. 122
Aristotle 111, 122
Arkadir, D. 63
Armony, J.L. 76, 345, 348
Armstrong, E. 417, 424
Arnoult, M.D. 219, 224
Aron, A.R. 82, 83, 85, 87, 241, 248
Asaka, Y. 429, 439, 441
Aschenbrenner-Scheibe, R. 438
Ashburner, J. 22, 23
Ashby, F.G. 100, 101, 102, 103, 104, 106, 107, 108
Ashe, J. 327
Aslan, A. 159
Astafiev, S.V. 279
Atchley, R. 294
Atkinson, R.C. 169, 190, 228, 229, 236, 248, 256, 260, 350, 353
Attneave, F. 219, 224
Awh, E. 181, 190, 210, 212, 217, 219, 224, 225, 226, 296
Ayers, M.S. 328
Azimian Faridani, N. 362, 377

Bachevalier, J. 271, 277
Baddeley, A.D. 7, 12, 131, 136, 146, 153, 155, 157, 169, 170, 172, 188, 190, 194, 213, 215, 219, 220, 223, 224, 225, 226, 229, 232, 233, 249, 256, 258, 261, 283, 291, 294
Badre, D. 186, 190, 257, 261, 446, 449
Bahlmann, J. 191
Baker, J.T. 243, 249
Baker, S.C. 188, 190, 277, 422
Ballard, D. 179, 191, 241, 250, 294
Balleine, B.W. 61, 62
Balota, D.A. 158
Balteau, E. 124
Baltes, P.B. 18, 23
Bandettini, P.A. 17, 24, 300, 327
Banfield, J.F. 416, 423
Banich, M.T. 138, 158, 292, 294
Barch, D.M. 190, 249
Barde, L.H.F. 241, 249
Baron, J.C. 124
Baron-Cohen, S. 414, 425
Barrett, L.F. 333, 345
Bartels, A. 399, 403
Bartlett, F.C. 305, 325
Barto, A.G. 45, 50, 51, 62, 63
Bauer, A. 438, 441
Bauer, H. 437, 438
Bauer, R.H. 271, 278, 291, 295